Study Guide to Accompany

Porth's Pathophysiology: Concepts of Altered Health States

SIXTH EDITION

Kathleen Schmidt Prezbindowski, PhD, MSN

Professor, Department of Biology
College of Mount St. Joseph
Cincinnati, OH

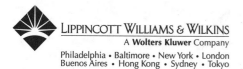

LIPPINCOTT WILLIAMS & WILKINS
A **Wolters Kluwer** Company

Philadelphia • Baltimore • New York • London
Buenos Aires • Hong Kong • Sydney • Tokyo

Managing Editor: Barclay Cunningham
Production Editor: Debra Schiff
Senior Production Manager: Helen Ewan
Art Director: Carolyn O'Brien
Manufacturing Manager: William Alberti

9 8 7 6 5 4 3 2

ISBN: 0-7817-2882-7

Care has been taken to confirm the accuracy of the information presented and to describe generally accepted practices. However, the authors, editors, and publisher are not responsible for errors or omissions or for any consequences from application of the information in this book and make no warranty, express or implied, with respect to the content of the publication.

The authors, editors, and publisher have exerted every effort to ensure that drug selection and dosage set forth in this text are in accordance with the current recommendations and practice at the time of publication. However, in view of ongoing research, changes in government regulations, and the constant flow of information relating to drug therapy and drug reactions, the reader is urged to check the package insert for each drug for any change in indications and dosage and for added warnings and precautions. This is particularly important when the recommended agent is a new or infrequently employed drug.

Some drugs and medical devices presented in this publication have Food and Drug Administration (FDA) clearance for limited use in restricted research settings. It is the responsibility of the health care provider to ascertain the FDA status of each drug or device planned for use in his or her clinical practice.

Introduction

The *Study Guide to Accompany Pathophysiology: Concepts of Altered Health States, Sixth Edition* is designed for use in conjunction with Carol Mattson Porth's text. Like the Porth text, this *Study Guide* broadens students' understanding of normal anatomy and physiology by exploring causes, alterations and adaptations, manifestations, and resolution of disease states. The emphasis in this guide is on active learning, not passive reading, as students bridge the gap from objectives to integration and application of knowledge. Examining concepts through a variety of approaches, students are helped not simply to study, but to learn, correlate, and apply to clinical settings.

The 61 chapters of the *Study Guide* parallel those of the Porth text. Students will find that the following features in each chapter enhance the effectiveness of this excellent text.

- Review Questions in each *Study Guide* chapter are grouped into sections according to those in the text chapter. At the start of each Review Question section, related pages in the Porth text are listed. Frequent references to text figures, tables, and charts encourage students to fully utilize the text.

- Review Questions include a variety of approaches to learning, such as multiple-choice, matching, arrange-in-correct-sequence, fill-in, discussion, and figure completion exercises. These exercises help students to "handle" concepts, almost as if they are working with clay, to achieve a depth of learning that comes through active participation.

- Answers to Review Questions are located at the end of the *Study Guide* where they can be bookmarked for easy access. For some answers, text page references are provided to stimulate further reading and discussion of specific text sections.

- Clinical correlations introduce application especially relevant for students in nursing and other areas of health science. These are based on my own experiences as an RN/MSN and on discussions with colleagues. Because Porth's text addresses a multitude of pathologies, clinical studies include many brief examples rather than just a few detailed case studies. These challenging exercises allow students to relate pathogenesis to actual clinical settings.

Acknowledgments

I offer thanks to students and colleagues at the College of Mount St. Joseph and the University of Cincinnati for many years of ongoing support of teaching, learning, and clinical practice. Special thanks to my family for their constant encouragement and caring: Maureen Schmidt Thielens and Alex Thielens; Amy Prezbindowski, Joost Claeys, and Stephanie Amy Claeys; and Laurie Prezbindowski. I am thankful for the expertise, enthusiasm, and patience of Lippincott Williams & Wilkins editors: Lisa Stead, Barclay Cunningham, and Debra Schiff.

About the Author

Kathleen Schmidt Prezbindowski holds a PhD in biological sciences, Purdue, and MSNs in Gerontological Nursing and Psychiatric–Mental Health Nursing, University of Cincinnati. Over the past 30 years, she has taught pathophysiology, anatomy and physiology, and biology of aging at Columbia Basin College, the College of Mount St. Joseph, and the University of Cincinnati. Dr. Prezbindowski is a professor of biology at the College of Mount St. Joseph, where she has been named Distinguished Professor of the Year. Through a grant from the U.S. Administration on Aging, Dr. Prezbindowski produced the first video series ever designed for older persons and coauthored a training manual on wellness in older adults. She is a delegate to the Health Promotion Institute of the National Council on the Aging. Dr. Prezbindowski has also authored four learning guides in anatomy and physiology.

Contents

CHAPTER 1

Concepts of Health and Disease

■ Review Questions

A. HEALTH AND SOCIETY (pages 3–5)

A1. List four or more advances made over the past century that have contributed to people's longer and healthier lives.

_____

_____

_____

A2. Circle the three most common causes of death in the United States today.

Cancer   Coronary artery disease

Digestive disorders   Stroke

Pneumonia   Tuberculosis

A3. Briefly discuss changes in perceptions of causes of illness over the course of history.

_____

_____

_____

A4. State one or more example of epidemics introduced to populations that lacked immunity to the diseases.

_____

_____

_____

A5. Defend or dispute this statement: "There is scientific evidence that emotions can cause specific diseases."

_____

_____

_____

A6. Give an example of how beliefs may contribute to disease.

_____

_____

_____

B. HEALTH AND DISEASE (pages 5–12)

B1. Write the name of the person from the following list that fits each description below. Not all answers will be used.

Aristotle   Ehrlich   Fleming

Galen   Harvey   Hippocrates

Hooke   Jenner   Koch

Lister   Nightingale   Pasteur

Röentgen   Salk   Vesalius

van Leeuwenhoek Wald

(a) Erroneously believed disease was caused by an imbalance of humors, but emphasized the importance of exercise, good diet, and rest to health: _____

(b) A 16th-century anatomist, his dissections contributed the major "encyclopedia of anatomy and physiology" for 1400 years:

_____

(c) Identified the "closed system of circulation" that forms the basis for blood pressure:

_____

(d) A Dutch lens maker, he refined the microscope: _____

(e) Carried out the first successful vaccination, specifically to protect against smallpox:

_____

(f) During the mid-19th century, identified the importance of sanitation and hygiene in controlling infection: _____

(g) As a result of studies of fermentation, laid the foundation for the "germ theory" of disease: _____

(h) Discovered x-rays: _____

(i) Laid a foundation for home care by sending nurses into tenement houses:

_____

(j) Discovered penicillin: _____

(k) Developed the polio vaccine widely used by 1955: _____

B2. Write a paragraph describing 20th century changes in health care. Incorporate these terms within your paragraph: *schools, rural, "magic bullets," digoxin and sulfa, dog pancreas, skin tests and chest x-rays, heart-lung machine, double helix, health risks.*

_____

_____

_____

B3. List several factors that have contributed to new health problems in the 21st century.

_____

_____

_____

B4. Briefly discuss some promising benefits and ethical dilemmas associated with completion of the human genome project.

_____

_____

_____

B5. Contrast the effectiveness of prevention with treatment of disease.

_____

_____

_____

C. PERSPECTIVES OF HEALTH AND DISEASE IN INDIVIDUALS (pages 12-16)

C1. Match definitions of health with the defining organization and date listed below.

WHO (1948)   WHA (1977)
USDHHS Healthy People 2010

(a) A state that allows people to live a socially and economically productive life:

_____

(b) A state of complete physical, social, and mental well-being, not merely the absence of disease: _____

(c) A state determined by interaction between a person's biology and behavior, environment, governmental policies and interventions, and access to quality health care:

_____

C2. State rationales for why these patients are likely to be more vulnerable to disease and have fewer adaptive (compensatory) mechanisms available.

(a) Tasha (2 days old and full-term) with normal health for a 2-day-old infant.

_____

(b) Joyce (age 42 years) has had rheumatoid arthritis in her hands and feet since age 18 years. _____

C3. Describe pathophysiology in this exercise by filling in the blanks or circling the correct option.

(a) Pathophysiology is the study of _____ and its effects on the structure and _____ of the body.

(b) Disease is a(n) _____ from normal structure and function with characteristic manifestations known as signs and _____, some of which derive from the disease itself, and some develop from the body's attempt to _____ to the disease.

(c) Etiology refers to the _____ of disease. Most disease states involve (one? more than one?) cause.

(d) Factors that predispose a person to a disease are known as _____ factors. Those that arise from events that occur after birth are known as (acquired? congenital?).

(e) _____ refers to the course that the disease takes (or its evolution) from start to finish.

(f) Histology, or the study of (tissues? entire organs?) plays an important role in diagnosis of the disease.

C4. Differentiate signs from symptoms in the following list by circling the signs.

Erythema (reddened skin)	Fever
	Headache
Pain	Skin lesions
Malaise (feeling generally yucky)	Nausea
	Emesis (vomiting)
Syncope (fainting)	

C5. Define the following two terms:

(a) Syndrome _____

(b) Sequelae _____

C6. How is a clinical diagnosis determined?

_____

_____

_____

C7. Natalie's diagnosis of anemia is based on a blood test that measures her red blood cell (RBC) count as "below a normal range." What percentage of the population has an RBC count that is "within the normal range"? ____ %

C8. Identify factors used to determine the accuracy of diagnoses by selecting answers that fit the descriptions below.

Reliability   Sensitivity
Specificity   Validity

(a) Whether a test measures what it is supposed to measure: _____

(b) The extent to which a test result can be repeated: _____

(c) The extent to which a test can identify those who do have the condition (the "true positives"): _____

C9. Match terms related to the clinical course of a disease to their descriptions.

Acute   Carrier
Chronic   Exacerbations   Subclinical

(a) Yaping's body contains the microorganism that causes a disease, but she shows no signs or symptoms of the condition: _____

(b) Mildred manifests no signs of tuberculosis, but tests positive on the skin test, meaning she has been exposed to the disease yet is not likely to develop it: _____

(c) When Therese is highly stressed, she has episodes in which her multiple sclerosis flares up: _____

(d) Diabetes and hypertension are _____ disorders, although they may have _____ episodes.

D. PERSPECTIVES OF HEALTH AND DISEASE IN POPULATIONS (pages 16-20)

D1. Circle the correct answers related to epidemiology.

(a) Epidemiology is more likely to study emphysema from the standpoint of:

(1) How lung tissue changes during the course of the disease

(2) Factors that lead to onset and development of the disease

(b) Prevalence refers to the number of ___ of an illness within a population in a certain time period.

(1) New cases

(2) Total existing cases

(c) ___ statistics measure the number of persons affected by a disease but still alive.

(1) Morbidity

(2) Mortality

(d) The mortality of diabetes is greatest among:

(1) American Indians

(2) Black people

(3) White people

D2. Describe famous health studies by completing this exercise.

(a) The Framingham and Nurses' Health studies that examine a specific group over an extended period of time are both examples of (case-control? cross-sectional? longitudinal or cohort?) studies.

(b) The Framingham study, named after _____, began in the year _____, and studied risk factors for _____ disease. The total number of participants was _____.

(c) The Nurses' Health Study followed a total of _____ female nurses over the past _____ years. The initial study focused on (heart disease? breast cancer?) but has since examined multiple factors.

D3. Describe these aspects of disease:

(a) "Natural history" of a disease _____
_____

(b) Prognosis _____
_____

D4. Write answers to indicate the levels of prevention in each health practice below aimed at a healthy heart.

Primary   Secondary   Tertiary

(a) Coronary bypass surgery: _____

(b) Exercising and low fat diet: _____

(c) Blood pressure checks: _____

(d) Blood cholesterol screening: _____

(e) Smoking cessation: _____

(f) Taking a diuretic: _____

Developmental Aspects: Concepts of Health and Disease in Children

■ Review Questions

A. INTRODUCTION (page 21)

A1. Choose the two true statements.

(a) Overall, infant mortality rates have **decreased** in the United States since 1900.

(b) Infant mortality among African-American babies is **higher** than among white babies.

(c) SIDS is an acronym meaning **serious infant disease syndrome.**

(d) To lower the risk for SIDS, an infant should be placed in the **prone** (i.e., face down) position at bedtime.

A2. Circle the correct answer in each statement.

(a) The overall infant mortality rate in the United States as of 1998 was *(6.0? 7.2? 143.3?)* per 1000 live births.

(b) Most infant deaths in the United States are due to:

(1) Prematurity and low birth weight

(2) Birth defects (congenital anomalies)

B. GROWTH AND DEVELOPMENT (pages 22–27)

B1. Circle the correct answer(s) or fill in the blanks in each statement.

(a) The head forms the greatest percentage of the body length at *(birth? age 10 years? age 25 years?).*

(b) One inch = *(0.254 cm? 2.54 cm? 25.4 cm?).* Therefore, Timmy who is 2 years old today and 3 feet tall is *(7.62? 72? 91?)* cm tall. Timmy is likely to reach a height of _____ by adulthood.

(c) Stephanie weighs 7 pounds at birth. She is most likely to weigh ___ pounds at 6 months of age and to weigh ___ pounds at 12 months.

(d) Billy is in the 95th percentile of height for his age group. His height is *(one? two? three?)* standard deviations above the mean.

(e) Typically, infant growth begins in the *(lower extremities and proceeds towards the head? head and proceeds towards the lower extremities?).*

B2. Arrange these stages in development in correct sequence from first to last:

Gastrula   Blastocyst
Morula   Zygote

B3. Choose the two answers that correctly match a term with its description.

(a) Human sperm: normally contains 23 chromosomes

(b) Trophoblast: typically forms the **embryo**

(c) Differentiation: increase in **number** of cells

(d) Mesoderm: forms **skeleton, muscles,** and **cardiovascular** structures

(e) Endoderm: forms **outer layers of skin** plus **brain** and **nerves**

B4. Choose the two true statements about human development:

(a) The notochord forms along the **midline** of the body.

(b) The embryonic heart normally begins to beat in about the **sixth** week of development.

(c) Limb buds normally begin to appear in about the **tenth** week of development.

(d) A developing baby who is in the eleventh week of gestation is considered a **fetus** rather than an **embryo.**

B5. Choose the two true statements:

(a) In embryonic and early fetal life, most red blood cells are formed in **bone marrow.**

(b) Formation of bone from cartilage tissue begins in the **sixth** month of fetal life.

(c) Brown fat contains **more** mitochondria than white fat.

(d) Normally during the **seventh** month of gestation, the diaphragm **is** functioning.

B6. Choose the two answers that correctly match a term with its description.

(a) Lanugo: **mature** hairs that form on skin during the **seventh** month of development

(b) Vernix caseosa: **cheese-like** covering that helps **protect** fetal skin from drying

(c) Brown fat: important in maintaining changes in body **temperature** at birth

(d) Surfactant: **mucus** that **lines airways**

B7. Choose the two true statements:

(a) The fetus gains most of its weight during the **first half** of the gestation period.

(b) The typical gestation period is 266 days **after fertilization**.

(c) A birth weight of 3500 g is considered **within the normal range** for a full-term baby.

(d) An infant born during the 37th week of gestation **is** considered **premature**.

B8. Newborn Crystal's weight is in the 8th percentile for gestational age. She *(is? is not?)* likely to be classified as SGA. List four or more factors that affect fetal growth and weight gain.

_____

_____

_____

_____

B9. Circle the correct answer(s) in each statement.

(a) Symmetric intrauterine growth retardation (IUGR) *(is? is not?)* likely to be reversible postnatally.

(b) In asymmetric IUGR, the following dimensions are likely to be smaller than normal: *(head circumference? body length? weight?)*.

(c) *(Symmetric? Asymmetric?)* IUGR is more likely to be related to intrauterine malnutrition.

(d) Meconium is a term for *(excess mucus in the respiratory tract? mucus-containing stool?)*

(e). Dubowitz and Ballard assessments involve assessments of *(cardiovascular? sensory? neurologic? muscular? skin?)* development. The *(Dubowitz? Ballard?)* method is more accurate for assessing infants born at 28 weeks' gestation.

B10. During Georgia's pregnancy, her blood glucose level frequently runs in the range of 300 to 400 mg/dL. This is a *(high? normal? low?)* blood glucose level. As a result of exposure to Georgia's blood glucose, Georgia's fetus is likely to have a *(higher? lower?)* than normal secretion of insulin. This will tend to cause the fetus to become *(hyper? hypo?)*-glycemic and to experience *(higher? lower?)* than normal fat deposition, resulting in a(n) *(LGA? SGA?)* size.

B11. Georgia's LMP was August 18. According to Nagele's rule, Georgia's baby should be due on _____ (what date?).

C. INFANCY (pages 27-33)

C1. Circle the correct answer(s) or fill in the blanks in each statement.

(a) Newborns typically lose *(5%-10%? 20%-25%?)* of birth weight within the first few days of life.

(b) Newborns are typically *(50? 65? 80?)* cm in length, which equals ___ inches.

(c) At birth, head circumference is typically _____ cm, and it is *(greater? less than?)* chest circumference. By age 1 year, head circumference is likely to be _____ cm.

(d) The cells of the nervous system that increase in number after birth are *(neurons? neuroglia?)*. Brain growth *(doubles? triples?)* in the first year of life.

(e) Infants are likely to have a *(faster? slower?)* respiratory rate at birth than at 3 months.

C2. Explain why infants are at higher risk than older children for:

(a) Airway obstruction

_____

_____

(b) Middle ear infections

_____

_____

C3. Choose the two true statements.

    (a) In the newborn, the **right** ventricle is typically thicker than the **left** ventricle.

    (b) Heart rate typically **increases** during the months following birth.

    (c) Head circumference of a newborn is a good indicator of **brain growth.**

    (d) The brain of a newborn typically **does** contain deep sulci.

C4. List two reasons that account for:

    (a) Frequent urination in the early months of life.

    _____

    (b) Need for frequent feedings in the early months of life.

    _____

C5. Choose the two true statements about the Apgar score.

    (a) Apgar evaluations are made at **1 minute** and **2 minutes** after birth.

    (b) The cardiovascular system is assessed in the Apgar test by both **heart rate** and **skin color.**

    (c) Infants can score overall within a range of 0 and 5 on the Apgar test.

    (d) A score of 4 to 5 indicates **severe distress.**

    (e) Most infants score 6 to 7 at 1 minute.

C6. Determine the Apgar score at 5 minutes for baby Alyssa who has a heart rate of 50 bpm, weak respiratory effort, limp muscle tone, no reflex irritability, and color indicating cyanosis. Score: _____

Should Alyssa's Apgar test be repeated at 10 minutes? _____

C7. Choose the two answers that correctly match a disorder with its description.

    (a) Linear skull fracture: does have palpable indentation

    (b) Cephalohematoma: a condition that **does not** cross suture lines

    (c) Caput succedaneum: edema and bruising caused by pressure on the scalp

    (d) Dystocia: difficult breathing

C8. Choose the two true statements about birth defects.

    (a) Morbidity and mortality tend to be **inversely** related to length of gestation.

    (b) The **occipital** is the bone most frequently fractured during labor and delivery.

    (c) Crepitus is a **crackling** sound heard as bones rub together.

    (d) **Vertex** birth is another term for **breech** birth.

C9. Choose the two answers that correctly match a term with its description.

    (a) The brachial plexus: includes portions of spinal nerves T2 through T6.

    (b) Erb-Duchenne paralysis: patient maintains the so-called **Waiter's tip** position of the upper extremity.

    (c) Klumpke's paralysis: caused by C5 through C6 spinal nerve injury and affects the **arm.**

    (d) Most babies born with injuries due to brachial plexus injuries **do** recover during the first several months of life.

C10. Choose the two true statements about premature infants:

    (a) Prematurity is **rare** among African-Americans.

    (b) Low birth weight (LBW) is responsible for about 22% of neonatal deaths in the United States.

    (c) Premature birth is more common among **teenagers,** and among women who **smoke** or are **malnourished.**

    (d) Premature infants tend to have **thin** skin and **less** than normal amounts of subcutaneous fat.

C11. Circle the correct answers or fill in blanks about baby Joost, who was born at 26 weeks and weighed 950 g at birth.

    (a) Joost's birth at 26 weeks and his weight *(increase? decrease?)* his risk for RDS, an acronym that refers to R_____, D_____, and S_____. Because Joost is a white boy, his risk for RDS is *(higher? lower?)* compared with that for African Americans and girls.

    (b) With RDS, Joost's lungs would be likely to produce a *(higher? lower?)* than normal amount of surfactant. Surfactant is needed to *(increase? decrease?)* lung compliance.

(c) Without ventilatory support, Joost frequently stops breathing for periods of 25 to 30 seconds, suggesting a diagnosis of *(apnea? periodic breathing?)*.

C12. Fill in blanks or circle correct answers about disorders affecting premature infants.

(a) The #1 and #2 causes of death among premature babies are (respectively): _____ and _____

(b) Write a possible cause for intraventricular hemorrhage (IVH) in premature infants: _____. Most infants *(do? do not?)* die because of IVH.

(c) NEC is an acronym for _____ _____. Babies who have enteral (tube) feedings are at *(increased? decreased?)* risk for NEC. This condition more commonly affects the *(small? large?)* intestine. NEC is thought to be initiated by *(bacterial infection? ischemia?)* of the intestine.

(d) Intramural air (which refers to _____) is a diagnostic characteristic of NEC.

C13. Choose the two true statements about nutrition in infants.

(a) The American Academy of Pediatrics **does** recommend breast feeding over use of cow's milk-based formula during the first year of life.

(b) Lactase is **milk sugar.**

(c) Soy-based formula **should** be introduced immediately if babies "spit up" breast milk- or cow's milk-based formula.

(d) Solid foods **should** normally be fed to an infant by a spoon, not as a thickener for milk in bottles.

C14. Fill in blanks or circle correct answers in this exercise related to nutrition of infants.

(a) Name two minerals that should be added to the diet of infants after 6 months of age: _____ and _____.

(b) The term "paroxysmal" means *(constant? comes and goes?)*.

(c) "Irritable infant syndrome" is also known as _____.

(d) Failure to thrive (FTT) due to parental neglect is an example of *(organic? nonorganic?)* FTT.

C15. For the following questions, select from the following list.

Nutritional deficiencies, including FTT
Respiratory problems   Injuries
Infectious diseases   SIDS

(a) The major cause of death in the United States in infants between the ages of 1 and 12 months is: _____

(b) The major cause of death in the United States in infants between the ages of 6 and 12 months is: _____.

C16. Circle all situations that increase risk for SIDS:

(a) Susan carefully places her baby on its stomach at bedtime.

(b) Cassandra is 16 years old when she gives birth to her baby.

(c) Dixie has stopped smoking now that she knows she is pregnant.

(d) Baby Jimmy's parents each smoke three packs of cigarettes a day.

(e) Juana gave birth to a baby at 32 weeks' gestation.

(f) Senda, a newborn, experiences prolonged periods of sleep apnea.

C17. The major cause of accidental death in the United States in children older than 12 months of age is *(falls? burns? poisoning? motor vehicle accidents?)*

C18. Name the communicable diseases against which each of the following immunizations protects:

(a) MMR: M_____
              M_____
              R_____

(b) DPT: D_____
              P_____
              T_____

D. EARLY CHILDHOOD (pages 33–35)

D1. Select the two true statements about early childhood.

(a) Christian is 2 years and 3 months old, so he is classified as a **toddler**.

(b) Stephanie, also described in Question B1(c), weighed 7 pounds at birth, so it is likely that she will weigh 36 pounds at 2-1/2 years of age.

(c) During early childhood, most of the increase in body length (height) is in the **trunk** rather than in extremities.

(d) According to psychologist Erik Erikson, **autonomy** and **initiative** are two important traits to be developed during the early childhood years.

D2. Select the best answer to each question.

(a) At age 6 years, height in inches and weight in pounds both measure about:

(1) 32

(2) 38

(3) 46

(4) 56

(b) Which answer best describes the condition *otitis media*?

(1) Aspiration pneumonia

(2) Barrel chest

(3) Middle ear infection

(4) Influenza

(5) A form of hepatitis

(c) The term that means an increase of tissue or organ mass by growth in cell size (not cell number) is:

(1) Atrophy

(2) Hypertrophy

(3) Aplasia

(4) Hyperplasia

(d) By the age of 2 years, brain size is about ___% of adult size.

(1) 30

(2) 50

(3) 70

(4) 90

D3. Explain one or more physical reasons why a 2-year-old child is more likely than a 1-year-old child to demonstrate complete control of urination and defecation.

_____

_____

_____

D4. Explain one or more physical reasons why toddlers and preschoolers are at an increased risk for injuries.

_____

_____

_____

E. EARLY SCHOOL YEARS TO LATE CHILDHOOD (pages 35–37)

E1. Select the two true statements about children between ages 6 and 12 years.

(a) In general, growth rate is **faster** during these years than in toddler and preschool years.

(b) Stephanie (also described in Questions B1[c] and D1[b]) who weighed 46 pounds when she started first grade at age 6, is likely to **almost double** her weight by age 12.

(c) A typical 6-year-old child (such as Stephanie) is likely to **double** her height by age 12.

(d) During early childhood years, center of gravity **lowers** as legs grow longer.

E2. Select the two true statements about children between ages 6 and 12 years.

(a) Children tend to look **leaner** with relatively **narrow** waists because these children gain lean muscle mass and lose body fat.

(b) Children in this age range have **lower** caloric requirements than adolescents do, reflecting the **slower** growth rate during early school years.

(c) Males move into puberty about **2 years earlier** than females.

(d) Children typically become **loners** (rather than forming relationships) during early school years.

E3. List several types of disorders that are likely to appear between ages 6 and 12 years.

_____

_____

_____

F. ADOLESCENCE (pages 37–41)

F1. Select the two true statements about adolescent growth spurts.

(a) These typically last for 4 to 6 years.

(b) They begin at an **earlier** age in girls than in boys.

(c) Boys typically gain **more** inches in adolescent growth spurts than females do.

(d) Typically, the growth spurt affects the trunk **before** the extremities.

F2. Circle the correct answers in these statements about typical adolescent changes.

(a) Heart rate *(increases? decreases?)*, blood pressure *(increases? decreases?)*, and hemoglobin level *(increases? decreases?)*.

(b) Sweat and oil gland activity *(increases? decreases?)*.

(c) Auditory function peaks at the age of *(13? 23? 33?)* years, and then declines.

(d) During adolescence, insulin secretion *(increases? decreases?)*.

(e) Growth of pubic and axillary hair is an example of *(primary? secondary?)* sex characteristics.

(f) Most adolescent deaths are attributed to *(accidents? cancer? infections? sports injuries?)*.

(g) The number one cause of accidental deaths among adolescents is *(falling? drowning? shootings with firearms? poisoning? being in automobile accidents?)*.

(h) The number one cause of cancer deaths among adolescents is *(leukemia? brain tumors? genital tumors?)*.

(i) The highest incidence of adolescent suicides is in *(African-American? white?)* *(males? females?)*.

F3. Select the two true statements related to adolescent health problems.

(a) **Falls** are the most common injuries that occur in high schools.

(b) Teen drug abuse is reported to have **increased** in the United States over the past 30 years.

(c) Of teens who become pregnant, it is reported that about 75% **do** deliver the babies.

(d) Of teens who become pregnant, about **one** in **five** does so during her first month of sexual activity.

CHAPTER 3

Developmental Aspects: Concepts of Health and Disease in Older Adults

■ Review Questions

A. THE ELDERLY AND THEORIES OF AGING (pages 43–46)

A1. Choose the two true statements.

(a) Aging is **inevitably** accompanied by disease.

(b) The average life expectancy has **increased** over the past several decades.

(c) The elderly population consists of more **women** than **men.**

(d) Older adults typically adjust **better** after retirement if their lives were dominated by **work** with little interest in **leisure pursuits.**

A2. Because Mrs. Thompson is 73 years old, she is likely to be classified as:

(a) Young-old

(b) Middle-old

(c) Old-old

A3. Choose the two true statements.

(a) About 1% of people over age 65 live below the poverty line.

(b) About 50% of people over 65 years of age live in long-term care including skilled nursing facilities.

(c) "Programmed changes" theories of aging propose that aging changes are **genetically programmed.**

(d) Both the free-radical theory and wear-and-tear theories are considered **stochastic** theories of aging.

A4. Define the term *telomerase* and describe its role in aging.

_____

_____

_____

B. PHYSIOLOGIC CHANGES OF AGING (pages 46–50)

B1. Circle the two typical aging changes of skin.

(a) Thickening of the dermis

(b) Decreased blood supply to skin and nails

(c) Increased activity of both oil and sweat glands

(d) Decreased melanin levels, the pigment that gives hair its color

B2. Circle the two answers that match conditions or processes with correct descriptions.

(a) Purpura: skin hemorrhages

(b) Pruritus: itching

(c) Xerosis: excessive moisture of skin

(d) Bone resorption: formation of new bone

B3. Choose the two true statements about normal aging changes.

(a) Older adults become "more solid citizens" as water content of the body **decreases** with age.

(b) Muscle cells that contribute to endurance are thought to remain **constant** with age.

(c) Aging men typically lose **more** of their bone mass than aging women do.

(d) Age-related bone loss begins primarily in **compact** bone, such as the shafts of long bones.

B4. Choose the two true statements.

(a) By age 65, about 40% of the population have some joint disease.

(b) Cartilage in joints typically becomes **thinner** in older adults.

(c) **Cardiovascular** disease is the number one cause of illness and death among the elderly population.

(d) Hypertension **is** considered a normal aging process.

B5. Choose the two typical aging changes of the cardiovascular system.

(a) Increases in diastolic blood pressure more than systolic blood pressure

(b) Increases in resistance to blood flow through the arteries

(c) Decreases in the maximal heart rate that can be achieved during exercise

(d) Decreases in the overall size of the heart, and especially the wall of the left ventricle

B6. Mrs. Jamison has been diagnosed with orthostatic hypotension. Write one practice that is likely to reduce consequences of her condition.

_____

_____

_____

B7. Circle all of the normal aging changes of the respiratory system.

(a) Decreased maximal oxygen consumption (VO_2max)

(b) Increased amount of work required for breathing

(c) Decreased amount of air left in lungs after maximal exhalation

(d) Increased vital capacity

B8. Indicate whether each of the following factors tends to increase or decrease with normal aging.

(a) Brain weight: _____

(b) Dendritic connections: _____

(c) Lipofuscin deposits: _____

(d) Rate of reflexes: _____

(e) Cognitive abilities: _____

B9. Write the normal aging change associated with each statement made by Ms. Linton, age 86.

(a) "Without my glasses, I wouldn't be able to read a thing."

_____

_____

(b) "I still have my car, but I never drive once the sun goes down."

_____

_____

(c) "My niece always comes with me when I go shopping for new clothes."

_____

_____

(d) "Come and sit down here close to me, look me in the face, and don't shout, thank you."

_____

_____

(e) "I always ask that nice nurse if she'll take a quick look in my ears."

_____

_____

(f) "These days I like my food with a touch of spice."

_____

_____

(g) "Those B_{12} shots I'm getting make me feel better."

_____

_____

B10. Circle all answers that match names of conditions with the correct descriptions.

(a) Presbycusis: visual loss of old age

(b) Edentia: toothlessness

(c) Xerostomia: dry mouth

(d) Achlorhydria: decreased secretions from the small intestine

(e) Diverticulosis: a condition of the colon associated with a low-fiber diet

B11. Choose the two true statements.

(a) Aging kidneys typically are **not** able to maintain normal fluid and electrolyte balance.

(b) Aging kidneys typically have decreased renal artery flow and decreased glomerular filtration rate (GFR).

(c) Low blood potassium levels in older adults are more likely the result of use of **diuretics** than on kidney dysfunction.

(d) Benign prostatic hyperplasia (BPH) is a **rare** condition among older men.

C. FUNCTIONAL PROBLEMS OF AGING (pages 50–57)

C1. Write ADL next to activities of daily living and IADL next to instrumental activities of daily living.

(a) Cooking, cleaning, and doing the wash: _____

(b) Using the telephone: _____

(c) Reading and writing: _____

(d) Bathing and dressing: _____

(e) Toileting and continence: _____

(f) Transferring from bed to chair and walking: _____

(g) Feeding: _____

C2. Match each type of incontinence with the related description. Choose from these answers:

Functional   Neurogenic   Overflow
Stress   Urge

(a) Mr. Washington: "I've got prostate problems." _____

(b) Mrs. Lorenzo: "I had nine kids, and now I have 'accidents' about every time I sneeze or even laugh." _____

(c) Mr. Kostovich: "I got 'sugar' (diabetes mellitus) about 15 years back." _____

(d) Ms. Lucci: " I know I have to 'go' and then I just can't get to the bathroom fast enough. My doctor's putting me on something that she says is for overactive bladder." _____

(e) Mr. Osborn: "I just can't get used to the layout in this new apartment; I forget which way it is to the bathroom." _____

C3. Choose the two true statements related to urinary incontinence.

(a) This condition is so common that it **is** considered a **normal** part of aging.

(b) Medications such as diuretics or sedatives are considered causes of **chronic** urinary incontinence.

(c) Kegel's exercises are designed to strengthen **pelvic floor** muscles.

(d) Estrogen replacement therapy (ERT) is most likely to help relieve **stress** incontinence rather than other types of incontinence.

C4. Give examples of how changes in the following organ systems increase risk for falls among elderly people.

(a) Special senses

_____

(b) Musculoskeletal system

_____

(c) Cardiovascular

_____

C5. Choose all of the true statements.

(a) Most elderly people who fall do so **at home.**

(b) Charles Bonnet syndrome is a condition involving **auditory** hallucinations associated with **hearing** impairment.

(c) Anhedonia refers to loss of **appetite** that may accompany depression.

(d) Pseudodementia associated with depression **does** generally improve with treatment for depression.

(e) The rate of suicide **increases** with age.

C6. Explain why diagnosis of depression among elderly people may be incorrectly attributed to aging changes.

_____

_____

_____

C7. Choose the two true statements related to depression.

(a) Depression **can** be induced by medications.

(b) Selective serotonin reuptake inhibitors (SSRIs) tend to have **more** cardiac side effects than other classes of antidepressants.

(c) Response to antidepressants usually occurs within 4 to 6 **days** of therapeutic dose levels.

(d) Depression is considered to be the **most** treatable psychiatric disorder among the elderly population.

C8. Choose all of the true statements about dementia.

(a) **Senility** is a term that refers to dementia.

(b) Alzheimer's disease is a **rare** form of dementia.

(c) Currently there is **no** specific diagnostic test and **no** cure for Alzheimer's disease.

(d) The progression of Alzheimer's disease has been slowed by drugs that inhibit **acetylcholine.**

(e) **Delirium** is a synonym for dementia.

C9. Rev. Davis has Alzheimer's disease. Write several signs and symptoms that are likely to occur over time.

_____

_____

_____

C10. Match each name with the related assessment tool, theory, or model.

Erikson   Folstein
Hall   Katz

(a) Mini-Mental State Examination (MMSE):

_____

(b) Elderly state of life development (ego integrity versus despair): _____

(c) Activities of daily living (ADLs): _____

(d) The PLST model of caring for older adults with Alzheimer's based on their increasing intolerance to stressors: _____

D. DRUG THERAPY IN THE OLDER ADULT (pages 57-60)

D1. Fill in blanks or circle correct answers to explain why drug protocols of older adults should "start low and go slow."

(a) Incidence of adverse drug reactions in the elderly is _____ times that found in younger adults.

(b) Absorption of oral drugs *(decreases? increases? stays about the same?)* with aging.

(c) Because older adults have *(more? less?)* total body fat than younger adults, fat-soluble drugs accumulate (have a prolonged half-life).

(d) Because of reduced total body water and lean mass, water-soluble drugs reach *(higher? lower?)* concentrations in blood.

(e) Another reason for higher blood concentration of drugs in older adults is related to *(increased? decreased?)* blood flow into the liver and *(increased? decreased?)* kidney function.

D2. Define the term *polypharmacy*, and discuss associated risks.

_____

_____

_____

D3. List several factors that can enhance client compliance for medication protocols.

_____

_____

_____

CHAPTER 4

Cell and Tissue Characteristics

■ Review Questions

A. FUNCTIONAL COMPONENTS OF THE CELL (pages 63–71)

A1. Explain why the study of cells is critical to understanding pathophysiology.

_____

_____

_____

A2. Arrange the chemical components of cells from highest to lowest concentration:

Carbohydrates   Lipids
Proteins   Water

_____

A3. Write names of chemicals from the following list next to their functions within cells:

Carbohydrates   Potassium   Lipids
Sodium   Proteins   Water

(a) Insoluble in water, this category of chemicals includes cholesterols and triglycerides: ____

(b) Form only a small amount of body tissues; are used primarily for cellular fuel: ____

(c) The major cation within cells (in intracellular fluid): ____

(d) Constitute(s) more than 70% of cells: ____

A4. List two or more functions of proteins synthesized by cells.

_____

_____

A5. Circle the correct answer within each statement.

(a) The type of RNA that moves amino acids to proteins that are forming on ribosomes is *(messenger? ribosomal? transfer?)* RNA.

(b) Histones are composed of *(DNA? RNA? proteins?)*.

(c) Sections of DNA that are meaningless because they are not copied in protein synthesis are known as *(exons? introns?)*.

(d) Ribosomal RNA is transcribed in *(ribosomes? the nucleolus?)*.

A6. Describe two methods by which cells actively involve in transcription (copying of DNA by mRNA) preceding cell division can be differentiated from inactive cells.

_____

_____

A7. Match the names of the following organelles with their descriptions.

Golgi   Lysosomes
Mitochondria   Peroxisomes
Rough ER   Smooth ER

(a) Proteins (which are the major components of enzymes) are synthesized here: _____

(b) Lipids are synthesized here: _____

(c) Carbohydrates that help to form glycoproteins are made here: _____

(d) Located close to the nucleus, these organelles modify proteins to prepare them for export from the cell: _____

(e) The inactive form of insulin is activated within these organelles in pancreatic cells: _____

(f) These organelles within sperm form the structure (acrosome) that contains enzymes capable of digesting the coverings over the female gamete: _____

(g) Enzymes that digest microbes are found in these sacs in phagocytic white blood cells: _____

(h) The fatal condition adrenoleukodystrophy is a disorder of these organelles that normally destroy harmful free radicals: _____

(i) These organelles contain their own DNA (inherited from the mother), so that they can self-replicate: _____

(j) These organelles extract energy from chemicals in foods and store the energy in ATP; large numbers are found in muscle cells that require much energy: _____

(k) Sarcoplasmic reticulum (SR) that releases calcium to activate muscle cells is a form of this organelle: _____

(l) Liver cells carry out their detoxification activities through these organelles: _____

A8. Circle all of the functions of lysosomes:

(a) Lipofuscin accumulates in lysosomes of aging cells.

(b) Pigments used in tattoos are retained in lysosomes of cells.

(c) They carry out heterophagocytosis when they digest aging parts of cells.

(d) They are called "powerhouses of the cell."

(e) They normally produce an enzyme that is missing in babies with Tay-Sachs disease.

A9. Choose an answer from the following list to fill in the blank.

The components of the cytoskeleton are primarily involved with _____ the cell.

(a) Shape and movements of

(b) Secretion by

(c) Protein synthesis within

A10. Write the name of the correct cytoskeletal structure next to the related description.

Actin and myosin   Basal bodies
Centrioles   Cilia
Flagella

(a) Provide motility for sperm: _____

(b) Move mucus and debris along respiratory membranes: _____

(c) Thin and thick filaments involved in muscle contraction: _____

(d) Form the mitotic spindle required for mitosis: _____

(e) Form the microtubules found in cilia and flagella: _____

A11. Write brief descriptions of the roles of microtubules in these clinical cases.

(a) Mrs. Jefferson, who has diabetes, has frequent respiratory infections.

_____

(b) Mr. Lewis is taking a form of colchicine for his gout.

_____

(c) Alex has progressive lung damage resulting from immobile cilia syndrome.

_____

(d) The autopsy of Sister Agnes' brain reveals the presence of neurofibrillary tangles associated with Alzheimer's disease.

_____

A12. Circle the two true statements about the cell (plasma) membrane.

(a) The bilayer of this membrane is composed of **lipid** through which lipid-soluble chemicals can be transported.

(b) The "tails" of the phospholipid molecules in this membrane are **hydrophilic.**

(c) Most of the specific functions of the cell membrane are carried out by **proteins,** including channels for transport of nonlipid-soluble chemicals.

(d) **Peripheral** proteins extend from inside to outside of the membrane.

A13. Name a disorder that is caused by a channelopathy of a chloride channel, which results in formation of excessively thick mucus in airways. _____

A14. Circle the correct answer. The A antigens that cause Katisha to have type A blood are found in the (cell coat? cell membrane?) of her red blood cells. The cell coat (is? is not?) involved in cell recognition.

B. INTEGRATION OF CELL FUNCTION AND REPLICATION (pages 72-77)

B1. Circle the correct answers or fill in the blanks within each statement.

(a) Hormones are considered (endocrine? paracrine? autocrine?) secretions, and they most often signal cells (distant from? close to?) where they are formed.

(b) If a hormone is present in excessive amounts, the body will normally (up? down?)-regulate by (increasing? decreasing?) the number of cell membrane receptors for that hormone.

(c) Receptors on nerve or muscle cells that respond to neurotransmitters are _____ channels, such as for sodium ions (Na^+).

(d) The microbial toxin that initiates the severe diarrhea of cholera acts as a *first messenger* that activates a(n) ___-protein and results in production of the second messenger named _____.

(e) Growth factors such as cytokines stimulate *(immunity? red blood cell formation?)*.

(f) Because they are lipids, steroid hormones *(can? cannot?)* pass across cell membranes. They then activate *(cAMP? the nucleus?)*, causing synthesis of proteins that alter cell function.

B2. Choose the answer that fits each description of a phase of the cell cycle.

G_0 G_1 G_2 M   S

(a) DNA is synthesized during this phase: ____

(b) This phase immediately precedes mitosis: ____

(c) Neurons remain in this phase throughout postnatal life: ____

B3. Choose the answer that fits each description of a phase of mitosis.

Anaphase   Metaphase
Prophase   Telophase

(a) The centrioles replicate and move to each end of the cell; the nuclear membrane disappears: _____

(b) Chromosome pairs are present at the midline of the cell: _____

(c) This phase follows anaphase: _____

B4. State the function of cyclins, cyclin-dependent kinases, and anaphase-promoting complex.

_____

_____

_____

B5. Circle the correct answers or fill in the blanks within each statement about metabolism.

(a) Synthesis of proteins from amino acids is an example of *(anabolism? catabolism?)*.

(b) ATP contains *(one? two? three?)* phosphates and *(one? two? three?)* high-energy bonds. *(ADP? ATP?)* contains more energy.

(c) Glycolysis is a process that *(does? does not?)* require oxygen. This process *(begins? completes?)* the catabolism of glucose which is converted into *(pyruvate? CO_2 and H_2O?)*. In the process, *(large? small?)* amounts of energy are captured in ATP.

(d) In the absence of oxygen, pyruvate is converted to _____ acid. Heart cells that lack oxygen can convert this acid back to _____ acid and use it as a fuel. Liver cells can reconvert lactic acid to _____ (a process known as _____).

(e) Aerobic metabolism is a process that *(does? does not?)* require oxygen. In this process, products of glycolysis move through the Krebs (or _____ acid) cycle within the *(cytoplasm? mitochondria?)*.

(f) Within the many steps of the Krebs cycle, hydrogens are removed and ionized so that their electrons can be conveyed along carriers in the electron _____ system (ETS). The ETS taps energy from these electrons to convert ADP to ATP by a process of oxidative phosphorylation. The chemical _____ causes death by poisoning the enzymes involved in oxidative phosphorylation.

(g) Aerobic metabolism provides sufficient ATP molecules to supply *(30? 60? 90?)*% of the body's energy needs.. The hydrogens and carbons from the original glucose combine with oxygen to form two byproducts of aerobic metabolism: ____ which is exhaled, as well as ____.

C. MOVEMENT ACROSS THE CELL MEMBRANE AND MEMBRANE POTENTIALS (pages 78-82)

C1. Explain why an understanding of cell membrane permeability is integral to the study of pathophysiology.

_____

_____

_____

C2. *(Active? Passive?)* transport processes of movement across membranes require expenditure of energy. Passive transport moves chemicals *("downhill" with? "uphill" against?)* the chemical or electrical gradient.

List three examples of passive transport processes.

_____

_____

_____

C3. Choose the answer that fits each description of transport processes.

Diffusion   Facilitated diffusion
Osmosis

(a) Movement of molecules or ions (related to their kinetic energy) from regions of high to low concentration of those chemicals: _____

(b) A process by which molecules such as glucose are transported because they are not lipid soluble and are too large to pass through protein pores: _____

(c) A process that requires a transport protein (carrier) but not ATP: _____

C4. Circle the correct answers or fill in the blanks within each statement about cell membrane transport.

(a) Lipid-soluble molecules such as the gases O_2 and CO_2, alcohol, and fatty acids pass across the *(phospholipid bilayer? proteins with pores?)* portions of cell membranes.

(b) A slight increase in temperature *(increases? decreases?)* the rate of diffusion.

(c) In osmosis, water moves from the region in which *(water molecules? other particles?)* are most concentrated to regions where they are less concentrated.

C5. Choose the two true statements about active transport mechanisms.

(a) These **do** require an energy source such as ATP.

(b) The Na^+/K^+ pump is responsible for keeping the concentration of Na^+ 14 times greater **inside** of the cell membrane than **outside.**

(c) Cotransport uses energy derived from **secondary** active transport.

(d) In antiport systems, sodium and a second chemical are transported in **opposite** directions.

C6. Circle the correct answers or fill in the blanks within each statement about active transport.

(a) Pinocytosis refers to cell *(eating? drinking?).*

(b) After phagocytosis, the ingested particle is transported to a *(mitochondrion? lysosome?)* where it is digested.

(c) One type of cell that engulfs bacteria by phagocytosis is a _____.

(d) Removal of cell debris is carried out by *(endo? exo?)*cytosis.

C7. Circle the correct answers within each statement about ion channels embedded in the cell membrane.

(a) Ion channels with negative charges attract and transport *(negative? positive?)* ions.

(b) Voltage-gated channels respond to *(electrical changes? presence of ligands?)* in the membrane.

(c) A neurotransmitter such as acetylcholine normally attaches to a receptor on a nerve or muscle cell. The *(acetylcholine? receptor?)* is known as a ligand and it is a chemical that has a *(high? low?)* affinity for a receptor.

C8. Choose the two true statements about membrane potentials.

(a) Potential difference and voltage **are** synonymous.

(b) Potential differences across cell membranes are measured in **volts.**

(c) Cell membranes typically have a **negative** charge on the **inside** of the membrane, created partly by **outflow** of potassium ions (K^+).

(d) To create a diffusion potential, a **semipermeable** membrane must have an **equal** concentration of a diffusible ion on **both sides** of the membrane.

(e) During an action potential of a neuron or a muscle cell, the membrane is very **impermeable** to sodium ions (Na^+).

D. BODY TISSUES (pages 82–94)

D1. Circle the correct answers or fill in the blanks within each statement.

(a) By the process of cell differentiation, cells become *(more? less?)* specialized.

(b) Highly differentiated cells such as neurons *(do not undergo? undergo active?)* mitosis.

(c) Stem cells are *(well? slightly?)* differentiated cells that are _____.

D2. Place in order, according to ability to undergo mitosis, from greatest to least.

Skeletal muscle cells   Blood-producing
Cancer cells   cells in bone marrow
Cells lining the stomach

_____, _____,

_____, _____

D3. Name the four basic types of tissues. Which of these develops mainly from ectoderm?

_____

_____

_____

_____

D4. Choose the two true statements about epithelium.

(a) Cells are held **tightly** together with **many** cell junctions.

(b) Epithelium is **highly vascular.**

(c) Epithelium lining the stomach and the intestine is derived from **mesoderm.**

(d) Glands (such as sweat glands and salivary glands) are composed of **epithelium.**

D5. Circle all answers that contain a type of epithelium and a correct location of that type of epithelium.

(a) Simple cuboidal: lines the intestine

(b) Keratinized stratified squamous: forms the epidermis of the skin

(c) Ciliated pseudostratified: lines the upper respiratory tract

(d) Transitional: forms the kidneys

D6. Circle correct answers or fill in blanks in the following statements.

(a) Glands that produce sweat or milk are classified as _____crine glands.

(b) Areolar connective tissue is *(loose? dense?)* connective tissue.

(c) The functioning cells of an organ are known as *(parenchymal? stromal?)* cells.

(d) Adipose is also known as _____ tissue. *(Brown? White?)* adipose tissue contains many mitochondria.

(e) Tendons are *(loose? dense regular? dense irregular?)* connective tissue that connect *(bone to bone? muscle to bone?).*

(f) Periosteum is *(loose? dense regular? dense irregular?)* connective tissue that covers *(cartilage? bone?).*

D7. Choose the two true statements about muscle tissue.

(a) **Smooth** muscle is found in the walls of blood vessels, stomach, urinary bladder, and in the iris of the eye.

(b) Skeletal and cardiac muscle **can** undergo a significant amount of mitosis.

(c) **Endomysium** surrounds a larger amount of muscle than **epimysium** does.

(d) It is the arrangement of **actin** and **myosin** that accounts for the striated appearance of skeletal and cardiac muscle.

D8. Circle all answers that match a term with a correct description.

(a) Sarcolemma: forms sarcoplasmic reticulum

(b) Myosin: thick, dark-staining myofilaments that form cross-bridges with actin

(c) Sarcomere: extends from one H zone to another

(d) Calsequestrin: regulates the location of Ca^{++} in muscle cells

(e) T tubules: convey action potentials from sarcolemma into the interior of muscle cells

(f) Tropomyosin: binds Ca^{++} so that myosin can form cross-bridges with actin

(g) Rigor mortis: due to lack of ATP needed to destroy connections between actin and myosin

(h) Smooth-muscle contraction: depends on Ca^{++} that enters cells from extracellular fluid

(i) Multiunit smooth muscle: found in walls of the GI tract where cells utilize gap junctions to signal contraction of adjacent cells

D9. Circle correct answers or fill in blanks in the following statements about nervous tissue.

(a) *(Axons? Dendrites?)* conduct impulses away from the cell body of the neuron.

(b) Sensory neurons are classified as *(afferent? efferent?).*

(c) *(Astroglia? Oligodendrocytes? Microglia? Ependymal cells?)* myelinate axons in the CNS, whereas _____ are phagocytic cells.

D10. Select the type of cell junction involved in each disease:

Continuous tight Desmosomes Gap (nexus) junctions

(a) Pemphigus with skin and mucosal blistering: _____

(b) Charcot-Marie-Tooth disease (a peripheral neuropathy): _____

D11. Circle correct answers or fill in blanks in these descriptions of extracellular matrix.

(a) One form of extracellular matrix is glycoaminoglycans (GAGs), which are *(simple sugars? polysaccharides?).* GAGs combine with proteins to form _____.

GAGs tend to form hydrated *(fibers? gels)* in connective tissues and allow great *(compression? stretching?)*.

(b) The GAG named_____ plays important roles in _____ and
_____.

(c) Of the three types of fibers in extracellular matrix, those made of *(collagen? elastin?)* are most common. Elastin fibers exhibit great *(strength? ability to stretch?)*.

(d) Integrins are _____ proteins. People with leukocyte adhesion deficiency tend to have a *(high? low?)* rate of infections because their white blood cells have too *(many? few?)* integrins.

CHAPTER 5

Cellular Adaptation, Injury, and Death and Wound Healing

■ Review Questions

A. CELLULAR ADAPTATION (pages 95-99)

A1. Explain why cells adapt.

_____
_____
_____

Circle the type of genes most involved in adaptations.

(a) "Differentiating" genes

(b) "Housekeeping" genes

A2. Choose the term or phrase that best fits each description of atrophy in the sentences below.

Decrease in hormones   Denervation
Disuse   Ischemia   Poor nutrition

(a) Decrease in size of breasts and thinning of vaginal lining in elderly women: _____

(b) Lack of adequate blood flow: _____

(c) Immobilization of a fractured leg:

_____

A3. Choose the term that best fits each description below.

Atrophy   Hypertrophy
Hyperplasia   Dysplasia   Metaplasia

(a) Enlargement of a tissue or organ related to increase in cell number: _____

(b) Enlargement of a tissue or organ related to increase in cell size: _____

(c) Reversible conversion of ciliated columnar epithelium lining the respiratory tract into stratified squamous epithelium in response to chronic irritation of smoking:

_____

(d) Enlargement of biceps brachii as a result of exercise: _____

(e) Increase in thickness of the heart wall in response to increased workload caused by hypertension: _____

(f) Formation of calluses on hands as a result of work with hands; wart formation; wound healing: _____

(g) The cellular adaptation in this list that is considered most "deranged" and most likely to lead to cancer: _____

A4. Removal of a large amount (up to 85%) of liver tissue (partial hepatectomy) *(will never? may?)* be followed by regrowth of most of the liver tissue. *Circle the correct phrase and explain why.*

_____
_____
_____

A5. Explain why benign prostatic hyperplasia/hypertrophy (BPH) might lead to hypertrophy of the bladder wall.

_____
_____
_____

A6. Select the condition from the following list that fits the related description.

Black lung disease   Fatty liver
Jaundice   Lead poisoning
Tay-Sachs disease   von Gierke's disease

(a) Due to excessive lipids that cause lethal brain deterioration in infants:

_____

(b) May be related to alcoholism, starvation, or diabetes: _____

(c) Involves accumulation of excessive amounts of glycogen in the liver: _____

(d) Indicated by formation of a blue line along gum margins in adults with this disorder:

_____

A7. List three or more possible causes of **jaundice**.

_____
_____
_____

A8. What does the term **lipofuscin** mean?
_____
Is it known to be harmful to cells? *(Yes? No?)*

A9. Name an occupation that is at high risk for causing black lung disease: _____.
What exactly accumulates in lungs of these workers? _____

B. CELL INJURY AND DEATH
(pages 99-107)

B1. Identify the category or cause of cell injury in each case. Choose from the following list.

Biologic agents   Chemical injury
Electrical injury   Ionizing radiation
Mechanical forces   Nonionizing radiation
Nutritional imbalances   Temperature extremes

(a) Visual effects related to vitamin A deficiency: _____

(b) Lead or alcohol toxicity: _____

(c) Exposure to gamma radiation: _____

(d) Lightning or electrocution by turning on a hair dryer while standing in pool of water: _____

(e) Fever of 107°F or being trapped in a blazing building: _____

(f) Jumping off of a high bridge: _____

B2. Circle the correct answer in each statement:

(a) Cold temperatures cause injury by *(vasoconstricting? vasodilating?)* blood vessels in skin.

(b) Heat tends to *(increase? decrease?)* metabolic rate.

(c) With injuries due to lightning, most severe injury tends to occur in *(skin at entrance and exit sites? internal organs?)*.

(d) Ultrasound and laser treatment involve *(ionizing? nonionizing?)* radiation.

B3. Choose the two true statements about radiation injuries:

(a) Nonionizing radiation is considered **more** lethal than ionizing radiation.

(b) Most radiation injury is related to exposure to **whole body irradiation**.

(c) Rapidly dividing cells (such as bone marrow or the lining of the GI tract) are **more** vulnerable to radiation than cells that undergo little or no mitosis (such as bone or muscle).

(d) The initial response to radiation is **edema** and **reddening of skin**.

B4. Which enzyme is lacking in the genetic order known as xeroderma pigmentosum? _____ As a result skin sensitivity to light is *(increased? decreased?)*, leading to *(increased? decreased?)* risk of skin cancer.

B5. Stanley attempts suicide by ingesting an entire bottle (100 tablets) of acetaminophen. Which of his organs is likely to be irreversibly damaged?
_____

B6. Circle the correct answer or fill in blanks in each statement about lead (Pb) toxicity.

(a) Children are most likely to be exposed to lead through _____.

(b) The most common age range for lead toxicity in children is *(1–2? 3–6? 6–12?)* years.

(c) The cardinal sign of lead toxicity in children is *(anemia? lead colic?)*, whereas the main sign of this disorder in adults is _____.

(d) Lead toxicity in children *(is? is not?)* likely to affect the nervous system and lower intelligence.

(e) Screening for lead toxicity involves a *(CT scan? finger stick? lumbar puncture?)* to check for the presence of erythrocyte protoporphyrin (EP).

B7. List three major mechanisms of cell injury:
_____,
_____, _____

Circle with which of those mechanisms, therapy with antioxidants such as vitamins E or C can be helpful.

B8. A free radical has one or more unpaired _____. List one or more sources of free radicals that you can avoid: _____.

B9. Identify the type of chemical that becomes damaged when the following cell parts are exposed to free radicals:

DNA   Lipid   Protein

(a) Enzymes: _____

(b) Genes: _____

(c) Bilayer of cellular membranes:

_____

B10. Circle the answers that have the correct definition following the term.

(a) Hypoxia: low blood level, possibly to the entire body

(b) Ischemia: low blood flow to certain tissues

(c) Infarction: tissue death when tissue is deprived of arterial blood

(d) Necrosis: reversible cell injury

(e) Edema: tissues with excessive fluid that increases diffusion distance between blood and cells

B11. Circle correct answers or fill in blanks to describe two major effects of hypoxia on cells.

(a) One product of anaerobic metabolism is _____ acid. Its accumulation in cells causes pH there to *(increase? decrease?)*, possibly damaging the nucleus and other cellular structures.

(b) *(Much? Little?)* ATP is produced by anaerobic metabolism, and ATP is especially needed for "fueling" the ____/____ pump. When that pump fails due to hypoxia, excessive *(Na⁺? K⁺?)* builds up in cells, affecting osmosis of water also, so that cells *(shrink? swell?)* dramatically. As a result, cell membrane permeability *(increases? decreases?)*, including membranes of lysosomes (that may release _____ enzymes).

B12. Dr. Benton writes "elevated serum levels of CPK, LDG, and GOT" on a patient's chart. What does this phrase suggest diagnostically?

_____

_____

_____

B13. Circle correct answers or fill in blanks to describe two other effects of hypoxia on cells.

(a) Normally intracellular calcium ion (Ca^{++}) levels are kept *(high? low?)* by *(active? passive?)* transport mechanisms.

(b) Hypoxia tends to cause *(increase? decrease?)* of intracellular Ca^{++}, which tends to *(activate? inhibit?)* enzymes that break down cell structure.

B14. Cellular swelling and accumulation of fat are likely to be examples of *(reversible? irreversible?)* cellular injury. Name two organs where fatty accumulation tends to occur._____

B15. Describe two or more examples of apoptosis in normal human function.

_____

_____

_____

B16. Apoptosis *(does? does not?)* appear to be involved in some pathologic conditions. List several examples.

_____

_____

_____

B17. *(Like? Unlike?)* apoptosis, necrosis does involve destruction of the cell membrane with release of cell contents that initiates an inflammatory response. Match the type of necrosis with descriptions below.

Caseous   Coagulative
Liquefactive

(a) Tissue develops the consistency of cottage cheese; normally occurs in lungs after tuberculosis: _____

(b) Occurs when enzymes pour out of dead tissue and digest that tissue, leaving a "hole" or abscess; can occur in brain or skin: _____

(c) Occurs as a result of ischemia, as in the heart following a myocardial infarction (heart attack): _____

B18. Gangrene refers to a *(small? large?)* mass of necrotic tissue. *Circle all characteristics more associated with moist gangrene than with dry gangrene.*

(a) Mr. Taylor, who has diabetes, has gangrene of four toes of the right foot; the tissue is black and swollen with blebs full of fluid on the surface of toes; amputation may be required.

(b) The gangrene on Ms. Jenkins' left leg has a **slowly** advancing pace with a **clear** line of demarcation of healthy versus gangrenous tissue.

(c) Nurse Hathaway notes that Ms. Jenkin's gangrene has no odor whatsoever.

(d) Dr. Carter finds during surgery that the client's colon feels cold to the touch, is swollen, and pulseless.

(e) Rev. Davis' gangrene is caused by disruption of blood flow through the anterior tibial artery to her right leg

B19. Answer these questions about gas gangrene.

(a) Which odoriferous gas is released and causes much of the malodor of gas gangrene?

(1) Nitrous oxide

(2) Methane

(3) Carbon dioxide

(4) Carbon monoxide

(5) Hydrogen sulfide

(b) Which microorganism lives in soil that may infect necrotic tissue and produce this gas? _____

(c) Gas gangrene tends to occur in several organs, namely the_____.

(d) Given that *Clostridia* are *(aerobic? anaerobic?)* bacteria, treatment may involve exposure to *(high? low?)* levels of oxygen within a hyperbaric chamber.

C. TISSUE REPAIR AND WOUND HEALING (pages 108–113)

C1. Arrange in correct sequence the degree to which these types of cells can regenerate, from most to least.

Labile   Permanent   Stable

Now identify which category of cells fits each of the following descriptions of tissues.

(a) Mature skeletal muscle, cardiac muscle, and neurons that will never regenerate:

_____

(b) Cells that have a daily turnover, such as skin, linings of the mouth, GI tract, much of the genitourinary tract, and blood-forming cells in bone marrow:

(c) Cells such as those in the liver that will grow if stimulated and if they have a supportive framework (stroma).

_____

C2. Choose the two true statements.

(a) Connective tissue that serves as a scaffolding for functional cells is known as **parenchymal tissue.**

(b) Cirrhosis is **more** likely than hepatitis to result in permanent liver damage.

(c) Healing by second intention is likely to occur **faster** with **better** results than healing by first intention.

(d) Inflammation **is** considered part of the normal wound-healing process.

C3. Complete these sequencing exercises about wound healing. First, arrange in correct sequence the phases of wound healing, from first to last.

Proliferative   Inflammatory
Remodeling

Next, arrange in correct sequence the events of the inflammatory phase, by number, from first to last. _____ _____ _____ _____.

(1) Migration of neutrophils or polymorphonuclear cells (PMNs) to the scene of the injury or infection

(2) Arrival of monocytes that will develop into powerful macrophages

(3) Constriction of injured blood vessels as platelets release vasoconstrictor chemicals

(4) Dilation and increased permeability of capillaries

C4. Describe the function of each of these cells or chemicals in the inflammatory and proliferative phases of wound healing:

(a) Macrophages

_____
_____
_____

(b) Tissue-angiogenesis factor (TAF)

_____
_____
_____

(c) PMNs

_____
_____
_____

(d) Fibroblasts

_____

_____

_____

(e) Endothelial cells

_____

_____

_____

C5. In general, determine whether each of the following is G (relatively good) or B (relatively bad):

(a) Granulation tissue and proud flesh: ____

(b) Keloid: ____

C6. Choose the two true statements.

(a) During the remodeling phase of healing, **both** formation and lysis of collagen fibers occur.

(b) In general, large wounds heal from the **outside** towards the **inside**.

(c) At the point when sutures are removed (about a week after the injury), wound strength is at about 70% of prewound strength.

(d) Usually wounds **do** ultimately heal to be 100% as strong as the prewound tissue.

C7. Match the vitamin with the related description.

Vitamin A   Vitamin B   Vitamin C

(a) Most are water soluble so it must be replaced daily to serve as cofactors for enzymes needed for healing: _____

(b) Helps to counteract anti-inflammatory effects of steroids in healing and facilitates formation of blood vessels: _____

(c) Needed for synthesis of the protein collagen: _____

C8. Choose the two true statements.

(a) Ischemic tissue is **more** likely to become infected during healing than tissue that is well supplied with blood.

(b) Chronic granulomatous disease is an **intrinsic** phagocytic disorder in which phagocytic cells **lack** the enzymes needed to do their jobs.

(c) Hyperglycemia **increases** effectiveness of phagocytes.

(d) Corticosteroids **enhance** inflammation and **accelerate** the healing process.

C9. Defend or dispute this statement: "Sutures enhance healing and help to prevent infection."

_____

_____

_____

C10. Contrast wound healing in the pediatric and elderly populations.

_____

_____

_____

CHAPTER 6

Genetic Control of Cell Function and Inheritance

■ Review Questions

A. GENETIC CONTROL OF CELL FUNCTION (pages 115–121)

A1. Circle the correct answer or fill in the blank within each statement.

(a) A gene is a section of _____ that codes for synthesis of a single _____.

(b) *(Transcription? Translation?)* is the first step in protein synthesis.

(c) The type of RNA formed by transcription of DNA is *(messenger? ribosomal? transfer?)* RNA.

(d) Liver cells contain *(the same? different?)* DNA that is present in skin cells. Their difference in structure relates to their transcribing *(all? only part?)* of their DNA.

A2. The organelles within the cytoplasm that contain DNA are named _____. Name one disorder that involves matrilineal inheritance transmitted by DNA in these organelles: _____

A3. Circle the correct answer or fill in blanks within each statement about DNA.

(a) A DNA nucleotide consists of one _____, one _____, and one _____.

(b) The "backbone" of DNA consists of alternating _____ and _____, with bases attached to *(deoxyriboses? phosphates?)*.

(c) In DNA, the base adenine is paired with *(cytosine? guanine? thymine?)*, whereas cytosine is paired with _____.

(d) Enzymes known as _____ases separate the double-stranded DNA when DNA is to be duplicated or transcribed. In transcription, *(only one strand is? both strands are?)* copied.

(e) Histones are *(RNA? proteins?)* that help to control the structure of DNA strands.

A4. Circle the correct answer or fill in blanks within each statement related to RNA.

(a) A codon is a series of *(one? two? three? four?)* bases found in *(mRNA? tRNA?)*. The codon indicates where a specific *(amino acid? rRNA?)* should be positioned.

(b) The codons AAA and AAG code for placement of *(leucine? lysine?)*. (Hint: see Table 6-1.) These two codons are called _____ because they code for the same amino acid.

(c) RNA and DNA differ in that *(RNA? DNA?)* is single stranded, RNA contains the sugar named _____, and RNA contains the base *(thymine? uracil?)*. During transcription, the triplet A T C in DNA would be transcribed as _____ in mRNA.

(d) The enzyme _____ is required for the transcription process. The sections of transcribed RNA that are spliced out before translation are known as *(exons? introns?)*. The mRNA molecules resulting from splicing of one section of DNA *(will be identical? may differ?)*.

(e) Transfer RNA (tRNA) is the *(largest? smallest?)* type of RNA. At least *(80? 64? 20?)* tRNAs exist, one for each type of amino acid. Transfer RNAs have sites that recognize amino acids and also _____.

(f) Ribosomal RNA makes up *(most? a small part?)* of ribosomes; ribosomes are formed in the *(cytoplasm? nucleus?)*. They are then attached to _____, where mRNA is "read" in the process of *(transcription? translation?)*.

(g) Polypeptides formed by translation each contain about *(10–30? 100–300? 1,000–3,000?)* amino acids.

A5. Circle all true statements.

(a) **All** genes are active in every cell.

(b) Gene expression is increased by gene **repression.**

(c) **Regulatory** genes stipulate amino acid sequence in proteins.

(d) An operon is a sequence of genes that includes **structural** genes for a particular protein plus **promotor** genes that initiate the synthesis of that protein.

(e) Operons are regulated by **negative feedback** mechanisms.

A6. Circle the correct answer or fill in the blank in these statements about mutations.

(a) Mutations are errors in _____, specifically in the *(base? phosphate? sugar?)* portion of a nucleotide.

(b) Most changes in base pairs *(do? do not?)* result in serious mutations.

(c) Mr. Jensen has one brown eye and one blue eye, an example of a poly-_____ that *(can? cannot?)* be transmitted to his children.

B. CHROMOSOMES (pages 121-124)

B1. Choose the two true statements about human chromosomes.

(a) Of the 23 pairs of chromosomes, 22 are known as **autosomes.**

(b) Autosomes are **different** in females and males.

(c) Normally, **females** receive an X chromosome from the mother and a Y chromosome from the father.

(d) A **Barr body** is an **inactive** X chromosome, meaning that is **does not** control genetic traits, and is present in **females** but not in males.

B2. Write **meiosis** or **mitosis** after each description below that fits that type of cell division.

(a) The process is preceded by replication of DNA (so that the 46 chromosomes are doubled): _____

(b) Involves two divisions: _____

(c) Includes pairing of homologous chromosomes (in tetrads or bivalents):

_____

(d) Results in two identical cells: _____

(e) Occurs only in ovaries or testes:

_____

B3. Describe one process in meiosis that leads to the possibility of an almost infinite variety of sperm or ova.

_____

_____

_____

B4. Each cell that begins meiosis (spermatogenesis) in males is likely to result in *(1? 2? 3? 4?)* mature sperm, whereas in females meiosis (oogenesis) produces ___ mature gamete(s) and ___ polar bodies.

B5. Answer these questions about chromosome structure.

(a) What is the division of genetics that studies the structure and characteristics of chromosomes? _____

(b) What is the source of human cells typically examined for chromosome structure?

_____

_____

(c) What is a karyotype?

_____

(d) What is an acrocentric chromosome?

_____

(e) How is the short arm of a chromosome designated? _____

(f) What function do telomeres play?_____

C. PATTERNS OF INHERITANCE (pages 125–127)

C1. Use each of the following answers once to fill in descriptions below.

Allele	Genotype	Locus
Multiple-gene	Multifactorial	Penetrance
Phenotype	Single-gene	

(a) "Type A" blood is a _____ , whereas "Ao" is the related _____.

(b) That 50% of people with a particular genotype will have the related phenotype is known as _____ of that gene.

(c) The specific location on a chromosome is known as the _____ of that gene, whereas the possible forms of genes at that site (such as A B or O for blood type) are known as _____s.

(d) Most human traits are determined by _____ inheritance; Mendelian laws govern _____ inheritance. _____ inheritance incorporates environmental effects.

C2. Genomic (or genetic) imprinting refers to genetic differences based on which _____ gives a particular gene to a child.

C3. Select the correct answers related to two parents, Annie and John, who have the following genotypes: Annie is AA and John is Aa.

(a) *(A? a?)* is the recessive gene.

(b) *(Mother's? Father's)* genotype is homozygous dominant. Which genotype is heterozygous?

(c) A carrier is *(homozygous? heterozygous?)* and *(does? does not?)* express the trait.

(d) In Mendel's work, "A" referred to *(round? wrinkled?)* peas.

(e) A graphic portrayal of Annie and John's family inheritance is known as a *(karyotype? pedigree?)*.

D. GENE TECHNOLOGY (pages 127–130)

D1. Describe the Human Genome Project and explain why it is an enormous undertaking.

_____

_____

_____

D2. In the "transcript mapping" method used in genome mapping, *(DNA? mRNA? tRNA?)* is isolated immediately after transcription. From this information, both the complementary DNA and the resultant gene product (_____) can be identified.

D3. Describe linkage studies in this exercise by circling the correct answer.

(a) These studies look at genes that are located on *(the same? different?)* chromosomes. They are located *(close together? far apart?)*, so they *(are? are not?)* likely to be linked during crossing-over of DNA in meiosis I.

(b) Two genes that are likely to be linked are genes for hemophilia and color-blindness, both located on the *(X? Y?)* chromosome. Because males have *(only one? two?)* X

chromosome(s), males are *(more? less?)* likely to inherit these conditions.

D4. Hemochromocytosis is a disorder that may be diagnosed by linkage studies. In this disorder, the person cannot metabolize _____ which accumulates in the _____.

D5. Using dosage studies in which the amount of an enzyme is measured, it is possible to determine whether _____ gave the gene to the child.

D6. Fill in blanks about hybridization studies.

(a) Somatic cell hybridization studies involve fusion of human somatic cells with cells of _____. These studies can identify the location of a specific _____ on a particular chromosome that codes for a specific enzyme.

(b) In situ hybridization uses "probes" consisting of _____ that can identify the location of a specific _____.

D7. Fill in blanks about recombinant DNA.

(a) Name two hormones that are available for pharmaceutical use as a result of recombinant DNA technology: _____ and _____.

(b) This technology involves the use of restriction enzymes (derived from _____) that cut _____ into many sections, a first step in isolating the _____ of interest.

(c) Ultimately, this DNA is introduced into a culture of _____ that express the gene by producing large amounts of the gene product (such as insulin).

D8. Describe how gene therapy can be used for persons with cystic fibrosis.

_____

_____

_____

D9. Explain how DNA fingerprinting can be used in forensics.

_____

_____

_____

CHAPTER 7

Genetic and Congenital Disorders

■ Review Questions

A. GENETIC AND CHROMOSOMAL DISORDERS (pages 131-140)

A1. Be sure that you understand the meaning of the following terms: *single-gene, multigene, and multifactorial inheritance; locus, allele; homozygous, heterozygous; genotype, phenotype; dominant, recessive.*

A2. Circle the two true statements.

(a) Signs and symptoms of **all** genetic defects **are** apparent at birth.

(b) Birth defects are the **leading** cause of infant deaths.

(c) **Blood group inheritance** is an example of a **codominance** in which **both** alleles in a gene pair may be fully expressed.

(d) A single-gene disorder (such as Marfan's syndrome) **will always affect only one part** of the body.

A3. The most common category of single gene disorder is:

(a). Autosomal dominant

(b) Autosomal recessive

(c) Sex-linked

A4. Refer to the pedigree chart presented in Figure 7-1 (text page 133), which depicts three generations of a family with an autosomal dominant disorder such as Huntington's disease (HD). Demonstrate your understanding of a pedigree chart by completing this exercise about this family.

(a) The grandparents (first generation) have *(2? 4? 6?)* children; of whom *(1? 2? 3?)* are male (squares) and *(1? 2? 3?)* are female (circles).

(b) In the second generation, *(2? 4? 6?)* individuals appear to be single; the other two are partnered, and each of these couples has *(2? 4?)* of their own children.

(c) Each individual receives chromosomes from each of his/her parents. Maternal chromosomes are represented by small *(circles? squares?)*; paternal chromosomes are shown by small *(circles? squares?)*.

(d) Given that the small colored circle represents the mutant autosomal dominant gene, the history of the HD gene in this family can be traced back to the *(grandmother? grandfather?)* who actually inherited the mutated gene from her own *(mother? father?)*.

(e) Do any of the four children in the second generation have the HD gene? *(Yes? No?)* If so, who? _____

(f) Can HD be transmitted from a mother to a son, or from a father to a daughter? *(Yes? No?)*

A5. Consult Table 7-1 (text page 133) and write names of four disorders *other than* HD that involve autosomal dominant inheritance. (Note that the pedigree chart in Fig. 7-1 could apply to these disorders as well.)

_____

_____

_____

A6. Circle the correct answer in each statement.

(a) For children to have autosomal dominant disorders, *(only one parent? both parents?)* must have the defective gene.

(b) It is probable that *(100%? 50%? 25%? 0%?)* of the children of a parent with an autosomal dominant disorder will inherit the condition.

(c) Asymptomatic individuals *(can? cannot?)* transmit autosomal dominant disorders to their children, thereby "skipping a generation."

A7. Complete this exercise about two autosomal dominant disorders.

(a) Marfan's syndrome is a __________ tissue disorder that primarily affects three systems, namely the *(skin? skeletal? muscular? cardiovascular? endocrine? special senses [eyes]?)*. Most life-threatening are effects on the ________ system. One readily observable effect is the *(short, obese? tall, thin?)* stature.

(b) Neurofibromatosis (NF) exists in *(two? three?)* forms located on *(the same? different?)* chromosome(s). *(NF-1? NF-2?)* involves skin lesions arising from peripheral nerves and also flat lesions on skin known as *(café-au-lait spots? Lisch nodules?)*. Also affected are *(eyes? ears?)* and skeleton. NF-2 exerts effects on *(vision? hearing?)*.

A8. Choose the two true statements about disorders of autosomal recessive inheritance.

(a) For children to have such disorders, **both parents** must have the defective gene.

(b) Carriers of such disorders **always** manifest signs or symptoms.

(c) Phenylketonuria is an autosomal recessive disorder that, if untreated, leads to **mental retardation.**

(d) Tay-Sachs disease results from faulty **mitochondrial** function.

A9. Circle the correct answers in these statements.

(a) Cystic fibrosis, sickle cell anemia, and Tay-Sachs disease are all autosomal *(dominant? recessive?)* disorders.

(b) All sex-linked disorders are carried on the *(X? Y? either X or Y?)* chromosome. These disorders affect more *(females? males?)*.

(c) Men with hemophilia *(can? cannot?)* transmit the defective gene for hemophilia to their sons.

A10. Determine the probability of phenotypes (and, where indicated, genotypes) of children of the following couples. Use Figures 7-1 to 7-3 below.

(a) Mr. Perez has the genotype for achondroplasia, and Mrs. Perez does not. (Note: "A = dominant; "a" = recessive for achondroplasia.) (Figure 7-1)

(b) Both Janet and Phillip are carriers for cystic fibrosis (CF). (Note: "C" = dominant; "c" is recessive for CF.) Complete the Punnett square. (Figure 7-2)

(c) Mimi is a carrier for hemophilia; Patrick does not have the mutant gene for hemophilia. (Note: "H" = dominant, or normal gene; "h" is recessive gene for hemophilia.) (Figure 7-3)

(Mrs.)	A	a (Mr.)
a	Aa	aa
a	Aa	aa

Probability of phenotypes:

Fig 7-1.

(Janet)	C	c (Phillip)
C	CC	___
c	___	___

Probable genotypes and phenotypes

Fig 7-2.

(Mimi)	X^H	Y (Patrick)
X^H	$X^H X^H$	$X^H Y$
X^h	$X^H X^h$	$X^h Y$

Probable phenotypes

Fig 7-3.

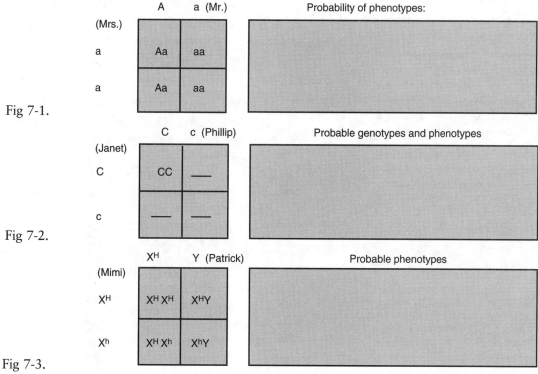

A11. Circle the disorders that are attributed to multifactorial inheritance.

Pyloric stenosis   Fragile X syndrome
Clubfoot   Diabetes mellitus
Tay-Sachs disease   Congenital heart disease
Congenital hip   Coronary artery disease
dislocation

A12. Circle the two true statements.

(a) Shorthand for a **female** with Down syndrome is 47,XY,+21.

(b) **Aneuploidy** refers to an abnormal chromosome number in cells.

(c) **Nondisjunction** is one cause of Down syndrome.

(d) Cells of people with Down syndrome typically contain a total of **21** chromosomes.

A13. Circle the correct answers or fill in the blanks in the following statements.

(a) Chromosomal disorders are *(frequently? rarely?)* associated with first trimester spontaneous abortions (miscarriages).

(b) Incidence of Down syndrome *(increases? decreases?)* with the age of the mother.

(c) Children with Down syndrome tend to have a *(larger? smaller?)* than normal head with *(larger? smaller?)* than normal tongue.

(d) Children with Down syndrome have a 10 to 20 times greater risk of the blood disorder _____. They are also at greater risk for _____ disease later in life.

A14. Circle the three answers that are the most accurate procedures for determining presence of Down syndrome in a fetus:

Amniocentesis   Alpha-fetoprotein
Chorionic villi   Human chorionic
sampling   gonadotropin
Percutaneous umbilical blood sampling

A15. Select the answers below that best fit descriptions below.

Fragile X syndrome   Klinefelter's
Turner's

(a) Monosomy X (or 45,X/0), a chromosomal disorder in which the female has only one X chromosome; she lacks ovaries and has other anatomical disorders: _____

(b) Polysomy X: males with extra X chromosome(s), such as genotype XXY or XXXY: _____

(c) A disorder that causes mental retardation, large testicles (macroorchidism), and highly flexible joints: _____

A16. Select the answers below that best fit descriptions of alterations in chromosome structure.

Deletion   Inversion
Robertsonian translocation   Translocation

(a) Results in a rare form of Down syndrome in which the individual has 46 chromosomes but a trisomy of the long arm of chromosome 21: _____

(b) A piece of a chromosome is broken off: _____

B. DISORDERS DUE TO ENVIRONMENTAL INFLUENCES (pages 140–144)

B1. Choose the two true statements.

(a) Formation of organs (organogenesis) normally occurs during the **middle** trimester (months **4** to **6**) of pregnancy.

(b) Development of the brain and the heart begin during the **third** week of human development. (*Hint:* refer to Figure 7-8, text page 141).

(c) Teratogens are **cancer**-causing agents.

(d) Thalidomide is an infamous teratogen that is known to cause **phocomelia** (meaning failure of the **extremities** to develop normally).

B2. Circle the correct answers in each statement.

(a) There *(is? is not?)* evidence that diagnostic levels of radiation cause congenital abnormalities.

(b) *(Most? Few?)* developmental defects are known to be caused by specific drugs or environmental agents.

(c) *(Water? Lipid?)*-soluble drugs such as alcohol and those with *(small? large?)* molecular weight are more likely to cross the placenta and expose the fetus.

(d) In the Food and Drug Administration's classification of drugs that may harm the fetus, those in class *(A? C? X?)* are contraindicated because they are known teratogens.

B3. Choose the two true statements.

(a) Megadoses of vitamin A have been found to **prevent** congenital defects

(b) Alcohol is harmful to the fetus **only** during the first **3 months** of gestation.

(c) Maternal smoking and abuse of alcohol and "crack" cocaine are all associated with **lower** than normal birth weight.

(d) Fetal alcohol syndrome (FAS) **can** often be detected by facial structures in the newborn.

B4. The U.S. Surgeon General's office recommends that pregnant women drink _____ servings of wine or beer per day.

(a) No more than four

(b) No more than two

(c) No

B5. Choose the two true statements about effects of cocaine on fetal development.

(a) Cocaine tends to **decrease** uteroplacental blood flow.

(b) Urine of babies whose mothers abused cocaine will test positive for cocaine for about the first **2 weeks** of the baby's life.

(c) Cocaine tends to **decrease** uterine contractions, **delaying** labor and delivery.

(d) Cocaine-induced **vasoconstriction** of fetal blood vessels is associated with urogenital birth defects of "crack babies."

B6. Fill in the blanks in this exercise.

(a) Increase in folic acid intake (such as 0.4 mg/d prenatally and more during pregnancy) has been found to decrease incidence of _____ defects such as _____.

(b) Folic acid is found in foods such as:

_____

(c) The antibiotic tetracycline is associated with defects in _____ development.

B7. Circle correct answers to these questions about TORCH-caused fetal anomalies.

(a) "TORCH" refers to *(chemicals? microorganisms?)* that are teratogenic.

(b) The "T" in "TORCH" stands for the *(bacterial? fungal? protozoan?)* disorder, *Toxoplasmosis*, which may be found in the excrement of *(dogs? cats?)*.

(c) "R" represents the *(bacterial? viral?)* infection *(mumps? German measles?)*, known as *Rubella*.

(d) "H" stands for *(hepatitis? herpes?)* infections.

C. DIAGNOSIS AND COUNSELING (pages 144–148)

C1. List components of a genetic risk assessment.

_____

_____

_____

C2. Fill in the blanks about serum markers that indicate increased likelihood of fetal anomalies.

(a) Analysis of maternal blood or amniotic fluid is likely to show an abnormal *(increase? decrease?)* in the serum marker named AFP (or _____) if the fetus has neural tube defects.

(b) Down syndrome is associated with a(n) *(increase? decrease?)* in AFP and a(n) *(increase? decrease?)* in the placental hormone HCG (or _____).

C3. Mrs. Hernandez, age 41, has given birth to one child with a neural tube defect. *Identify the diagnostic tests that she may receive during her current pregnancy.*

Amniocentesis   Alpha-fetoprotein
Chorionic villi sampling   testing
Dermatoglyphic analysis   Ultrasound

(a) Which of the above tests can be performed at about 10 weeks of gestation?

_____

(b) Which test is noninvasive and uses high-frequency sound? _____

(c) Which test studies patterns on palms and soles? _____

(d) Which procedure involves inserting a needle through the mother's abdominal and uterine wall? _____

C4. Complete this exercise about diagnostic fetal karyotyping by filling in the blanks or selecting the correct answers.

(a) This process studies fetal _____. What is the source of fetal cells studied in karyotyping?

(b) Karyotyping *(can? cannot?)* be used for prenatal diagnoses of genetic defects; the process *(can? cannot?)* reveal the gender of the fetus.

CHAPTER 8

Alterations in Cell Differentiation: Neoplasia

■ Review Questions

A. CONCEPTS OF CELL GROWTH (pages 149–153)

A1. Complete the table below on common cancer sites based on Figure 8-1, page 150 of the text.

(a) Cancer incidence

Males	Females
1. Prostate	1.
2. Lung	2.
3. Colorectal	3.
4. Bladder	4.

(b) Cancer deaths

Males	Females
1.	1.
2.	2.
3.	3.
4.	4.

A2. Choose the two true statements.

(a) **Cancer** is currently the leading cause of death in the United States.

(b) The term **proliferation** means specialization of cells.

(c) The G_0 phase is the **least active** phase of the growth cycle.

(d) **Apoptosis** is an attempt by the body to regulate cell number and type.

A3. Arrange in correct sequence these phases of the growth cycle following the "M" phase:

G_1 G_2 S

——, ——, ——

A4. Methotrexate, a particular type of drug used in chemotherapy (see p. 172), interferes with replication of DNA required to double chromosome numbers before cell division occurs. This drug attacks cancer cells while they are in the _____.

(a) G_1 or G_2 phase

(b) M phase

(c) S phase

A5. Arrange these categories of cells by letter in correct sequence from most to least differentiated.

(a) Pluripotent stem cells as in bone marrow

(b) Progenitor cells that can be recruited to form new cells of the same cell line

(c) Highly specialized cells such as neurons

——, ——, ——

A6. Circle the correct answers in these statements.

(a) As cells increase specialization, they *(lose? increase?)* their ability to divide.

(b) Neoplasms *(do? do not?)* serve useful purposes because they grow at the expense of other healthy tissues of the host.

B. CHARACTERISTICS OF BENIGN AND MALIGNANT NEOPLASMS (pages 153–161)

B1. Choose the two true statements.

(a) **All** tumors are cancerous.

(b) Sarcomas are cancers that derive from **epithelial** tissues.

(c) Leukemias are **malignant** tumors of **blood.**

(d) A leiomyosarcoma is a **malignant** tumor of **smooth muscle.**

B2. Write *M* for malignant and *B* for benign next to correct descriptions.

(a) An osteoma: ____

(b) Most likely to be encapsulated: ____

(c) Tumor grows by crab-like infiltration and is likely to metastasize: ____

(d) Cells are poorly differentiated: ____

(e) Hemangiosarcoma: ____

B3. Circle correct answers or fill in the blanks in each statement.

(a) When cancer cells mutate early in differentiation, they are likely to be *(more? less?)* highly malignant than cancer cells that mutate late in differentiation.

(b) Highly anaplastic cells are likely to resemble *(each other? cells from the site of origin?)*.

(c) Malignant cells exhibit a *(greater? lesser?)* degree of contact inhibition than normal cells. This is one reason why cancer cells have *(increased? decreased?)* cohesiveness and tend to *(stay in one place? infiltrate other regions?)* in the body. Another factor that contributes to spread of cancer is release of _____ by cancer cells that break down matrix between cells.

(d) Shedding of fetal antigens by cancer cells serve as _____ for cancer and indicate that these cells are *(more? less?)* differentiated than normal cells.

B4. Mrs. Wren has a chest x-ray that reveals a lesion. A biopsy of the lesion identifies these cells as cancer cells that originated in Mrs. Wren's kidney. Explain.

_____

_____

_____

B5. Mrs. Chan's endometrial cancer has metastasized to several sites in her large intestine.

(a) Explain how this is likely to have occurred: _____

_____

_____

(b) Cancer cells that spread into her lymph vessels and nodes are more likely to gain access to blood in *(arteries? veins?)*.

B6. Tell which cancer is more likely to metastasize to **liver** and which to **lungs**. Explain why.

(a) Mr. Thomas' testicular cancer:

_____

_____

_____

(b) Mr. Chase's colon cancer:

_____

_____

_____

B7. For every 10,000 cancer cells that leave a primary tumor, *(1? 100? 1,000? 9,999?)* is/are likely to survive and start a secondary tumor. Circle the correct answer and explain why.

_____

_____

_____

B8. Identify the factors that help cancer cells to succeed and survive at a secondary site.

Laminin   NM 23
Platelets   Tumor-angiogenesis
Type IV collagenase   factors

(a) Combined with cancer cells, they form tumor emboli within the bloodstream: _____

(b) Enzymes that help cancer cells to make their way through basement membranes to move into new areas: _____

(c) Chemicals secreted by tumor cells that stimulate growth of new blood vessels around the cancer cells: _____

(d) High levels of this tumor suppressor gene appear to reduce risk of breast cancer metastasis: _____

B9. Complete this exercise about tumor growth.

(a) Circle the answer that is true of cancer cells.
(1) They have a shorter cell cycle, so divide at a faster rate.
(2) They live longer than normal cells because they do not die on schedule.

(b) List three factors that increase rate of tumor growth.

_____

_____

_____

(c) A tumor is normally undetectable until it contains more than _____ cells.

B10. Explain how Mrs. Garcia's signs and symptoms of her end-stage colon cancer may be caused by the pathogenesis of cancer.

(a) Severe constipation with impaction, and blood in the stool

(b) Difficulty urinating

(c) Severe abdominopelvic pain

(d) Weight loss of 50 pounds even though she retains large amounts of fluid in her abdomen

(e) Fractured hip and hypercalcemia

C. CARCINOGENESIS AND CAUSES OF CANCER (pages 161-167)

C1. *Carcinogenic* is a term that means:

(a) RNA

(b) Blood-vessel-forming

(c) Cancer-causing

(d) DNA

(e) Cachectic (cachexia-causing)

C2. Choose the two true statements about carcinogenesis.

(a) Most cancers are probably caused by **one** factor.

(b) Proto-oncogenes are **normal** sections of DNA that have the potential of being transformed into **cancer-causing** sections of DNA called **oncogenes**.

(c) Most cancers are known to be caused by viruses.

(d) Because the p53 gene is an **anti-oncogene**, deficient activity of this gene (as in Li-Fraumeni cancer syndrome) **increases** the risk of breast and other kinds of cancer.

(e) Typically a normal cell can be converted into a cancer cell by the presence of **one** oncogene.

C3. Choose the two true statements about carcinogenesis.

(a) The initiation step in carcinogenesis is a **reversible** mutation of DNA.

(b) The **initiation** step in carcinogenesis must precede the promotion step in carcinogenesis.

(c) Promotors do **not** alter DNA but change its expression.

(d) Promotion **is not** reversible, even if the promotor is removed.

(e) The progression step of carcinogenesis is **the same as** the promotion step.

C4. Circle the correct answers in each statement.

(a) Direct-acting carcinogens *(do? do not?)* require activation by the body to become carcinogenic.

(b) Vitamins A, C, and E are *(free radicals? antioxidants?)* that *(cause? inhibit?)* damaging effects of carcinogens on DNA.

(c) Inheritance of retinoblastoma, familial adenomatous polyposa (FAP), and

Li-Fraumeni cancer syndrome tends to follow autosomal *(dominant? recessive?)* patterns.

C5. BRCA1 and BRCA2 refer to genes that increase a person's risk for _____ cancer.

C6. Jimmy, age 42, is having a history and physical taken. He states to the nurse that he "live(s) on hot dogs and barbecued pork, fries, beer, cigarettes, and playing cards with my buddies." Describe the aspects of Jimmy's lifestyle that increase his risk for cancer.

_____

_____

_____

C7. A town of Native Americans in northern Alaska smokes fish as its primary industry. Speculate about causes for the high incidence of GI cancers and liver problems in middle-aged and elderly members of that population.

_____

_____

_____

C8. Match the type of cancer with the patient likely to be at greatest risk for it. Select from these answers:

Leukemia   Lung
Skin   Vaginal

(a) Julia's mother took DES while she was pregnant with Julia: _____

(b) Jesse, age 38, has done fieldwork in southern Arizona since he was a child; he experienced three severe sunburns between ages 7 and 10: _____

(c) Henry, age 68, is a survivor of the bombing of Hiroshima: _____

(d) Paul, age 53, is retiring after 30 years as uranium mine worker: _____

C9. Describe roles played by viruses in carcinogenesis.

_____

_____

_____

C10. Match the virus with the correct description below.

Epstein-Barr virus   Hepatitis B virus
Human T-cell   Human papillomavirus
  leukemia virus-1

(a) Associated with liver carcinoma as well as cirrhosis and hepatitis B:

_____

(b) An RNA virus carried in CD4 cells and associated with a form of leukemia:

_____

(c) Over 60 different types include those that cause warts (papillomas) and squamous cell carcinomas of the cervix:

_____

(d) Associated with four human cancers including some lymphomas:

_____

D. DIAGNOSIS AND TREATMENT (pages 167–175)

D1. Answer these questions about early detection of cancer.

(a) Explain why cervical dysplasia cells are more likely to shed and be detected during a Papanicolaou (Pap) smear than normal cells are.

_____

_____

_____

(b) List several methods besides the Pap smear that are methods of secondary prevention (screening) for cancer.

_____

_____

_____

D2. Mr. Rhodenberger's nurse practitioner discusses with her patient that his PSA level is higher than it was 3 months ago. What information is the nurse practitioner conveying?

_____

_____

_____

D3. Indicate the types of cancer with which the following antigens (tumor markers) are linked.

Alpha-fetoprotein   Carcinoembryonic
Human chorionic   antigen
 gonadotropin
Prostate specific antigen

(a) Associated with most colorectal and pancreatic tumors: _____

(b) Normally formed in the fetal liver and yolk sac, this antigen may also be elevated with primary liver cancers:

_____

D4. Polymerase chain reaction (PCR) tests exhibit _(high? low?)_ sensitivity to specific types of tumor cells, and a _(high? low?)_ percentage of false-positives (meaning that is not specific).

_____

D5. Identify whether the following results of diagnostic tests on Mr. Rhodenberger's chart (from Question D2) are indicative of grading (G) or staging (S) of his cancer. Also answer related questions by filling in the blanks.

(a) T2, N3, M1: ____ To what does "N" of "N3" refer? Involvement of _____.

(b) Moderately undifferentiated cells: ____ Which carries a worse prognosis: grade I or grade IV? _____.

D6. About ____% of all cancer patients will have surgery related to their cancers. List several factors that determine the type of surgery indicated.

_____

_____

_____

D7. State one example of a prophylactic use of surgery related to cancer.

_____

_____

_____

D8. Circle the correct answer. Cryosurgery involves use of:

(a) High frequency current

(b) Corrosive paste

(c) Cold liquid nitrogen

(d) Laser beam

D9. Complete this exercise about Ms. Bonner's radiation for breast cancer.

(a) She receives radiation for 5 weeks pre-surgery. This is an example of _(adjuvant? palliative? primary?)_ use of radiation.

(b) Her radiation is _(ionizing? nonionizing?)_, which especially targets _(slowly? rapidly?)_ dividing cells. Fast-growing cells are typically more _(radiosensitive? radioresistant?)_ than slow-growing cells.

(c) Ms. Bonner is likely to receive _(one large dose? multiple fractionated doses?)_. Explain why.

_____

_____

(d) Her red blood cell count drops after several radiation treatments. How does the resulting hypoxia *help* cancer cells to survive?_____

_____

_____

_____

(e) Explain why Ms. Bonner's skin over the site of the radiation is reddening (erythema) and why her blood counts are checked frequently. _____

_____

D10. Match the type of radiation with the related description below. Choose from these answers:

Brachytherapy
External beam radiation
Unsealed internal radiation

(a) Mr Bennett takes iodine-131 by mouth for his thyroid cancer:

_____.

(b) Ms. Murray has a sealed container of cesium-137 inserted into her uterus for 24 hours: _____.

(c) Radiation from a linear accelerator is pinpointed to Louis's tumor:

_____.

D11. Complete this exercise about use of chemotherapy for cancer patients. Fill in the blanks or circle the correct answers.

(a) Explain why multiple courses of treatment are required for effective chemotherapy.

_____

_____

(b) *(Combination? Single drug?)* chemotherapy is generally most effective.

(c) Methotrexate is a cell-cycle *(specific? nonspecific?)* anticancer drug. It is most effective during the *(G₁? M? S?)* phase of the cycle. It is a component of the *(CHOP? CMF?)* drug regimen for breast cancer.

(d) Most chemotherapy is administered directly into *(arterial blood? venous blood? skeletal muscles?)*.

D12. Describe side effects of Georgia's chemotherapy treatment in this exercise.

(a) The **nadir** for thrombocytopenia for her specific drug regimen is 21 days.

_____

(b) The drug has a **high emetic potential** and causes **increased gastric motility**.

(c) It is likely to cause **stomatitis**.

_____

(d) **Amenorrhea** is a likely side effect.

_____

(e) It is associated with a **risk of second malignancies**.

_____

D13. Mrs. Jordan has been receiving intensive chemotherapy for several months for her ovarian cancer. Explain why it is likely that she may:

(a) Wear a bandana over her bald head

_____

_____

(b) Have lost 40 pounds

_____

_____

(c) Decline an invitation to go out with a friend who has a bad cold.

_____

_____

(d) Feel so weak that she sleeps much of her day

_____

_____

D14. Describe the action of the anticancer drug, tamoxifen.

_____

_____

_____

D15. Define **biotherapy.**

_____

_____

_____

Now contrast the two major categories of cancer biotherapy by writing "A" for active or "P" for passive forms of immunotherapy.

(a) Introduction of antigens such as BCG that stimulate the patient's immune system: ____

(b) Vaccines composed of antigens derived from the patient's own tumor cells that activate immune responses: ____

(c) Introduction of natural killer (NK) cells activated by lymphokines such as interleukin-2 (IL-2); these directly attack cancer cells (as well as normal cells): ____

(d) Use of T cells taken from the person's tumor (tumor-infiltrating lymphocytes or TIL cells) and grown to form large numbers before reinfusion; TILs attack tumor cells but not normal cells: ____

D16. Match the biologic response modifiers (BRMs) with descriptions below.

Hematopoietic growth   Interferons
    factors   Interleukins
Monoclonal antibodies

(a) Mrs. Jordan (see Questions D13 [c] and [d]) is receiving CSFs and erythropoietin to reverse the side effects of her chemotherapy drugs: _____.

(b) These antibodies were used to detect the presence of Mrs. Jordan's ovarian cancer: _____.

(c) Matthew's Kaposi's sarcoma (KS) is treated by these BRMs that stimulate his own NK cells and T lymphocytes to combat this AIDS-related cancer: _____.

(d) Mrs. Kern received this class of chemicals to activate many aspects of her immune system to attack metastasizing cells from her kidney tumor: _____.

D17. Complete this exercise concerning bone marrow transplantation (BMT) for Lynn, who has leukemia.

(a) Lynn is going to receive an allogenic BMT, meaning that the marrow cells are from *(her own harvested and treated cells? an HLA-matched donor's cells?)*.

(b) Before the graft is made, she receives high doses of chemotherapy. Why?

_____

_____

(c) Supportive therapy to reduce side effects of the BMT includes growth factors such as neutropin, erythropoietin, and thrombopoietin, which will increase production of _____, _____, and _____, respectively.

(d) Explain why PBSTC might have lower procedure-related morbidity for Lynn than BMT._____

_____

_____

D18. *(Somatic cell? Germ-line?)* gene therapy inserts genes into ova or sperm to eliminate a genetic defect in future generations. This form of gene therapy *(has? has not?)* been approved by the FDA and NIH. List several examples of uses of *somatic* cell gene therapy.

_____

_____

_____

E. CHILDHOOD CANCERS (pages 175–178)

E1. Choose the two true statements about childhood cancers.

(a) Cancer is the **leading** cause of death among children.

(b) Most childhood cancers involve cells of **epithelial** origin.

(c) Families with one child with cancer are at **increased** risk to have another child who develops cancer.

(d) Children with hereditary disorders such as Down syndrome have an **increased** risk for developing cancer.

E2. Circle the correct answers in these statements about childhood cancers.

(a) Cancer is *(more? less?)* frequently found among children than adults, contributing to the *(ease of? difficulty in?)* diagnosing childhood cancer.

(b) Acute lymphocytic leukemia (ALL) has a *(higher? lower?)* survival rate among children under age 15 than acute myeloid leukemia (AML). Hodgkin's disease has an extremely *(high? low?)* survival rate among this population.

(c) Sequelae of radiation treatment on growth and cognitive development are greater if the child is *(of preschool age? of school age or older?)* when the treatment is given.

(d) Radiation and chemotherapy *(virtually never? are known to?)* cause damage to heart and lungs.

_____

_____

CHAPTER 9

Stress and Adaptation

■ Review Questions

A. HOMEOSTASIS (pages 181-183)

A1. Match the following theorist researchers with descriptions of their work.

Claude Bernard   Hans Selye
Walter Cannon

(a) Identified the *milieu intèrieur* as the fluid environment around cells:

_____

(b) Described homeostasis as a stable internal environment achieved by mechanisms that resist various disturbances that he described as "fight or flight" responses:

_____

(c) In the early 1930s, he described mechanisms of adaptation to stress: _____

A2. Complete this exercise about control mechanisms of the body.

(a) When David runs a mile, his muscles release heat, which causes his body temperature to increase. In efforts to return his temperature back to normal, his sweat glands are likely to *(increase? decrease?)* secretions, and blood vessels of his skin are likely to *(dilate? constrict?)*. These mechanisms are examples of *(positive? negative?)* feedback control mechanisms because they alter a parameter such as temperature in the *(same? opposite?)* direction as it had originally been changed.

(b) Most control systems of the body are *(positive? negative?)*. They introduce *(stability? instability?)* into a system. An example is release of the pancreatic hormone insulin in response to *(elevated? decreased?)* blood glucose level. The effect of insulin is to *(raise? lower?)* blood glucose level.

B. STRESS (pages 183-189)

B1. Briefly describe possible roles of stress in disease causation.

_____
_____
_____

B2. List the three specific anatomic changes that Hans Selye described in rats exposed to various stressors.

_____
_____
_____

B3. Write the meaning of the acronym GAS described by Hans Selye:

G _____ A _____ S _____.

Answer these questions about the GAS. Use the following answers.

Alarm   Exhaustion   Resistance

(a) Arrange in correct sequence the three phases of the GAS: _____, _____,

_____

(b) Which phase involves action of pituitary and both adrenal medulla and adrenal cortex hormones, as well as sympathetic nerves? _____

(c) In which phase does the body try to fight back or "resist"? _____ But if these mechanisms fail, then the stage of _____ (with possible death) occurs.

B4. List several conditions likely to result from emotional disturbances (stress) and the body's adaptive mechanisms.

_____
_____
_____

B5. Discuss stressors and their impact by completing this exercise about Mrs. Robinson, whose daughter's wedding is this week.

(a) The joy Mrs. Robinson feels for her daughter's happiness is considered *(eustress? distress?)*, whereas her concerns about the reception for 400 people is ____stress. The stressors associated with planning the wedding are _____genous stressors.

(b) Mrs. Robinson is recovering from hip replacement and her husband has prostate cancer. These are likely to be *(internal? external?)* conditioning factors that *(increase? decrease?)* her adaptive capacity.

B6. Identify the three major systems that interact in response to stressors.

_____
_____
_____

B7. Defend or dispute this statement: "Stress can lead to growth."

_____
_____
_____

B8. Match the parts of the brain with stress-related functions below.

Cerebral cortex   Hypothalamus
Locus ceruleus-   Limbic system
  norepinephrine pathway   Thalamus
Reticular activating system

(a) Conveys sensory information about stressors to different parts of the brain: _____

(b) Facilitate mental alertness and vigilance during stress responses (2 answers): _____, _____

(c) Involved primarily with emotional aspects of stress responses: _____

(d) Coordinate autonomic and endocrine responses to stressors: (2 answers): _____, _____

(e) A site of neurons in the brain stem that release norepinephrine (NE): _____

(f) CRF made here stimulates release of ACTH that triggers adrenal cortical production of cortisol: _____

B9. Refer to Figure 9-2 in the text and complete this exercise about roles of chemical mediators in stress responses.

(a) NE, see B8(d)-(e), is a *(sympathetic? parasympathetic?)* neurotransmitter and is chemically classified as a *(catecholamine? glucocorticoid?)*. NE prepares the body for stress by *(increasing? decreasing?)* heart and respiratory rates, *(increasing? decreasing?)* salivation and digestive activity, *(increasing? decreasing?)* sweat (to cool the body), and *(constricting? dilating?)* the pupils.

(b) Cortisol, see B8(f), is a *(catecholamine? glucocorticoid?)* that *(increases? decreases?)* blood glucose level, *(increases? decreases?)* production of thyroid hormone, and *(increases? decreases?)* growth, metabolism, and immunity, as the body focuses on efforts to regain balance.

(c) A high blood level of cortisol leads to a *(high? low?)* level of CRF and ACTH; this is an example of a *(positive? negative?)* feedback mechanism.

(d) CRF *(stimulates? inhibits?)* the locus ceruleus which then *(increases? decreases?)* release of CRF; this is a *(positive? negative?)* feedback loop.

(e) Through several mechanisms, chronic stress *(stimulates? inhibits?)* release of growth hormone; this fact may help to explain failure to _____ (FTT) in children.

(f) Antidiuretic hormone (or _____) released in stress helps the body to *(retain? eliminate?)* water and *(increase? decrease?)* blood pressure.

(g) Effects of stress-related CRF on the pituitary gland as well as gonads can cause a(n) *(increase? decrease?)* in estrogen in women, leading to failure to ovulate and _____. Chronic stress in men can cause a(n) *(increase? decrease?)* in testosterone production as well as a(n) *(increase? decrease?)* in sperm production.

B10. Describe relationships between neuroendocrine and immune function in this exercise.

(a) Two classes of hormones that inhibit immune function are _____ and _____. See B9 (a) and (b). The fact that at least eight hormones influence lymphocytes is evidenced by presence of

_____ for these hormones on lymphocytes.

(b) It is known that cytokines such as interleukins released by _____ activate the hormones of the HPA system. This system includes cells of the hypothalamus as well as the _____ and _____ glands.

B11. Consider how each of the following factors would be likely to have an impact on your own adaptation to the stress of your being diagnosed with an illness such as diabetes, multiple sclerosis, or a brain tumor. Select one diagnosis and discuss with a friend or a colleague.

(a) Your life experiences

_____

_____

(b) Your nutritional patterns and status

_____

_____

(c) Your overall health status

_____

_____

(d) Your hardiness

_____

_____

B12. Circle the person who is likely to adapt better in each case. Then identify from the following list the type of factor involved in each case of adaptation. Write the factor on lines provided.

Age   Health status
Psychosocial factors   Timing of onset

(a) Loss of 25% of total blood volume in:

_____

(1) Jeanette, by arterial hemorrhage within a period of 3 minutes

(2) Irma, by bleeding from a peptic ulcer over the course of 3 months

(b) Prolonged diarrhea in: _____

(1) Jamie, who is 2 months old

(2) Cassandra, who is 20 years old

(c) A respiratory infection in: _____

(1) Terrence, who has cystic fibrosis

(2) Paula, whose lungs are healthy

(d) Diagnosis of HIV-positive status in:

_____

(1) Lee, who has a supportive significant other and caring siblings

(2) Sandy, who is homeless and suffers from alcoholism

B13. Contrast these two sleep disorders: *insomnia* and *increased somnolence*.

_____

_____

_____

C. DISORDERS OF THE STRESS RESPONSE (pages 189–194)

C1. Identify the pattern of stressors in each case below.

Acute time-limited   Chronic intermittent
Chronic sustained

(a) Jamal, age 5, has had middle ear infections four times in the past 2 years:

_____

(b) Chris, age 40, was diagnosed with amyotrophic lateral sclerosis (ALS, or Lou Gehrig's disease) when he was 37. He can still speak and swallow, but most of the rest of his body is paralyzed: _____

C2. Mr. Clement, who has diabetes and significant renal impairment, is involved in an auto accident and brought to an emergency room. His blood pressure is 192/112 mm Hg. Speculate about the impact of this acute stress on him.

_____

_____

_____

C3. Define **premorbid stress** and state an example of it in your own life.

_____

_____

_____

C4. Jennifer, age 19, is the only survivor of a boating accident 3 months ago in which both her fiancé and her brother drowned. Write the related sign or symptom next to each of Jennifer's statements that characterize her post-traumatic stress disorder (PTSD). Select from these terms:

Avoidance   Alcohol or drug abuse
Depression   Intrusions
Memory problems   Sleep disturbances
Survival guilt

(a) "I just want to be alone and drink; I shouldn't even be alive." _____

(b) "Three nights this week I woke up and lived it all over again." _____

C5. Complete this exercise about PTSD.

(a) List several other events besides boating accidents that might lead to PTSD.

_____
_____
_____

(b) Physiologic mechanisms of PTSD include activation of _____-related systems in several brain parts, exaggerated *(sympathetic? parasympathetic?)* nerve responses, and *(increased? decreased?)* levels of cortisol. The factor that differs from typical stress responses is _____.

(c) Studies suggest that strong family relationships may *(increase? decrease?)* risk for PTSD among children exposed to violent events.

(d) List several methods other than antidepressant or antianxiety medications that may be used in the treatment of PTSD.

_____
_____

C6. One example of biofeedback therapy is based on the finding that during stress, temperature *(increases? decreases?)* in fingers or toes, as a result of sympathetic vaso*(constriction? dilation?)* of blood vessels in the extremities. Such changes can be monitored by the patient as a result of *(electromyodermal? electrodermal? electrothermal?)* detection.

C7. List two factors that present obstacles to research on physiologic responses to stress in humans.

_____
_____

Now list specific examples of noninvasive stress-measurement techniques:

(a) Cardiovascular changes: _____,
_____

(b) Sweating: _____

(c) Hormonal levels in urine: _____

(d) Hormonal levels in saliva: _____

C8. Defend or dispute this statement: "Stress *does* cause disease."

_____
_____
_____

CHAPTER 10

Alterations in Temperature Regulation

■ Review Questions

A. BODY TEMPERATURE REGULATION
(pages 195–198)

A1. Circle the two true statements.

(a) Core body temperature is normally about 42°C.

(b) Body temperature is typically highest in the **morning**.

(c) Core body temperature is typically **lower** than skin temperature.

(d) Rectal temperature is typically **higher** than oral temperature.

(e) Because fat conducts heat **poorly**, adipose tissue is a **good** insulator.

A2. Circle the correct answers or fill in the blanks in these statements about Timmy, age 3, who has a fever and otitis media (middle ear infection).

(a) The nurse measures Timmy's temperature by ear-based thermometry that usually *(does? does not?)* correlate well with rectal temperature. Factors that might alter the accuracy of this method in Timmy's case include _____.

(b) His core body temperature is 40°C, which is about *(102.2°F? 104.0°F? 105.8°F?)*. Every 1°C rise in body temperature equals a ____°F rise in body temperature.

(c) One mechanism that can help lower Timmy's temperature is vaso*(constriction? dilation?)* of blood vessels in his skin.

A3. Write *L* next to mechanisms by which the body loses heat, and write *G* next to mechanisms related to heat gain (or heat production).

(a) Release of catecholamines such as epinephrine produced during stress: ____

(b) Shivering: ____

(c) Strenuous exercise: ____

(d) Sweating: ____

(e) Use of a cooling blanket: ____

(f) Diuresis (for example, by use of diuretics): ____

A4. Select answers from the following list of heat loss mechanisms that fit descriptions below.

Conduction   Convection
Evaporation   Radiation

(a) George feels a chill as a breeze from an open window reaches him while taking a shower: _____

(b) The backs of Julia's thighs feel cool as she sits on a metal bench in her running shorts: _____

(c) Emilio runs a 10K race on a 105°F day: _____

(d) This mechanism is likely to account for most of Lucy's heat loss as she sits outside on a 60°F day: _____

B. INCREASED BODY TEMPERATURE
(pages 198–205)

B1. Circle correct answers or fill in the blanks in each statement about fever.

(a) Fever is caused by *(resetting the temperature set point in the hypothalamus? ineffectual temperature-regulating mechanisms?)*.

(b) The human temperature set point typically has an upper limit of ____°C (or ____°F). List two factors that might cause the core body temperature to exceed this.

(c) Fever is also known as _____. Antipyretic agents *(increase? decrease?)* body temperature by *(causing vasodilation? resetting the temperature set point?)*.

(d) Bacteria that cause fever release chemicals called *(endo? exo?)*genous pyrogens. These chemicals stimulate body cells to release _____genous pyrogens, such as _____-1 or -6 or TNF, which stands for _____.

B2. Suggest a likely mechanism for fever in each of the following cases. Note: none of these clients has an infection.

(a) Mrs. Graham has had a myocardial infarction (heart attack).

_____

_____

(b) Mr. Giovanni has Hodgkin's disease.

_____

_____

(c) Infant Jeremy has increased intracranial pressure (ICP) following head trauma. He is not responding to antipyretic therapy.

_____

_____

B3. Defend or dispute this statement: "Fever is beneficial."

_____

_____

_____

B4. Select the class of fever that fits each description below.

Intermittent   Relapsing
Remittent   Sustained

(a) Billy had a fever for 3 days, then a normal temperature for 2 days, and then the cycle repeated: _____

(b) Cicely's temperature has varied between 101°F and 104°F for 5 days:

_____

B5. During a fever, heart rate and metabolic rate are both likely to *(increase? decrease?)*. As a result, the person has a(n) *(increased? decreased?)* need for hydration.

B6. Arrange these phases of a fever in correct sequence from first to last:

Chill   Defervescence
Flush   Prodrome

_____ → _____ →
_____ → _____.

Now write the correct phase (chosen from the list above) next to each related description.

(a) Shivering and goose bumps signal an attempt by the body to conserve heat to meet the body's new temperature set point:

_____

(b) Stages that decrease body temperature back towards normal (two answers):

_____ , _____

B7. Lawrence has a history of herpes simplex type I (HSV-I). He breaks out with a fever blister now as he has a fever. Explain.

_____

_____

_____

B8. Ms. Johnson's chart indicates that she has an "FUO." Define FUO and list several possible causes.

_____

_____

_____

B9. Body temperature is *(better? more poorly?)* regulated in infants than in adults. Fever in children under the age of 3 years is defined as a temperature greater than ____°C = ____°F.

B10. During a history and physical examination, Mr. Baker, age 87, reports to the nurse that he takes medicine for "my Parkinson's disease and a water pill for my heart." The nurse records his oral temperature at 100.2°F. Explain why his temperature should be further monitored.

_____

_____

_____

B11. Arrange these conditions from least to most serious forms of hyperthermia:

Heat cramps   Heat exhaustion
Heat stroke   Heat syncope

_____ → _____ →
_____ → _____

Now select from the same answers shown above to identify conditions that fit descriptions given below.

(a) Larry and Laurie (both age 28) have just run 15 miles one hot day in Arizona. Larry suddenly faints as blood pools in his skin in an attempt to cool his body: _____ Laurie's body is depleted of salt by prolonged sweating followed by drinking water: _____

(b) Ms. Dawson, age 92, and Ms. Waters, age 88, live in a house that has no air conditioning. The temperature outside has reached 101°F. Ms. Waters calls 911 to say that Ms. Dawson has fallen. When paramedics arrive they find that Ms. Dawson's core temperature is 104.6°F and her skin is hot and dry: _____

B12. Treatment of heat stroke must be done *(rapidly? slowly?)* because organ damage occurs when core temperature reaches ____°C (____°F). List three vital organs that are especially vulnerable to the effects of hyperthermia: _____, _____, _____

B13. Fill in blanks and circle correct answers in these statements about drugs that can induce fever.

(a) Thyroid hormone *(increases? decreases?)* metabolism and heat production.

(b) Drugs that *(increase? decrease?)* sweating or cause vaso_____ can induce fever, as do those that cause the body to release endogenous _____.

(c) Drug fevers *(are? are not?)* typically accompanied by tachycardia.

B14. What is the meaning of the term "malignant" in "malignant hyperthermia"? _____ This condition *(is? is not?)* hereditary. People with this condition experience *(gradual? rapid?)* rise in body temperature related to excessive _____ activity.

Explain why patients with this condition may be high surgical risks.

_____

_____

_____

C. DECREASED BODY TEMPERATURE (pages 205–207)

C1. Answer these questions about Sven, a construction worker who fell into icy water.

(a) Hypothermia occurs more rapidly when someone is exposed to cold *(air? water?)*.

(b) Sven's core temperature is currently 84°F, indicating *(mild? moderate? severe?)* hypothermia. Oral thermometry *(is? is not?)* likely to accurately measure his temperature.

(c) *Circle the signs and symptoms that Sven is likely to manifest.*
Shivering
Rapid heart rate
Low blood pressure
Decreased metabolic rate and oxygen consumption
Loss of consciousness
Hypoglycemia

(d) Treatment efforts for Sven are likely to involve *(active? passive?)* rewarming because Sven is *(able? unable?)* to increase his body heat at this point by shivering.

CHAPTER 11

Alterations in Nutritional Status

■ Review Questions

A. NUTRITIONAL STATUS (pages 209–220)

A1. Describe how the adage "You are what you eat" applies to pathophysiology.

_____

_____

_____

A2. List four routes by which foods can reach body cells.

_____

_____

_____

A3. Arrange these food types by caloric value (from greatest to least):

Alcohol   Carbohydrates or proteins
Fats

_____, _____, _____

A4. Select the chemical category that best fits each correct description below.

Carbohydrates   Fats   Proteins

(a) Glucose and glycogen are both examples:

_____

(b) Present in two forms (brown and white); more than 90% of body energy (or fuel) is stored in this form within the body:

_____

(c) Insulates and protects organs: _____

(d) The nervous system, including the brain, depends almost exclusively on this type of chemical as a fuel source: _____

(e) When these chemicals are catabolized in excessive amounts (as in starvation or complications of diabetes mellitus), they lead to formation of ketoacids:

_____

(f) Composed of combinations of the 20 different amino acids sequenced correctly:

_____

(g) Typically accounts for about one third of the calories in the U.S. diet; serves as carriers for vitamins A, D, E, and K:

_____

(h) Typically accounts for almost two thirds of the calories in the U.S. diet: _____

(i) Much is stored as triglycerides, which can be broken down by the action of lipases for use as fuel: _____

(j) Linoleic acid is the one chemical in this category that is required in the diet:

_____

(k) Form about 75% of solids in the human body, including much of muscles and bones, hemoglobin, antibodies, and enzymes: _____

(l) Contain about 16% nitrogen, so their adequacy is measured by positive or negative nitrogen balance: _____

A5. Circle the correct answers or fill in blanks in the following statements about metabolism.

(a) Anabolism involves the (_breakdown? synthesis?_) of chemicals, a process that (_uses? releases?_) energy in the form of the high-energy chemical named _____. Such chemical reactions require catalysts known as (_enzymes? substrates?_).

(b) The breakdown of glucose to CO_2 and H_2O is a(n) (_anabolic? catabolic?_) process. Normally the brain requires _____ g (_____ kcal) of glucose per day to meet its energy needs. This fuel (_must be provided as glucose? can be supplied by amino acids and the glycerol portion of triglycerides that are converted to glucose?_).

(c) As Elissa eats excessive amounts of carbohydrates each day, her body modifies these and stores them as _____ and as _____.

(d) When Elissa's blood glucose level drops between meals, glucose can be formed from stored glycogen by the process of (*glycogenolysis? gluconeogenesis?*) or from amino acids, lactate, or glycerol by the process of _____. Name a hormone that can catalyze either of these two processes within the liver. _____

(e) *Circle all hormones that increase blood glucose level (and also glucose availability to cells) by processes described in (d) or by mobilization of fats.*

Cortisone	Epinephrine
Glucagon	Growth hormone
Insulin	Thyroid hormone

A6. Explain why much weight is typically lost in the first several days of a weight-loss program, after which the rate of weight loss slows.

_____

_____

_____

A7. Describe the conditions under which BMR is calculated.

_____

_____

_____

A8. Thermogenesis refers to _____ production, for example when heat is released by catabolism of foods or by exercise.

A9. Bill, who weighs 154 pounds (70 kg), has a 600-calorie sandwich for lunch and a 100-calorie drink. Approximately how many hours of the following activities will Bill need to do to "burn" the calories in that lunch?

(a) Sitting in class: _____ hours

(b) Walking leisurely (20 to 25 minutes per mile): _____ hours

(c) Running (11 minutes per mile): _____ hours

A10. Defend or dispute this statement: "Because there is no specific dietary requirement for carbohydrates, the FDA recommends that carbohydrates be eliminated from the diet."

_____

_____

_____

A11. Circle the correct answers in the following statements about nutritional needs.

(a) The RDA refers to an amount of a nutrient required for _____ healthy persons of a specific group.
(1) Almost all
(2) Half of

(b) _____ are likely to require more kcal/kg body weight.
(1) Preschoolers
(2) Fifth graders

(c) _____ is likely to require more kcal/kg body weight.
(1) Maureen, not pregnant
(2) Norine, 7 months pregnant

(d) _____ amino acids are classified as "essential."
(1) 9
(2) 20

(e) _____ is protein (but not calorie) malnutrition
(1) Marasmus
(2) Kwashiorkor

(f) _____ fats tend to raise blood cholesterol.
(1) Polyunsaturated
(2) Saturated

(g) _____ carbohydrates are recommended for the diet.
(1) Simple
(2) Complex

(h) Vitamins _____ directly provide energy.
(1) Do
(2) Do not

(i) Because _____ vitamins are stored in the body, it is more likely that excessive dietary amounts of these will lead to toxicity.
(1) A, D, E, K (fat soluble)
(2) B complex and C (water soluble)

(j) Calcium, phosphorus, and magnesium are all _____
(1) Macrominerals
(2) Trace minerals

(k) A daily intake of _____ of fiber is recommended.

(1) 20 to 30 g

(2) 200 to 300 g

A12. Match the following components of a nutritional assessment with their descriptions.

Anthropometric   Dietary intake
    measurement   Health history
Laboratory studies Physical examination

(a) 24-hour dietary recall: _____

(b) Current weight compared with weight 5 years earlier; ability to complete activities of daily living: _____

(c) Condition of skin, hair, and gums: _____

(d) BMI, skinfold thickness, waist to hip ratio, and bioelectrical impedance: _____

(e) Assessment of serum levels of albumin, vitamins, and minerals: _____

A13. Calculate your own body mass index (BMI) in this exercise.

(a) Your weight = _____ pounds divided by 2.2 pounds/kg = _____ kg.

(b) Your height = _____ inches × 2.54 cm/inch = _____ cm divided by 100 = _____ meters. Now square that number = _____ m².

(c) Calculate BMI = your weight in kg (_____) divided by your height squared (_____ m²).

(d) A BMI of 32 kg/m² indicates that the person is (underweight? normal weight? overweight? obese?). What does your BMI indicate about your weight?

B. OVERNUTRITION AND OBESITY (pages 220–224)

B1. Answer these questions about overnutrition and obesity.

(a) The World Health Organization describes "being overweight" as a BMI that exceeds (25? 30? 35? 40?).

(b) About (15? 35? 55? 75?)% of the U.S. population is estimated to be overweight, and about one in (2? 3? 4?) of these persons is classified as obese.

(c) Obesity is attributed to (genetic? environmental? both genetic and environmental?) factors.

(d) Obesity is more prevalent among (women? men?) who live below the poverty level.

B2. Write a short essay about factors that contribute to overnutrition and obesity. Include these terms: *automobile, computer, energy density, portions, anxiety,* and *comfort.*

_____
_____
_____

B3. Research indicates that *(presence of fat? fat distribution?)* is the more important factor for morbidity and mortality. Mrs. Santangelo weighs 225 pounds. Her waist is 42″ and her hips are 45.″ Answer these questions about her fat distribution.

(a) Her waist to hip ratio is *(0.8? 0.933? 1.07?)*, which indicates *(upper? lower?)* body obesity. Women are more likely to exhibit *(upper body or abdominal? lower body or gluteal-femoral?)* obesity.

(b) Her excessive abdominal fat has a higher risk of impairing liver function if the fat is *(visceral? subcutaneous?)*. List several other health conditions for which she is at increased risk.

_____
_____
_____

B4. Theresa, age 24, who is Mrs. Santangelo's daughter, is 5′5″ and weighs 155 pounds. She consults the nutritionist for ideas that may help keep her from becoming obese. Make several suggestions.

_____
_____
_____

B5. Complete this exercise about Mr. Hastings, age 48, who is 6′ tall and weighs 220 pounds.

(a) Circle the following characteristics of Mr. Hastings that are health risk factors:

(1) His age

(2) His waist measurement: 41 inches

(3) HDL of 32 mg/dL and LDL of 184 mg/dL

(4) Blood pressure of 136/82 mm Hg

(5) He has never smoked.

(6) He is able to exercise but limits his activity to a golf game about once a month.

(7) His BMI

(b) Mr. Hastings talks with a nutritionist about his goal to lose 20 pounds over the next 6 months. To do this, it is recommended that he reduce caloric intake by *(300-500; 500-1000?)* kcal/day. His diet should contain less than *(10? 30? 50?)*% fat calories.

(c) His exercise goal should include ____ hour(s) or more of moderate activity *(once a day? most days each week?)*.

(d) Suggest techniques for behavioral modifications to help with his weight loss.

_____

_____

_____

(e) Based on his BMI, Mr. Hastings *(is? is not?)* a candidate for a surgical intervention for his weight.

B6. Obesity is a *(rare? common?)* disorder among children and adolescents. Concurrently, about ____% of children in the United States are overweight. Two common methods of assessing childhood obesity are a measurement of higher than 85th percentile for the _____ skinfold and weight for height of greater than ____%. State two major concerns about childhood obesity.

_____

_____

B7. Circle all risk factors for obesity for children. Having:

Active lifestyle   Highly educated parents
Parents in poverty   Obese parents
Many siblings

C. UNDERNUTRITION (pages 224–229)

C1. Match descriptions below with these categories of causes of undernutrition:

Lack of food availability
Physical health problem
Willful eating behaviors

(a) Crohn's disease: _____

(b) Anorexia nervosa: _____

(c) Kwashiorkor and marasmus: _____
    _____

C2. Identify characteristics below as those pertaining to **kwashiorkor** or **marasmus.**

(a) Deficiency of both calories and protein:
    _____

(b) The child looks wasted with stunted growth but has relatively normal skin and hair:
    _____

(c) This condition occurs when a child is displaced from the mother's breast after birth of another child: _____

(d) The child manifests an enlarged abdomen with hepatomegaly, edema, and skin lesions:
    _____

C3. Edward, a healthy 32-year-old man, is stranded in his sailing boat with virtually no food or fresh water for 5 weeks before he is rescued. Answer these questions about him. Select from these answers:

Carbohydrate   Fat   Protein

(a) Most of Edward's body's available sources of calories are likely to be those stored as
    _____.

(b) Breakdown of large amounts of _____ is likely to cause Edward to develop ketosis.

(c) Loss of lean mass causing his "wasting" appearance results mostly from breakdown of _____.

(d) Poor wound healing comes primarily from _____ deficiency.

(e) Identify the correct sequence in which each type of body chemical is called on as a fuel source (from first to last): _____, _____, _____.

C4. Antonio is in the final stages of AIDS and Julia is dying of ovarian cancer. Describe systemic effects of tissue wasting that are likely to take place in the cases of Antonio and Julia.

_____

_____

_____

C5. Treatment of severe protein-calorie malnutrition should be undertaken *(rapidly? slowly?)*. Edema *(is? is not?)* likely to occur, and diuretics *(should? should not?)* be used.

C6. Complete this exercise about eating disorders.

(a) The incidence of eating disorders is greater among *(females? males?)*. About ____ of 1000 cases of anorexia nervosa are fatal.

(b) Besides including an eating disorder, "female athlete triad" affects the _____ and _____ systems.

C7. Circle the characteristics listed below that would contribute to a DSM-IV-TR diagnosis of anorexia nervosa for Amelia, aged 16.

   (a) Amelia maintains her weight at 87% of the expected BMI for her height.

   (b) She has an intense fear of gaining weight.

   (c) Although she reached menarche at age 13, Amelia has not menstruated for the past 18 months.

   (d) Amelia does not think that she has a problem with low body weight.

   (e) She has fine body hair (lanugo).

   (f) Her ECG result is abnormal, her BP is 76/46 mm Hg, and she has electrolyte imbalances.

C8. Explain how amenorrhea associated with anorexia can be linked to osteoporosis.

   _____

   _____

   _____

C9. Complete this exercise by filling in the blanks or circling the correct answers about Marianne, age 21, who measures 5'2" and weighs 105 pounds. She intentionally vomits several times a week after binge eating. Her teeth are severely eroded and her dentist has recommended extraction of all of her teeth with fitting for dentures. She has esophageal reflux with heartburn and has developed pneumonia twice this year.

   (a) Which DSM-IV-TR criteria of bulimia nervosa does Marianne meet?

   _____

   _____

   (b) Her bulimia is classified as *(purging? nonpurging?)*.

   (c) What is the likely cause of her dental problems and her heartburn?

   _____

   _____

   (d) How are her episodes of pneumonia likely to be related to her eating disorder?

   _____

   _____

   (e) Her body weight is more typical of *(bulimia? anorexia?)*.

C10. List several therapy goals for binge eaters.

   _____

   _____

   _____

CHAPTER 12

Alterations in Activity Tolerance

■ Review Questions

A. ACTIVITY TOLERANCE (pages 231–236)

A1. Contrast "activity," "exercise," and "rest."

_____

_____

_____

_____

A2. Mr. Peterson, the nurse in the diabetes education program, explains the benefits of an exercise program to Ruth, age 58, who was recently diagnosed with Type 2 diabetes mellitus and who has moderate coronary artery disease. Complete this exercise about statements that Mr. Peterson makes.

(a) "Regular exercise helps to *(raise? lower?)* your blood levels of the 'bad cholesterol' (low-density lipoproteins, or LDLs), and *(raise? lower?)* your 'good cholesterol,' (high-density lipoproteins, or HDLs)."

(b) "Exercise is likely to *(improve? have no effect on?)* your control of your sugar."

(c) "Staying with your exercise can make your heart and lungs work *(better? worse?)* and *(increase? decrease?)* your reserves to call on if you are sick."

(d) "I think you'll find that moving around more will just make you feel better." (List three pyschosocial benefits that Ruth is likely to gain by regular exercise.)

_____

_____

_____.

A3. Contrast aerobic versus isometric exercise by circling the correct answer or filling in the blanks.

(a) Running or jogging a mile is an example of *(aerobic? isometric?)* exercise, which is also known as *(endurance? resistance?)* exercise. Muscle fibers responsible for this exercise are *(red? white?)* because they have myoglobin and *(many? few?)* mitochondria to carry out aerobic metabolism. Training in aerobic exercise helps muscles to use _____ more efficiently.

(b) Weight lifting and water-skiing are *(aerobic? isometric?)* exercise because muscle length *(does? does not?)* change *(iso* = same) during the activity. This is also known as *(endurance? resistance?)* exercise because *(strength? stamina?)* develops. *(Red, slow-twitch? White, fast-twitch?)* fibers with *(many? few?)* mitochondria carry out these anaerobic, intense (but time-limited) activities.

(c) In which type of exercise is muscle mass more likely to hypertrophy and require more oxygen? *(Aerobic? Isometric?)*

A4. Match the requirement lacking for physical activity in each of these cases. Choose from these requirements, and use each only once.

Cardiopulmonary fitness
Muscle strength, flexibility, and endurance
Energy sources
Motivation and mental endurance

(a) Ms. Timmons, age 18, is hospitalized for severe depression:

_____

(b) Mr. Benson, age 72 and a former professional boxer, has congestive heart failure with reduced "maximal oxygen consumption": _____

(c) Jonathan, age 12, has Duchenne's muscular dystrophy: _____

(d) Susannah, age 15, weighs 70 pounds as a result of her anorexia nervosa:

_____

A5. Answer these questions about the body's adaptive mechanisms during exercise. (It may help to look ahead at Figures 21-1 and 27-1 in the Study Guide.)

(a) The rate at which oxygen is consumed by muscles depends on factors 1-4. Describe each of these factors in a few words

1) _____

2) _____

3) _____

4) _____

(b) Cardiac output refers to the amount of blood pumped out by the heart *(each minute? with each heartbeat or contraction?)*. At rest, this value is about ___ liters/minute. During exercise, a healthy heart can increase cardiac output to about *(1.5? 2–6? 8–10?)* times resting values.

(c) Cardiac output is determined by the calculation:

(1) Stroke volume + heart rate

(2) Stroke volume × heart rate

(d) During exercise, increase in *(sympathetic? parasympathetic?)* nerve impulses as well as hormones epinephrine and _____, will increase heart rate and strength of contraction.

(e) Contraction of leg muscles *(increases? decreases?)* venous return to the heart, stretching the heart. (Visualize a thick balloon stretching as it is filled with water.) According to Frank-Starling's law, a stretched muscle will contract *(more? less?)* forcefully. Therefore, increased venous return *(increases? decreases?)* stroke volume and cardiac output.

(f) During exercise, which component of blood pressure (BP) increases more? *(Systolic? Diastolic?)*. This is due to high cardiac output with rapid movement of blood into vessels within *(skeletal muscles? GI tract and kidneys?)* (which keeps diastolic BP relatively low). As a result, the difference between systolic and diastolic BP (known as _____ pressure) typically *(increases? decreases?)*. An example: Tim's BP goes from 120/72 to 156/86 mm Hg as he exercises. His pulse pressure goes from ____ to ____ mm Hg.

(g) Pulmonary blood flow (or _____) increases with higher cardiac output during exercise. As a result, gas exchange between air and blood in lungs is likely to *(increase? decrease?)*.

(h) As the brain senses a rise in arterial CO_2 during exercise, the brain sends nerve impulses to the diaphragm to *(increase? decrease?)* rate and depth of ventilation.

(i) To assure that active muscles get about 90% of cardiac output, the brain and local controls signal vessels into muscles to *(constrict? dilate?)* as vessels into GI tract and kidneys are *(constricted? dilated?)*. One benefit of athletic training is the *(increased? decreased?)* growth of capillaries around muscles.

(j) Delivery of O_2 and nutrients to active muscles also depends on an adequate *(red? white?)* blood count.

A6. Match terms about muscle activity to related descriptions below. Use these terms:

Endurance   Flexibility   Strength

(a) Range of motion: _____

(b) Ability of muscles to forcefully pull on bones: _____

(c) Ability of muscles to act over extended periods: _____

A7. Choose the correct answers about resources needed for muscle activities.

(a) For relatively short periods (under 40 minutes) of exercise, ___ provides energy.

(1) Aerobic metabolism

(2) ATP, creatine phosphate, and/or muscle glycogen

(b) A balanced diet to meet exercise needs should contain mostly:

(1) Protein

(2) Fats

(3) Complex carbohydrates

(c) The food type that is most needed to rebuild muscles is:

(1) Protein

(2) Fats

(3) Carbohydrates

(d) During prolonged exercise, intake of ____ must also be maintained.

(1) Pure water

(2) Fluids and electrolytes

A8. Draw in arrows to indicate whether the following activities increase (↑) or decrease (↓) as adaptive mechanisms during exercise.

(a) Blood flow into skin: _____

(b) Sweating with need for replacement of fluid and electrolytes: _____

(c) Shift of proteins and fluids from interstitial spaces into blood plasma: _____

(d) Contractions and secretions of the GI tract: _____

(e) Immune system function following regular, moderate exercise: _____

A9. Match terms associated with activity assessments with their descriptions.

Ergometric tests   Fatigue severity scale
Human activity profile   Maximal heart rate
Metabolic equivalents   Rating of perceived
                          exertion

(a) A rating of 13 means that the heart rate is 130 beats/minute, and that the person experiences the activity as "somewhat hard": _____

(b) Multiples of the basal metabolic rate; vary with types of activities: _____

(c) Rate is likely to be 160 beats/minute for a 60-year-old: _____

(d) A paper and pencil test with nine statements that rate fatigue from 1 to 7:

_____

(e) An assessment of 94 common daily activities that assess quality of life: _____

(f) Treadmill and stationary bicycle assessments of activity tolerance: _____

B. ACTIVITY INTOLERANCE AND FATIGUE
(pages 236–240)

B1. Contrast terms in each pair:

(a) Tiredness/fatigue _____

_____

_____

_____

(b) Situational stressors that cause fatigue/ developmental stressors that cause fatigue

_____

_____

_____

(c) Central fatigue/peripheral fatigue

_____

_____

_____

(d) Effects of exercise on persons who are: conditioned /deconditioned

_____

_____

_____

B2. Choose the correct characteristics of chronic fatigue.

(a) Has a rapid onset

(b) Lasts longer than 1 month

(c) Is relieved by cessation of activity.

(d) Serves a protective purpose

B3. List several areas of life that are likely to be affected by chronic fatigue.

_____

_____

_____

List eight or more categories of people who are at increased risk for chronic fatigue.

_____

_____

_____

B4. Complete this exercise about Laurie, who appears to have chronic fatigue syndrome (CFS).

(a) To meet criteria for CFS, Laurie must have had her condition for at least 6 *(weeks'? months'?)* duration. Community surveys indicate that ___ to ___ persons out of 100 have CFS.

(b) Laurie reports the following symptoms. Circle all that meet CDC criteria for CSF.
   (1) "I never wake up feeling rested."
   (2) "My joints are swollen and they hurt."
   (3) "My muscles ache."
   (4) "I'm depressed all the time."
   (5) "My throat hurts and my glands are swollen here (points to neck)."
   (6) "I can't do anything in the evening because I just feel awful after a full day."

(c) The cause of CFS is _____. Briefly discuss theories of causation of CFS.

_____

_____

_____

(d) How is CSF diagnosed?
  (1) Specific, definitive tests for CSF
  (2) History, physical, and tests to rule out other disorders.

(e) Identify the nature of the tests that are likely to be performed on Laurie:

Blood glucose   BUN   CBC
Serum Na⁺ and K⁺   Guaiac test
Lyme disease

  (1) Check for blood in the stool:

  _____

  (2) Serum electrolytes: _____
  (3) Check for anemia or infections:

  _____

  (4) Test for bacterial disease caused by tick bite that can have systemic effects:

  _____

  (5) Check for diabetes mellitus:

  _____

  (6) Test for renal function:

  _____

(f) Briefly describe management of CFS.

  _____
  _____
  _____
  _____

C. BED REST AND IMMOBILITY (pages 240-247)

C1. Describe the beneficial effects of gravity that occur in the standing position.

  _____
  _____
  _____

C2. Ms. Valentine, age 34, requires 4 days of total bed rest after a serious accident. Before the accident, she was in good health. Describe changes likely to occur by completing the following exercise.

(a) When Ms. Valentine first required bed rest on Monday, her blood flow shifted to her *(legs and thighs? thorax, arms, and head?)*. Her stroke volume *(increased? decreased?)* to about ___ L/min, and her heart rate *(increased? decreased?)*.

(b) Baroreceptors sensed the changes in fluid volume and *(increased? decreased?)* production of ADH and aldosterone. As a result, urine output *(increased? decreased?)* causing *(de? over?)*hydration as well as a(n)

(increase? decrease?) in hematocrit and blood viscosity.

(c) By Wednesday, her veins *(increased? decreased?)* their reservoir function, *(increasing? decreasing?)* venous return, stroke volume, and cardiac output. Her heart began a compensatory *(increase? decrease?)* in rate.

(d) By Friday, when Ms. Valentine was first able to get up, she experienced _____ hypotension, partly related to her dehydration and also to altered _____ nerve responses as well as some heart muscle *(a? hyper?)*trophy.

(e) List likely manifestations of Ms. Valentine's orthostatic hypotension.

  _____
  _____
  _____

C3. Explain why two other major alterations in cardiovascular responses are likely to accompany Ms. Valentine's prolonged bed rest.

(a) Increased cardiac

  _____
  _____
  _____

(b) Venous _____ with risk for _____ formation. Note that the three major factors that lead to thrombus formation (Chapter 7) are present. These are:
  (1) _____
  (2) _____
  (3) _____

C4. Explain why prolonged bed rest increases potential for the following alterations in other systems.

(a) Respiratory infections

  _____
  _____

How can coughing and deep breathing (C&DB) help?

  _____
  _____
  _____

(b) Urinary tract infections and kidney stones

  _____
  _____
  _____

How can increased fluid intake help?

_____
_____
_____

(c) Disuse atrophy of muscles and demineralization of bones

_____
_____
_____

(d) Increased protein breakdown and negative nitrogen balance related to insulin resistance

_____
_____
_____

(e) Constipation and fecal impaction

_____
_____
_____

C5. Choose the three true statements related to prolonged bed rest.

(a) For each week of bed rest, muscles lose about 1% of their mass.

(b) Weight loss during this period is related to loss of **lean muscle mass** and **fat.**

(c) Well-trained athletes tend to lose weight **more slowly** than deconditioned persons do during this time.

(d) Contractures may occur causing muscles to **shorten** and develop **decreased** range of motion.

(e) During prolonged bed rest, **osteoclasts** continue to function but **osteoblasts** do not.

(f) Bones become **rigid** and **more** prone to fracture.

C6. List three factors that increase risk for pressure sores (decubiti) during bed rest with immobility.

_____
_____
_____

C7. Draw in arrows to indicate likelihood of increased (↑) or decreased (↓) changes in response to long-term bed rest.

(a) Awareness of muscles and body position (kinesthesia): _____

(b) Visual and auditory hallucinations:

_____

(c) Anxiety, depression, and fear: _____

(d) Ability to learn and retain new material:

_____

(e) Ability to carry out usual social roles:

_____

C8. List several tenets of a care plan for a client on prolonged bed rest.

_____
_____
_____

CHAPTER 13

Blood Cells and the Hemopoietic System

■ Review Questions

A. COMPOSITION OF BLOOD AND FORMATION OF BLOOD CELLS (pages 251–256)

A1. Complete this exercise about blood that has been centrifuged in a tube with an anticoagulant, such as heparin (as in Figure 13-1 of your text).

   (a) Arrange these layers from top to bottom in the tube:

      Buffy coat   Plasma
      Red blood cells

      _____, _____, _____

   (b) Which of these layers contains white blood cells and platelets? _____

   (c) Which layer forms about 42% to 47% of blood? _____

A2. In assessing Mr. Gregory, the ER nurse notes the following: productive cough and abnormal lung sounds indicating a severe respiratory infection; edema (extra fluid between cells) of his legs and ankles, and ascites (extra fluid in the peritoneal cavity). Laboratory test results indicate that Mr. Gregory has poor clotting function and low blood protein levels. Relate these manifestations to his diagnosis of cirrhosis of the liver.

   _____

   _____

   _____

A3. Circle the correct answer in each statement about blood cells.

   (a) Erythrocytes are *(red blood cells? white blood cells? platelets?)*. Their main function is in *(carrying O_2? infection control? clotting?)*.

   (b) White blood cells are also known as *(thrombocytes? leukocytes?)*. They function in *(carrying CO_2? infection control? clotting?)*.

   (c) The most common type of white blood cell is a *(neutrophil? lymphocyte?)*. These WBCs originate in *(bone marrow? lymph tissue?)* as *(myeloblasts? metamyeloblasts?)*. Presence of myeloblasts in circulating blood *(is normal? indicates a blood disorder?)*.

   (d) "PMNs" or "segs" are terms used to describe *(mature? immature?)* neutrophils, whereas "bands" are *(mature? immature?)* neutrophils. Neutrophils that line walls of small blood vessels are known as *(circulating? marginating?)* PMNs. Neutrophils arrive *(early? late?)* in the inflammation process, where their granules function as *(chromosomes? lysosomes? ribosomes?)*.

A4. Select the type of white blood cell (WBC) that fits the related description.

    Basophils   Eosinophils
    Lymphocytes   Monocytes

   (a) Comprise 24% to 40% of WBCs; nucleus is spherical and takes up most of the cell; has two main types (B and T); function in immunity: _____

   (b) The largest WBCs, they become macrophages and function in chronic inflammations: _____

   (c) Contain histamine involved in allergic responses: _____

   (d) Increase in number during parasitic infections: _____

   (e) Agranulocytes (2 answers): _____ and _____

A5. Jill's platelet count of 15,000/μL indicates that she is at greater risk for excessive *(clot formation? bleeding?)*. A normal platelet count is _____/μL.

A6. The term *hematopoiesis* means _____. Fill in this blank and then complete this exercise about this process by filling in blanks or circling the correct answer.

(a) Before birth, hematopoiesis takes place primarily in *(bone marrow? liver and spleen?)*; after birth, blood cells form mainly in _____.

(b) Red marrow indicates presence of *(RBC? WBC?)*-forming cells; yellow marrow contains mostly _____ cells. Name the bones in which most red marrow is found in adults: _____.

(c) All blood cells originate from *(progenitor? pluripotent stem?)* cells that *(do? do not?)* have the capacity for self-renewal throughout life. Progenitor cells such as CFUs or BFUs can *(self-renew? differentiate?)* to form specific types of blood cells.

(d) Name two types of disorders of hemopoietic stem cells. _____
One treatment for stem cell disorders is a stem cell _____.

(e) Hormone-like growth factors called _____ normally stimulate hematopoiesis. Examples are erythropoietin (EPO), which stimulates production of _____ blood cells and _____ that stimulates production of neutrophils and other granulocytes. Interleukins are useful clinically for AIDS patients because these chemicals stimulate _____ production.

B. DIAGNOSTIC TESTS (pages 256-257)

B1. A complete blood count (CBC) is performed on Angelique's blood. Identify the component of the CBC most likely to be indicated by her results. (See Table 13-2 in the text.)

Blood smear   Differential WBC
Platelet   Red blood cell
White blood cell

(a) 12,000/μL: _____ count

(b) 3.6 million/μL: _____ count

(c) Percentage of each type of WBC:
_____ count

(d) Presence of microcytic (small) RBCs:
_____

B2. Angelique's ESR (or "sed") rate is measured at 25 mm/hour. This rate is *(high? normal? low?)*, suggesting the presence of _____.

B3. Tommy, age 3, has a bone marrow aspiration. From which bone is his marrow likely to be drawn? _____. For what purposes is such a procedure likely to be performed?

_____
_____
_____

CHAPTER 14

Alterations in Hemostasis

■ Review Questions

A. MECHANISMS OF HEMOSTASIS (pages 259-263)

A1. "Hemostasis" literally means _____ of blood flow.

A2. Arrange the five steps/stages of hemostasis in correct sequence from first to last:

Coagulation   Clot retraction
Fibrinolysis   Platelet plug formation
Vasospasm

_____ → _____ →
_____ → _____ → _____

A3. Circle the correct answers in each statement about initial stages of hemostasis.

(a) In vasospasm, blood vessels *(constrict? dilate?)*, usually for *(less than a minute? several days?)* after the injury.

(b) *(Thromboxane A$_2$? Prostacyclin?)* is a vasoconstrictor released from *(platelets? the lining of blood vessels?)*. *(TXA$_2$? Prostacyclin?)* is a vasodilator that inhibits platelet aggregation.

(c) Platelets are derived from large cells known as *(megakaryocytes? thrombocytes?)* in bone marrow. Because they contain mitochondria, platelets *(can? cannot?)* produce ATP and they can synthesize prostaglandins needed for platelet function. They also provide *(ADP? growth factors?)* that stimulate growth of smooth muscle and fibroblasts which can maintain vessel walls or cause overgrowth as in atherosclerosis.

(d) Platelets typically exist for just over *(a week? 3 months? 8-9 years?)*. Their production is regulated by the chemical named *(erythro? thrombo?)poetin*.

(e) When platelets bind to injured vessels, their receptors become *(smooth? spiny?)* so they adhere to exposed *(elastin? collagen?)* in the vessel by way of *(TXA$_2$? vWF?)*.

(f) Platelet release of chemicals such as TXA$_2$ cause a "snowball effect" as platelet aggregation *(increases? decreases?)*. The platelet plug is later stabilized by *(fibrin? prothrombin?)* formed in the process of coagulation.

A4. Fill in the blanks about normal blood clotting (coagulation).

(a) The intrinsic coagulation pathway begins as _____ comes into contact with injured _____ walls.

(b) The extrinsic coagulation pathway begins outside the _____.

(c) A vitamin necessary for normal blood clotting is vitamin ___.

(d) A mineral needed for normal blood clotting (coagulation) is _____.

A5. Match the coagulation factor with the correct description.

IV   VIII   X

(a) Citrate chelates this factor so that blood stored for transfusions will not clot: factor _____

(b) This is the endproduct of both the intrinsic and extrinsic coagulation pathways: activated factor _____

(c) This factor is most often deficient in hemophilia; normally carried by the von Willebrand factor (vWF): factor _____

A6. Contrast terms in each pair:

(a) Fibrinogen/fibrin

_____
_____
_____

(b) Thrombin/plasmin

_____
_____
_____

(c) An anticoagulant/a fibrinolytic agent

_____
_____
_____

A7. Dr. Chen is transported to University Hospital with a "rule out MI" (RO MI) directive. Within 30 minutes of his arrival at the ER, Dr. Chen is given a dose of t-PA. Does his receiving this medication *suggest* that he was experiencing a heart attack? _____

A8. Match each chemical with the related description.

Heparin	Plasminogen
Plasminogen-activator inhibitor	Tissue plasminogen activator
Warfarin	

(a) A vitamin K antagonist, it decreases prothrombin production; can be taken orally: _____

(b) Produced by some blood cells (basophils) and connective tissue cells (mast cells); helps to inactivate thrombin; most forms cannot be taken orally: _____

(c) Typically found in blood; once activated, it causes breakdown of fibrin (fibrinolysis):

_____

(d) May be administered to heart attack (myocardial infarction) patients to dissolve fibrin clots before they become extensive:

_____

(e) If present in the body in excessive amounts, this chemical may lead to a heart attack:

_____

A9. Classify the following chemicals according to their functions; write answers on lines provided. (Note: some chemicals fit into more than one category.)

Antithrombin III	Calcium ions
Coagulation factors VII to XII	Fibrinogen
Protein C	Heparin
Tissue-plasminogen activator	Thrombin
	Warfarin (Coumadin)

(a) Procoagulation factors: _____

_____

(b) Anticoagulation factors: _____

_____

(c) Fibrinolytic agents: _____

_____

B. HYPERCOAGULABILITY STATES (pages 263-264)

B1. Respond to this statement: "Blood clotting is good news and bad news."

_____
_____
_____

B2. Thrombi in *(arteries? veins?)* are composed of platelets and fibrin clots. Select correct answer, then list several factors that can lead to excessive clot formation due to:

(a) Increased platelet function

_____
_____
_____

(b) Increase in coagulation factors

_____
_____
_____

B3. Select the category of factors that leads to hypercoagulability associated with each condition below. In some cases, more than one answer is appropriate.

Damaged blood vessel lining
Increased clotting factors
Platelet adhesiveness and aggregation
Stasis of blood flow

(a) Atherosclerosis: _____

_____

(b) Smoking: _____ _____

(c) Diabetes: _____ _____

(d) Thrombocytosis: _____

(e) Immobilization after childbirth or surgery:

_____

(f) Heart failure: _____

(g) Pregnancy or use of oral contraceptives:

_____

(h) Cancer: _____

B4. Mr. Longstreth, age 72, 5'11", 232 lbs, is in an ER in Sarasota, Florida. He and his partner drove from Cincinnati to Florida within 24 hours, trying not to "dawdle" (Mr. Longstreth's term) along the way. Mr. Longstreth's chest pain, severe dyspnea (difficulty breathing), and rapid breathing suggest the presence of a pulmonary embolism (PE). Explain why Mr.

Longstreth might be a candidate for a PE. (For more info on PE, see pages 656–658)

_____
_____
_____

C. BLEEDING DISORDERS (pages 264-269)

C1. Claudia has a platelet count of 20,000/μL. Answer these questions about Claudia's condition by circling the correct answers:

(a) This count:
    (1) Is normal
    (2) Indicates thrombocytosis
    (3) Indicates thrombocytopenia

(b) Claudia has **petechiae** on her arms; these are:
    (1) Large bruises
    (2) Pinpoint red areas

(c) She also has frequent occurrences of **epistaxis,** which is:
    (1) Abnormal menstrual bleeding
    (2) Bleeding from gums
    (3) Nosebleeds

C2. Explain probable mechanisms for low platelet counts in the following persons.

(a) Mr. Lewis has cirrhosis of the liver.

_____
_____
_____

(b) Ms. Schmidt has been taking sulfa drugs for an infection.

_____
_____
_____

(c) Mr. Stanford is halfway through his chemotherapy protocol for cancer.

_____
_____
_____

(d) Mrs. Fernandez has widespread thrombi in small vessels of her brain and kidneys; she has severe headaches and seizures; she is undergoing "plasma-cleaning" (plasmapheresis).

_____
_____
_____

C3. Jennifer, the neonatal nurse, administers vitamin K to newborn baby Kareenya. Explain why Kareenya may require vitamin K.

_____
_____
_____

C4. Discuss the likely cause of bleeding in each case.

(a) Mr. Lewis (see **C2.**[a] above) has had alcoholism for over 20 years.

_____
_____
_____

(b) In providing information for her history and physical, Mrs. Snyderman tells the nurse that that she has taken "pain medicine" for her arthritis for many years. She notes that whenever she has a cut or she scratches a sore, she "bleeds forever."

_____
_____
_____

(c) Terry has been taking antibiotics for recurrent infections.

_____
_____
_____

(d) Timmy and Tommy, 10 years of age, are identical twins who each have 1% of normal blood levels of factor VIII. Both boys have sufficient damage to joints of their legs that their mobility is limited. Tommy has developed hepatitis C.

_____
_____
_____

(e) Samantha's vWF deficiency was diagnosed after she had her wisdom teeth removed.

_____
_____
_____

C5. Circle the factors in the following list that are likely to lead to hypocoagulability.

Aneurysm	Dehydration
Lack of Factor VIII as in the most common form of hemophilia	Smoking
	Splenomegaly
	Smoking and taking oral contraceptives
Diabetes mellitus	Taking 0.5 aspirin each
Lack of vitamin K	day
Heparin or coumadin	

C6. DIC is an acronym for _____.
Complete this exercise about the disorder.

(a) List several causes or triggers of DIC.

_____
_____
_____

(b) Explain why DIC is called a "paradoxical" disorder.

_____
_____
_____

(c) Which signs are more observable in DIC? *(Bleeding? Ischemia?)* List several examples.

_____
_____
_____

(d) Which organs are likely to become necrotic as a result of ischemia?

_____
_____

C7. Define these two forms of vascular disorders that may lead to bleeding.

(a) Telangiectasia

_____
_____
_____

(b) Senile purpura

_____
_____
_____

CHAPTER 15

The Red Blood Cell and Alterations in Oxygen Transport

■ Review Questions

A. THE RED BLOOD CELL (pages 271-276)

A1. State the primary role of red blood cells (RBCs). _____

Now write the secondary role of RBCs.

_____

Explain how the structure of RBCs is well designed for these functions.

_____

A2. Circle the type of hemoglobin that has a greater tendency (affinity) to bind to oxygen (O_2).

(a) HbA

(b) HbF

Explain the significance of this fact.

_____
_____
_____

A3. Discuss how iron (Fe) functions in blood by completing this exercise. Fill in the blanks or circle the correct answer.

(a) Typically, most iron is ingested in foods such as _____. Iron is transported within plasma to bone marrow in the form of *(transferrin? ferritin?),* and stored in the liver as _____. Low levels of *(transferrin? ferritin?)* indicate a need for an iron supplement.

(b) At any given time, most of the Fe of the body is:
(1) Stored in the liver
(2) Suspended in plasma
(3) Present in hemoglobin

A4. Complete this exercise about erythropoiesis.

(a) Arrange these stages in development of RBCs in sequence from first to last.

Erythroblasts   Erythrocytes
Normoblasts   Pluripotent stem cells
Reticulocytes

_____ → _____ →
_____ → _____ →
_____

(b) In which stage do most potential RBCs move out of bone marrow and into circulating blood?_____

(c) Because RBCs live about ____ days, about ___% of RBCs are replaced each day. One reason that a mature RBC lives a relatively short life span is that it lacks a

_____.

(d) Where is almost all erythropoietin produced within the human body? Circle the correct answer from the following list.

Bone marrow   Kidneys
Liver   Spleen
Thymus

(e) What serves as the trigger for production of erythropoietin? _____
_____

A5. LaVerne Jackson, age 47, has had diabetes for 32 years. She manifests a common effect of long term diabetes, renal failure, and takes dialysis treatments (to clean her blood). She feels debilitating fatigue much of the time. Her hemoglobin (Hb) level is currently 6.5 g/dL. Explain what is likely to cause her fatigue, and what treatment may help.

_____
_____
_____

A6. Mrs. Jackson's husband, Rev. George Jackson, has serious liver disease that causes jaundice, which is due to excessive _____ in blood. The Reverend has black skin. How can the nurse best assess the presence of jaundice in Rev. Jackson?

_____

_____

What other conditions besides liver disease can lead to jaundice?

_____

_____

_____

A7. Although erythrocytes transport oxygen, RBCs cannot utilize oxygen for ATP-production as virtually all other body cells do. Why not?

_____

_____

_____

One product of anaerobic metabolism in RBCs is 2,3-DPG. How does this chemical "help tissues"?

_____

_____

_____

A8. Select correct numbers in this list as answers for below.

1	2	4	6	9	14
20	42	75	98	120	

(a) Number of hemes and also Fe atoms in each hemoglobin molecule: ____

(b) Typical hemoglobin value: ____ g/dL

(c) Normal RBC count for women: ____ million/mm³

(d) A likely value for MCV in megaloblastic anemia: ____ fL

A9. Susan F. gave birth to a healthy baby boy. However, Susan hemorrhaged so much that her hematocrit dropped to 12%. Answer these related questions.

(a) Write a value for a normal hematocrit: _____%.

(b) Susan receives treatment to stimulate RBC production. Which test is the best indicator of successful anti-anemic therapy? Circle the correct answer.

(1) Total RBC count

(2) Hematocrit

(3) Reticulocyte count

(c) Which value for this test most indicates success of the therapy? Circle the correct answer.

1   15   150   1200

A10. Choose the two true statements.

(a) Hypochromic anemia indicates a **lower** than normal concentration of Hb in blood.

(b) Jaundice is a classic sign of **anemia.**

(c) Overall, normal RBC values tend to be **higher** for women than for men.

(d) In general, the value for hemoglobin can be expected to be **one third** the value of hematocrit.

B. ANEMIA (pages 276–283)

B1. Causes of anemia fall into two major categories. Fill in the blanks.

(a) Blood loss, for example by: _____ or by _____.

(b) Inadequate replacement of normal RBCs, for example by _____ deficiency or _____ failure.

B2. Complete this exercise by filling in the blanks about signs and symptoms of anemia that fit into three major categories:

(a) Hypoxia that may manifest by

_____.

Compensatory mechanisms lead to *(increased? decreased?)* heart rate; vasoconstriction of blood vessels in skin, nail beds, and gums, causing *(pallor? cyanosis?)*; and *(increased? decreased?)* RBC production which may cause bone pain.

(b) Changes in RBC _____ or color, as seen in microcytic or megaloblastic anemias, or in hypochromic anemias.

(c) Manifestations of the underlying cause of anemia, such as _____ accompanying hemorrhagic anemia resulting from an automobile accident.

B3. Circle correct answers about different types of anemia.

(a) Hypovolemic shock is more likely to accompany *(acute? chronic?)* blood loss. Fluid shifts from intercellular spaces into blood plasma, causing blood to be more *(concentrated? dilute?)*. These RBCs have *(normal? reduced?)* hemoglobin level.

(b) Loss of blood due to gastric irritation associated with chronic aspirin use is more likely to lead to *(acute? chronic?)* anemia. This *(is? is not?)* iron-deficiency anemia. These cells have *(normal? reduced?)* hemoglobin level, so are said to be *(normochromic? hypochromic?)*.

B4. Choose the two true statements.

(a) Sickle cell anemia is classified as a(n) **autosomal recessive** hereditary disorder.

(b) About 1 in 1200 African Americans carries the sickle cell trait.

(c) A person with *sickle cell trait* is **more** likely than one with *sickle cell anemia* to experience sickle cell crises.

(d) Sickle cell anemia is likely to be a **progressive** ("gets worse over time") disease.

B5. Answer these questions about sickle cell anemia (SCA).

(a) Describe sickle cell "crises."

_____
_____
_____

(b) List several situations that trigger hypoxia that patients with SCA should avoid.

_____
_____
_____

(c) Circle what is typically the most serious complication of SCA in the following list.
(1) Fatigue
(2) Bleeding into joints with limitation of mobility and confinement to wheel chair
(3) CVA (cerebrovascular accident = stroke)
(4) Malaria

(d) Children with SCA typically start showing signs and symptoms at about age 4 to 6 ___. Fill in the blank with an answer from the following list.
(1) Hours
(2) Days
(3) Weeks
(4) Months
(5) Years

(e) Which organ is especially at risk for destruction in SCA children by age 5 years? _____ How can such organ injury contribute to serious infections and septicemia? _____
_____

(f) Circle the correct answer. Currently there *(is? is not?)* a cure for SCA. Screening tests for SCA *(are? are not?)* available.

B6. Match the type of anemia that fits each description.

Aplastic	B_{12} deficiency
Chronic disease	Folic acid deficiency
Hemolytic	Hemorrhagic
Iron-deficiency	Sickle cell
Spherocytosis	Thalassemia

(a) A megaloblastic anemia caused by gastritis with decreased production of intrinsic factor; accompanied by neurologic changes:

_____

(b) A megaloblastic anemia associated with malnutrition, for example, in elderly people or people with alcoholism; not accompanied by neurologic changes: _____

(c) A cause of acute anemia with risk of hypovolemic shock; cells are of normal size and color: _____

(d) End-stage renal failure, AIDS, or cancer are most likely causes of: _____

(e) Accompanies gastric irritation associated with chronic aspirin use for control of arthritis pain: _____

(f) RBCs are injured and destroyed, for example by transfusion reactions, toxins, venoms, malaria, or by mechanical injury with burns or heart valve defects; RBCs are normal size and color: _____

(g) Signs and symptoms include increased risk of bleeding, infections, and fatigue:

_____

(h) Hereditary anemia affecting blacks; hemoglobin HbS causes abnormally shaped RBCs, which leads to hypoxia:

_____

(i) Hereditary anemia in various racial and ethnic groups; errors occur in synthesis of hemoglobin chains; children with the disorder may have severe growth retardation: _____

(j) An autosomal dominant disorder in which RBCs form tight spheres that are easily destroyed in vessels of the spleen; may be treated by splenectomy: _____

B7. Worldwide, *(women? men?)* are at greater risk for iron-deficiency anemia.

(a) Explain why._____

_____

_____

(b) List several categories of persons also at increased risk for this type of anemia.

_____

_____

_____

B8. Discuss two forms of nutritional anemias in this exercise.

(a) Vitamin B_{12} deficiency decreases production of _____ cells as well as _____ surrounding neurons. Absorption of this vitamin requires production of intrinsic factor (IF) from the _____ lining. This is needed to "ferry" vitamin B_{12} through the GI tract to the *(large? small?)* intestine, where it is absorbed into blood and then passes to bone marrow.

(b) Explain why cancer patients are at risk for folic acid anemia._____

_____

_____

(c) Folic acid supplements are recommended in pregnant women to prevent _____ defects (NTDs).

B9. Choose the two answers that match a form of anemia with a description of a person at high risk for that anemia.

(a) Pernicious anemia: postgastrectomy or postileectomy patient

(b) Folic acid anemia: patient with long-term alcoholism

(c) Aplastic anemia: newborn baby

(d) Hemolytic anemia: postsplenectomy patient

C. TRANSFUSION THERAPY
(pages 283–285)

C1. Circle the two true statements about blood transfusions:

(a) Transfusions are typically given only when a person's **hematocrit** level reaches 8% to 10%.

(b) Whole blood rather than packed red blood cells should be administered to people who have had a **slow** hemorrhage or **chronic** anemia.

(c) **Predeposit** blood is an autologous transfusion in which the patient's blood is collected weeks before an elective surgery.

(d) In crossmatching blood, donor's RBCs are incubated with recipient's **serum** to check for compatibility.

C2. Choose the two true statements about blood types.

(a) Because Annie has type A blood, she is likely to have A antigens on her RBCs.

(b) Annie's genotype for her Type A blood is likely to be either AA or AO.

(c) Because Oliver has Type O blood, it is expected that he has **both** the A antibody and the B antibody in his serum.

(d) It **is** likely that Oliver would have had the A and B antibodies in his serum at the **time of his birth**.

C3. Choose the two true statements about blood types:

(a) Rh-positive blood normally **does** have the D antigen on RBCs.

(b) Most people with Rh-negative blood **do** have D antibodies.

(c) The most feared reaction with an incompatible blood transfusion is destruction of **recipient's** RBCs by the donor's related **antibodies.**

(d) The recipient's vital signs **should** be monitored before and during the transfusion.

C4. Circle the signs and symptoms of a transfusion reaction.

Sensation of icy cold along the vein into which blood is being infused

Bradycardia	Chills
Difficulty breathing	Pale face
Fever	Hives

Extremely high blood pressure

Nausea and vomiting

D. POLYCYTHEMIA (pages 285–286)

D1. Note the ratios between hematocrit and Hb. Circle the answer that best suggests polycythemia.

(a) 42:14

(b) 30:10

(c) 12:4

(d) 66:22

D2. Mr. Miller, a 58-year-old man, has a diagnosis of polycythemia vera. Answer these questions about him.

(a) Circle all of the following that are likely to increase:

(1) Red blood cell count

(2) Hematocrit

(3) Hemoglobin

(4) Platelet count

(5) White blood cell count

(6) Plasma

(b) Circle all of the following that are likely to increase:

(1) Blood volume

(2) Blood viscosity

(3) Blood pressure

(4) Risk of thrombus formation

(c) Mr. Miller's skin, fingernails, and gums are likely to have what sort of appearance:

(1) Pale

(2) Dusky or cyanotic

D3. Identify the type of polycythemia likely to occur in each case below. For reference purposes, refer to Figure 13-1, page 252 in the text, showing normal RBC count (hematocrit) and plasma (no polycythemia).

(a) Mr. Miller's polycythemia vera. Type: _____

(b) Mrs. Sweet, age 88, became dehydrated over the course of a scorching hot week; her hematocrit level is high, but her RBC count is normal. Type: _____

(c) Alexis moves from Philadelphia to Aspen, Colorado. Type: _____

(d) Mrs. McLaughlin, age 64, has advanced chronic obstructive pulmonary disease with cor pulmonale, associated with 50 years of smoking. Type: _____

E. AGE-RELATED CHANGES IN RED BLOOD CELLS (pages 286–287)

E1. Answer these questions about Jarred and Cassandra, both 2 months of age, by circling the correct answer.

(a) Jarred was full term and weighed 8 pounds at birth. From birth until about 2 months of age, Jarred's RBC count, hematocrit, and hemoglobin levels were likely to have *(elevated? declined?)*. His body is increasing the production of *(HbF? HbA?)* which has a great capacity for giving up oxygen to tissues.

(b) Cassandra weighed 4 pounds when she was born at 32 weeks' gestation. Her mother had smoked two packs of cigarettes per day throughout the pregnancy. Cassandra's blood is likely to have *(more? less?)* HbA (and more HbF) than Jarred's. Protein supplements *(are? are not?)* likely to help Cassandra raise her HbA levels. Cassandra had jaundice at birth. Jaundice is *(rare? common?)* among preterm infants.

E2. Fill in the blanks or circle the correct answers about hemolytic disease of the newborn (HDN):

(a) HDN is more likely to occur in the *(first? second or third?)* Rh-positive baby delivered of an Rh-_____ mother.

(b) As the baby's RBCs are destroyed by the mother's anti-Rh antibodies, the newborn's blood level of bilirubin is likely to be *(higher? lower?)* than usual. The condition known as _____ may occur, in which bilirubin deposits injure the _____. Treatment typically includes _____-therapy, which is exposure of skin to _____. Bilirubin in skin is broken down to a chemical that can be excreted by _____ and _____ systems.

(c) If this baby needs a transfusion, (s)he should receive Type O Rh-_____ blood. The baby will still be Rh-positive, but the Rh-neg blood (not vulnerable to the mother's anti-Rh antibodies) will help the child survive until its mother's anti-Rh antibodies are diluted from the baby's blood.

(d) Prevention of future HDN can be afforded by injection of Rh *(antigens? antibodies?)* to the Rh-negative mother during and following pregnancy with an Rh-positive baby.

E3. Hemoglobin levels typically *(increase? decrease?)* slightly with aging. Which type of anemia is most common among elderly people? _____

Disorders of White Blood Cells and Lymphoid Tissues

■ Review Questions

A. HEMATOPOIETIC AND LYMPHOID TISSUE (pages 291–293)

A1. Complete this exercise about formation of white blood cells (WBCs).

   (a) White blood cells (WBCs) are all formed in bone marrow, which is also known as _____ tissue.

   (b) Some WBCs, namely _____, mature and circulate in the lymphatic system. Name the organs that comprise this system.

   _____

   (c) B lymphocytes mature in the *(bone marrow? thymus?)*, whereas T lymphocytes mature in the _____.

   (d) One other category of lymphocyte is the _____ cell.

A2. Contrast roles of *pluripotent stem cells* and *progenitor cells* in WBC formation.

   _____

   _____

   _____

A3. Describe functions of the following cytokines: *GM-CSF, erythropoietin, interleukin-1, and c-kit ligand.*

   _____

   _____

   _____

A4. Arrange the following structures in the pathway of lymph fluid in correct sequence from first to last:

   Afferent lymphatic channels
   Collecting trunk
   Efferent lymphatic channels
   Lymph node
   Neck veins

Fluid in blood plasma → interstitial fluid → lymph in lymph capillaries → _____ → _____ → _____ → _____ → _____ .

A5. Describe the "good news" and "bad news" of lymph channels and lymph nodes.

   _____

   _____

   _____

B. DISORDERS OF WHITE BLOOD CELLS (pages 293–295)

B1. Complete this exercise about WBC deficiency.

   (a) Circle the correct answer. A normal WBC count is *(600? 6,000? 60,000? 6 million?)*/μL. A low WBC count is known as *(leukocytosis? leukopenia?)*.

   (b) Typically, more than 50% of WBCs are *(neutrophils? lymphocytes?)*.

   (c) Neutrophils normally live in the circulating blood for about ____ day(s). Because of this short life span, interference with neutrophil production quickly leads to neutro_____.

B2. Select the factor leading to neutropenia that matches the related description. One answer will be used twice.

   Aplastic anemia
   Bacterial or viral infection
   Congenital neutropenia
   Drugs that interfere with normal marrow function
   Felty's syndrome
   Hemopoietic cancer
   Metastatic solid tumor cancer

   (a) A form of rheumatoid arthritis in which large amounts of neutrophils are destroyed in the spleen: _____

(b) Hereditary disorders such as Kostmann's syndrome and cyclic neutropenia:

_____

(c) Chemotherapy or irradiation: _____

_____

(d) Cause of most cases of neutropenia: _____

_____

(e) Condition that decreases production of RBCs, platelets, and most WBCs: _____

_____

(f) WBCs used up faster than they can be replaced: _____

(g) Spread of breast carcinoma to bone marrow, which prevents normal marrow function:

_____

(h) Leukemia in which normal bone marrow function is displaced by unregulated formation of immature (and useless) cancerous WBCs: _____

B3. Julie reports that her mother has been taking a series of chemotherapy treatments for cancer over the past 8 months. Her mother also has developed sores in her mouth that are so painful that she cannot eat and she has recurrent bouts of nausea and vomiting. As a result, Julie's mother is extremely tired and emaciated; and her self-esteem is low related to loss of most of her body hair (alopecia). She has recurrent respiratory infections. Explain why she is likely to have these signs and symptoms.

_____

_____

_____

C. INFECTIOUS MONONUCLEOSIS (pages 295–296)

C1. The microbe that causes infectious mononucleosis (IM) is the EBV virus; this abbreviation stands for: E_____ B_____ V_____.

C2. Arrange in correct sequence these phases in the pathogenesis of infectious mononucleosis (IM):

Incubation period (4 to 8 weeks)
Manifestations (2 to 3 weeks)
Prodromal (several days)
Recovery phase (2 to 3 months)

_____ → _____ →

_____ → _____

C3. Arrange these events in the course of pathogenesis of IM in the correct order.

(a) Atypical T-cell proliferation result from stimulation by infected B cells; such cells are useful diagnostically; they also cause lymphadenopathy, and eventually destroy infected B cells.

(b) Some B cells die and release virus into blood causing fever and production of IgM and IgG antibodies, as well as heterophil (Paul-Bunnell) antibodies used to diagnose IM.

(c) The Epstein-Barr virus invades B lymphocytes in tissues lining the mouth and throat.

_____ → _____ → _____

C4. The nurse asks Sarah how she has been feeling and Sarah makes the statements listed below. Circle the three statements that indicate presence of the typical triad of manifestations of infectious mononucleosis (IM).

(a) "I have a pounding headache."

(b) "My glands are so swollen on both sides of my neck; I feel like I can hardly move my neck."

(c) "My throat is killing me; it hurts to even **think** of talking."

(d) "My temperature was 102.5°F this morning."

(e) "I have terrific pain in my hip joints."

C5. In infectious mononucleosis, lymphocytes may proliferate so much that they account for 95% of the total WBCs. In normal blood, _____ % of all WBCs are lymphocytes. Explain why the condition is named infectious *mono*nucleosis when it is *not* the monocytes that increase in number.

_____

_____

_____

C6. Explain why lymph nodes, spleen, and liver tend to enlarge in response to blood disorders such as IM (and also leukemia).

_____

_____

_____

C7. Circle the two true statements about infectious mononucleosis (IM).

(a) Infectious mononucleosis (IM): most common among welfare and Medicaid patients

(b) The virus that causes IM **can be transmitted** through saliva.

(c) IM more commonly affects **children** and **adolescents** than **old people.**

(d) Most persons who survive infectious mononucleosis **do** experience significant impairment after the disease.

(e) IM is spread **only** by clients with **current symptoms** of IM.

D. NEOPLASTIC DISORDERS OF HEMATOPOIETIC AND LYMPHOID ORIGIN (pages 296–301)

D1. Summarize the basic problem in leukemia. *Circle the correct answer in the later sentence.*

_____

_____

_____

Leukemia occurs *(only in children? only in adults? in persons of all ages?)*. It is a *(common? rare?)* cause of cancer deaths in children.

D2. Circle correct answers or fill in blanks in these statements about leukemia:

(a) The "A" in ALL and AML stands for *(acquired? acute?)*. Write P, R, or W next to the following warning signs of acute leukemia to indicate whether the sign indicates deficiency in RBCs, platelets, or WBCs:

(1) Fatigue, lethargy, dyspnea, pallor: ___

(2) Repeated infections, such as genitourinary: ___

(3) Easy bruising and nosebleeds (epistaxis): ___

(b) Chronic leukemias have a more *(sudden? gradual?)* onset than acute leukemias.

(c) Lymphocytic leukemia involves accelerated production of immature _____ cells that infiltrate organs such as _____. *(Myelocytic? Lymphocytic?)* leukemia affects pluripotent stem cells in *(bone marrow? lymph tissue?)*, preventing normal hematopoiesis.

(d) Causes of leukemia *(are? are not?)* known. Write several factors that are associated with increased incidence of leukemia.

D3. Write the pathophysiologic rationale for each of these factors related to acute leukemia or its treatment.

(a) "Blasts" forming 60% to 100% of circulating blood cells. _____

_____

(b) Leukostasis requiring leukapheresis

_____

(c) Nausea and vomiting, headache, papilledema

_____

(d) High levels of uric acid in blood that can lead to renal damage

_____

(e) Tumor lysis syndrome

_____

(f) Graft-versus-host disease following allogeneic transplantation

_____

D4. Arrange in correct sequence from first to last in chemotherapy treatment of leukemia:

Intensification or consolidation
Induction
Maintenance

_____ → _____ →
_____

D5. Explain why the following regimens may accompany chemotherapeutic treatment of leukemia.

(a) CNS prophylaxis

_____

_____

_____

(b) Antibiotic therapy

_____

_____

_____

(c) Allopurinol

_____

_____

_____

D6. Select the type of leukemia that fits each description below.

ALL   AML   CLL   CML

(a) The most common type of leukemia in children and young adults, this form of leukemia now has a higher cure rate (70%) than other types of leukemia: _____

(b) The most common type of cancer that follows treatment for a primary cancer; also the type of leukemia associated with Down syndrome; has less than a 20% cure rate: _____

(c) Most likely to affect elderly persons; the slow course permits a normal life for many years; often diagnosed by enlarged lymph nodes: _____

(d) Hairy cell leukemia (HCL) is a rare form of this type of leukemia with lymphocytes that have fine, hairlike projections; most often occurs in older men and has a median survival rate of 6 years: _____

(e) Patients often present with a feeling of abdominal fullness related to splenomegaly; clients with high counts of leukocyte blast cells have a poor prognosis: _____

E. MALIGNANT LYMPHOMAS
(pages 301–303)

E1. Circle the correct answer.

Whereas leukemias are cancers initiated in (bone marrow? lymph tissue?), lymphomas primarily involve (bone marrow? lymph tissue?). The abnormal lymphocytes produced lead to (increased? decreased?) immunity and (increased? decreased?) risk of infections.

E2. Contrast the two major types of lymphomas by writing H for Hodgkin's or N-H for non-Hodgkin's lymphoma next to related descriptions. For one case, both answers are used.

(a) Begins with a single enlarged lymph node, usually above the diaphragm, and typically in the neck: ___

(b) Begins with several enlarged lymph nodes in various locations: ___

(c) Enlarged lymph nodes are typically painless: ___

(d) Much more common and typically more lethal form of lymphoma: ___

E3. Although the cause of lymphomas is unknown, this form of cancer has been associated with the _____ virus. Lymphomas have been found to occur more in persons who have a history of the EBV-associated disorder _____.

E4. Diagnosis of Hodgkin's lymphoma requires the presence of _____ cells in biopsy of lymph nodes. Describe these tumor cells.

_____
_____
_____

E5. (a) Explain why the staging of Hodgkin's disease is critical.

_____
_____

(b) List several "B" symptoms associated with stage B lymphomas.

_____
_____
_____

E6. Describe the meaning of "CHOP" therapy in non-Hodgkin's lymphoma treatment.

_____
_____
_____

E7. At age 27, Margaret was diagnosed with non-Hodgkin's lymphoma. Massive radiation cured her lymphoma. At age 37, myocardial ischemia required a quadruple bypass. At age 47, she experienced a myocardial infarction (MI) and shortly thereafter went into clinical trials for an angiogenic medication to increase coronary perfusion (blood flow). Explain the likely connection between the lymphoma and the cardiac disease.

_____
_____
_____

F. MULTIPLE MYELOMA (pages 303–305)

F1. Describe multiple myeloma by completing this exercise. Circle the correct answers or fill in the blanks.

(a) Multiple myeloma is a cancer that leads to huge numbers of plasma cells derived from (B? T?) lymphocytes. Plasma cells excrete antibodies known as _____ (____).

(b) Myeloma cells secrete chemicals that stimulate (osteoblasts? osteoclasts?) that cause bone (synthesis? destruction?) and fractures.

(c) Abnormal plasma cells can also secrete amyloid which can cause damage to _____ and _____. Other abnormal proteins cause injury to _____ and CRF.

F2. Helen was diagnosed at age 42 with multiple myeloma. She had to go on disability from her job as a mathematician to undergo treatments with profound side effects. After 44 months of chemotherapy and/or radiation, she had to stop treatments owing to effects of *pancytopenia*. She experienced extreme *pain* in her back, hips and extremities. She died at age 47 of complications of *chronic renal failure (CRF)*. Explain reasons for the *italicized* conditions.

_____

_____

_____

CHAPTER 17

Mechanisms of Infectious Disease

■ Review Questions

A. TERMINOLOGY (pages 309–310)

A1. Select terms from the following list that complete the exercise below. Use each term once.

Colonized   Host
Mutualism   Normal microflora
Opportunistic infection   Pathogenic
Virulent

  (a) Matthew, a newborn, has not yet established a _____ in his large intestine. After he ingests nutrients, bacteria will take up residence in his GI tract, produce vitamin K, and have a relationship of _____ with Matthew.

  (b) Shawn has pneumonia. She is serving as _____ to a highly _____ strain of bacteria that have _____ her lungs.

  (c) Peter has an infection caused by *Pneumocystis carinii* microbes that are not typically _____ in healthy persons. But in Peter's immunocompromised state, because he has AIDS, these microbes establish an _____.

B. INFECTIOUS DISEASE (pages 310–318)

B1. Select the type of infectious agent that matches each description. Answers may be used more than once.

Bacteria   Chlamydiae
Fungi   Mycoplasma
Parasites   Prions
Rickettsiae   Viruses

  (a) Some are oncogenic; some cause illnesses such as chickenpox, shingles, genital herpes, or AIDS: _____

  (b) Contain no DNA or RNA, only proteins; cause Creutzfeld-Jacob disease in humans and BSE ("mad cow disease") in animals: _____

  (c) RNA or DNA core surrounded by a protein envelope derived from the membrane of the host cell; may remain latent in human cells for years, and then become activated; incapable of replicating outside of living cells: _____

  (d) Classified as prokaryocytes because they lack a true nucleus and organized organelles; they do contain DNA and RNA, and can reproduce outside of human cells:

_____

  (e) The rigid cell wall (composed of peptidoglycan) of these microbes makes them vulnerable to antibiotics such as penicillin that attack this wall, but the antibiotic does not injure human cells because they lack this wall: _____

  (f) Considerably smaller than bacteria, these microbes lack the rigid cell wall, so are resistant to penicillin; known to cause some pneumonias and genital infections:

_____

  (g) Include yeasts such as *Candida* and molds; cause athlete's foot, jock itch, and ringworm; produce a cell wall that is not made of peptidoglycan, so that the organism is not vulnerable to penicillin: _____

  (h) Manifest characteristics of viruses (can reproduce only within a living cell) and of bacteria (have rigid peptidoglycan cell wall); depend on a vector such as a tick for transmission; cause Rocky Mountain spotted fever: _____

  (i) Cause common genital infections; may cause blindness (trachoma) if the eyes of a baby are exposed to this microbe within the birth canal: _____

  (j) Include protozoans (such as water-borne *Giardia lamblia*), worms (such as tapeworms), and arthropods (such as head or pubic lice, fleas, mites, and chiggers):

_____

B2. Circle the correct answers or fill in the blanks in each statement about bacteria.

(a) Spherical bacteria are classified as *(bacilli? cocci? spirochetes?)*. The bacteria that cause syphilis, *Treponema pallidum*, are classified as *(bacilli? cocci? spirochetes?)*.

(b) *Staphylococci* are bacteria arranged in *(clusters? single lines? pairs?)*, whereas diplococci are arranged in _____. In the name *Staphylococcus aureus*, "*aureus*" is the *(genus? species?)* name.

(c) Some bacteria form spores that *(increase? decrease?)* their resistance in unfavorable environments. *Mycobacterium tuberculosis* bacteria that cause tuberculosis are distinctive because of how they respond to an _____ stain.

(d) Bacteria that cannot survive in the presence of oxygen are called:

(1) Aerobes

(2) Anaerobes

(3) Facultative anaerobes

(e) Gram-positive bacteria take a ___ stain with the Gram's stain procedure.

(1) Red (safranin)

(2) Purple (crystal violet)

B3. Answer these questions about fungal infections.

(a) Paul's dermatophyte infections, commonly known as athlete's foot and jock itch, are caused by *(superficial? deep?)* pathogens that require relatively *(cool? warm?)* temperatures.

(b) Melissa just completed intensive antibiotic therapy for a respiratory infection; now she has a "yeast infection" (*Candida*) of her urethral and vaginal mucous membranes. Explain the connection.

_____

_____

B4. Complete this exercise about parasitic infections.

(a) Amebic dysentery is a GI infection caused by *(protozoa? worms? arthropods?)*. List three mechanisms by which protozoan infections can be transmitted.

_____

_____

_____

(b) List three categories of worms that can infect humans.

_____

_____

Such infections are a health problem primarily in *(the United States? developing nations?)*.

(c) Mites, chiggers, lice and fleas are all called _____-parasites because they infest the body through external surfaces, such as skin. Clothing, bedding, combs or brushes are common modes of transmission for fleas and _____.

C. MECHANISMS OF INFECTION (pages 318–323)

C1. Ms. Leonard is a nurse-specialist in epidemiology for the Public Health Department. Write an appropriate job description for this position.

_____

_____

_____

C2. Select the term that best fits each description. Choose from these terms.

Endemic	Epidemic
Incidence	Pandemic
Prevalence	

(a) Number of new cases of influenza in Detroit over a period of 3 winter months:

_____

(b) Sudden outbreak of dysentery in a county in western Kentucky such that the prevalence exceeds normal rates for that county:

_____

(c) Goiter was considered _____ to the Midwest before the general availability of fresh fish or iodized salt.

C3. Identify the mode of transmission in the following cases. Choose from these answers.

Direct contact	Ingestion
Inhalation	Penetration

(a) Jill, who was born with cystic fibrosis, currently has viral pneumonia: ____

(b) Manuelo eats pork that is not fully cooked; he develops a tapeworm infection: ____

(c) Patrick comes down with a case of *Shigella* infection after eating a salad prepared by a worker whose hands had fecal contamination: ____

(d) Raphael receives a tetanus infection after stepping on the sharp edge of a piece of farm equipment coated with soil containing *Clostridium tetani*: ____

(e) Sandra contracts genital herpes after unprotected sex: ____

(f) Mary Sue develops Lyme disease after she is bitten by an infected tick: ____

C4. List three examples of vertical transmission of infection (from mother to child).

_____

_____

_____

C5. Cite examples of factors that normally protect against infection of the:

(a) Respiratory tract

_____

(b) GI tract

_____

(c) Skin

_____

C6. Select the source of infections that fits the related description.

Endogenous agents   Fomites
Nosocomial   Zoonoses

(a) Shared brushes or hats (as vectors for lice eggs); improperly washed spoons or forks: _____

(b) Rabies, Rocky Mountain spotted fever from a tick bite, or saliva from a cat bite: _____

(c) An impetigo infection contracted during Danny's stay in the pediatric department of the hospital: _____

C7. Arrange the following stages in the course of a disease from first to last.

Acute   Convalescence and recovery
Incubation   Prodromal

_____ → _____ →
_____ → _____

Now identify the stage that fits each description:

(a) Microbes are actively replicating in the host, but no signs or symptoms are present: _____

(b) A general feeling of malaise (slight fever, headaches, muscle aches, and fatigue) appears, but not signs highly specific to this disease: _____

(c) Following the period of maximal impact of the disease, resolution occurs: _____

(d) This phase is prolonged in an insidious disease: _____

C8. Circle the correct answer about each disease.

(a) Celeste has a viremia which refers to a viral disease in *(blood? urine?)*.

(b) Mrs. Jefferson's *(diverticulosis? diverticulitis?)* is a condition that involves inflammation.

(c) A disease with an abrupt onset is a(n) *(fulminant? insidious?)* illness.

(d) *Shigella* and *Giardia* typically cause infections of *(digestive? urinary?)* systems.

(e) *Helicobacter pylori* is associated specifically with Nancy's *(gastric ulcers? foot abscesses?)*.

C9. Complete this exercise about factors that increase virulence of microbes. Choose from the following answers:

Adhesive factors   Evasive factors
Invasive factors   Toxins

(a) Capsules or enzymes that cause clot formation are both mechanisms that protect microbes from WBCs: _____

(b) Leukocidins produced by microbes destroy WBCs: _____

(c) Enzymes (eg, phospholipidases) enable microbes to break through cell membranes: _____

(d) Ligands (or adhesins) on microorganisms bind to specific receptors on target host cells: _____

(e) Examples are chemicals produced by the bacteria that cause diphtheria, pertussis, and tetanus (DPT), as well as traveler's diarrhea and many forms of food poisoning: _____

D. DIAGNOSIS AND TREATMENT OF INFECTIOUS DISEASES (pages 323–329)

D1. Write the two requirements for diagnosis of an infectious disease:

(a) Finding of a specific _____

(b) Presence of _____ and _____ consistent with the specific diagnosis

D2. Match the diagnostic technique with the related description. Select from these answers:

Antigen detection   Culture
Genome sequences   Serology

(a) Checking antibody (IgG or IgM) titer from Naomi's blood to verify her suspected case of hepatitis B: _____

(b) Collection of microbes in Tom's sputum for growth on agar, followed by staining and microscopic examination: _____

(c) Use of DNA probes; polymerase chain reactions (PCR) to quantify the amount of HIV virus (viral load) in Barry's blood: _____

(d) Use of fluorescent antibodies that identify the specific pathogen causing Jerry's meningitis: _____

D3. List three major categories of treatments for infectious diseases.

_____
_____
_____

D4. Explain how ideal antimicrobial medications work.

_____
_____
_____

D5. Select the antibiotic that fits each description.

Aminoglycosides   Cephalosporins
Sulfonamides

(a) Broad-spectrum antibiotics that work by disrupting the bacterial cell wall: _____

(b) Interfere with bacterial protein synthesis; may have nephrotoxic or ototoxic side effects: _____

(c) Interfere with normal metabolism of bacteria; may cause allergic effects: _____

D6. List several mechanisms by which bacteria develop resistance to antibiotics.

_____
_____
_____

D7. Select the antimicrobial medication that fits each description.

Antibiotic   Antifungal
Antiparasitic   Antiviral

(a) Penicillin that targets the cell wall of bacteria: _____

(b) Reverse transcriptase inhibitors and protease inhibitors: _____

(c) Antimicrobials needed especially in poor, developing nations: _____

(d) Targets membrane lipid ergosterol, an essential component of cell membranes of certain microbes: _____

D8. Fill in the blanks about immunotherapy treatment for infections. (See also Chapter 18.)

(a) Vaccines are used as _____ against many preventable infections such as MMR and DPT.

(b) Cytokines are chemicals produced by human _____ blood cells. These stimulate body defenses against infections; for example, _____.

(c) Interferons (IFNs) and interleukins (ILs) are examples of _____ made by WBCs.

(d) IVIG is an acronym for _____, and consists of anti-_____ that can boost immune capabilities of an infected host.

D9. Identify the appropriate surgical intervention or condition requiring surgery.

Appendectomy   Debridement
Gas gangrene   Infected heart valve

(a) Infection of second- and third-degree burns required removal and cleaning of sections of Jimmie's skin: _____

(b) Mrs. Romanowski's hysterectomy led to ischemia of abdominal organs and infection that required removal of sections of her intestine and urinary bladder: _____

(c) Susannah's streptococcal infection as a child resulted in endocarditis that caused heart murmurs and related surgery: _____

(d) Billy required surgery to prevent organ rupture and possible peritonitis: _____

CHAPTER 18

Immunity and Inflammation

■ Review Questions

A. IMMUNE SYSTEM (pages 331–349)

A1. Contrast components of body defenses by writing "NS" next to nonspecific and "S" next to specific defenses.

   (a) B lymphocytes that lead to production of antibodies: ___

   (b) T lymphocytes that destroy a specific type of microbe: ___

   (c) Intact skin that serves as a barrier against microbial infection: ___

   (d) Inflammation involving "swollen glands" (lymph nodes with phagocytes) in the neck: ___

A2. Discuss these two essential features of specific human defenses.

   (a) Recognition of "intruders" versus self

   _____

   _____

   _____

   (b) Memory response

   _____

   _____

   _____

A3. Complete this exercise about immunity.

   (a) *(Antigens? Antibodies?)* are foreign to the host, and they *(stimulate? inhibit?)* an immune response.

   (b) Circle the antigens in the following list.

     Bacteria   Fungi
     Penicillin   Pollen
     Protozoans   T lymphocytes
     Transplanted organs   Viruses

   (c) A site on an antigen that is recognized by a specifically shaped lymphocyte or antibody (see Figure 18-1) is called an antigenic determinant or an _____.

   (d) A single bacterium is likely to present *(only one? three? hundreds of?)* antigenic determinant(s) to human immune cells.

A4. Circle the answers that correctly match a type of cell with a correct description.

   (a) Lymphocytes: the primary cells of the specific immune system

   (b) B lymphocytes: associated with cell-mediated immunity

   (c) T cells: normally outnumber B cells three or four to one

   (d) Helper T cells: regulatory cells that enhance responses of other lymphocytes

   (e) Cytotoxic T cells: effector cells that actually destroy antigens

A5. Refer to textbook Figures 18-4 and 18-5 and complete this exercise about activation of immune cells.

   (a) The trigger for both B and T lymphocytes is the recognition of an anti-_____ by B- or T-cell receptors. Antigens are presented to lymphocytes by APCs or a_____ p_____ cells. Give one example of an APC: _____

   (b) Further activation of lymphocytes with chemicals known as cyto_____ causes B or T cells to _____.

   (c) In B cells, the receptors are immunoglobulins, also known as anti-_____. Activated B cells produce effector cells known as _____ cells that secrete antibodies (Igs) that bind to the intruding antigen and assure its removal. Antibody-mediated immunity (or AMI) is also known as *(cytotoxic? humoral?)* immunity because antibodies are small and suspended in blood (a "humor").

   (d) T cells are involved in _____-mediated immunity (or CMI), which is also known as *(cytotoxic? humoral?)* immunity because T cells exert toxic effects directly on antigens.

A6. Explain how T and B cells can specifically respond to the diverse microbes and other antigens to which the human body is exposed each day.

———————————————————————
———————————————————————
———————————————————————

How does the immune system "remember" to respond to antigens that have been "seen" before?

———————————————————————
———————————————————————
———————————————————————

A7. Describe Kate's MHCs in this exercise.

(a) MHC stands for a M_____ H_____ complex molecules. These chemicals are coded for by DNA on Kate's chromosome ___. Because Kate's cells have unique MHCs, a kidney transplanted from Susan to Kate is likely to be recognized as *(self? nonself?)* because Susan's MHCs differ from Kate's. Because MHC molecules do play a role in transplant rejection, these chemicals are classified as anti*(gens? bodies?)*.

(b) Kate's MHCs should allow her immune system to recognize her own cells as "self," not "nonself." Errors in such recognition lead to _____ diseases (eg, some forms of arthritis or diabetes) in which Kate's immune system would *(destroy? tolerate?)* her own cells. (See Chapter 19.)

A8. Now distinguish the two categories of MHCs in this exercise.

(a) MHC I molecules are found on *(nearly every cell of the body? APCs and B cells?)*. As a result, they can flag the immune system if the body cell is altered by cancer or by viral invasion. The virus or cancer cell is degraded, and portions of it (antigens) complex with MHC I molecules. This complex is then recognized by *(helper? cytotoxic?)* T cells as an "intruder" that must be destroyed.

(b) MHC II molecules are found on _____ and _____ cells. MHC IIs bind to antigens from microbes that have been phagocytosed and digested within macrophages. *(CD4 helper? CD8 cytotoxic?)* T cells recognize antigens complexed with MHC II complexes.

A9. Circle the correct answer or fill in the blanks.

Human MHC proteins are also known as HLA (or h_____ l_____ antigens) because they were first detected on _____ blood cells. MHC I molecules are divided into subtypes HLA-A, _____, and _____. Because of the diversity in MHC molecules, it *(is? is not?)* likely that each person's MHC (or HLA) antigens will be unique. For transplant compatibility, it is critical that donor and recipient MHC (or HLA) antigens be *(very similar? dissimilar?)*.

A10. Circle the correct answers or fill in the blanks.

Macrophages develop from *(neutrophils? monocytes?)*. Kupffer's cells are macrophages in the *(liver? lungs?)*, whereas microglial cells are macrophages in the _____. Their functions are to serve as _____ that present antigen-MHC II complexes to *(CD4? CD8?)* cells; they also secrete _____ such as TNF and IL-1 that produce fever and help to activate T and B cells. Macrophages also remove antigen-antibody complexes by the process of _____.

A11. What function do dendritic cells share with macrophages?

———————————————————————
———————————————————————
———————————————————————

Dendritic cells are found in _____ tissue and also in skin where they are known as _____ cells.

A12. A third type of cell that can serve as an APC is a *(B? T?)* lymphocyte. Complete this exercise about these cells.

(a) B cells are more associated with destruction of *(bacteria and their toxins? fungi, protozoans, and viruses?)*. They do this by *(direct killing action? causing production of antibodies?)*, which is *(cytotoxic? humoral?)* immunity. (See A5.)

(b) As B cells mature, they develop receptors that are _____. In lymph tissue, B cells that encounter complementary antigens and T-cell/cytokine stimulation will transform into _____ cells (and produce antibodies) or _____ cells. (See A5 and A6.)

A13. Refer to the textbook figure of an antibody (Fig. 18-8 and Table 18-3) as you describe significant components of antibodies. Circle the correct answer or fill in the blanks.

(a) Antibodies or immunoglobulins are *(lipids? proteins?)* with *(1? 2? 4?)* polypeptide chains (2 light, 2 heavy) with at least ___ antigen-binding sites.

(b) Three classes of antibodies have shapes that resemble the letter "Y." These are Ig__, Ig__, and Ig__.

(c) The function of the antibody is to bind to an _____. These sites are found at the ends of the *(forked? tail?)* portion of the antibody; this region is known as the Fab or _____-binding fragment. This Fab end is *(constant? variable?)* in shape because this portion of all antibodies must conform to diverse antigens. Each B cell clone produces antibodies with one specific antigen-binding variable region or _____. The tail end (Fc fragment) is *(constant? variable?)* for the particular class of immunoglobulin (such as IgD or IgG).

A14. Identify the type of antibody likely to be secreted in each case.

IgA IgD IgE IgG IgM

(a) These antibodies are detected in baby Cleo's blood. Because these are the first antibodies to be secreted in response to an antigen and because they do not cross the placenta, it is determined that Cleo must have the related antigens (and infection that caused them): ___

(b) Baby Leo received these immunoglobulins from his mother because this type does cross the placenta and provide Leo with at least temporary immunity against many bacterial and viral infections; these Igs typically make up three quarters of all circulating antibodies: ___

(c) Paul has conjunctivitis, which is normally prevented with the help of antibodies in tears in the eyes; these antibodies are also found in other secretions, such as saliva and the mucus of airways, GI tract, and vagina. They help to prevent adhesion of bacteria to epithelial linings: ___

(d) Dorothy has allergies to pollen and several foods that are mediated by antibodies that trigger release of histamine from her mast cells and basophils: ___

(e) Found on B lymphocytes as antigen receptors: ___ (See Figure 18-4 in the text.)

A15. You have now looked at functions of macrophages, dendritic cells, and B lymphocytes. Complete this exercise about T lymphocytes by circling the correct answers or filling in the blanks. (See A5 and A12.)

(a) T cells are more associated with control of *(bacteria? viral?)* infections. They do this by *(direct killing action? causing production of antibodies?)*, which is *(cell-mediated or CMI? humoral or AMI?)* immunity. (See A5 above.)

(b) T cells also activate other ___ cells and also ___ cells. They are involved in _____ of grafts and in *(immediate? delayed?)* hypersensitivity reactions (see Chapter 19).

(c) T cells form in *(bone marrow? lymph tissue?)* and mature in the *(thymus? thyroid?)* where helper T cells develop CD4 receptors and cytotoxic T cells develop ____ receptors.

(d) Helper T (CD__) cells activated by recognition of an antigen complexed with MHC *(I? II?)* molecules play key regulatory roles in immunity. Helper T cells secrete _____, such as interleukins (ILs), that activate most other types of immune cells; for example, attracting more _____ cells to the infected area.

(e) Cytotoxic T (CD__) cells are activated by MHC *(I? II?)* molecules complexed with cells infected with viruses or cancer (antigens); this process ensures that neighboring cells with MHC I but *not* infected with antigen will be spared from attack by CD8 cells. List several mechanisms by which cytotoxic T cells destroy infected cells. _____

_____

(f) NK (or n_____-k_____) cells *(are? are not?)* lymphocytes. They destroy cancer cells or virus-infected cells *(directly? by releasing antibodies?)*. They differ from T cells in that NK cells *(do? do not?)* need to be activated by the specific antigen. How do NK cells know not to kill normal human cells?

_____

_____

A16. Hussein is 20 years old and in excellent health. Complete this exercise concerning his lymphoid organs.

(a) Circle all of his central lymphoid organs.

Bone marrow   Lymph nodes
MALT tissues lining passageways into the body
Peyer's patches in GI organs   Spleen
Thymus   Tonsils

(b) Hussein's thymus is likely to be located in his *(neck? thorax, anterior to his heart?)*.

His thymus is likely to be *(larger? smaller?)* now than when he was 10 years old.

(c) Normally, as T cells mature under the influence of cytokines and thymic hormones, they move from thymic *(cortex to medulla? medulla to cortex?)*. Most of these cells *(do? do not?)* leave the thymus. Normally, only T cells that recognize _____ antigens are selected to leave the thymus and circulate in blood or lymph.

(d) Most of Hussein's lymph nodes are likely to be located in his *(hands and feet? trunk and proximal ends of his extremities?)*. Refer to text Figure 18-10. Maturing *(B? T? both B and T?)* cells are located in lymph nodes.

(e) Hussein's spleen is likely to be located just posterior to his *(liver? stomach?)* on the upper *(right? left?)* of his abdomen. Old red blood cells are destroyed within *(red? white?)* pulp. White pulp serves as another site for activation of ___ and ___ cells.

(f) Microbes inhaled into Hussein's airways will be greeted (and attacked) by immune cells in two sites, namely _____ and _____.

A17. Complete this exercise about cytokines.

(a) Cytokines *(are made by? act on?)* immune cells, primarily *(B? T?)* lymphocytes and macrophages. These chemicals act on cells *(distant from? nearby?)* the cells that produce them where they bind to specific _____. Most cytokines affect *(only one? more than one?)* type of cell, and may lead to cascade effects.

(b) Name several cytokines that mediate inflammation by producing fever and mobilizing neutrophils._____
_____
_____ `

(c) Name several cytokines that stimulate hematopoiesis. _____

_____
_____

(d) Name an interleukin and its receptor that are critical for sustained T-cell proliferation; without them, severe combined immunodeficiency (SCID) results. _____
_____
_____

(e) Explain how interferons (IFNs) help protect the body. _____
_____
_____

(f) Name a cytokine that is responsible for tissue wasting in "wasting diseases" such as AIDS: _____
_____
_____

A18. Write "S" (specific or acquired) or "NS" (nonspecific or innate) to indicate the type of immunity in each example.

(a) Immunization: ___

(b) Infection with a specific microbe (and its antigens): ___

(c) Inflammation: ___

(d) Skin or mucous membrane (barriers): ___

A19. Now write "A" (active) or "P" (passive) to indicate the type of acquired immunity in each example.

(a) Immunization with injection of antigens to which the body develops immunity: ___

(b) Infection with a specific microbe (and its antigens): ___

(c) A dose of gamma-globulin: ___

(d) Transfer of IgG antibodies from mother to baby across the placenta: ___

A20. Production of antibodies in humoral immunity depends more directly on *(B? T?)* lymphocytes. List several mechanisms by which antibodies are able to combat infection.

_____
_____
_____

A21. Anastasia receives her DPT immunization and somewhat later receives a "booster." To which dose is she likely to mount a greater immune response (produce more antibodies)?

_____
_____
_____

A22. Cell-mediated immunity depends more directly on *(B? T?)* lymphocytes and macrophages. *(Helper? Cytotoxic?)* T cells play a critical role in producing IL-2, which then stimulates killing activity by *(helper? cytotoxic?)* T cells and macrophages.

A23. Circle the correct answer or fill in the blanks. Parts (b) through (d) describe the overall effects of the complement system in this exercise. (*Hint:* refer to Table 18-5 and Figure 18-14 in the textbook.)

(a) The complement system consists of *(lipids? proteins?)* numbered C1 to ____ plus other factors in blood that act in a cascade of reactions to mediate *(cytotoxic? humoral?)* immunity.

(b) Release of chemicals such as histamine from mast cells and basophils, causing blood vessels to *(constrict? dilate?)* and have *(increased? decreased?)* permeability. This process, called _____, brings more phagocytic cells to the infected area.

(c) Coating of microbes to make them more inviting to phagocytes is a process called _____; as a result, phagocytes are more attracted to these "tasty morsels," a process called _____.

(d) Finally, punching of holes in cell membranes of intruders and destroying them so that phagocytes can ingest the "tasty morsels." This process is _____.

A24. List two factors that exert checks and balances (self-regulation) on the immune system.

_____

_____

B. DEVELOPMENTAL ASPECTS OF THE IMMUNE SYSTEM (pages 349–350)

B1. Discuss immunity in infants by completing this exercise. Circle the correct answer or fill in the blanks.

(a) Sara, a full-term newborn, has antibodies in her blood that protect her from a number of diseases for several months. These are *(IgAs? IgGs? IgMs?)*.

(b) Annie, born prematurely at 7 months, is likely to have *(normal? deficient?)* immunity. Explain why. _____

_____

(c) Celia, a newborn whose mother has the HIV virus, *(will? might? will not?)* have IgGs against the HIV virus in her blood. Is Celia infected with HIV? _____

(d) IgM antibodies *(can? cannot?)* cross the placenta. What does the presence of IgM antibodies in 2-month-old Jill's blood indicate? _____

(e) IgA antibodies are transferred from mother to baby Miji *(across the placenta? through breast milk?)*. How can these antibodies help Miji? _____

B2. Circle those factors that are likely to be *decreased* in elderly persons.

Incidence of autoimmune disease
Cell-mediated immunity
Antibody-mediated immunity
T cell count   Infections   Cancers
Range of antibodies that can be recognized
IL-2 cytokine production

C. THE INFLAMMATORY RESPONSE (pages 350–355)

C1. Describe the "good news" and "bad news" of inflammation.

_____

_____

_____

C2. Explain the mechanisms that lead to the five cardinal signs and symptoms of an acute inflammation:

(a) Redness and warmth

_____

_____

_____

(b) Swelling (edema)

_____

_____

_____

(c) Pain and loss of function

_____

_____

_____

C3. In a sunburn, edema occurs *(immediately? a number of hours?)* after the injury.

_____

C4. Answer these questions about the cellular stage of inflammation by circling the correct answers or filling in the blanks. (See also Chapters 13 and 16.)

(a) First cells to arrive on the scene are *(monocytes? neutrophils?)*. These cells produce chemicals known as _____ molecules that cause them to slow down and stick to the inner walls of vessels, a process known as _____.
Neutrophils are likely to arrive at the injured area within *(1.5? 5?)* hours of the injury.

(b) Neutrophils move out of dilated blood vessel by the process of _____.
The cytoplasmic granules in these cells contain _____ that destroy the phagocytosed particles.

(c) To make sufficient neutrophils available during inflammation, the white blood cell count *(increases? decreases?)*; this process is called leuko*(cytosis? penia?)*. As a result, immature neutrophils known as *(segs? bands?)* may appear in circulating blood. This condition is known as a "shift to the _____."

(d) Two other types of leukocytes known as _____phils and _____phils increase during allergic reactions or parasitic infections. *(Basophils? Eosinophils?)* release histamine that *(constricts? dilates?)* vessels during acute inflammation.

(e) _____cytes are leukocytes that play important roles in chronic infection. Their lifespans are considerably *(longer? shorter?)* than those of neutrophils. Monocytes mature into cells known as _____. These may migrate to _____ where they act as APCs.

C5. Arrange in correct sequence the stages of phagocytosis:

Adherence/opsonization   Chemotaxis
Engulfment   Intracellular killing

_____ → _____ →
_____ → _____

C6. List several chemicals that attract leukocytes to infected or inflamed areas.

_____

_____

_____

C7. Indicate whether each of the following factors increases or decreases during systemic responses to inflammation.

(a) Plasma proteins such as fibrinogen or C-reactive protein made by the liver:

_____

(b) Body temperature in response to release of cytokines such as IL-1 and IL-6:

_____

(c) Erythrocyte-sedimentation rate (ESR):

_____

(d) Breakdown of skeletal muscle with release of amino acids from muscle proteins:

_____

(e) Energy level: _____

C8. Fill in the blanks with names of the chemicals that fit each description.

Bradykinin   Leukotrienes
Platelet-activating factor Prostaglandin

(a) Aspirin reduces inflammation and pain by inhibiting production of _____.

(b) _____ increase(s) capillary permeability, causing edema and pain.

(c) _____ cause(s) a wheal-and-flare reaction that accompanies some allergic reactions.

(d) _____ and _____ contribute to bronchial asthma.

C9. Serous exudates are *(viscous? watery?)* fluids resulting from inflammation; purulent exudates contain pus, which consists of _____.

C10. *(Acute? Chronic?)* inflammation is more likely to lead to production of fibroblasts that lead to scarring and deformity. A *(nonspecific? granulomatous?)* inflammation occurs in response to presence of foreign bodies such as splinters, sutures, or asbestos. Tuberculosis is an example of a *(nonspecific? granulomatous?)* inflammation in which the center of the granuloma is *(cheesy? coagulated and hard?)*.

CHAPTER 19

Alterations in the Immune Response

■ Review Questions

A. IMMUNODEFICIENCY DISEASE (pages 357–365)

A1. List three major categories of functions of the immune system.

_____

_____

A2. Now list four major categories of dysfunction of the immune system

_____

_____

A3. Identify the nature of immunodeficiencies by writing "P" for primary (hereditary or congenital) or "S" for secondary (or acquired) next to each case. (The second lines are provided for answers to Question A4.)

(a) Tracy has frequent respiratory infections related to her radiation and chemotherapy treatments for cancer: _____ _____

_____

(b) Peter has a shingles infection associated with his AIDS diagnosis: _____ _____

_____

(c) Pete's thymus has failed to develop (DiGeorge syndrome): _____ _____

_____

(d) Mrs. Jefferson, a patient with diabetes, has frequent infections of her urinary tract and her feet: _____ _____

_____

(e) Phoebe, age 20, has received a kidney transplant. To reduce her risk for organ rejection, she will take immunosuppressant medications for the rest of her life: __ ___

_____

(f) Timmy, age 3 years, has repeated middle ear infections as a result of lack of maturation of B-lymphocyte stem cells and resulting IgG deficiency: _____ _____

_____

A4. Now classify the immunodeficiencies above according to the following categories. (Write these answers on the extra lines in the previous questions.)

B-cell (humoral) deficiency
Combined B-cell and T-cell deficiencies
Complement disorders
Phagocytic dysfunction
T-cell (cellular) deficiency

A5. Select the three true statements in the following list.

(a) Genes that cause immunodeficiency are typically present on **autosomes,** and **few** are on **X-chromosomes.**

(b) Maternal antibodies that protect the newborn from infections are IgMs.

(c) The first antibodies that infants produce are typically IgMs.

(d) By about the age of **2 years,** a child's antibody production level typically matches adult levels.

(e) Humoral immunodeficiencies are **more** likely to lead to fungal and protozoan infections than to bacterial infections.

(f) People with agammaglobulinemia are likely to have **fewer** antibodies than those with hypogammaglobulinemia.

A6. Circle correct answers or fill in blanks in each statement.

(a) *(IgA? IgG? IgM?)* is the most common selective immunoglobulin deficiency. About *(10%? 25% 50%?)* of these individuals have some form of allergy related to lack of these Igs in respiratory or digestive mucous membranes (See text Table 18-3). Administration of IgA *(does? does not?)* help these individuals.

(b) There are four subclasses of *(IgA? IgG? IgM?)* antibodies. IgG2 antibodies are directed against *(protein? polysaccharide?)* antigens, for example, against microbes with capsules made of _____.

(c) Pat's nephrotic syndrome results in abnormal blood filtration with loss of IgA and IgG (but not IgM) antibodies in urine. Why not IgM? _____

A7. Most people with T-cell immunodeficiencies have *(primary? secondary?)* deficiencies. Explain why.

_____

_____

One example of a primary immunodeficiency is DiGeorge syndrome, which is an *(autosomal? X-linked)* disorder. Circle signs and symptoms of this disorder.

Eyes set closely together
Large jaw (macrognathia)
Failure of thymus to develop
Failure of parathyroid gland to develop
Hypercalcemia
Heart defects
Increased risk of infections

A8. Describe secondary T-cell immunodeficiencies in this exercise.

(a) List several causes of such deficiencies: _____.

One sign of T-cell deficiencies is _____ infections, which are caused by normally harmless pathogens. Another sign is *anergy*. Describe this condition.

_____

(b) Write the meaning of the acronym SCIDS: _____.

In this condition, *(B-? T-?)* cell deficiency occurs. Without treatment, SCIDS patients are likely to die by the age of ___ years. Treatments include _____ transplantation.

(c) The condition known as ataxia-telangiectasia involves ataxia, which is _____, and telangiectasias, which are _____. Intellectual development *(is? is not?)* likely to be diminished. *(Helper? Cytotoxic?)* T cell levels are especially affected, as well as Ig levels, which lead to increased _____ infections.

(d) Wiskott-Aldrich syndrome involves excessive *(bleeding? clotting?)* and increased risk of cancers such as _____. The chickenpox virus known as _____ may be lethal to these children.

A9. Most disorders of the complement system are *(X-linked? autosomal dominant? autosomal recessive?)*. For severe symptoms to occur, the patient must be *(homozygous? heterozygous?)* for the disorder. Currently, treatments *(can? cannot?)* cure primary disorders of the complement system.

Describe several effects of complement disorders.

_____

_____

_____

A10. Explain how cirrhosis of the liver can lead to secondary disorders of the complement system.

_____

_____

_____

A11. Describe primary phagocytic disorders in this exercise. Fill in the blanks or circle the correct answers.

(a) Samuel experiences recurrent *Pseudomonas* and *Aspergillus* pulmonary infections as well as *Candida* oral infections (thrush) associated with CGD, or _____ _____ disease. These infections occur because Samuel's phagocytes *(are not attracted to? do not kill ingested?)* microbes. Diagnosis for CGD involves checking ability of Samuel's phagocytic cells to change a dye's color from yellow to _____.

(b) Timothy has Job's syndrome, which involves excessive Ig___ synthesis and reduced *(chemotaxis? engulfment?)* by PMNs. Most commonly, infections with *(Staphylococcus aureus? Streptococcus pyogenes?)* occur.

A12. List two examples of illnesses associated with secondary phagocytic disorders.

_____

_____

A13. Briefly describe stem-cell transplantation procedures.

_____

_____

_____

B. ALLERGIC AND HYPERSENSITIVITY DISORDERS (pages 365–372)

B1. Allergens are defined as any foreign substance that can _____. Describe allergens in this exercise by filling in the blanks or circling the correct answer.

(a) List four methods by which allergens can enter the body.

_____

_____

_____

_____

(b) *(Large, complex compounds such as proteins? Simple inorganic or organic chemicals or metals?)* more commonly trigger immediate hypersensitivity responses, and these are mediated by *(antibodies [Igs]? T lymphocytes?).*

(c) Symptoms of hay fever are likely to be *(the same? different?)* in response to different allergens such as mold spores or ragweed pollen.

B2. Refer to Figures 19-4 through 19-7 and Table 19-1 in the textbook and contrast classes of hypersensitivity responses in this exercise.

(a) In which classes are antibodies (Igs) involved? *(I? II? III? IV?).* These responses all involve *(B? T?)* lymphocytes. Which type involves IgE? ___ Which types involve IgG and IgM? _____

(b) In which class are T cells, not antibodies, involved? ___ The T cells directly destroy the antigen or secrete _____ that do the deed. These are *(immediate? delayed?)* hypersensitivity reactions because they occur 1 to 3 *(minutes? hours? days?)* after exposure to the antigen.

(c) Which classes involve complement? ___ and ___

(d) Which class involves formation of immune complexes (involving IgG) that can lead to vasculitis and edema with localized necrosis and severe organ damage? ___ Such an immune effect on blood vessels is known as an _____ reaction. List several examples of organs damaged by such antigen-antibody complexes: _____ .

B3. Brenda has allergies to ragweed pollen. Complete this description of her experience.

(a) When Brenda breathes in air containing the pollen, the _____ cells (with ____ attached) in walls of her airways are exposed to the environmental antigens, in this case, _____.

(b) The antigens then trigger release of allergy-producing mediators from granules in her mast cells, leading to an _____ response. Name several of these mediators.

_____

(c) Which type of hypersensitivity reaction is Brenda experiencing? *(I? II? III? IV?)* This is a(n) *(immediate? delayed?)*-type of hypersensitivity.

(d) Brenda has a runny nose and watery eyes, signs of _____. Because her allergies occur annually in the same 2 months of the year, she has *(perennial? seasonal?)* allergies.

(e) Like Brenda, several of her family members have allergies to ragweed pollen and several other allergens. Their allergies are likely to be *(atopic? nonatopic?).* Brenda and family members with similar allergies probably have *(high? low?)* levels of basophils, mast cells, and IgEs.

(f) Brenda takes desensitization treatments for her allergies. These are injections of small doses of *(antigens? antibodies?)* which cause her to build up Ig__ that blocks the pollen from combining with IgEs on her cells.

B4. April, age 10, has a number of food allergies. Complete this exercise about April's allergies.

(a) She is allergic to milk, eggs, and several types of nuts and fish These foods are primarily *(proteins? carbohydrates?).* The foods interact with Ig__ bound to cells lining the digestive tract, making this a type __ allergic response.

(b) Food allergies more commonly manifest in *(adults? children?).* List several types of manifestations of food allergies.

_____

(c) Because no one else in her family has these allergies, April's allergies are likely to be *(atopic? nonatopic?).*

(d) Suggest how April might best manage her allergies. _____

_____

_____

B5. Sondra, a newborn, is Rh positive; she has a 2-year old brother, Jason, who is also Rh positive. Their mother is Rh negative. Sondra has HDN, an abbreviation for _____ disease of the _____. In this type ___ hypersensitivity reaction, mother's *(Rh-positive RBCs? Rh antibodies?)* crossed the placenta to enter Sondra's blood. Specifically, these are Ig___ antibodies that can bind to and destroy Sondra's RBCs, leading to conditions such as _____.

B6. Bob, a student nurse, is being tested to see whether he has tuberculosis. A dose of PPD (or _____ _____ _____) is injected *(intravenously? subcutaneously?)* at 2 PM on Tuesday. By 2 PM on Thursday, Bob has a small (less than 0.2 cm) reddened area at the site of the injection, indicating that Bob *(has tuberculosis? has enough sensitized T cells to cause a hypersensitivity reaction?)*. This is an example of a type ___ hypersensitivity reaction.

B7. Contact dermatitis is a type ___ hypersensitivity.

  (a) List three or more examples of causes of contact dermatitis.

  _____
  _____
  _____

  (b) Suggest how you might determine exactly what did cause the contact dermatitis.

  _____
  _____
  _____

  (c) The affected area typically becomes *(pale and cool? swollen, red, and warm?)*. What treatments would you suggest?

  _____
  _____
  _____

B8. State several reasons why latex allergies are so common in the United States.

  _____
  _____
  _____

Which types of hypersensitivity reactions result from repeated latex exposure? Types _____ or _____. Which is less common but far more serious? Type ___. Management should involve *(repeated exposure to latex for desensitization? avoidance of latex?)*.

C. TRANSPLANTATION IMMUNOPATHOLOGY (pages 372–373)

C1. Phoebe, age 20, has received a kidney transplant. See question A3(e). Answer these questions related to Phoebe.

  (a) Phoebe's new kidney came from a female accident victim, age 38, who was unrelated to Phoebe. This is an example of a(n) ___ cadaver graft. Fill in the blank from the following list.
  (1) Allogeneic
  (2) Autologous
  (3) Syngeneic

  (b) Over the past decade, the 1-year survival rate for kidney transplants has reached about *(15%? 45%? 70%? 95%?)*. The survival rate is highest when donor-host HLA antigens *(match closely? are unmatched?)*.

  (c) Within 36 hours of the transplant surgery, Phoebe's immune system began to mount a response against the donor kidney tissues. This is known as ___ disease. Fill in the blank from the following two choices.
  (1) Graft-versus-host-disease (GVHD)
  (2) Host-versus-graft-disease (HVGD)

  (d) HVGD required activation of Phoebe's *(B? T?)* lymphocytes which then activated her ___ lymphocytes. As a result, Phoebe's antibodies initially attacked graft *(B or T cells? kidney tubule cells? blood vessels?)*, diminishing blood flow to the transplanted organ. This is known as an _____-type reaction, and it is classified as a *(cellular? humoral?)* rejection because Phoebe's antibodies destroyed donor kidney tissue. See question B2(d).

  (e) Eventually the transplanted kidney fails, as indicated by a(n) *(increase? decrease?)* in creatinine levels in Phoebe's blood.

C2. Arrange types of transplant rejections in correct sequence from first to last.

Acute   Chronic   Hyperacute
_____ → _____ → _____

Phoebe's transplant rejection (in C1) is classified as _____.

C3. Circle the two true statements about graft-versus-host-disease (GVHD).

  (a) Immunosuppressed graft recipients are **more** likely to mount a GVHD than persons with normal immunity.

(b) The risk of GVHD is greater if donor and host have very **different** HLA antigens.

(c) In GVHD, T cells within the donated tissue attack **recipient** (host) cells.

(d) The recipient's skin is **rarely** a target of GVHD.

C4. List typical signs and symptoms of GVHD as it affects these organs.

(a) Intestine

_____

_____

(b) Liver

_____

_____

(c) Skin

_____

_____

_____

C5. Identify treatments that are designed to prevent GVHD.

_____

_____

_____

D. AUTOIMMUNE DISEASE (pages 373–377)

D1. Explain self-tolerance in this exercise.

(a) Write a brief definition of *self-tolerance*.

_____

_____

_____

(b) Describe the key to developing self-tolerance.

_____

_____

_____

(c) Explain how self-reactive (or autoreactive) lymphocytes are normally eliminated.

_____

_____

_____

D2. List several examples of autoimmune diseases.

_____

_____

_____

D3. Now write rationales for roles of the following in development of autoimmune disease.

(a) Heredity

_____

_____

_____

(b) Trigger factors such as a chemical substance or virus

_____

_____

_____

(c) Gender

_____

_____

(d) Decreased level of suppressor T cells

_____

_____

_____

(e) Superantigens such as *Staphylococcus* in toxic shock syndrome

_____

_____

_____

D4. Wolfgang Amadeus Mozart may have died from heart failure associated with rheumatic fever. Fill in blanks to explain how this may have occurred.

(a) Mozart may have suffered a _____coccal infection. A protein in the cell wall of these bacteria is very similar to the role of antigens in the endocardial lining of the _____, which forms heart valves.

(b) The streptococcal infection caused production of antibodies that should have been directed to _____ bacteria, but in a case of "mistaken identity" or molecular _____, were instead directed to the antigens in Mozart's heart valves in association with his own specific _____. With failure of valves to direct blood properly, heart workload (*increased? decreased?*) leading to heart _____. (See more in Chapter 26.)

D5. Blood (or serum) testing for diagnosis of an autoimmune disease involves identification of auto-_____ against tissues or cells. One example of such a test is the ELISA test, which refers to: _____-_____ _____ assay.

CHAPTER 20

Acquired Immunodeficiency Syndrome

■ Review Questions

A. THE AIDS EPIDEMIC AND TRANSMISSION OF HIV INFECTION (pages 379-382)

A1. Circle the two true statements about AIDS.

(a) About 70% of the world's HIV infections are in the United States.

(b) In the United States, blacks and Hispanics have a **lower** rate of HIV infection than whites.

(c) The first cases of what we now term **AIDS** were first reported in the United States in 1971.

(d) Most HIV infection worldwide is caused by the HIV-1 **virus.**

(e) Worldwide, most HIV infections are transmitted through **unprotected heterosexual sex.**

A2. Circle the three main fluids that serve as "vectors" for almost all HIV transmission. Then underline the one other fluid that has been documented as a vector for HIV transmission.

Blood	Breast milk
Feces	Mosquito venom
Nasal secretions	Saliva
Semen	Sweat
Tears	Urine
Vaginal fluids	Vomitus (emesis)

A3. Explain how alcohol and cocaine use are related to HIV transmission.

_____

_____

A4. Circle the two true statements about HIV/AIDS.

(a) The "A" in the acronym AIDS stands for **autoimmune.**

(b) Since 1985, blood donations **have** routinely been tested for HIV.

(c) Between 70% to 80% of patients with hemophilia who received blood factors before 1985 became infected with the HIV virus.

(d) About 90% of pregnant women who have the HIV virus give birth to infected babies.

A5. Circle one of the following phrases to show what "seroconversion" means.

(a) Having a virus (or other antigen) in the bloodstream

(b) Having antibodies (developed against this antigen) in the bloodstream

A6. Samantha is an HIV-negative nurse who accidentally sticks herself with a needle contaminated with HIV-positive blood. The chances are about ___ that Samantha will seroconvert (become HIV-positive) from this single occurrence. *Insert the correct answer from the following list.*

1 in 3	1 in 33
1 in 66	1 in 136
1 in 333	1 in 1 million

A7. Circle the three true statements about HIV/AIDS.

(a) That Jonathan has a history of two STDs (genital herpes and chlamydia) **increases** his risk for having HIV infection.

(b) Although Gary has been infected with HIV, because he has no signs or symptoms of HIV means that he **cannot** transmit the virus.

(c) On 1/1/02, Patrick had unprotected sex during which he was infected with HIV. On 2/15/02, he was **likely** to be in the "window period" for HIV seroconversion.

(d) HIV transmission **can** occur by oral sex.

(e) It is **very likely** that a person infected with HIV virus in 1992 will still not test HIV-positive a decade later.

B. PATHOPHYSIOLOGY OF AIDS (pages 382–392)

B1. Circle the correct answer. How does AIDS kill? Primarily by destruction of:

(a) Many types of body cells, as in liver, kidneys, and lungs

(b) Immune cells so that the body succumbs to infections and/or cancer

B2. Circle the two types of cells that are most commonly infected by the HIV virus.

B lymphocytes   CD4$^+$ T lymphocytes
CD8$^+$ T lymphocytes   Macrophages
Neutrophils

B3. Choose the three true statements.

(a) CD4$^+$ T cells are also known as **T-helper** cells.

(b) A retrovirus is one that carries its nucleic acid as DNA.

(c) The HIV virus carries its nucleic acid in the form of DNA.

(d) One normal function of CD4$^+$ T cells is to **activate B-lymphocytes** so that antibody production will occur.

(e) CD4$^+$ cells **are** involved in regulating cytotoxic CD8$^+$ T cells and NK cells.

B4. Arrange in correct sequence (from first to last) the steps in replication of HIV within human CD4$^+$ T cells.

(a) Assembly of protein-coated RNA leads to release of new HIV viruses

(b) Attachment of HIV to a receptor on a CD4$^+$ T cell occurs.

(c) Cleavage (with help of a protease) of the polyprotein into smaller viral proteins occurs.

(d) With the help of the enzyme integrase, viral-like DNA is integrated into the original DNA of the CD4$^+$ cell.

(e) Reverse transcription occurs as viral RNA is copied to form viral-like DNA.

(f) Translation of viral-like mRNA forms a polyprotein.

(g) Transcription of the viral-like DNA results in formation of viral-like mRNA.

(h) Uncoating takes place as the protein coat is removed from the HIV virus.

__ → __ → __ → __ → __ → __ → __ → __

B5. Contrast infected CD4$^+$ T cells that remain *latent* with those that release *virions*.

_____

_____

B6. Circle the correct answer(s). HIV-infected persons typically begin to show symptoms of HIV:

(a) As soon as the CD4$^+$ T cell level drops slightly

(b) Only when the CD4$^+$ T-cell level drops dramatically

B7. Choose the two true statements about HIV diagnosis.

(a) The Western blot test is the **first** test normally performed to detect HIV status.

(b) Both **ELISA** and Western blot test for HIV antibodies (not HIV antigens).

(c) PCR tests identify the presence of the HIV **virus** rather than the **antibody** to HIV.

(d) Newborns whose mothers have HIV infections can be better diagnosed for HIV infection by the **ELISA** and **Western blot tests** than by PCR.

B8. Home testing for HIV identifies the *(HIV virus? antibody against HIV?)*. Circle the correct answer then briefly describe these tests.

_____

_____

_____

B9. Identify the CD4$^+$ T-cell category (1 to 3) and the clinical category (A to C) of each client listed in the table below. All three clients have experienced persistent swollen lymph nodes in neck or axillae, sore throat, and night sweats. Their CD4$^+$ counts listed are values as they were before treatment. (*Hint*: Refer to textbook Chart 20-2.)

Client	CD4$^+$ Count	CD4$^+$ Category	Signs or Symptoms	Clinical Category
Carl	202 cells	____	Has had one AIDS-defining illness (PCP), shingles, and foot infections	____
Terry	512 cells	____	Headaches, malaise, athlete's foot	____
Kelsey	32 cells	____	Has had many AIDS-defining illnesses (esophageal candidiasis; recurrent pneumonia, including PCP and TB; CMV; invasive cervical cancer; HIV-wasting syndrome), and peripheral neuropathy	____

(a) Determine which client(s) has/have AIDS according to the CDC definition:

_____

_____

(b) Which three illnesses listed in the table tend to occur more often in women and were included in the 1993 expanded CDC definition of AIDS-defining illnesses?

_____

_____

_____

B10. Identify typical phases of HIV infection and fill in the blanks below.

Acute   Latent
Overt AIDS (or symptomatic)

(a) Phase in which viral load is high, approximately 2 to 4 weeks after infection:

_____

(b) Symptoms may mimic those of a flu: fatigue, fever, night sweats, lymphadenopathy, pharyngitis, GI problems, muscle and joint pain:

_____

(c) Viral load is down, CD4$^+$ T-cell count is dropping, and the person has either no symptoms or only mild ones:

_____

(d) The CD4$^+$ T cell count may approach zero; signs and symptoms include opportunistic infections, cancers, AIDS dementia, CMV blindness, and wasting syndrome: _____

B11. Complete the table describing opportunistic infections (OIs) that are more likely to occur in AIDS clients than in persons with normal immune function. Use the bold symbols for systems:

D-E. Digestive (esophageal)
D-I. Digestive (intestinal)
N-S. Nervous/Sensory
R. Respiratory

Name of Microbe	Class of Microbe	System(s) Commonly Infected
Candida albicans	Fungus	D-E, NS
Cryptosporidium		
Cytomegalovirus (CMV)		
Herpes simplex (HSV)	Virus	
Mycobacterium avian complex (MAC)		
Mycobacterium tuberculosis	Bacterium	R
Pneumocystis carinii (PCP)		
Toxoplasma gondii		

B12. Now identify the opportunistic infection from the table that matches each description.

(a) Common cause of diarrhea that may lead to serious dehydration and electrolyte imbalances: _____

(b) Cause of the yeast infection "thrush" of the esophagus (also of mouth, vagina):

_____

(c) The most common presenting sign of AIDS during the 1980s; common once CD4$^+$ T-cell levels drop below 200 cells/μL and rare in persons with normal immunity; diagnosis includes identification of the microbe in sputum or lavage specimens:

_____

(d) Leading cause of death from HIV globally; multidrug-resistant (MDR) forms pose special threats to persons with HIV; may also cause meningitis: _____

(e) Symptoms include painful swallowing:

_____

(f) OI of the brain involving headaches, lethargy, confusion, and seizures:

_____

B13. List three types of neurologic disorders for which persons with AIDS are at greater risk.

_____

_____

_____

B14. Name one type of opportunistic cancer that affects small blood vessels in mouth, GI tract, lungs, and leads to violet lesions on skin; linked to a herpesvirus: _____

List two other types of cancers for which persons with AIDS are at increased risk:

_____, _____

B15. Bill has had AIDS-defining illnesses over the course of 7 years. His HAART regimen includes two reverse-transcriptase inhibitors, a protease inhibitor, and several prophylactic medications. Identify Bill's HIV-related disorders.

(a) Bill is 6'1" tall. His weight has dropped from 182 lbs before HIV was diagnosed to his current weight of 142: _____

(b) Although his weight is down, and his face and extremities appear lean, Bill has a noticeable "belly." His cholesterol and triglyceride levels are elevated:

_____

(c) Bill's chart includes the following notations: "N/V, abd pain, palpable liver" and his blood work lists "elevated lactate" levels: _____

B16. Refer to Question B4. Identify which of the eight phases of HIV replication is interrupted by the following anti-HIV drugs.

(a) Protease inhibitors (PIs) such as indinavir (IDV) or saquinavir (SAQ): ___

(b) NRTIs such as AZT, ddI, or ddC: ___

B17. Explain why vaccines and prophylactic medications are also taken by many AIDS clients. _____

_____

Live-virus vaccines *(should? should not?)* be given to persons with HIV/AIDS. Circle the correct answer and then list several types of vaccines that should be taken by HIV-infected persons.

_____

_____

_____

B18. Robert has just tested positive for HIV. He identifies himself as gay but has not come out to any of his family members.

(a) List some of the feelings that he is likely to be experiencing.

_____

_____

_____

(b) List several psychosocial resources that may offer support to Robert.

_____

_____

_____

(c) Describe your own feelings about working with an HIV-infected client.

_____

_____

_____

C. PREVENTION OF HIV INFECTION (page 392)

C1. Choose the two true statements.

(a) "Natural" or "lambskin" condoms are **more** effective than latex condoms against HIV transmission.

(b) It **is** advisable that petroleum-based lubricants be used with latex condoms.

(c) Full-strength household bleach **is** effective in killing the HIV virus.

(d) Use of crack cocaine **is** likely to increase risk of HIV infection.

C2. Brian is 14 years old and has asked for information on HIV prevention. Write a paragraph describing your response to Brian.

_____

_____

_____

D. HIV INFECTION IN PREGNANCY AND HIV IN INFANTS AND CHILDREN (pages 392–395)

D1. Choose the two true statements.

(a) Most infants who have the HIV virus have received it through **blood transfusions.**

(b) If a newborn's mother is HIV-positive, the newborn **will also** test positive for the HIV antibody.

(c) Administration of the RTI zidovudine (sometimes abbreviated AZT) **does** decrease risk of HIV transmission during pregnancy, labor, or delivery.

(d) The U.S. Public Health Department recommends HIV counseling and testing **only** if a pregnant woman is considered at "high risk" for HIV infection.

D2. Circle the factors that increase risk of perinatal transmission from an HIV-positive mother to her baby:

(a) A high maternal HIV viral load

(b) High maternal CD4+ count

(c) Exposure of the fetus to a large amount of maternal blood during the birth process

(d) Short time from rupture of the amnion to delivery of the baby

D3. Newborns infected with HIV are likely to demonstrate a pathogenesis that is *(similar to? different from?)* that of adults with HIV. For example, PCP is likely to occur relatively *(early? late?)* in the course of the child's condition. HIV-infected babies typically weigh *(more? less?)* than their non-HIV counterparts, and *(do? do not?)* experience failure to thrive (FTT) and developmental delays.

CHAPTER 21

Control of the Circulation

■ Review Questions

A. ORGANIZATION OF THE CIRCULATORY SYSTEM (pages 399–402)

A1. List the components of the circulatory system.

_____

_____

_____

A2. Choose the two true statements.

(a) The aorta is a **systemic** artery.

(b) Blood moves **faster** and under **greater pressure** through the aorta than through the pulmonary artery.

(c) The main function of valves of the heart is to **pump blood.**

(d) The right ventricle pumps blood into the **aorta.**

(e) The average (mean) arterial blood pressure (BP) is **greater** in pulmonary vessels than in systemic blood vessels.

A3. Arrange answers in correct sequence.

(a) Amount of blood (from greatest to least) at any given time.

Arteries and arterioles   Venules and veins
Heart

_____ → _____ →

_____

(b) Blood pressure (from greatest to least):

Arteries   Veins   Capillaries

_____ → _____ →

_____

(c) Pathway of blood (from first to last):

Pulmonary artery   Superior vena cava
Right side of the heart

_____ → _____ →

_____

A4. Compared with the right side of the heart, the left side normally pumps (*more? less? the same amount of?*) blood with each contraction.

B. THE HEART AS A PUMP (pages 402–410)

B1. Circle correct answers about the heart.

(a) The (*left? right?*) side of the heart is more anterior in location.

(b) (*Atria? Ventricles?*) have thicker walls, which is consistent with their functions as (*pumps? reservoirs?*). Atria serve primarily as (*pumps? reservoirs?*).

(c) Most of the heart wall is formed of (*endo? myo? peri?*)cardium.

B2. Arrange in correct sequence from outermost to innermost.

Endocardium   Fibrous pericardium
Myocardium   Pericardial cavity
Parietal pericardium   Visceral pericardium

_____ → _____ →

_____ → _____ →

_____ → _____

B3. Write "C" for cardiac muscle and "S" for skeletal muscle next to descriptions of each type of muscle.

(a) Contractions are voluntary: ___

(b) Contractions are of longer duration: ___

(c) Muscle cells are separated from each other by intercalated disks that permit muscle cells to contract as a unit (or syncytium): ___

(d) Calcium channel blockers particularly inhibit this type of muscle, which stores less calcium in its cells: ___

B4. Describe the "fibrous skeleton" of the heart and state its importance.

_____

_____

_____

B5. Select descriptions that fit each valve. Use the following answers:

Aortic   Bicuspid   Pulmonary
Tricuspid

(a) Located immediately inferior to the openings into the coronary arteries: _____

(b) Also known as the mitral valve: _____

(c) Prevent retrograde blood flow from the ventricles into the atria: _____and _____

(d) Also known as semilunar valves: _____and _____

(e) Anchored by chordae tendineae and papillary muscles that prevent these valves from everting: _____and _____

B6. Refer to textbook Figure 21-10, and answer these questions about the cardiac cycle.

(a) The ECG is a recording of *(electrical? contractile?)* activity of the heart. The P wave is associated with impulses that lead to contraction of the *(atria? ventricles?)*, whereas the *(QRS complex? T wave?)* heralds ventricular contraction.

(b) Arrange the following events in the cardiac cycle in correct sequence from first to last, beginning with the QRS complex:

(A) AV valve closure as ventricular pressure surpasses atrial pressure

(B) Opening of semilunar valves as ventricular pressure surpasses pressure in the great arteries (pulmonary artery and aorta)

(C) Start of ventricular contraction

(D) Dramatic drop in ventricular pressure to less than atrial pressure causing AV valves to open; rapid ventricular filling follows

(E) Ejection period

(F) Semilunar valve closure as ventricular pressure drops below that in the great arteries

(G) T wave signaling the start of ventricular relaxation

(H) P wave signaling atria to give blood an "extra push" into ventricles

___ → ___ → ___ → ___ → ___ → ___ → ___ → ___

(c) Identify events listed in Question B6(b) that are most closely associated with heart sounds:

(1) First heart sound ("lubb"): ___

(2) Second heart sound ("dup"): ___

(3) Third heart sound (if present): ___

(4) Fourth heart sound (if present): ___

(d) Which valves remain open all during ventricular diastole (so ventricles can fill during this time)? *(AV? Semilunar?)* Which valves are open only during ventricular systole? *(AV? Semilunar?)*

(e) Ventricles pump out most of their blood volume *(early? late?)* in ventricular systole. The total volume of blood pumped out with each ventricular contraction is known as _____ volume (SV).

(f) At its highest level, ventricular pressure reaches the same level as pressure within the *(atria? great arteries?)*. In Figure 21-10, that value is ____ mm Hg.

(g) What factor determines pressure in the aorta during ventricular diastole? _____ Figure 21-10 indicates that diastolic BP in the aorta is ___ mm Hg.

(h) Circle the correct answers. Write in normal values to validate your answers.

(1) Stroke volume is calculated as:
   A. SV = ESV − EDV
   B. SV = EDV − ESV
   SV = _____ mL − _____ mL = _____ mL/beat

(2) Ejection fraction is calculated as:
   A. SV/EDV   B. SV/ESV
   C. ESV/EDV
   EF = _____ mL/ _____ mL = _____ %

(i) Because Mrs. Lewis has a diagnosis of congestive heart failure, she is likely to have a(n) *(increase? decrease?)* in both stroke volume and ejection fraction, leading to a(n) *(increase? decrease?)* in EDV.

B7. Answer these questions about right atrial pressure (RAP).

(a) Suzanna's RAP is 0 mm Hg. This value is *(high? normal? low?)*.

(b) Mrs. Pope's RAP is 9 mm Hg, suggesting *(strong? weak?)* pumping of the right side of the heart. A sign of this RAP is likely to be *(bulging? sunken?)* veins in the neck.

B8. Answer these questions about heart function. Refer to the left side of Study Guide Figure 21-1, page 94.

(a) Determine the average cardiac output (CO) of a resting adult:
Cardiac output (CO) = stroke volume × heart rate
= _____ mL × _____ beats/min
= _____ mL/min = ____ L/min

(b) At rest, Tony has a cardiac output of 6 L/minute. During a strenuous cross-country run, his maximal cardiac output is 18 L/minute. Tony's cardiac reserve is _____.

(c) As he runs, Tony's muscles surrounding his leg veins squeeze *(more? less?)* blood back to his heart, therefore *(increasing? decreasing?)* his venous return and his end-diastolic volume (EDV) or preload. As a result, his myocardial fibers have stretched *(more? less?)*.

(d) Within limits, a stretched muscle (much like a stretched rubber band or balloon) contracts with *(greater? less?)* force as stretching causes maximal overlap of _____ and _____ filaments in muscles. This is a statement of the _____-Starling mechanism.

(e) List several reasons why venous return might be reduced, leading to decreased stretching of the heart, RAP, preload, stroke volume, and cardiac output._____
_____
_____

(f) Mr. Stinson has hypertension and aortic valve stenosis; both of these factors tend to *(increase? decrease?)* afterload and *(increase? decrease?)* stroke volume. Stroke volume is *(directly? inversely?)* related to afterload.

B9. Answer these questions about Mrs. Rosenthal, age 76.

(a) Mrs. Rosenthal's resting cardiac output is 1.2 L/minute, and her heart is "enlarged." Explain the connection. _____

(b) She is taking digoxin, a drug with positive inotropic effects. Such a drug is designed to increase the heart's *(contractility? rate?)*.

(c) Mrs. Rosenthal's resting heart rate is 120 beats/minute. At this rate, the length of one cardiac cycle is ____ second(s). When Mrs. Rosenthal becomes anxious, her heart rate

increases to 180 beats/minute, allowing only ____ second(s) for each cardiac cycle. Such rapid heart rates especially shorten the time allotted for ventricular *(systole? diastole?)* which is the period when ventricles *(eject? fill?)*. This factor contributes to her *(high? low?)* cardiac output.

C. BLOOD VESSELS AND THE SYSTEMIC CIRCULATION (pages 410-420)

C1. Arrange layers of the wall of an artery or vein in correct sequence from outermost to innermost.

Externa   Intima   Media
Tunica: _____ → _____ → _____

Which layer contains smooth muscle that permits constriction of the vessel? Tunica _____

C2. Match types of blood vessels to descriptions below. Use these answers.

Arterioles   Arteries   Capillaries
Veins   Venules

(a) Site of gas, nutrient, and waste exchange: _____

(b) Act as site of greatest resistance (and drop in blood pressure): _____

(c) Have thick, muscular walls that can withstand a high level of blood pressure: _____

(d) Connect capillaries with veins: _____

(e) Thin-walled, distensible vessels; most have valves to prevent backflow: _____

C3. Describe the characteristics of smooth muscle that permit blood vessels to maintain a constant state of muscle tone (see page 411) and also contract to return blood to the heart.
_____
_____
_____

State the function of calmodulin in smooth muscle.
_____
_____
_____

C4. Describe factors that determine blood flow through body tissues and maintain blood pressure (BP).

(a) According to Poiseuille's law, when a blood vessel is narrowed to half of its original diameter, resistance to flow through that vessel increases *(2? 4? 8? 16? 32?)* times. List three mechanisms by which blood vessels may become narrowed. _____

_____

(b) Blood flow through vessels is directly related to *(blood pressure? resistance?)* in those vessels, and inversely related to *(blood pressure? resistance?)* in those vessels. This can be expressed by the equation F = _____/_____.

(c) Dawn's hematocrit is 62, which is *(higher? lower?)* than normal. As a result, Dawn's blood has a *(high? normal? low?)* viscosity, which *(increases? decreases?)* resistance to flow.

(d) Blood flows most rapidly (i.e., with greatest velocity) through *(the aorta? capillaries? veins?)*, and it flows most slowly through _____. Explain how these differences in velocity are advantageous to your own body. _____

(e) Blood flow is most rapid *(within the center? against the wall?)* of a blood vessel. Smooth blood flow is known as *(laminar? turbulent?)* flow. Turbulent flow (which increases risk of clot formation) is more likely to occur *(in curving or branching? at straightaway?)* sections of blood vessels.

(f) An aneurysm is a section of a vessel that has "ballooned out." Such an area has *(more? less?)* wall tension than a vessel of normal diameter. This factor *(increases? decreases?)* risk of rupture. Relationships between vessel diameter (or radius) and wall tension are described by _____'s law.

(g) Which vessels have greatest distensibility and compliance, meaning that these vessels can hold large amounts of blood with only slight changes in pressure? *(Arteries? Capillaries? Veins?)*

C5. Refer to textbook Figure 21-2 and discuss blood pressure in different parts of the circulatory system by completing the following exercise.

(a) Systolic BP in the aorta and other arteries is about _____ mm Hg, whereas diastolic BP in these vessels is about _____ mm Hg. The difference between these two pressures is

known as _____ pressure, and is typically about _____ mm Hg.

(b) How is the concept of pulse pressure applied clinically? _____

_____

_____

(c) A normal value for pulse pressure in the left ventricle is: _____ mm Hg. Explain why this value is so high. _____

_____

_____

(d) Pulse pressure *(becomes greater? dissipates?)* as blood passes through arterioles, capillaries, venules, and veins. As a result, "a pulse" *(can? cannot?)* normally be palpated on these vessels.

C6. Which two factors determine arterial blood pressure? _____ and _____. List three or more factors that contribute to development of SVR (systemic vascular resistance)

_____

_____

_____

On Study Guide Figure 21-1, fill in blanks and complete arrows to show how nervous, hormonal, and other factors increase blood pressure.

C7. Classify the following factors as those involved in *L* (long-term) or *S* (short-term) regulation of BP and blood flow through tissues.

(a) Dr. Lang, age 83, has chronic hypertension. Her kidneys sense the high BP and attempt to lower it by eliminating more water (diuresis) and sodium (natriuresis) in urine: ___

(b) As Mrs. Lister stands up quickly, blood accumulates in her lower body. Baroceptors in her neck sense low BP there and signal the brain stem to raise her BP: ___

(c) Growth of collateral blood vessels in lower extremities as a response to Mr. Fulbright's atherosclerosis: ___

(d) Ms. Foster, age 68, has osteoporosis. A fall on her porch fractures a wrist, which leaves Ms. Foster shrieking in pain. Her blood pressure shoots up: ___

(e) Hyperemia in Juliet's legs during her 10-K run causes release of lactic acid and other products of muscle metabolism: ___

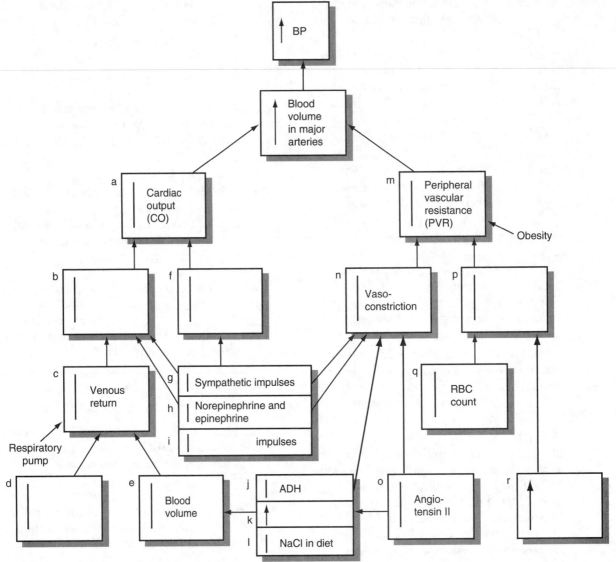

Figure 21-1.

(f) Release of aldosterone from Mr. Nunez's adrenal cortex causes his kidneys to retain sodium and water: ___

C8. The RAA (renin-angiotensin-aldosterone) mechanism (*increases? decreases?*) BP.

Fill in the blanks as you arrange RAA events in correct sequence from first to last:
_____ → _____ → _____ → _____

(a) The enzyme ACE made by lungs converts angiotensin I to angiotensin II.

(b) The enzyme renin converts the plasma protein angiotensinogen into angiotensin I.

(c) Angiotensin II exerts two effects that raise BP: stimulates aldosterone production, and increases systemic vascular resistance (SVR)

by vasoconstricting arterioles in skin, GI tract, and kidneys.

(d) Renin is released from JG cells in kidneys in response to low BP in renal vessels.

C9. Classify the following chemicals as constrictors or dilators that regulate blood flow.

(a) ADH (vasopressin) released from the posterior pituitary: _____

(b) Angiotensin II (part of the RAA):

_____

(c) Histamine, bradykinin, and prostaglandin E released during inflammation: _____

(d) Serotonin that is associated with migraine headaches: _____

(e) Epinephrine and norepinephrine:

_____

Functions of Autonomic Nervous System (ANS) Nerves

		Parasympathetic (P) (Vagus) Nerves	Sympathetic (S) Nerves
(a)	Heart rate (pulse)		IN
(b)	Heart contractility		
(c)	Vasoconstriction of arterioles in skin, GI tract, and kidneys (shunting blood to major arteries)		

(f) Nitric oxide (NO) derived from endothelial lining of blood vessels: _____

D. NEURAL CONTROL OF CIRCULATORY FUNCTION (pages 420-424)

D1. Compare and contrast *chemoreceptors* with *baroreceptors*.

_____

_____

_____

D2. Discuss the response of Mrs. Lister, mentioned in Question C7(b), to a sudden drop of BP caused by her standing up by completing the following exercise when you select the correct answer or fill in the blanks.

(a) If baroreceptors sense decreased BP, they send impulses to Mrs. Lister's *(cerebellum? cerebrum? medulla?),* where neurons in her *(vasomotor? cardioinhibitory?)* center will initiate *(sympathetic? parasympathetic?)* impulses. These will then will *(elevate? lower?)* her blood pressure by two mechanisms. Name them._____

_____

(b) If Mrs. Lister's BP-regulating reflexes do not respond quickly, she may become dizzy and fall as a result of _____ hypotension.

D3. Fill in the table above contrasting autonomic effects on factors that influence blood pressure (BP). Write "IN" for increase, "DE" for decrease, or "NA" (not applicable or no effect). One example has been done for you.

D4. Write "ACH" (acetylcholine) or "NE" (norepinephrine) next to related descriptions below.

(a) Also known as noradrenaline, this neurotransmitter is produced by most sympathetic nerves, which are therefore called "adrenergic nerves": ___

(b) Similar chemically to the hormone adrenalin made by the adrenal medulla: ___

(c) Classified chemically as a catecholamine: ___

(d) L-DOPA and dopamine are chemicals made during the series of reactions that lead to formation of this neurotransmitter: ___

(e) Once used, this neurotransmitter is either recycled into the neuron that produced it or destroyed by enzymes MAO or COMT: ___

(f) Drugs that block alpha- or beta-adrenergic receptors (such as "beta blockers") will inhibit action of this neurotransmitter: ___

(g) Produced by parasympathetic nerves such as the vagus—which are called "cholinergic nerves": ___

(h) Drugs that are classified as "anticholinergics" block action of this neurotransmitter: ___

D5. Identify the type of receptor which, when stimulated by norepinephrine (NE), will result in each effect listed below. Select from these answers:

Alpha-1 (α_1)   Alpha-2 (α_2)
Beta-1 (β_1)   Beta-2 (β_2)

(a) Bronchodilation (widening) of airways: ___

(b) Vasoconstriction: ___

(c) Increase heart rate and strength of contraction: ___

D6. Mr. Giattino arrives at the ER after a severe head injury. His blood pressure is 264/118 mm Hg. The emergency department staff suspect that Mr. Giattino is having a "CNS ischemic response" or a "Cushing reflex." Explain the mechanism.

_____

_____

_____

D7. The nurse is checking Mr. Baker's baroreceptor function and cardiovascular reflexes by means of the Valsalva maneuver. She asks Mr. Baker to "bear down" as if trying to push out a bowel movement. Select the sequence of responses that should occur after Mr. Baker initiates bearing down.

(a) Mr. Baker ceases bearing down.

(b) Increased pressure within his thorax leads to decreased venous return, stroke volume, and systolic BP; the nurse notes an increase in pulse (a compensatory mechanism).

(c) Venous return increases, causing stroke volume and blood pressure to rise.

(d) Reflex vagal impulses lead to a detectable decrease in heart rate.

_____ → _____ → _____ → _____

E. THE MICROCIRCULATION AND LYMPHATIC SYSTEM (pages 424-428)

E1. Select answers that fit the following descriptions. Choose from these answers.

Interstitium	Lymphatic vessels
Metarterioles	Nutrient flow
Nonnutrient flow	Precapillary sphincters

(a) Control blood flow into arterial ends of capillaries: _____

(b) Capillaries that do involve exchange of gases and nutrients between blood and tissues:

_____

(c) Fibers along with water and proteins that form a thin gel between cells; edema involves excessive amounts: _____

E2. Circle the correct answers in each statement.

(a) Plasma colloidal osmotic pressure (PCOP) is a *(pushing? pulling?)* force that tends to move fluid and particles from *(plasma into interstitium? interstitium into plasma?)*.

(b) Intracapillary fluid pressure is a *(pushing? pulling?)* force that is *(directly? inversely?)* related to arterial blood pressure. This force tends to move fluid and particles from *(plasma into interstitium? interstitium into plasma?)*.

(c) The combined pushing and pulling forces across capillary membranes tend to push substances out of blood at the *(arterial? venous?)* end of capillaries and to pull substances back into blood at the *(arterial? venous?)* end of capillaries. Fluid and proteins not returned to blood immediately are eventually "picked up" by _____ vessels and returned to plasma.

(d) Movements of substances from blood into interstitium is likely to *(increase? decrease?)* in the presence of hemorrhage because blood pressure is *(higher? lower?)* than normal.

(e) In a standing position, blood pressure in veins of the legs tends to *(increase? decrease?)* as a result of gravity.

E3. Mr. McGrath has cirrhosis of the liver. As a result, his production of plasma proteins is likely to be *(increased? decreased?)*, leading to *(edema? high blood pressure?)*. Which plasma protein is normally most abundant in plasma? *(albumin? fibrinogen? globulin?)*

E4. Six years ago, Mrs. Reese had a right mastectomy in which 10 axillary lymph nodes were removed. She has since experienced several infections related to *Staphylococcus aureus* that were serious enough to require hospitalization. Her right arm is constantly swollen to about three times the size of her left arm. Explain.

_____

_____

_____

E5. Identify the two locations on yourself where all lymph fluid flows into blood plasma.

_____

_____

E6. List four factors that can cause edema.

_____

_____

_____

_____

CHAPTER 22

Alterations in Blood Flow in the Systemic Circulation

■ Review Questions

A. DISORDERS OF THE ARTERIAL CIRCULATION (pages 429-445)

A1. Match each term with its correct definition.

Infarction	Ischemia
Patent	Perfusion

(a) Death of tissue or organ due to inadequate blood flow: _____

(b) Lack of adequate blood flow: _____

(c) Blood flow to a region: _____

(d) Open (normal), as in blood vessel or duct:

_____

A2. Describe the "good news" and "bad news" of fats in the body.

_____

_____

A3. Describe lipoproteins by completing the following exercise.

(a) Which type of lipoprotein is the main carrier of cholesterol that is released into the bloodstream and settles in blood vessels? *(HDL? LDL? VLDL?)* For this reason, these lipoproteins are called the *(good? bad?)* cholesterol. *(Low? High?)* blood levels are associated with atherosclerosis leading to heart disease. What does the abbreviation LDL stand for? _____

(b) Explain why persons with a genetic form of hypercholesterolemia (Type IIA) have high blood levels of LDLs. _____

_____

(c) Which type of lipoprotein consists of a relatively high percentage of protein? *(HDL? LDL? VLDL?)* These lipoproteins are called the *(good? bad?)* cholesterol because they transport cholesterol back to the liver for excretion. *(Low? High?)* blood levels tend help to prevent heart disease.

Smoking and diabetes both tend to *(increase? decrease?)* HDLs.

(d) Which lipoproteins transport most triglycerides that are made in the body? _____

(e) The proteins that make up part of lipoproteins are known as _____-proteins. (See textbook Figure 22-1.) Explain their importance. _____

A4. Choose the two true statements about high cholesterol.

(a) High blood cholesterol levels caused by complications of diabetes or obesity are examples of **primary** hypercholesterolemia.

(b) High-calorie diets, even if not high in fats, **do** increase LDL levels.

(c) Excessive dietary intake of triglycerides, cholesterol, and other saturated fats **depress** LDL receptor numbers or function.

(d) The Expert Panel on Detection and Treatment of High Blood Cholesterol in Adults targets **triglycerides** as the primary target for lowering cholesterol.

A5. Complete this exercise about Amy, age 33, whose mother (but not father) has familial hypercholesterolemia (type IIA).

(a) Because this is an autosomal *(dominant? recessive?)* genetic disorder and one of her parents has the defective gene, Amy *(can? cannot?)* inherit this disorder. In fact, she has a *(0? 25? 50? 100?)%* chance of having this disorder. The incidence of this disorder is about ___ persons per 1000.

(b) Amy's total cholesterol level is 298 mg/dL with an LDL of 170 ml/dL. These values are *(high? normal?)*. Her LDL level is related to the *(high? low?)* level of effective LDL receptors on her cells.

(c) Amy's physical examination by her cholesterol specialist includes palpation of

her Achilles tendons. Explain why._____
_____

(d) The nutritionist suggests that Amy's management of her cholesterol disorder should include:

(1) *(Increased? Decreased)?* exercise which is likely to *(increase? decrease?)* her HDLs above her current level of 45 mg/dL.

(2) Increased intake of foods such as _____.

(3) Decreased dietary intake of _____ and _____ especially *(saturated? unsaturated?)* fats. With a 2000-calorie-daily diet, this would mean ____ calories of saturated fat.

(4) Decrease in caloric intake to reduce Amy's current body mass index of 28 to less than ____.

A6. Match the type of cholesterol-lowering drug with the following descriptions.

Cholestyramine and colestipol
Clofibrate and gemfibrozil
Niacin
Statins (Lipitor, Zocor, Mevacor)

(a) Block hepatic synthesis of cholesterol by inhibiting an enzyme (HMG-CoA reductase) in the pathway: _____

(b) Prevent absorption of cholesterol from foods in the intestine: _____

(c) Block hepatic synthesis of VLDLs which therefore lowers LDL synthesis: _____ and _____

A7. Sean is a 21-year-old whose mother died of a heart attack at age 42. Sean smokes two packs of cigarettes a day; eats a cheeseburger, chips, and a shake for lunch and dinner almost daily; and has not exercised in a year. His cholesterol is 242 mg/dL and his blood pressure is 134/84 mm Hg.

(a) Identify Sean's risk factors for coronary heart disease that **are** modifiable.
_____
_____

(b) Identify those that are **not** modifiable.
_____
_____

(c) Explain how cigarette smoking may increase Sean's risk of coronary disease.
_____

(d) Is it likely that Sean's blood vessels would demonstrate any atherosclerotic changes at his current age?
_____
_____

A8. Answer these questions about additional risk factors for atherosclerosis.

(a) Homocysteine is associated with *(increased? decreased?)* risk of blood clots as well as damage to the lining of _____. This chemical is derived from *(meats? vegetables?)*. Plasma levels of homocysteine may be lowered by intake of _____.

(b) Lipoprotein(a) appears to mimic *(HDLs? LDLs?)* in *(increasing? decreasing?)* risk for coronary disease. CRP (or _____ _____ protein) is a sign of inflammation that may damage blood vessels.

(c) Name several microbes that may be associated with atherosclerosis _____
_____.

A9. Refer to Figure 22-6 in the textbook and circle all factors in the following list that appear to contribute to development of atherosclerosis.

(a) Damage to endothelium with recruitment of inflammatory cells

(b) Formation of foam cells as monocytes in blood vessel walls ingest lipids

(c) Smooth muscle proliferation in vessel walls under the influence of growth factors

(d) Development of yellow streaks in the intima

A10. Describe four possible effects of atherosclerosis by filling in each blank with one of the following terms:

Aneurysm   Emboli
Ischemia   Obstruction

(a) Hemorrhage or rupture of atherosclerotic plaque may lead to vessel _____.

(b) Narrowing of the lumen can reduce blood flow to tissues, a condition known as _____.

(c) Thrombi that catch on damaged endothelium may lead to formation of _____.

(d) Atherosclerosis can cause weakening of the vessel wall, leading to _____.

A11. Fill in the blank, then use the list to answer the questions below to identify the etiologic category of each example of vasculitis.

The term *vasculitides* is plural for blood vessel inflammation, or _____.

Direct injury   Infectious agent
Immune process   Physical agent
Secondary to other disease

(a) One manifestation of Genevieve's lupus (SLE) is skin sensitivity to sunlight; she has a characteristic "butterfly rash" on her face: _____

(b) Peter has hives (urticaria) which is a group II hypersensitivity vasculitis: _____

(c) Ms. Alvino developed frostbite on toes of both feet after she was stranded in a snow storm: _____

A12. Match the condition with the related description of clients seen by an emergency room nurse.

Acute arterial occlusion
Atherosclerotic occlusive disease
Giant cell temporal arteritis
Polyarteritis nodosa
Raynaud's phenomenon
Thromboangiitis obliterans

(a) Anna-Maria, age 30, came to the ER after a hand injury in a restaurant kitchen where she works. Anna-Maria states her concern about recent episodes in which fingers of both hands developed numbness and tingling. At first pale, they then turned deep red and began to throb. These attacks occurred especially when she was anxious and working in the "cold room" of the kitchen: _____

(b) Mr. Knight, age 60, presents with acute pain and paresthesia (numbness and tingling) in his left leg; the leg is pale and cool. He has a left femoral pulse, but left popliteal and dorsalis pedis pulses are absent. Mrs. Knight reports that her husband has a history of atrial fibrillation (with resulting stasis of blood in the left atrium that increases risk of embolus formation): _____

(c) Gilbert Scanlon, age 68, has a history of two strokes. Today, his BP is 180/106. His skin manifests a bluish mottling (livedo reticularis) and he reports numbness. Blood work reveals a serum creatinine level of 4.8 mg/dL, which indicates about 25%

of normal kidney function: _____

(d) Jack Whitehead, age 38, is a chain-smoker. Skin on his hands and feet appears thin and shiny with noticeable ulcer formation on his right foot. Capillary refill time on his toes is 5 to 6 seconds. (*Hint*: his condition is also known as Buerger's disease.): _____

(e) Mrs. Sonneborn, age 70, presents with severe pain and tenderness on the right side of her head, blurred vision, and an elevated "sed rate." Blood work reveals an elevated ESR: _____

(f) Mr. Vonnahme, age 74, was diagnosed with type 2 diabetes mellitus 10 years earlier. All pulses in his lower extremities are diminished and bruits are noted over his femoral arteries. He reports calf pain "whenever I walk even out the driveway to the mailbox." With his feet on the floor, his legs appear red (dependent rubor); when his legs are raised above heart level they develop pallor. (*Hint*: this condition is also called arteriosclerosis obliterans.): _____

A13. Fill in the blanks to indicate which four conditions listed in question A12 are called peripheral vascular diseases because they primarily affect circulation in the extremities.

_____, _____, _____, and _____

A14. Which client in question A12 has signs of intermittent claudication? _____

A15. Explain why cigarette smoking is contraindicated for clients with arterial disease.

_____

_____

_____

A16. Choose the three true statements about aneurysms.

(a) Aneurysms involve abnormal **narrowing** of blood vessels.

(b) The **aorta** is the most common site of aneurysms.

(c) Berry aneurysms most commonly occur in arteries that supply the **legs**.

(d) **Atherosclerosis** is a common cause of aneurysms.

(e) Clot formation is **more** likely to occur in aneurysms than in vessels with normal diameter.

(f) Dissecting aneurysms most commonly affect **cerebral** arteries.

A17. Mr. Fey experiences an intense, ripping pain, "like a sword slashed down my back." Within a few moments, he faints (syncope), has pallor and poor capillary refill, and within 4 hours, he dies. Mr. Fey had a history of hypertension. What type of aneurysm did Mr. Fey most likely experience? _____

On autopsy, the site of the primary tear of Mr. Fey's aneurysm was located in the ascending aorta; the tear extended to 8 cm below the point where the aorta pierces the diaphragm. His aneurysm is more likely to be classified as a Stanford Type *(A? B?)*.

A18. State the greatest risk involved with aneurysms that can lead to fatality.

_____

_____

What treatment can prevent such an outcome?

_____

_____

B. DISORDERS OF THE VENOUS CIRCULATION (pages 445-450)

B1. List three factors that normally assist veins with the job of returning blood from lower extremities to the heart.

_____

_____

B2. Describe the three types of veins in lower extremities by completing the following exercise.

(a) List the three types of veins from most superficial to deepest. _____

_____

(b) Explain how blood in deep veins is normally prevented from moving to superficial ones when calf muscles contract. _____

_____

(c) Over 80% of blood normally flows through _____ veins. When deep veins are blocked, blood is forced out into superficial veins, leading to *(primary? secondary?)* varicose veins. The most

common cause of this type of varicose veins is DVT (d_____ v_____ t_____).

B3. Circle all factors that are likely to increase risk of varicose veins.

Male gender   Pregnancy
Obesity   Age over 50 years
A family history of varicose veins
Working in a job that involves long-term standing

B4. Varicose veins are more likely to affect *(deep? superficial?)*. Circle the answer and then explain why:

_____

_____

_____ .

B5. List several healthy behaviors that can help prevent harmful effects of varicose veins.

_____

_____

_____ .

B6. Circle the correct answer in each statement.

(a) The saphenous vein is a *(deep? superficial?)* vein in the *(upper? lower?)* extremity.

(b) Edema is a major sign of chronic *(arterial? venous?)* insufficiency, whereas ischemia is a major sign of chronic *(arterial? venous?)* insufficiency.

(c) A thrombus that is in the posterior tibial vein is more likely to pass directly to the *(liver? lung?)*.

B7. Match the vascular condition with the most likely signs and symptoms:

Chronic venous insufficiency
Deep venous thrombosis
Peripheral arterial disease
Varicose veins

(a) Unsightly appearance, aching, and possibly edema that subsides when legs are elevated: _____

(b) Ischemia: _____ _____

(c) Often asymptomatic, but may manifest pain, swelling, and other signs of inflammation, such as fever, malaise, and high white blood cell count; may lead to pulmonary embolism: _____

(d) Stasis dermatitis, edema, necrosis of subcutaneous tissue, skin atrophy, and possibly ulcers of tissues covering the inner ankle: _____

B8. The three major factors that lead to venous thromboses are listed here. Identify which factor is involved in each of the following cases of thromboses.

Hypercoagulability   Vessel injury
Venous stasis

(a) Congestive heart failure or heart attack:

_____

(b) Pregnancy: _____

(c) Hip surgery: _____

(d) Indwelling venous catheter: _____

(e) A smoker taking oral contraceptives:

_____

(f) Sitting on a plane ride from Boston to Los Angeles and drinking only one glass of water: _____

B9. The most serious potential outcome of DVT is a _____ .

B10. List several effective treatments for DVT.

_____
_____
_____

C. DISORDERS OF BLOOD FLOW DUE TO EXTRAVASCULAR FORCES (pages 451–457)

C1. The term "compartment" in the condition named "compartment syndrome" refers to:

(a) The abdomen

(b) The thorax

(c) The cranial cavity

(d) Muscle regions of arms or legs

(e) The vertebral canal

C2. Potential causes of compartment syndrome are listed below. Refer to textbook Figure 22-13 and visualize more causes in each category; write several here.

(a) Decreased compartment size: circumferential eschar in burns area; casts;

_____

(b) Increased compartment volume: bleeding; swelling after thrombosis or burns;

_____

C3. Circle the three true statements about compartment syndrome.

(a) Compartment syndrome is likely to cause changes in sensation **before** muscle dysfunctions such as contractures occur.

(b) Pain **is not** typically a symptom of this syndrome.

(c) Capillary refill time and peripheral pulses are often **normal** with this syndrome.

(d) Elevation of the extremity **is** part of the typical treatment plan for compartment syndrome.

(e) Skin changes **do** commonly accompany this syndrome.

C4. Complete this exercise about pressure ulcers.

(a) Pressure ulcers are also known as _____ . Describe the basic problem. _____
_____
_____

(b) Identify the locations on yourself where this skin condition would be most likely to occur._____
_____
_____

(c) List several factors that increase risk for decubiti. _____
_____
_____

(d) Define "shearing forces" that can lead to decubiti. _____
_____
_____

C5. Write specific interventions that nurses can take in efforts to prevent decubiti in each of these clients.

(a) Mrs. Albertson, age 88, has Alzheimer's disease and is in bed; she is dehydrated, anemic, and incontinent of bowel and bladder. _____
_____
_____

(b) Mr. Little, age 34, suffered a brain injury 5 years ago. He is in a wheelchair and requires assistance with all activities of daily living (ADL). _____
_____
_____

C6. Identify the stage of decubitus indicated in each case below.

Stage I   Stage II
Stage III   Stage IV

(a) Depth of necrosis extends into subcutaneous tissue; ulcer is a deep crater: _____

_____

(b) Black skin appears bluish-purple; no blistering or ulceration visible:

_____

CHAPTER 23

Alterations in Blood Pressure: Hypertension and Orthostatic Hypotension

■ Review Questions

A. ARTERIAL BLOOD PRESSURE (pages 459–463)

A1. Choose the two true statements.

(a) High blood pressure **rarely** contributes to death and disability.

(b) The term "patent blood vessels" refers to **occluded** vessels.

(c) Systolic pressure occurs when the heart is **contracting**.

(d) About 70% of the total stroke volume leaves the heart during the **first third of systole**.

(e) The dicrotic notch in a blood pressure tracing occurs just **before** the peak of systolic pressure.

A2. Complete this exercise about blood pressure (BP). (Refer to Figure 21-1, page 94 of the Study Guide.)

(a) Circle the factors that are likely to increase systolic blood pressure.

   (1) Aorta with highly elastic walls

   (2) Large stroke volume

   (3) High velocity of ejection of stroke volume

(b) Most of the peripheral vascular resistance (PVR) that controls BP is built up in:

   (1) Arterioles and small arteries

   (2) Venules

   (3) Capillaries

(c) Circle the factors that are likely to increase diastolic BP.

   (1) Arteriosclerosis of small arteries

   (2) Sympathetic nerve impulses

   (3) Aortic valve regurgitation

(d) Pulse pressure is likely to increase with:

   (1) A rise in systolic BP

   (2) Decreased diastolic BP

   (3) Aortic valve regurgitation

(e) Mean arterial BP (MABP) is equal to diastolic BP plus ⅓ of:

   (1) Systolic BP

   (2) Diastolic BP

   (3) Pulse pressure

(f) The MABP for a blood pressure of 160/100 mm Hg is:

   (1) 120

   (2) 130

   (3) 140

   (4) 153

A3. Mrs. Shaw, age 58, weighs 240 pounds. Answer the following questions about her BP measurement at the clinic.

(a) The circumference of Mrs. Shaw's arm is 12″. The width of the BP cuff should be at least:

   (1) 3″

   (2) 4.8″

   (3) 7.2″

   (4) 9.6″

If the cuff is too small for her arm, BP is likely to be *(over? under?)*estimated.

(b) Mrs. Shaw tells the clinic nurse that her BP "usually runs about 140 over 90." The nurse should inflate the cuff to about _____ mm Hg, and then deflate the cuff at about ___ mm every 5 seconds.

(c) The nurse begins to hear sounds at 162 mm Hg, which is Mrs. Shaw's *(systolic? diastolic?)* BP. The nurse hears the last sound at 92 mm Hg, which is Mrs. Shaw's *(systolic? diastolic?)* BP, or *(K1? K4? K5?)* sound. The "K" stands for _____ sound.

(d) Mrs. Shaw's BP is categorized as:

(1) High-normal

(2) Hypertension (stage 1)

(3) Hypertension (stage 2)

(4) Hypertension (stage 3)

(e) Mrs. Shaw states that her BP is "never this high when I take it at home." Comment.

_____

_____

_____

(f) When a repeated BP results in similar values, the nurse should recommend that Mrs. Shaw have her BP checked again on another occasion within:

(1) 2 years

(2) 1 year

(3) 2 months

(4) 1 week

A4. Mr. Murray is in the recovery room after same-day surgery. His BP cuff is set to inflate automatically every 10 minutes. Such equipment is likely to be somewhat *(more? less?)* accurate than manual BP measurements.

B. ESSENTIAL HYPERTENSION (pages 463–473)

B1. Circle the factor that carries a higher risk for hypertension.

(a) 25-year old *(woman? man?)*

(b) *(Higher? Lower?)* socioeconomic group

(c) *(African? European?)* American ancestry

B2. Circle the two true statements.

(a) Between 1980 and 1990, mortality rate from heart disease and stroke **decreased**.

(b) Hypertension **is** a significant risk factor for heart disease, renal failure, and stroke.

(c) An early sign of essential hypertension is **decreased** urinary output.

(d) A recent report from the National Institutes of Health recommends that adult

BP optimally should be less than 140/90 mm Hg.

B3. To obtain accurate BP readings, it is recommended that the patient have rested for at least 5 minutes at the BP site. List several other recommendations to ensure accuracy.

_____

_____

_____

B4. Essential hypertension is chronic high blood pressure with *(a? no?)* known cause. One factor likely to be involved is pressure natriuresis, which may contribute to increased risk of hypertension for African Americans. Describe.

_____

_____

_____

B5. List at least 12 other mechanisms or factors that are likely to contribute to essential hypertension. (*Hint:* refer to Questions A2 and B1.)

_____

_____

_____

B6. Complete this exercise about BP.

(a) Jeremy is a healthy newborn who was born this morning. Write a typical BP for him: ___/___ mm Hg. Two weeks from now his systolic BP is likely to be about ____ mm Hg. His systolic BP will probably reach 120 mm Hg by the time he reaches age ___ years.

(b) Describe the salt-thrifty gene of African Americans. Then list other factors that may relate to the high incidence of hypertension among blacks. _____

_____

_____

(c) Describe the antihypertension "DASH plan." _____

(d) Circle correct answer to show which body shape is more associated with hypertension.

(1) "Apple" shape (fat in abdomen)

(2) "Pear" shape (fat in hips and thighs)

(e) Cells may develop resistance to insulin in type ___ diabetes mellitus, in obesity, and in other instances. As a result, the body is likely to produce *(higher? lower?)* amounts of insulin. Hyperinsulinemia tends to *(increase? decrease?)* cardiac output, PVR, and sodium retention, all of which *(increase? decrease?)* risk of hypertension.

(f) BP is typically lowest at about *(4 AM? 10 AM? 4 PM?)*. The term "dippers" refers to persons whose BP falls during the *(night? afternoon?)*. Being a "dipper" is associated with *(more? less?)* organ disease in hypertensive persons.

B7. Circle the factors that have been shown to decrease BP.

(a) Reduction of alcohol intake

(b) Weight loss of 10 pounds (if overweight)

(c) Snacks of fruits or vegetables rather than chips or ice cream

(d) Decreased insulin resistance

(e) Discontinuing use of oral contraceptives

(f) Potassium supplements (in hypertensive persons)

B8. Complete this exercise about systolic BP.

(a) With normal aging, elasticity of vessels *(increases? decreases?)*, especially among *(larger? smaller?)* arteries. The left ventricle must *(increase? decrease?)* its force, pumping into a stiffened aorta. As a result, *(systolic? diastolic?)* BP increases between the fourth and ninth decades. This type of hypertension refers to a systolic BP greater than ____ mm Hg with a diastolic BP less than ____ mm Hg.

(b) How is diastolic BP likely to change with age? _____

(c) Because systolic BP increases with aging and diastolic BP does not, pulse pressure is likely to *(increase? decrease?)*.

(d) Explain how these changes can lead to myocardial ischemia and heart failure.

_____
_____
_____

B9. Describe effects of hypertension in the following exercise.

(a) List organs that are usually "target organs" of chronic hypertension.

_____
_____

(b) Risk of strokes is greater with *(systolic? diastolic?)* hypertension.

(c) Can hypertensive therapy reduce the left ventricular hypertrophy (LVH) described in question A8(d)? _____

_____

(d) Explain how effects of high blood pressure on kidneys can exacerbate the hypertension.

_____
_____
_____

B10. *(Many? Few?)* diagnostic tests are available for diagnosing essential hypertension. Explain the significance.

_____
_____
_____

B11. Mr. Lanter tries to adopt a lifestyle that will reduce his stage 1 hypertension. Answer these related questions.

(a) Mr. Lanter considers eating a soup with a label that lists 1200 mg of sodium per serving. This serving would include *(2%? 20%?)* of a sodium intake of 6 g/day.

(b) Would reduction of saturated fats directly decrease his BP? _____

(c) He would like to drink two 6-ounce glasses of wine at dinner. This *(does? does not?)* exceed the daily limit recommended by the JNC-VI report.

(d) Which form of exercise would be more beneficial for Mr. Lanter? *(Swimming? Weight-lifting?)*

B12. Select the antihypertensive medication that fits each description by selecting from the list and filling in the blanks with your answers.

Angiotensin converting enzyme inhibitors	α_1-receptor antagonists
β_1-blockers	β_2-blockers
Central adrenergic inhibitors	Calcium channel blockers
Diuretics	

(a) Directly inhibit sympathetic nerves; have high incidence of side effects:

_____

(b) Decrease contractility of the heart and dilate blood vessels which decreases venous return and workload of the heart:

_____

(c) Selectively affect heart, decreasing rate and contractility: _____

(d) Directly reduce blood volume:

_____

(e) Interfere with conversion of angiotensin I to II: _____

(f) Dilators that reduce peripheral vascular resistance (PVR): _____

B13. Mr. Lanter's BP is still hypertensive after 4 months of attempts at lifestyle changes. Complete this related exercise.

(a) He is likely to be started on a *(low? high?)* dosage of medication and build up *(rapidly? step-wise?)*. His compliance is likely to be greater with a prescription for *(one? three?)* dose(s) per day.

(b) Select the two medications from the list in question B12 that are most likely choices for initial drug treatment for Mr. Lanter's hypertension. These drugs have also been shown to decrease risk for heart disease.

_____, _____

C. SECONDARY HYPERTENSION (pages 473–477)

C1. Choose the two true statements about secondary hypertension.

(a) **Almost all** hypertension is of this type.

(b) Many of the conditions causing secondary hypertension **can** be cured or corrected.

(c) Secondary hypertension is **rarely** seen in persons under age 30.

(d) The largest single cause of secondary hypertension is **kidney** disease.

C2. Complete this exercise about several types of secondary hypertension.

(a) Define renovascular disease. _____

_____

_____

The most common form of renovascular disease is narrowing of the renal artery by the condition known as _____.

(b) Reduced renal flow associated with hypertension can initiate release of _____ from kidneys. This chemical triggers the renin-angiotensin-aldosterone (RAA) mechanism, which further increases BP. Angiotensin II is a powerful vaso*(constrictor? dilator?)* that increases PVR. Angiotensin II also stimulates release of the hormone _____ that causes kidneys to *(eliminate? retain?)* Na^+ and H_2O. Aldosterone also leads to *(hyper? hypo?)*kalemia.

(c) Besides the RAA mechanism, aldosterone levels can be increased by:

(1) Addison's disease

(2) Primary hyperaldosteronism

(3) Cushing's disease

(4) Excessive intake of European licorice

(d) A salt-restricted diet *(is? is not?)* likely to help persons with high aldosterone levels.

(e) Epinephrine and norepinephrine are the two major hormones produced by the adrenal *(cortex? medulla?)*. These chemicals are classified as _____. A tumor of cells that make these hormones is known as a _____oma. These tumors can also arise in *(sympathetic? parasympathetic?)* ganglia, sites of nerve cells that release the catecholamines. The most common symptom is _____. Circle other signs from the following list:

(1) Decreased sweat

(2) Palpitations

(3) Pallor

(4) Weight gain

(f) Coarctation of the aorta is a *(dilation? narrowing?)* of the vessel. Affected persons are likely to have high BP and strong pulses in the *(arms? legs?)*.

C3. Choose the three true statements about malignant hypertension.

(a) Malignant hypertension is caused by chemicals released by **cancer** cells.

(b) For a diagnosis of this type of hypertension, diastolic pressure must be greater than 160 mm Hg.

(c) Associated spasms of cerebral vessels can lead to **encephalopathy**.

(d) Azotemia (high blood levels of BUN and creatinine), acidosis, hypocalcemia, and proteinuria are **all** indicators of renal dysfunction that can be caused by malignant hypertension.

(e) Malignant hypertension can usually be treated **gradually at home**.

(f) Treatment for malignant hypertension is likely to include **vasodilators**.

C4. Identify the type of hypertension in each of the following pregnancies. Fill in the blanks using terms in the following list.

Chronic hypertension
Gestational hypertension
Preeclampsia/eclampsia

(a) A normal level of protein in a 24-hour urine is less than 300 mg. Faith's 24-hour urine protein level is 1,100 mg. Her BP (at 24 weeks of gestation) has elevated dramatically to 162/98 mm Hg. This is her first pregnancy: _____

(b) Betty Sue, 17, has no history of hypertension, but her BP now (at 24 weeks' gestation) is 142/84 mm Hg. Results of tests for protein in her urine are negative. If her BP returns to normal by about 3 months postpartum, this will confirm her diagnosis: _____

(c) Mrs. Swedeland, 39, has a history of hypertension, stage 1. Her BP actually decreased during her first trimester. Now at 30 weeks' gestation, her BP is 160/102 mm Hg: _____

C5. Choose the three true statements about hypertension in pregnancy.

(a) Incidence of hypertension in pregnancy is **greater** among African American women than among white women.

(b) Incidence of hypertension in pregnancy is **greater** among younger mothers than among older mothers.

(c) Severe preeclampsia/eclampsia is **more** likely to involve thrombocytosis than thrombocytopenia.

(d) Persistent headache and visual problems **are** signs of preeclampsia/eclampsia.

(e) **Decreased** liver enzymes such as ALT and AST are signs of preeclampsia/eclampsia.

(f) Decreased glomerular filtration rate (GFR) is a sign of preeclampsia/eclampsia.

C6. Edema *(never? sometimes? always?)* accompanies pregnancy-induced hypertension (PIH or eclampsia). Circle the correct answer and then explain.

_____

_____

C7. Circle the factors that increase risk for preeclampsia.

(a) Single (rather than multiple) fetuses

(b) Women with a history of chronic hypertension

(c) Presence of a hydatidiform mole (cystic, pathologic ovum)

(d) Diabetes mellitus

(e) Proteinuria early in pregnancy

C8. Contrast preeclampsia with eclampsia.

_____

_____

_____

C9. Explain possible mechanisms of PIH or preeclampsia in this exercise.

(a) It is normal for pregnant women to have a(n) *(increase? decrease?)* in circulating blood volume and a related *(increase? decrease?)* in cardiac output.

(b) Early in a normal pregnancy BP *(does? does not?)* increase. This is probably caused by a(n) *(increase? decrease?)* in peripheral vascular resistance (PVR). Later in the course of a normal pregnancy, BP *(does? does not?)* increase, probably related to a(n) *(increase? decrease?)* in PVR.

(c) Women who develop PIH are thought to have an abnormally *(high? low?)* sensitivity to vasoconstrictors such as _____ or _____. As a result, their PVR does not decrease and BP does increase.

C10. Circle the helpful interventions for PIH or preeclampsia.

(a) Avoidance of alcohol and tobacco use

(b) Bed rest

(c) Birth of the fetus

(d) ACE-inhibitors

(e) Dietary salt restriction

D. HIGH BLOOD PRESSURE IN CHILDREN AND THE ELDERLY (pages 477–480)

D1. Circle the correct answers in each statement.

(a) That Donnie's parents both are hypertensive places Donnie at *(higher? lower?)* risk for high BP. That he was also born with a low Apgar score (a score of 5 at 10 minutes) places him at *(higher? lower?)* risk.

(b) In infancy or early childhood, hypertension is more likely to be *(essential? secondary?)*, with the most common cause being *(coarctation of the aorta? kidney disorders?)*.

(c) At age 3, Donnie's BP averages 113/67 mm Hg. This classifies his BP in the *(25th? 75th? 95th?)* percentile for his age. This is *(significant? severe?)* hypertension, which means that Donnie *(need not? should?)* be evaluated and treated.

D2. Choose the two true statements.

(a) Incidence of hypertension for older adults (older than 65 years) is 7 in 10 for African Americans and 6 in 10 for whites.

(b) The most common type of hypertension among elderly is **diastolic**.

(c) For a 70-year old, systolic BP should be **less than** 170 mm Hg (100 + the age).

(d) With aging, baroreceptor sensitivity is likely to **decrease**.

D3. List several factors that can help to ensure accurate measurement of BP in the elderly.

_____

_____

_____

E. ORTHOSTATIC HYPOTENSION (pages 480-485)

E1. Describe the normal mechanism of regulating BP when a person stands up. Circle the correct answers or fill in the blanks.

(a) On standing, blood shifts to *(upper? lower?)* parts of the body. As a result, BP *(increases? decreases?)* in the upper body.

(b) State the normal locations of baroreceptors: _____ and _____. When these sense a drop in BP, which responses are typically initiated: *(Increase? Decrease?)* in heart rate and vaso_____. Contraction of leg muscles to support the standing position also *(increase? decrease?)* venous return (review Figure 21-1, page 94 of the Study Guide).

E2. Define orthostatic hypotension.

_____

_____

_____

Describe factors that can lead to this condition in this exercise.

(a) List several mechanisms by which circulating blood volume might be reduced.

_____

_____

(b) List examples of medications that can lead to this condition.

_____

_____

_____

(c) Explain how diabetes or stroke can cause orthostatic hypotension.

_____

_____

_____

E3. Gladys, age 85 years, has been in bed with a severe respiratory infection for most of the past 4 days. Complete this exercise

(a) Today Gladys has gotten out of bed three times. Each time she feels weak and dizzy just after she stands up; to date she has not fainted on standing. Her classification of orthostatic hypotension is Class ___.

(b) Explain the probable causes of her dizziness.

_____

_____

(c) List several interventions that can help reduce risk of falls for Gladys._____

_____

_____

CHAPTER 24

Alterations in Cardiac Function

■ Review Questions

A. DISORDERS OF THE PERICARDIUM (pages 487–491)

A1. Describe the pericardial cavity in this exercise.

(a) The pericardial cavity is located between the _____ and the _____. (Choose from the following options)

Fibrous pericardium   Myocardium
Parietal pericardium   Visceral pericardium

(b) _____ mL (or _____ tbsp) of serous fluid is normally present in this cavity.

(c) State the major concern about pericardial disorders. _____

_____

_____

A2. Select pericardial disorders that fit the following descriptions.

Acute pericarditis   Cardiac tamponade
Constrictive pericarditis   Pericardial effusions

(a) Scar tissue binding visceral and parietal layers of the pericardium that interferes with cardiac filling: _____

(b) Life-threatening condition in which the heart cannot fill adequately because it is compressed by excessive pericardial fluid:

_____

(c) Characterized by this triad of signs and symptoms: chest pain, "leathery" pericardial friction rub, and ECG changes of T wave and ST segment: _____

_____

(d) Exudate within the pericardial cavity; especially dangerous if volume is large or when it accumulates rapidly: _____

_____

(e) Inflammation in which pericardial capillaries dilate and become more permeable: _____

_____

A3. Choose the two answers with a term matched with a correct description.

(a) Pain due to acute pericarditis is best described as a **suffocating pressure.**

(b) A **purulent** exudate is one that contains "**pus**" (consisting of WBCs and microbes).

(c) Constrictive pericarditis **can** occur from pericardial effusions that lead to pericardial scarring.

(d) In cardiac tamponade, excessive fluid **expands the chambers of the heart.**

(e) Pericardiocentesis refers to **excessive fluid in the pericardial cavity.**

A4. Mrs. Barrett has pulsus paradoxus. Describe her condition in the following exercise.

(a) During inspiration, lung volume normally *(increases? decreases?)*, and pressure within lungs *(increases? decreases?)*, "inviting" increased venous return to the heart. As the right side of the heart fills and exerts pressure on the septum, the volume of the left side of the heart *(increases? decreases?)*. As a result, stroke volume normally *(increases? decreases?)* by about _____ mm Hg during inspiration.

(b) Mrs. Barrett's systolic blood pressure decreases by about 10 mm Hg during her inspiration. This alteration leads to *(more? less?)* than normal stroke volume during inspiration. This *(is? is not?)* an indicator of pulsus paradoxus which can indicate cardiac tamponade. Explain.

_____

_____

_____

B. CORONARY HEART DISEASE (pages 491–507)

B1. Circle correct answers in each statement.

(a) The circumflex artery is a branch of the *(left? right?)* coronary artery.

(b) In most persons, the posterior portion of the interventricular septum is supplied with blood by the *(right? left?)* coronary artery.

B2. Mr. Adilifu has a pulse of 160 beats/minute and a blood pressure of 120/50 mm Hg. As a result, his coronary artery perfusion (blood supply) is likely to be *(higher? lower?)* than normal. Explain.

_____

_____

_____

B3. Circle the three true statements.

(a) Normally heart muscle meets its energy needs through burning of **glucose** in **anaerobic** pathways.

(b) Adenosine and other metabolites resulting from myocardial contractions cause **vasodilation** of coronary vessels.

(c) Endothelial-relaxing factor (EDRF) is produced by cells lining **coronary vessels**.

(d) EDRF and endothelins **both** cause **vasoconstriction** of coronary arteries.

(e) Coronary heart disease (CHD) **is** highly associated with atherosclerosis.

B4. Circle the correct answers in each statement.

(a) Signs and symptoms of coronary heart disease do not typically occur until a branch of a coronary artery is at least *(25%? 50%? 75%?)* occluded.

(b) Atherosclerotic lesions occur most often in *(proximal? distal?)* areas of coronary arteries.

(c) Rupture of atherosclerotic plaques occurs most often just *(after arising in the morning? before bedtime?)*, and when stress levels are *(high? low?)*—both related to *(sympathetic? vagal?)* activity.

(d) Atherosclerotic plaque *(increases? decreases?)* risk of thrombus formation and coronary occlusion.

(e) Aspirin *(stimulates? inhibits?)* platelet aggregation; high dosages *(do? do not?)* increase its effectiveness.

B5. Match the technique for assessing coronary blood flow with the related descriptions by filling in the blank with choices from this list.

Cardiac catheterization
Electrocardiography
Exercise stress testing
Nuclear imaging

(a) An invasive technique that can be used to produce images of the heart, measure cardiac output, take samples for blood gases, or view coronary arteries:

_____

(b) The most frequently used device for detecting myocardial infarction; a Holter monitor is a continuous ambulatory unit used to detect such changes that accompany ischemic episodes over a 24-hour period: _____

(c) One example is measurement of regional myocardial perfusion by scintigraphy with thallium or technetium; depending on the specific test, "hot spots" or "cold spots" can indicate ischemia or infarction:

_____

(d) Monitor of heart rate, blood pressure, and ECG changes that indicate ischemia during bicycle or treadmill exercise: _____

_____

B6. Mr. Sawyer is having a coronary angiogram performed. Circle the vessels that are appropriate sites for retrograde insertion of the coronary catheter.

(a) Left femoral artery

(b) Left femoral vein

(c) Right femoral artery

(d) Right femoral vein

B7. Discuss chronic ischemic heart disease in this exercise.

(a) Clot (thrombus) formation is one of the *three* main mechanisms by which cardiac ischemia is likely to occur. List the other two. (*Hint*: one is included in Question B4.)

_____,

_____.

(b) List several reasons why Mrs. Caruso, who has *normal* coronary blood flow, may have inadequate coronary perfusion to meet needs of her heart muscle.

_____

_____

_____

B8. Mr. Clark, age 72, reports to Dr. Connors that over the past month he has been having "bouts of pain in my chest whenever I walk up to the top floor (two flights) to go to bed, but the pain stops just about as soon as I stop." Complete this exercise.

(a) The consistency of Mr. Clark's chest pain on exercise suggests chronic *(stable? unstable?)* angina. "Angina pectoris" literally means _____. Angina indicates myocardial *(ischemia? infarction?)*. The pain is most likely *(sharp or stabbing? squeezing or suffocating chest pain?)*.

(b) Mr. Clark's angina over the past month fits into the Canadian Cardiovascular Society Class *(I? II? III? IV?)*. If he could routinely walk up only one flight of stairs without pain, he would fit into class ___ and would have *(stable? unstable?)* angina. (See text page 498.)

(c) An angiogram indicates that Mr. Clark has advanced coronary atherosclerosis, but he states that he has never experienced angina until "this past month." Explain.

_____

(d) When Mr. Clark experiences angina, it is probably better that he *(sit? lie?)* down. Explain. _____

_____

_____

(e) List several interventions other than medications that may reduce Mr. Clark's frequency of angina.

_____

_____

_____

(f) Dr. Connors prescribes nitroglycerin pills. Explain why Mr. Clark must place these pills under his tongue but not swallow them.

B9. Match the anti-anginal medication with the related description by filling in the blanks with choices from the following list.

Antiplatelet drugs
β-adrenergic-blocking drugs
Calcium antagonists
Long-acting nitrates
Lipid-lowering drugs
Nitroglycerin

(a) Decrease venous return, and thus decrease preload (amount of blood that the heart needs to pump); may also inhibit platelet activity so as to decrease thrombus formation: _____

(b) Fast-acting vasodilator that decreases preload; available sublingually, by spray, or topically (patch or paste):

_____

(c) Decrease myocardial contraction, vasodilate coronary and peripheral arteries; effect of the latter is to decrease preload:

_____

(d) The "statins" that reduce LDLs and lower risk for atherosclerosis: _____

(e) Decrease cardiac contractions by blocking B_1 receptors on the heart:

_____

(f) Aspirin is an example: _____

B10. Complete this exercise about myocardial ischemia and myocardial infarction (MI).

(a) Mrs. Holly sometimes experiences angina at rest, often at night. This is classified as *(stable? unstable?)* angina. It is associated with *(vasospasm? thrombus formation?)*. Dysrhythmias that accompany pain *(increase? decrease?)* risk of sudden death.

(b) Mr. Ravin has symptoms similar to those of Mrs. Holly except that he has elevated cardiac enzyme levels (see question B11 below). These findings indicate *(no? some?)* myocardial injury. Mr. Ravin's diagnosis is likely to be:

(1) Unstable angina

(2) Non–ST-segment elevation (non–Q-wave) MI

(3) ST-segment elevation (non–Q-wave) MI

(4) ST-segment elevation (Q-wave) MI

(c) Arrange the diagnoses listed in B10(b) according to amount of myocardial damage likely, from most to least damage:

____, ____, ____, ____

(d) Which two diagnoses in B10b are commonly known as *heart attacks* or *acute myocardial infarctions* (AMIs)? ___, ___

(e) Which diagnosis is most likely to be most responsive to fibrinolytic therapy because the thrombus is fibrin-rich? ___

B11. Serum cardiac markers are helpful in diagnosis of MIs because these chemicals, which are normally found in *(intact myocardial cells? blood serum?)*, are released as a result of damage or death of heart cells. The level of these "markers" in blood is *(directly? inversely?)* related to the extent of myocardial injury. The box on textbook page 501 indicates that blood levels of most of these markers rise and then decline within about 3 *(hours? days? weeks?)* of onset of the MI. Now select markers that fit the following descriptions from the following list.

Total creatine kinase   Lactic dehydrogenase
Myoglobin   Troponin I

(a) A low molecular weight molecule, it is the first of these chemicals to be released post-MI: _____

(b) A chemical that regulates calcium in muscles, it is ideal for diagnosis of an MI 3 days after onset: _____

(c) An enzyme that helps provide ATP to cardiac cells: _____. Explain why assessment of MB isoenzyme is performed. _____

B12. Choose the two true statements about myocardial infarctions (MIs)

(a) MIs more commonly involve the **right** coronary artery than the **left**.

(b) The onset of an MI is **abrupt** and typically involves **severe, crushing pain**.

(c) Pain of an MI **is** typically relieved by nitroglycerin.

(d) Early hospitalization after onset of symptoms of an MI **does** reduce the risk of sudden death from the MI.

B13. Explain by writing a short description why a heart attack may be accompanied by:

(a) Nausea and vomiting

_____

_____

_____

(b) Tachycardia and pale, cool, moist skin

_____

_____

_____

B14. Circle the correct answers or fill in the blanks in each statement about heart attacks and complications.

(a) Irreversible myocardial cell death occurs within about *(a half hour? 6 hours? a day?)* after onset of severe myocardial ischemia.

(b) Early reperfusion by fibrinolytic therapy, within *(20? 60? 180?)* minutes of the onset of ischemia can prevent cell death. The reperfused and recovering area of myocardium is known as *(necrotic? stunned?)* myocardium. It *(will? may?)* regain full function.

(c) After an MI, which area is most likely to recover most? *(Necrotic? Injured? Ischemic?)* zone (see textbook Figure 24-11). Post-MI inflammation of the necrotic tissue along with newly formed granulation tissue leads to *(soft? scar?)* tissue within a *(day? week?)* after the MI. This soft tissue is at greater risk for _____ compared with healthy heart muscle.

(d) Necrotic myocardial tissue is usually completely replaced with scar tissue by 2 *(months? years?)* after the MI. This tissue *(is? is not?)* able to conduct impulses and contract normally. The extent of damage determines heart function and can be readily detected by changes in the _____. This scar tissue is at risk for a potentially fatal outpouching known as a ventricular _____.

(e) A sharp chest pain within 1 day to several weeks afer the MI may indicate the complication of *(endo? peri?)*carditis.

B15. Complete this exercise about treatment modalities for heart patients.

(a) Immediate treatment for all emergency cardiac patients includes anticoagulant therapy such as _____ and

_____. Workload of the heart is also reduced by drugs such as _____ and _____.

(b) ECG changes (such as elevation of the _____ segment and changes in the __ wave) contribute to the diagnosis of myocardial infarction. Describe or explain chemical interventions for persons with a diagnosis of acute myocardial infarction (AMI):

  (1) _____ by nasal prongs

  (2) Morphine given *(by mouth? intramuscularly? intravenously?)*. Morphine controls pain and is also a vaso*(constrictor? dilator?)* that *(increases? decreases?)* preload.

  (3) Methods to reestablish blood flow include _____ that directly breaks down clots, or _____ that activates plasminogen to form plasmin which breaks down clots.

  (4) Stool softener: _____
  _____

  (5) Low-salt diet:
  _____
  _____

(c) Note that *(none? some?)* of the interventions for MI is/are similar to those for angina (question B9).

(d) Revascularization procedures include the following. Briefly describe each one.

  (1) PTCA (also known as a "_____ angioplasty") with or without stent
  _____

  (2) Brachytherapy using _____ within coronary arteries
  _____

  (3) Atherectomy: _____ removal of the atherosclerotic plaque
  _____

  (4) CABG, an acronym for c_____ a_____ b_____ g_____. Vessels used to reperfuse the heart usually include the _____ vein and/or the _____ artery. (See textbook Figure 24-15.)

B16. List several lifestyle changes that are incorporated into a post-MI rehabilitation protocol.
_____
_____
_____

C. MYOCARDIAL DISEASE (pages 507–510)

C1. Differentiate myocarditis and cardiomyopathies from MI.
_____
_____
_____

C2. Circle the two true statements about myocarditis.

  (a) This condition is most often caused by **viral infection.**

  (b) ECG changes and elevated cardiac marker levels **are** used to diagnose myocarditis.

  (c) Most cases of myocarditis are **fatal.**

  (d) Treatment focuses on **active exercise** immediately after diagnosis.

C3. What is the major cause of primary cardiomyopathies? _____. Add the correct answer then select the type of the cardiomyopathy that fits the related description from the following list.

Dilated   Hypertrophic
Peripartum   Restrictive

  (a) Ventricular muscle walls thicken; microscopic examination of heart muscle tissue indicates abnormal organization of muscle fibers: _____

  (b) As indicated in textbook Figure 24-16, this cardiomyopathy involves the greatest ventricular radius or diameter:
  _____

  (c) Ventricle walls become rigid, limiting their filling and stroke volume; may involve amyloid infiltration; uncommon form of cardiomyopathy in the United States:
  _____

  (d) Probable or definite cause of more than one third of young athletes who die suddenly: _____

  (e) Occurring during pregnancy: _____
  _____

  (f) Likely to involve dyspnea, decreased stroke volume, and possibly heart failure:
  _____

D. INFECTIOUS AND IMMUNOLOGIC DISORDERS (pages 510–514)

D1. Complete this exercise about Lucy, age 16, who has infective endocarditis as a complication of a serious infection from *Staphylococcus aureus*. She has no known history of heart problems and does not use IV drugs.

(a) Most cases of infective endocarditis are caused by *(bacteria? fungi? viruses?)*. Most persons who develop this condition *(do? do not?)* have a history of previous valve disorders or congenital heart defects. Because Lucy does not have such a history, she is likely to have *(acute? subacute?)* bacterial endocarditis.

(b) This condition requires two independent factors, which are a damaged _____ and a _____.

(c) Vegetative lesions on heart valves are composed of _____

(d) Arrange in correct sequence (from first to last) the events likely to occur in the course of bacterial endocarditis:

(1) Initiation of immune responses to bacteria that can cause systemic injury

(2) Formation of vegetative lesions that damage heart valves

(3) Release of emboli containing microbes from free edges of valve surfaces

___ → ___ → ___

(e) Lucy's acute bacterial endocarditis *(is? is not?)* likely to be accompanied by fever and chills. List other signs and symptoms that Lucy is likely to have._____

_____

D2. Complete this exercise about Antonio, age 9, who has been diagnosed with rheumatic fever (RF) almost a month after a "strep sore throat" with headache, swollen neck glands, and fever.

(a) RF follows a GAS infection, which refers to g_____ A s_____; it *(can? cannot?)* be prevented by antibiotics for streptococcal infections. This condition is more likely to occur in persons with *(poor? excellent?)* health care.

(b) This condition *(affects only heart valves? is systemic?)*. Circle the organs of the body besides the heart that are most likely to be affected:

Central nervous system   Joints
Kidneys   Liver   Skin

(c) Now select the organ (from D2[b]) that fits the sign or symptom of RF:

(1) Erythema marginatum and subcutaneous nodules: _____

(2) Sydenham's chorea: _____

(3) Polyarthritis that responds to aspirin therapy: _____

(d) The manifestations described in D2c are likely to be *(permanent? temporary?)* effects of RF.

(e) If Antonio moves into a chronic phase of RF, it is likely to involve *(temporary? permanent?)* valve damage that occurs *(within the next month? decades?)* after the triggering event. Circle the valve that most often stenoses as a result: *(aortic? mitral? pulmonary? tricuspid?)*.

(f) If valve disease persists, Antonio should have prophylactic therapy with the antibiotic _____ for about 10 *(days? weeks? years?)*, and especially before _____ procedures.

D3. Match the condition with the description from the following list.

Bacterial endocarditis   Kawasaki's disease
Rheumatic fever

(a) Aschoff's bodies are a characteristic of: _____

(b) A disorder of inflamed blood vessels in many parts of the body; most serious effects are on coronary arteries that may lead to heart failure in young children; probably of immune origin: _____

(c) Up to 20% of cases follow surgery for prosthetic valve replacement: _____

(d) The Duke diagnostic system for this disorder includes positive blood cultures for the causative microbe, and indication of heart valve involvement: _____

(e) The most common cause of acquired heart disease in young children: _____

D4. Circle all answers that are signs or symptoms of the *acute* phase of Kawasaki disease.

(a) Spiking a fever of 104°F over the course of 5 days

(b) Itchy skin rash

(c) Conjunctivitis with yellowish discharge

(d) Swollen, red palms and soles

(e) Red throat and strawberry tongue

(f) Peeling of skin on fingers and toes

E. VALVULAR HEART DISEASE (pages 515–520)

E1. Discuss heart valve disorders in this exercise.

(a) The most common cause of most acquired valve disorders is _____.

(b) Which two heart valves are most likely to be damaged in valve diseases? _____ and _____ Explain. _____
_____

(c) State the major problem resulting from heart valve disorders.
_____

(d) Stenosis is a problem with (opening? closing?) a valve, whereas regurgitation is a problem with (opening? closing?) the valve. Valve incompetence is an alternative term for valvular (regurgitation? stenosis?)

E2. Identify the valve disorders that fit the related descriptions.

Aortic valve regurgitation
Aortic valve stenosis
Mitral valve prolapse
Mitral valve regurgitation
Mitral valve stenosis

(a) The left atrium enlarges as blood accumulates there and increases risk for mural (wall) clot and embolus formation; anticoagulation therapy is used:
_____

(b) Most likely to lead to dyspnea related to pulmonary congestion and edema:
_____

(c) Because the valve acts as a swinging door, blood sloshes back and forth between the left atrium and left ventricle. Results: the S_1 sound is prolonged, and left atrial overload and pulmonary congestion occur:
_____

(d) Also known as floppy mitral valve syndrome; more common in women, and usually asymptomatic; symptoms may be controlled by avoidance of caffeine, alcohol, and tobacco: _____

(e) The left ventricle hypertrophies as it works to pump out blood; this may lead to heart failure; slower pulse because left ventricular systole takes longer: _____

(f) Because coronary arteries perfuse during ventricular diastole, perfusion of these vessels decreases as diastolic pressure drops in this condition: _____

(g) Pulse pressure widens as diastolic pressure decreases when the aortic valve allows blood to flow back into the left ventricle during diastole; stroke volume and systolic pressure increase as the left ventricle pumps out that same blood repeatedly: _____

(h) Water-hammer pulse and head bobbing with each heart beat (Musset's) sign are indicators of this valve disorder:
_____

E3. List several techniques used to diagnose valve disorders. _____
_____

F. HEART DISEASE IN INFANTS AND CHILDREN (pages 520-530)

F1. Circle the correct answers or fill in blanks in these statements about heart development.

(a) Most heart development occurs between the third and eighth (week? month?) of prenatal development.

(b) The truncus arteriosus ultimately bifurcates into the two vessels named the _____ and the _____.

(c) Endocardial cushions form (AV? semilunar?) valves as well as parts of the atrial and ventricular _____.

(d) The septum primum and septum secundum contribute to formation of the (atrial? ventricular?) septum. The opening in the atrial septum that allows fetal blood to pass from right atrium directly to left atrium is known as the foramen _____.

F2. Select the structure in fetal circulation that fits each description.

Ductus arteriosus   Ductus venosus
Foramen ovale   Placenta
Umbilical arteries   Umbilical vein

(a) Carry/ies "red" blood (low in CO_2, high in O_2) from fetal internal iliac arteries to placenta: _____

(b) Carries blood from umbilical vein to inferior vena cava: _____

(c) Two structures that allow fetal blood to bypass the deoxygenated lungs; normally close within days after birth:

_____, _____

F3. A red blood cell (RBC) is in the fetal descending aorta. Arrange in correct sequence (from first to last) the structures that the RBC will pass through in the most direct route to the fetal brain. Use answers from question F2. (One structure will not be used.)

_____ → _____ →
_____ → _____ →
_____

F4. Circle the correct answers or fill in the blanks in these statements about fetal and postnatal circulation.

(a) Fetal PO_2 and O_2 saturation are typically *(higher? lower?)* in fetal life than postnatally.

(b) During fetal life lungs are filled with *(air? fluid?)* and are *(well oxygenated? hypoxic?)*. As a result, pulmonary vessels vaso*(constrict? dilate?)* causing fetal lungs to have *(high? low?)* resistance to flow. For this reason, most blood in the fetal pulmonary artery flows into lower pressure *(lungs? ductus arteriosus?)*.

(c) At birth, the baby's first breath causes lung volume to *(increase? decrease?)* and pressure there to *(increase? decrease?)*. This *(raises? lowers?)* pulmonary resistance and *(increases? decreases?)* pulmonary blood flow which contributes to closure of both the ductus arteriosus and the _____. Premature babies whose lungs do not inflate well are more likely to have these fetal structures *(close early? remain open?)*.

(d) *(Thickening? Thinning?)* of smooth muscle in walls of pulmonary vessels normally occurs over the first weeks of postnatal life, *(lowering? raising?)* pulmonary resistance even further. But if a baby has a congenital heart defect (e.g., a septal defect) that increases pulmonary artery flow, this flow stimulates pulmonary vaso*(constriction? dilation?)* that maintains pulmonary vascular resistance and for 1 to 3 months and masks the symptoms of the congenital defect.

(e) Such excessive pulmonary artery flow can injure pulmonary vessels. To prevent this, a procedure known as pulmonary _____

can limit pulmonary flow and protect those vessels.

F5. Complete this exercise about congenital heart defects.

(a) Most congenital heart defects are caused by *(one? many?)* factor(s). Children with Down syndrome have a ____% chance of having a heart defect. Ultrasound can detect different heart defects in a fetus as early as ____ weeks.

(b) Most congenital heart defects are _____ defects.

(1) Left-to-right shunt

(2) Right-to-left shunt

Explain your answer.

_____

(c) Which type of shunt leads to right ventricular hypertrophy (RVH) with possible RV failure?

(1) Left-to-right shunt

(2) Right-to-left shunt

(d) Which type of congenital heart defect is classified as "with cyanosis"?

(1) Left-to-right shunt

(2) Right-to-left shunt

Explain your answer. _____

_____

F6. Explain why infants with congenital heart defects are at risk for "failure to thrive."

_____

_____

F7. Select types of congenital heart defects listed here that fit the following descriptions.

Atrial septal defect   Coarctation of the aorta
Endocardial cushion defects
Patent ductus arteriosus
Pulmonary stenosis
Tetralogy of Fallot
Transposition of the great vessels
Ventricular septal defect

(a) Which two of these defects lead to cyanosis (i.e., "blue babies")? _____,

_____

(b) In this defect, the foramen ovale does not close, leading to a left-to-right shunt because of low pulmonary resistance; more common in "preemies" whose lungs are hypoxic:

_____

(c) Involves four defects, among them, pulmonary stenosis, ventricular septal defect, and right ventricular hypertrophy:

_____

(d) Narrowing of the aorta, almost always distal to the ductus arteriosus; as a result, blood pressure is considerably higher in the brachial artery than in the femoral artery:

_____

(e) The aorta and the pulmonary artery have their locations and roles "switched"; may be corrected by an "atrial switch" surgery:

_____

(f) In this defect, some of the neonate's aortic blood flows back into pulmonary artery, overloading lungs, possibly causing left-sided failure; may be caused by excessive prostaglandin production because these are vasodilators: _____

(g) The most common congenital heart defect; symptoms depend on the size of the defect, and typically begin to appear at 1 to 6 months: _____

(h) Common heart defect in children with Down syndrome; likely to affect tricuspid or mitral valve: _____

(i) Because blood flow to lungs is limited, treatment may include use of prostaglandin E to maintain patency of the ductus arteriosis (two answers):

_____

_____

F8. Describe causes and symptoms of "tet" spells in infants with tetralogy of Fallot.

_____

_____

_____

CHAPTER 25

Disorders of Cardiac Conduction and Rhythm

■ Review Questions

A. CARDIAC CONDUCTION SYSTEM
(pages 531–537)

A1. Complete this exercise about the cardiac conduction system.

  (a) Most myocardiac cells *(can? cannot?)* initiate and conduct impulses. Specialized pacemaker and conduction tissues generate impulses at a *(faster? slower?)* rate than other heart tissues.

  (b) Arrange in correct sequence from first to last in the conduction pathway:

    AV node   Bundle and
    Purkinje fibers   bundle branches
    SA node

    _____ → _____ →
    _____ → _____

  (c) Which structure is the normal "pacemaker"? (Choose from answers for A1[b].) _____ It is located in the wall of the *(right? left?)* atrium.

  (d) Internodal pathways connect between the _____ and _____. (Choose from answers for A1[b].) The middle one of these pathways is known as _____ internodal tracts.

  (e) Conduction through the AV node and bundle is *(rapid? slow?)*. State an advantage of this fact.

    _____

    _____

  (f) Which structure provides the only connection between conductile tissue of atria and ventricles? (Choose from answers for A1[b].) _____ State an advantage of this arrangement.

    _____

    _____

  (g) Where are the bundle branches located?

    _____

  (h) Purkinje fibers have *(rapid? slow?)* transmission. State an advantage of this fact.

    _____

    _____

A2. Complete this exercise about the cardiac conduction system.

  (a) Define an action potential.

    _____

    _____

  (b) The inside of a resting cardiac muscle cell membrane typically has a charge of *(+90? -90?)* mV with many more *(Na^+? K^+?)* located inside the membrane and more *(Na^+? K^+?)* located outside of the cell membrane.

  (c) A stimulus triggers entrance of *(Na^+? K^+?)* into the cell. Fast Na^+ channels open at about ____ mV, a point known as "threshold." Electrical potential then rises to a peak of about ____ mV and spreads *(rapidly? slowly?)* across the cell membrane. This period is known as phase *(0? 1?)* or _____ polarization. It also corresponds to the *(P wave? QRS complex?)* of the ECG.

  (d) Repolarization starts with a(n) *(downward? upward?)* slope (phase 1) as the inside of the membrane develops a more *(positive? negative?)* potential.

  (e) The slope flattens out in phase 2 (the _____ phase). What accounts for this plateau, and what is its impact?

    _____

    _____

    Phase 2 corresponds to the *(QRS complex? ST segment?)*.

  (f) The phase 3 slope forms *(dramatically? gradually?)* as K^+ ions move *(into? out of?)* the cell and the influx of Na^+ and Ca^{+2} *(begins? ceases?)*.

(g) Phase 4 *(does? does not?)* require ATP to pump out Na$^+$ and return the cell to its original (resting) state. Phase 4 corresponds to *(systole? diastole?)*.

A3. Choose the correct answers about the refractory period.

(a) The heart is unresponsive to any stimuli whatsoever during:

(1) Absolute refractory period

(2) Relative refractory period

(3) Supernormal excitatory period
As a result, a second myocardial contraction *(can? cannot?)* normally be superimposed over a first one.

(b) The heart can respond to a weak stimulus during the _____ period. In heart disease, ischemia can generate extra _____ beats during this period.

A4. Mrs. Pohlmann is having a clinical ECG performed. Complete this exercise about her ECG.

(a) It is likely that ____ leads will be placed on her body. Draw a normal ECG in the space below.

(b) Select the part of her ECG that best fits each description below. Choose from these answers.

P wave   PR interval
QRS complex   RR interval
ST segment   T wave

(b1) Represents repolarization of ventricles: ____

(b2) Represents depolarization of ventricles: ____

(b3) Represents depolarization of the AV node, bundle of His, and Purkinje fibers: ____

(b4) A measure of the length of one cardiac cycle: ____

(c) Mrs. Pohlmann's PR interval should be less than ___ sec:

(1) 0.02

(2) 0.04

(3) 0.2

(d) Her T wave should rise about ____ mV.

B. DISORDERS OF CARDIAC RHYTHM AND CONDUCTION (pages 537–546)

B1. Choose from the following answers as you describe properties of myocardium.

Automaticity   Conduction
Excitability   Refractoriness

(a) Certain heart muscle cells are normally responsive to external stimuli; injured cells can develop this property: _____

(b) Normal properties of all myocardial cells: _____ and _____

(c) Responsible for the heart's regular initiation of contractions: _____ and _____

B2. The normal heart is paced at a rate of _____ beats/min by the *(SA? AV?)* node. If this normal pacemaker fails, the *(AV node? Purkinje fibers?)* is/are likely to pace at _____ beats/min. As a last resort, the Purkinje system can pace at _____ beats/min.

B3. Define ectopic pacemakers and explain what may cause them.

_____
_____
_____

B4. List two factors that must be present for "reentry" that leads to certain dysrhythmias.

_____
_____
_____

B5. Normal "sinus rhythm" refers to a heart rhythm in which the ____ node serves as pacemaker. Defend or dispute this statement: "Sinus rhythm should be regular with all RR intervals equal."

_____
_____
_____

B6. Complete this exercise about sinus dysrhythmias.

(a) Todd's resting pulse rate is 54 beats per minute (bpm), and his PR interval is 0.16 sec. He has _____cardia. List several factors that can lead to this condition.

_____
_____

(b) Mrs. Edelstone's resting heart rate is 110 bpm with a normal P wave and PR interval. She has a fever of 102°F. Her cardiac dysrhythmia is _____cardia. Explain.

_____
_____

(c) Write one mechanism of "escape" likely to occur in sinus arrest.

_____
_____
_____

B7. Supraventricular dysrhythmias originate within the *(atria? ventricles?)*. Select the condition that fits each description.

Atrial fibrillation   Atrial flutter
Premature atrial   Paroxysmal atrial
  complexes   tachycardia
Sick sinus syndrome

(a) "Sawtooth pattern" of P waves is due to the reentry phenomena; ventricles may contract after a certain number of atrial systoles, such as 4:1. Example: 400 atrial bpm:100 ventricular bpm. (textbook Fig. 25-10 top tracing): _____

(b) Bradycardia-tachycardia syndrome is the most common form; usually caused by AV node damage: _____

(c) Occurs when atrial cells cannot repolarize in time for the next stimulus; no discernible P waves—only oscillations of the baseline known as fibrillatory waves (Fig. 25-10, second tracing): _____

(d) Refers to all tachycardias that are supraventricular (arise above the division of the bundle of His): _____

B8. Choose the two true statements.

(a) With premature atrial complexes (PACs), the closer the ectopic focus is to the SA node, the more **normal** the PAC is.

(b) Type I atrial flutter typically involves a heart rate that is **more** rapid than Type II atrial flutter.

(c) Both atrial flutter and atrial fibrillation may be seen in persons with no apparent disease.

(d) In junctional dysrhythmias, the **Purkinje fibers** act as pacemaker.

B9. Mr. Joseph, age 81 years, has been diagnosed with atrial fibrillation.

(a) This dysrhythmia is *(common? rare?)* among elderly.

(b) His ECG is likely to appear with:

(1) Grossly disorganized atrial activity

(2) Frequent P waves but otherwise organized

(c) He states that he is taking a "blood thinner." Explain.

_____
_____

B10. Circle the factors that have been implicated in dysrhythmias.

Aging   Tobacco use
Coronary artery disease   Digitalis toxicity
Electrolyte imbalances   Open heart surgery
Stress   Caffeine
Infection such as rheumatic fever

B11. Complete this exercise about ventricular dysrhythmia.

(a) Mrs. Aster, age 42 years, has "PVCs," which refers to _____ _____ contractions. Circle correct answers about her condition.

(1) Likely to be caused by ectopic pacemakers within ventricular walls

(2) Although Mrs. Aster has no apparent heart disease, her PVCs are still clinically significant.

(3) Her ECG is likely to show "pauses" following the PVCs.

(b) Mr. Blackburn's ventricles are "quivering," and his ECG is "grossly disorganized." It is more likely that his diagnosis is ventricular *(tachycardia? fibrillation?)*.

(c) The QRS complexes in Mrs. Calafia's ECG ranges from 0.12 to 0.16 sec with a rate of 160 to 180 bpm; there are no discernible P waves. Her diagnosis is likely to be ventricular *(tachycardia? fibrillation?)*. Such a rapid heart rate *(increases? decreases?)* diastolic filling time, causing a(n) _____ *(increase? decrease?)* in her stroke volume and cardiac output.

B12. Choose the two true statements.

(a) Dysrhythmias that arise in ventricles typically are **less** serious than those that originate in atria.

(b) A QRS complex that is 1.0 sec long is considered a **normal** length.

(c) A bundle branch block involves a QRS complex that is **wider** than normal.

(d) Lengthening of the PR interval indicates **delayed** conduction through the AV node or the His-Purkinje system.

B13. Arrange these forms of heart block from least serious to most serious.

First-degree
Second-degree: Mobitz type II
Second-degree: Wenckebach's phenomenon
Third-degree

_____→_____ →

_____→_____

Now select the type of heart block that best fits each description.

(a) Complete heart block in which atrial and ventricular conduction pathways are not linked; decreases cardiac output and may cause fainting episodes known as Stokes-Adams attacks: _____

(b) Characteristic lengthening of the PR interval until the impulse is blocked and the cycle repeats: _____

(c) Isolated heart blocks of these types usually are not symptomatic: _____ and _____

B14. Describe the following types of diagnostic techniques for dysrhythmias in this exercise.

(a) Contrast Holter monitoring with a surface ECG.

_____

_____

(b) State the purpose of exercise stress testing.

_____

_____

(c) Explain how intracardiac ECGs are performed.

_____

_____

B15. Match the class of antidysrhythmic drug with the correct description. Use these answers.

Class I   Class II
Class III   Class IV
Cardiac glycosides

(a) Block excessive sympathetic activity:

_____

(b) Treat ventricular fibrillation by extending the action potential and refractory period:

_____

(c) Calcium channel blockers that reduce cardiac workload: _____

(d) Block fast sodium channels; several types decrease conductivity: _____

(e) Digitalis drugs that slow rapid atrial contractions: _____

B16. Choose the two true statements.

(a) Electronic pacemakers **can** be temporary or permanent.

(b) Defibrillation is known as **synchronized** cardioversion.

(c) The purpose of a defibrillator is to **shock the SA node to start.**

(d) Ablation therapy **destroys** or **removes** dysrhythmic tissue.

B17. AICDs are automatic _____ cardioverter-_____ that are used to reverse (*atrial? ventricular?*) tachydysrhythmias.

CHAPTER 26

Heart Failure and Circulatory Shock

■ Review Questions

A. PHYSIOLOGY OF HEART FAILURE (pages 547-560)

A1. Review the concepts listed here by returning to Study Guide Chapter 21, Questions B6(h), B8, and B9, and Figure 21-1.

Cardiac output   Cardiac reserve
Stroke volume   Venous return
Frank-Starling   End-diastolic volume
  mechanism   (EDV) or preload
Afterload   Ejection fraction
Cardiac contractility   Inotropic effects

A2. Test your understanding of these concepts as you circle correct answers or fill in blanks in these statements.

(a) Indicate whether preload and EDV are likely to increase or decrease in each case:

    (1) When venous return increases, for example, during exercise: _____

    (2) When stroke volume is reduced, as in heart failure or aortic valve regurgitation: _____

    (3) With fluid retention, as in renal failure: _____

(b) Afterload increases when systemic vessels vaso-*(constrict? dilate?)*. It also increases in *(hyper? hypo?)*tension and in aortic *(stenosis? regurgitation?)* because the heart must do more work if any of these factors are present.

(c) Circle the factors that have positive inotropic effects on the heart.

Digitalis   Epinephrine
Myocardial infarction   Sympathetic nerve
  or ischemia   impulses
Vagus nerve impulses

A3. Describe alterations associated with heart failure by completing this exercise.

(a) In heart failure, the heart is likely to be *(overstretched? not stretched adequately?)*, so that the diameter of the heart *(increases? decreases?)*. Contractility of the heart then *(increases? decreases?)* as actin and myosin filaments are *(better? inadequately?)* juxtaposed.

(b) Circle the factors that are likely to decrease in heart failure.

Afterload   Cardiac output
Ejection fraction   Myocardial wall
Preload   tension
Stroke volume

(c) Circle the answers that are likely to be compensatory mechanisms that the body will carry out to try to "fix" heart failure.

    (1) Vasodilation

    (2) Increased vagus nerve impulses

    (3) Increased heart rate

    (4) Release of renin and aldosterone

    (5) Release of the vasoconstrictor endothelin-I

    (6) Hypertrophy of the ventricular wall

    (7) Increased blood flow to kidneys

(d) Explain how the RAA mechanism affects heart failure by circling the correct answers or filling in the blanks.

    (1) Angiotensin II is a powerful vaso*(constrictor? dilator?)*. One of its effects is to *(increase? decrease?)* renal perfusion, which *(increases? decreases?)* urine output and *(increases? decreases?)* blood volume. This *(improves? exacerbates?)* heart failure.

    (2) Angiotensin II stimulates release of _____ from the adrenal *(medulla? cortex?)*. This hormone causes kidneys to retain _____ and _____.

(3) Both these effects cause preload and afterload to (*increase? decrease?*) even further.

(4) Angiotensin II is a factor that contributes to ventricular _____trophy, which may temporarily improve heart function but may also lead to _____.

A4. Contrast *heart failure* with *congestive heart failure* (CHF).

_____

_____

_____

A5. Write "ICF" next to causes of heart failure that result from impaired cardiac function, and "EWD" next to those related to excess work demands of the heart.

(a) Excessive production of thyroid hormone: ___

(b) IV fluid overload: ___

(c) High blood pressure: ___

(d) Tetralogy of Fallot: ___

(e) Heart attack: ___

(f) Heart valve disease: ___

A6. Most forms of CHF are (*high? low?*) output. Write examples of causes of CHF in which output is normal but still inadequate for body needs.

_____

_____

_____

A7. Contrast systolic and diastolic heart failure in this exercise by circling the correct answers and filling in the blanks.

(a) Systolic failure is also known as (*backward? forward?*) failure in which the heart has a problem with (*ejection? filling?*). Major symptoms are related to (*edema? ischemia?*).

(b) Diastolic failure is also known as (*backward? forward?*) failure in which the heart has an impaired (*ejection? filling?*). Signs and symptoms all involve (*edema? ischemia?*)

(c) Write *D* for diastolic failure and *S* for systolic failure next to each disorder to indicate likely effects on the heart.

(1) Mitral stenosis: ____

(2) Hypertension: ____

(3) Aortic valve regurgitation: ____

(4) Tachycardia, for example, during the stress of exercise of a diseased heart: ____

A8. Write a sign or symptom on each line below to indicate manifestations of each type of CHF.

AA: Abdominal discomfort and anorexia
APE: Acute pulmonary edema
Asc: Ascites
DN: Dyspnea at night
F: Fatigue
HS: Hepatomegaly and splenomegaly
ICP-P: Increased capillary pressure in pulmonary capillaries
ICP-S: Increased capillary pressure in systemic capillaries
JVD: Jugular vein distention
SA: Swollen ankles
PSOB: Perceived shortness of breath

(a) Left-sided CHF: ____, ____, ____, ____, ____

(b) Right-sided CHF: ____, ____, ____, ____, ____, ____

A9. Define each of these terms and explain why they are frequent signs of CHF:

(a) Orthopnea: _____

_____

(b) Diaphoresis: _____

_____

(c) Cool, clammy skin: _____

_____

(d) Nocturia: _____

_____

(e) Cheyne-Stokes breathing: _____

_____

_____

(f) Exertional dyspnea:_____

_____

A10. Mrs. Griffin was diagnosed with CHF eight years ago. She is now in skilled nursing care on oxygen by nasal cannula 24 hours a day. Mrs. Griffin remains in bed or in a wheel chair because she has episodes of angina even at rest. Her weight has dropped from 160 lb to 93 lb over the past 2 years. Recently she had a "PEG" (percutaneous esophageal gastrostomy) feeding tube inserted. Circle the correct answers or fill in the blanks.

(a) Mrs. Griffin's condition is categorized as Class (*I? II? III? IV?*) CHF according to the New York Heart Association Functional Classification.

(b) Explain how her weight loss is related to CHF. _____

_____

(c) Explain what a sudden gain of 2 pounds may mean. _____

_____

A11. Match the technique used for CHF diagnosis with the related description.

Echocardiography
History and physical examination
Pulmonary capillary wedge pressure
Thermodilution method

(a) Uses a Swan-Ganz catheter with an inflatable balloon-tip: _____

_____

(b) Demonstrates motion of atria and ventricles during the cardiac cycle:

_____

(c) Cardiac output and SvO$_2$ can be measured by injection of a solution of known temperature followed by measurement of blood temperature change:

_____

(d) Identifies dyspnea, enlarged liver, fluid in the abdomen (ascites), and edema of legs and feet: _____

A12. Select the treatments for CHF that fit the following descriptions.

Angiotensin converting enzyme inhibitors
Dietary modifications
Digitalis   Diuretics

(a) Restriction of sodium and fat intake:

_____

(b) Interrupts part of the renin-angiotensin-aldosterone (RAA) pathway:

_____

(c) Slows conduction through the heart, reducing heart rate in a tachycardic heart; may improve cardiac contractility:

_____

(d) Decreases preload: _____

A13. Circle the signs and symptoms that are likely to accompany acute pulmonary edema:

(a) Nonproductive cough

(b) Bradycardia (slow heart rate)

(c) Calm demeanor

(d) Dyspnea

(e) Dry skin

(f) Crackles heard upon auscultation

(g) Pink, frothy sputum

(h) Confusion and lethargy

A14. Mrs. Griffin (Question A10) has an episode of acute pulmonary edema. Her blood pressure is 98/48 mm Hg. Answer these related questions.

(a) This condition is the most dramatic effect of *(right? left?)*-sided heart failure.

(b) Why might lipstick or nail polish on Mrs. Griffin interfere with assessment of this condition?

_____

_____

(c) Describe a simple measure that can relieve some of her orthopnea. _____

_____

_____ `

(d) What effect would a powerful diuretic such as furosemide (Lasix) be likely to have on her? _____

_____

_____

(e) How can morphine help Mrs. Griffin?

_____

_____

A15. Cardiogenic shock is shock that results from a _____ problem. Fill in the blank, then choose the two true statements about cardiogenic shock.

(a) The most common cause of this type of shock is **heart attack**.

(b) In **all** cases of cardiogenic shock, cardiac output is **inadequate**.

(c) Myocardial depressant factor is a medication that **helps to reverse** effects of cardiogenic shock.

(d) As in heart failure, CVP and PCWP **decrease** in cardiogenic shock.

A16. Complete this exercise about treatments for cardiogenic shock.

(a) Nitroprusside (Nipride) and nitroglycerin are vaso*(constrictors? dilators?)* that will *(increase? decrease?)* venous return, *(increase? decrease?)* preload, and *(increase? decrease?)* systemic vascular resistance (SVR). As a result, blood is likely to be moved *(into? out of?)*

pulmonary vessels and *(into? out of?)* systemic circulation.

(b) Catecholamines such as epinephrine may be helpful because they *(increase? decrease?)* cardiac contractility; however, they are also vaso*(constrictors? dilators?)* that will *(increase? decrease?)* SVR.

(c) *(Continuous hemofiltration? An intro-aortic balloon pump?)* increases diastolic blood pressure which *(increases? decreases?)* coronary perfusion.

(d) Define refractory heart failure.

_____

_____

Identify techniques utilized in attempts to prolong survival of refractory heart patients

Cardiomyoplasty
Heart transplantation
Ventricular assist device

(1) A latissimus dorsi muscle is wrapped around the heart to augment cardiac contraction: _____

(2) A donor heart is sutured to the recipient's atria: _____

B. CIRCULATORY FAILURE (pages 560-568)

B1. Shock can be defined as _____ List four factors required for adequate oxygenation of tissues.

_____

_____

_____

B2. Review Study Guide Figure 21-1 (page 94) as you describe compensatory mechanisms designed to reverse shock by increasing cardiac output and blood pressure.

(a) Sympathetic nerve activity *(increases? decreases?)*. Effects include *(brady? tachy?)*cardia and *(increased? decreased?)* strength of contraction (dependent on current cardiac ability).

(b) Another is vaso*(constriction? dilation?)* of veins and venules, which is helpful because veins store *(much? little?)* of the body's blood volume. As a result, venous return *(increases? decreases?)*, which (according to the _____-Starling mechanism) should *(increase? decrease?)* stroke volume and cardiac output.

(c) Circle vessels that are typically constricted by sympathetic nerve activity.

(1) Cerebral

(2) Coronary

(3) Vessels to skin, kidneys, and abdominal muscles

(d) Another sympathetic effect is *(increased? decreased?)* sweat production, which together with vasoconstriction leads to *(warm, flushed? cool, clammy?)* skin in most forms of shock.

(e) Describe three mechanisms that are physiologic attempts to restore blood volume and increase cardiac output and blood pressure.

(1) Shift of fluid from *(blood into interstitium = third spacing?)* *(interstitium into blood?)*.

(2) Renal retention of fluid caused by renal vasoconstriction related to _____ nerves and the chemicals _____ and _____, and also caused by hormones _____ and _____.

(3) Hypothalamic responses that include _____ as well as release of the hormone _____.

(f) These compensatory mechanisms for shock tend to *(increase? decrease?)* preload and *(increase? decrease?)* afterload; if prolonged, they are likely to "become more trouble than they are worth."

B3. Describe effects of shock at the cellular level.

(a) Buildup of _____ acid in cells; this acid is a product of *(aerobic? anaerobic?)* metabolism.

(b) ATP levels *(increase? decrease?)*. One effect is failure of the _____-potassium pump. *(Na^+? K^+?)* tends to leak into cells, pulling water along. As a result, cells are injured by *(dehydration? swelling?)*. Lysosomal rupture releases _____ that further injure or kill cells.

B4. Refer to textbook Table 26-3. Circle signs and symptoms of mild or moderate shock due to blood loss.

(a) *(Brady? Tachy?)*cardia

(b) Vaso*(constriction? dilation?)* of vessels in GI tract and kidneys, as well as in skin that appears *(flushed? pale?)* and is *(dry? moist?)*

(c) *(Hypo? Hyper?)*tension

(d) *(Agitation? Stupor or coma?)*

(e) *(Increased? Decreased?)* urinary output

(f) *(Hunger? Thirst?)*

B5. Now underline answers to questions B4(a) through (f) that result from compensatory mechanisms rather than problems originating in the hypovolemic shock itself.

B6. Complete this exercise about Donald, age 24, who has lost about 1500 mL (about 3 pints) of blood in a motorcycle accident that occurred 2 hours earlier.

(a) Donald's hypovolemic shock is due to *(hemorrhage? third-spacing?)*. Because his total blood volume is reduced by ___%, he is likely to be in *(mild? moderate? severe?)* shock.

(b) Refer to textbook Figure 26-12. Which drops at a slower pace in hypovolemic shock? Donald's *(cardiac output? mean arterial pressure [MAP]?)*. Explain.

_____

_____

(c) Circle the treatment that would be **least** helpful for Donald?

(1) Antishock garments

(2) Administration of IV fluids

(3) Oxygen

(4) Vasodilators such as dopamine

(5) Elevation of his legs

(d) Drugs that stimulate vasoconstriction tend to *(mimic? oppose?)* sympathetic responses and affect *(α? β_1? β_2?)* receptors on blood vessels

B7. In distributive shock, total blood volume is *(increased? decreased? normal?)* but venous return *(increases? decreases?)* as blood vessels *(constrict? dilate?)* excessively. This type of shock results from *(increased? decreased?)* sympathetic nerve activity or from release of vaso-*(constrictor? dilator?)* chemicals.

Circle the types of shock that are forms of distributive shock.

Anaphylactic	Cardiogenic
Hypovolemic	Neurogenic
Obstructive	Septic

B8. Ms. Fern is a nurse who has developed hypersensitivity to latex. Complete this exercise about her.

(a) Exposure to latex causes her cells to release the chemical _____, which is a vasodilator. It also *(increases? decreases?)* permeability of blood vessels. As a result, her blood pressure *(increases? decreases?)* and blotchy red spots appear on her skin. These are _____.

(b) Ms. Fern experiences bronchospasm and dyspnea. Explain.

_____

(c) Epinephrine is administered quickly. How does this help?

_____

B9. Identify the type of shock in each case below. Choose from the list of answers to question B7.

(a) Severe burns with "third-spacing":

_____

(b) Brain injury that injures sympathetic nerves: _____

(c) Prolonged vomiting or diarrhea:

_____

(d) The most common form of distributive shock, it has a mortality rate of about 40%: _____

(e) Allergic reaction to shrimp or bee stings:

_____

(f) MI leading to congestive heart failure (CHF): _____

(g) Cardiac tamponade: _____

(h) Pulmonary embolism: _____

(i) Low blood glucose (hypoglycemia) resulting from an insulin reaction:

_____

B10. Mr. Chabot, age 92, has sepsis involving gram-negative bacteria probably introduced to his blood stream through an infection from his indwelling catheter. The microbes trigger release of cytokines from his immune system, including _____, _____, and _____.

Fill in these blanks, then circle all of the signs or symptoms that are likely to be seen in Mr. Chabot.

(a) Temperature of 96.0°F

(b) Skin pallor

(c) Cool, clammy skin

(d) Inappropriate behavior

(e) Hypotension

(f) Blood cultures positive for bacteria

(g) Hyperventilation

(h) Leukocytopenia

C. COMPLICATIONS OF SHOCK (pages 568–570)

C1. Betsy, age 32, has third-stage hypovolemic shock resulting from severe burns suffered in a house fire 10 days ago. Describe her complications of shock in this exercise.

(a) Ischemia of kidneys for _____ is known to destroy renal function.

(1) 1 to 2 minutes

(2) 15 to 20 minutes

(3) 12 to 18 hours

(4) 3 to 4 days

Explain why acute renal failure often accompanies shock. _____

_____

How can Betsy's renal function be assessed?

_____

_____

(b) Betsy has developed a bleeding peptic ulcer. Explain. _____

_____

_____

(c) ARDS is an acronym for a_____ r_____ d_____ s_____.
Typically signs of it begin about 1 to 2 *(hours? days? weeks?)* after the original trauma. ARDS damage to Betsy's lungs makes them *(stiffer? more compliant?)*. ARDS *(is? is not?)* usually fatal. See Study Guide Chapter 29, question D10, for more on ARDS.

(d) Betsy is at increased risk for DIC which occurs in about _____% of septic clients. See Study Guide Chapter 14, question C6, on DIC.

C2. MODS is an acronym for m_____ o_____ d_____ s_____. This condition is most likely to occur in the state of *(compensated? decompensated?)* shock. Mortality due to MODS *(is? is not?)* directly related to number of organs affected. List several factors associated with shock that lead to MODS.

_____

_____

_____

D. CIRCULATORY FAILURE IN CHILDREN AND THE ELDERLY (pages 570-574)

D1. Ashley, age 2 months, has right-sided failure resulting from a ventricular septal defect (VSD). Currently, she has no respiratory infection.

(a) Circle the signs and symptoms likely to be present in Ashley.

(1) Ascites

(2) Bradycardia

(3) Ankle edema

(4) Dyspnea

(5) Oliguria

(6) Fatigue

(7) Gallop rhythm

(8) Use of her accessory muscles while breathing

(9) Jugular vein distention

(10) Grunt on inspiration

(11) Warm hands and feet

(12) Slow feeding

(13) Hepatomegaly

(b) Ashley is weighed daily. Explain why.

_____

(c) Circle those treatments that are likely to be used to treat Ashley.

Digoxin   Dilators
Diuretics   Oxygen
Small, frequent meals by tube feeding
Supine (lying flat, face up) positioning

D2. Choose the two true statements.

(a) Congenital heart defects are the **most common** cause of congestive heart failure (CHF) in children.

(b) Congestive heart failure is a **rare** cause of disability in elderly.

(c) With aging, blood vessels tend to become **stiffer**, which **increases** afterload.

(d) **Complete bed rest** is usually advised for elderly persons with CHF.

(e) Age-related cardiovascular changes **are** in themselves sufficient to cause heart failure.

CHAPTER 27

Control of Respiratory Function

■ **Review Questions**

A. STRUCTURAL ORGANIZATION OF THE RESPIRATORY SYSTEM (pages 577–583)

A1. Refer to Figure 27-1 below and label steps 1 to 3 in respiration. Use these terms:

Diffusion of gases   Pulmonary perfusion   Ventilation

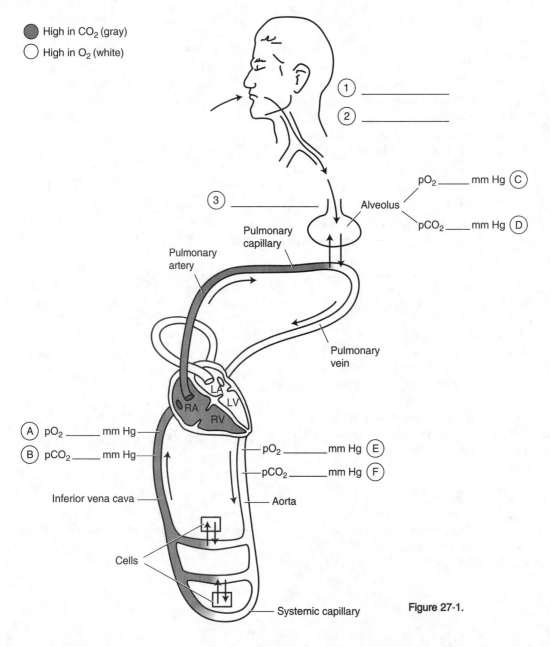

● High in CO_2 (gray)

○ High in O_2 (white)

① _____

② _____

③ _____

pO_2 _____ mm Hg Ⓒ

pCO_2 _____ mm Hg Ⓓ

Alveolus

Pulmonary capillary

Pulmonary artery

Pulmonary vein

LA

LV

RA

RV

Ⓐ pO_2 _____ mm Hg

Ⓑ pCO_2 _____ mm Hg

pO_2 _____ mm Hg Ⓔ

pCO_2 _____ mm Hg Ⓕ

Inferior vena cava

Aorta

Cells

Systemic capillary

Figure 27-1.

A2. Arrange in correct sequence the structures through which the air you breathe normally passes as you inhale.

Alveolar ducts	Alveolar sacs
Bronchi	Bronchioles
Larynx	Nose or Mouth
Pharynx	Trachea

_____ → _____ →
_____ → _____ →
_____ → _____ →
_____ → _____

A3. Dr. Kirkland has a tracheostomy tube through which air enters his trachea. What functions of his upper airways must mechanical equipment replace for Dr. Kirkland?

_____
_____
_____

A4. Alan smokes 2.5 packs a day (ppd). Write two or more effects of cigarette smoke on Alan's airways.

_____
_____
_____

A5. Which structure listed in Question A2 is common to both the respiratory system and the digestive system? Explain the significance of this anatomical arrangement.

_____
_____
_____

A6. Which structure listed in Question A2 functions both in speech and as the "watchdog of the lungs?" _____ The space between the vocal folds is known as the *(glottis? epiglottis?).* The *(cricoid? epiglottis? thyroid?)* cartilage is a leaf-shaped structure that normally prevents food or liquids from entering airways during swallowing.

A7. Choose the two true statements.

(a) Vocal cords are located in the **pharynx**.

(b) During the Valsalva maneuver, bradycardia **precedes** tachycardia.

(c) In the tracheobronchial tree there are typically **23** levels of branching.

(d) The **carina** is the point at which the trachea divides into the two primary bronchi.

A8. Lorie has aspirated a small piece of candy. Dr. Lennon expects to find it in the right bronchus rather than the left. Why?

_____
_____
_____

A9. The walls of bronchioles *(do? do not?)* have cartilage rings. How is this fact significant during an asthma attack?

_____
_____
_____

A10. Choose the two true statements about lungs.

(a) The **base** of each lung lies on the diaphragm.

(b) Lungs produce angiotensin-converting enzyme (ACE) that helps to **raise** blood pressure.

(c) Respiratory bronchioles are part of the **conducting zone** of the respiratory system.

(d) **Type I** alveolar cells produce surfactant that tends to cause alveoli to **collapse**.

A11. *(Bronchial? Pulmonary?)* arteries supply lungs with blood that is high in O_2 and low in CO_2.

A12. Ms. Espada has a diagnosis of "pleural effusions." This means that she has an abnormal amount of fluid in her:

Pleural cavity	Parietal pleura
Visceral pleura	

Now arrange the three answers above from most superficial to deepest:
_____ → _____ → _____

B. EXCHANGE OF GASES BETWEEN THE ATMOSPHERE AND LUNGS (pages 583-592)

B1. Complete this exercise about gases.

(a) The atmosphere around you contains enough gaseous molecules to exert pressure on a column of mercury (Hg) to make it rise _____ mm. The atmosphere is said to have a pressure of 760 mm Hg (or about _____ inches).

(b) Air is almost 80% nitrogen and about 20% _____. Calculate the PO_2 in the atmosphere: 760 mm Hg $\times$ 0.20 = _____ mm Hg. To what does the "P" in PO_2 refer? _____

(c) Heidi is placed on 60% oxygen to help her get adequate oxygen while she has pneumonia. She will now breathe (2? 3? 5?) times the amount of oxygen in environmental air, or a pressure of _____ mm Hg. Paul has an anaerobic bacterial infection for which he is placed in a hyperbaric chamber with 3 atmospheres of pressure. The amount of pressure on his body will be 760 mm Hg per 1 atmosphere × 3 atmospheres = _____ mm Hg.

(d) Besides nitrogen and oxygen, which other gas normally comprises a major amount of alveolar air? 47 mm Hg worth of _____ and a negligible amount of CO_2. Jillian is sitting outside on a hot, humid day. The air has 90% humidity. Which is likely to have a higher humidity? (The atmosphere? Alveoli in Jillian's lungs?)

B2. Answer these questions about pressure by inserting one of the two following terms. Intrapleural or Intrapulmonary (or intraalveolar)

(a) Which pressure is inside of airways and alveoli? _____

(b) Which pressure is that found between the parietal and visceral pleurae? _____ This value is normally always (positive? negative?). Explain why. _____ _____

(c) Which pressure is likely to be the higher value? _____

(d) Which pressures increase during forced expiration? _____

B3. Answer these questions about ventilation.

(a) The chest cavity is a(n) (open? closed?) cavity. Name the structures that form it. _____ _____ Normally the one opening into this cavity is the _____.

(b) Circle the principal muscle(s) involved in ventilation. (Diaphragm? Intercostals?) The nerve supply to this muscle mass consists of the (phrenic? intercostal?) nerves, which are derived from the mid(cervical? thoracic?) portion of the spinal cord. Contraction of this muscle causes the diaphragm to move (superiorly? inferiorly? laterally?) about (1 mm? 1 cm? 10 cm?) with each normal inspiration.

(c) As these muscles contract, the volume of the thorax and lungs (increases? decreases?), whereas the pressure within these closed spaces (increases? decreases?). As a result, air is (pushed out of? sucked into?) lungs; this process is ___spiration.

(d) Expiration is a(n) (active? passive?) process in which the diaphragm (contracts? relaxes?) and moves (down? up?), causing pressures within the chest to (increase? decrease?), and air is (pushed out of? sucked into?) lungs. This process is normally assisted by elastic _____ of lungs.

(e) (External? Internal?) intercostal muscles aid in (ex? in?)spiration because they help to (lift? lower?) ribs. ___ternal intercostals have the opposite effect during ___spiration.

B4. Mrs. Villella has advanced emphysema. She sits on the side of her bed, with arms braced on a bedside table, breathing with pursed lips, and using her accessory muscles to help her exhale. Name the accessory muscles that aid expiration. _____ _____

B5. Complete this exercise about lung compliance.

(a) Compliance means (ease of? resistance to?) inflation. Which type of balloon has more compliance? A balloon that:

(1) Is new and has never been inflated

(2) Has been inflated 50 times

(b) Explain why lungs are likely to be less compliant than normal in the following persons.

(1) Baby Anastasia is born at 27 weeks' gestation rather the normal 38 to 40 weeks:_____ Anastasia's condition is known as _____

(2) Mr. Wzolek, a coal miner for 35 years, has "black lung" with carbon particles and fibers in his lung interstitium. _____

B6. Choose the two true statements about surfactant in lungs.

(a) Surfactant **lowers** surface tension, and **increases** lung compliance.

(b) Surfactant is made primarily of **carbohydrates**.

(c) This chemical has hydrophilic ends pointing toward the **inside** of alveoli.

(d) Surfactant causes alveoli to be **wetter**.

(e) Without surfactant, alveoli with the **smallest** diameter would collapse sooner than larger alveoli.

B7. Circle the correct answers or fill in the blanks about air flow within lungs.

(a) Resistance to air flow is greater in *(small? large?)* airways. This is a statement of *(Laplace's? Poiseuille's?)* law.

(b) Resistance to air flow is normally greater during *(in? ex?)*spiration; it is also greater if airways are partially blocked by mucus. For these reasons, asthmatics typically have more difficulty during ___spiration.

(c) Turbulence is likely to be greater in *(bronchioles? trachea and bronchi?)* because of the *(larger? smaller?)* diameter there. As a result of this turbulence, respiratory sounds are heard when a stethoscope is placed over the *(bronchioles? trachea and bronchi?)*.

(d) Airways collapse when *(compressing? distending?)* pressure is excessively high.

B8. Choose the term from this list that best fits each description. (The second blank line will be used for Question B9). (*Hint*: it may help to refer to Figure 27-18 and Table 27-1 in the textbook.)

Expiratory reserve volume
Inspiratory reserve volume
Functional residual capacity
Minute volume
Residual volume
Total lung capacity
Tidal volume
Vital capacity

(a) A normal breath: _____; 500 mL

(b) The maximal amount of air that a healthy adult can exhale after taking in the largest possible breath (IRV + TV + ERV): _____; _____ mL

(c) The volume of air remaining in lungs at the end of a normal exhalation that can be used to oxygenate blood prior to the next inhalation: _____; _____ mL

(d) Tidal volume × respiratory rate: _____; _____ mL

B9. Fill in the normal volumes for each answer in B8. The first one is done for you.

B10. Choose the two true statements.

(a) A **spirometer** is used primarily to measure **heart rate**. _____

(b) $FEV_{1.0}$ is measured in seconds (or fractions of seconds) rather than in volume (mL or liters)

(c) An emphysemic (who has difficulty with exhalation) is likely to have a **decreased** $FEV_{1.0}$.

(d) Persons with stiff, noncompliant lungs tend to breathe at a **faster** rate, taking more **shallow** breaths.

C. EXCHANGE AND TRANSPORT OF GASES (pages 592–599)

C1. Discuss ventilation and perfusion in this exercise.

(a) As you sit in a chair, which part of each of your lungs is likely to ventilate better? *(Apex? Base?)*. Explain.

_____

_____

(b) If you lie on your back, which parts of your lungs will inflate better? *(Posterior or dependent? Anterior or nondependent?)* Explain. _____

_____

(c) Perfusion refers to *(air? blood?)* flow through a capillary bed. Based on gravity, which part of the lungs is likely to perfuse better? *(Apex? Base?)*

(d) Pulmonary blood vessels offer *(greater? less?)* resistance to flow than systemic vessels do. Explain why. _____

_____

(e) Consequently, the pulmonary vessels have much *(more? less?)* pressure than systemic vessels. A typical pulmonary artery BP is ____/____ mm Hg versus ____/____ mm Hg for major systemic arteries.

(f) For blood to move through lungs, BP must be greater in the pulmonary *(artery? vein?)* than in the pulmonary *(artery? vein?)*. Which is more likely to increase pressure in pulmonary veins and lead to pulmonary edema? Failure of the *(right? left?)* ventricle. Explain._____

_____

_____

C2. When lung tissue is hypoxic, pulmonary blood vessels vaso-*(constrict? dilate?)*. Circle the correct answer in the preceding sentence and then describe the "good news" and "bad news" of this response.

(a) Good news:

_____

_____

_____

(b) Bad news:

_____

_____

_____

C3. Match the clinical cases below that relate to each of the four factors from Fick's law describing diffusion across the alveolar-capillary membrane.

Diffusion distance
Partial pressure of gases
Surface area for gas exchange
Solubility and molecular weight of gases

(a) Mrs. Westerfield was diagnosed with emphysema 6 years ago:

_____

(b) Mr. Frederick has interstitial viral pneumonia: _____

(c) Nina is hiking at 10,000 feet:

_____

(d) Senator Reider has left-sided heart failure causing pulmonary edema. Her arterial PO_2 is greatly decreased, but her PCO_2 is only slightly elevated: _____

C4. In a normal breath, Jules, a healthy 19-year-old, inspires 500 mL; this is a normal _____ volume. Typically, about *(150? 350?)* mL will reach his alveoli (alveolar ventilation). The remaining _____ mL, known as _____ dead space, never gets into his conducting airways.

C5. In Question C1, you examined the ventilation and perfusion of lungs. Match either **dead air**

space or **shunt** with related descriptions below in which these two volumes are mismatched. (Refer to textbook Figure 27-21)

(a) Ventilation without perfusion (air without blood). Example: pulmonary embolism:

_____

(b) Perfusion without ventilation (blood without air). Example: atelectasis:

_____

C6. Nina's newborn has the congenital heart defect known as tetralogy of Fallot. The baby is a "blue baby" because blood is passing from right to left ventricle through a defect in the ventricular septum without passing through pulmonary vessels. This baby has *(ventilation without perfusion? perfusion without ventilation?)*.

C7. Refer to Figure 27-1 and complete this exercise about gas transport within blood.

(a) By the time blood leaves the pulmonary capillary bed to enter pulmonary veins, the left side of the heart, the aorta and then other large arteries, the levels of PO_2 and PCO_2 are *(higher than? lower than? about the same as?)* levels of those gases in alveoli.

(b) Fill in values for PO_2 and PCO_2 on the figure at (A-F).

(c) When Jeremy has arterial blood gases (ABG) checked, blood is likely to be drawn from the _____ artery in his wrist. His arterial PO_2 is 50 mm Hg, and his is PCO_2 48 mm Hg. Are these typical values for a healthy adult?

(d) Normally, more than ____% of O_2 is carried in blood attached to hemoglobin (Hb) in red blood cells. Each Hb has ____ sites known as hemes, where O_2 can bind. If all Hbs had 3 of the 4 Hbs "saturated" with O_2, then the O_2 saturation (SO_2) would be ____%. This is a normal SO_2 for *(arterial? venous?)* blood. SO_2 for arterial blood is typically ___%.

(e) Only about 1% of O_2 is dissolved in _____. This amount can be increased when a person is exposed to a _____ chamber, for example, when Hb is permanently bound to CO (_____).

(f) Visualize your muscles when you are actively exercising. List several changes in active muscle tissue that will cause O_2 to detach from Hb, enter plasma, and soon reach your active muscles. Refer to textbook

Figure 27-22. _____
_____

In exercising muscles, the O_2-Hb dissociation curve shifts to the *(left? right?)*, indicating that *(more? less?)* O_2 is detaching from Hb and oxygenating tissues at any given level of PO_2.

(g) Figure 27-22 points out that *(PO_2? SO_2?)* may reach lower levels that are still compatible with life than are possible for *(PO_2? SO_2?)*. Which value can reach levels greater than 100? *(PO_2? SO_2?)*

C8. Complete this exercise about transport of carbon dioxide (CO_2).

(a) Most CO_2 is typically carried in blood:

   (1) As dissolved CO_2

   (2) As bicarbonate

   (3) On hemoglobin (Hb)

(b) Write the chemical formulas for:

   (1) Carbonic acid: _____

   (2) Bicarbonate: _____

(c) Show how bicarbonate is formed in blood by filling in the blanks in Study Guide Figure 27-2 below.

(d) What is the role of the enzyme carbonic anhydrase in the reaction shown in that figure?

_____
_____

(e) The reactions in that figure demonstrate that the increase in CO_2 in the body (as in most respiratory disorders) will tend to cause a(n) *(increase? decrease?)* in acid (H^+) in the body.

(f) What percentage of CO_2 is carried in blood as carbaminohemoglobin (Hb-CO_2)? ___ %

D. CONTROL OF BREATHING (pages 599-604)

D1. Choose an answer from the following list to show the primary location of the respiratory control.

(a) Basal ganglia

(b) Brain stem

(c) Cerebral cortex

(d) Limbic system

D2. Choose the two true statements:

(a) The **pneumotaxic** center stimulates inspiration and tends to cause prolonged inspirations.

(b) Hypoxia serves as the **main** stimulus of respiration in normal, healthy persons.

(c) Chemoreceptors that sense elevation in CO_2 are **central** (rather than **peripheral**) receptors.

(d) Chemoreceptors that sense hypoxia are those that are in the **aortic** and **carotid bodies**.

D3. Mr. Friday has chronic obstructive pulmonary disease (COPD). His chart indicates that his oxygen should be administered at 1 to 2 L/minute. Why not administer oxygen at 5 L/minute so that Mr. Friday will feel better faster?

_____
_____
_____

D4. Complete this exercise on reflexes involving the respiratory system.

(a) As you take a deep breath, visualize the *(irritant? J? stretch?)* receptors in your airways that are being stimulated. These will inhibit *(in? ex?)*spiration and promote *(in? ex?)*spiration. This is called the _____ reflex.

(b) The cough reflex is triggered by receptors in the *(alveoli? pharynx? trachea and bronchi?)*. Irritating substances there initiate nerve impulses along the _____ nerves to the cough center located in the *(hypothalamus? medulla? midbrain?)*.

D5. List several reasons that might account for Roseanna's lack of a cough reflex.

_____
_____
_____

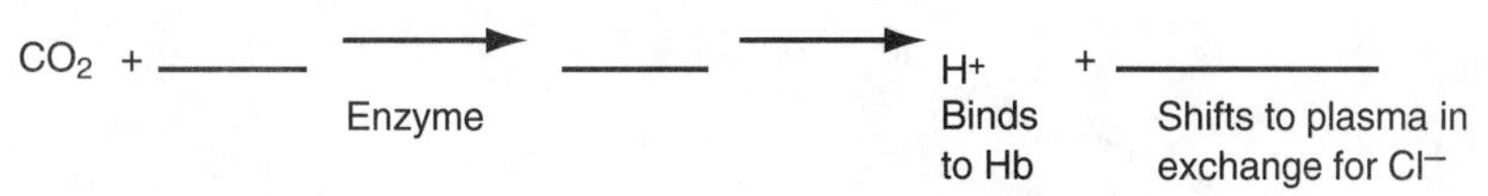

CO_2 + _____ $\xrightarrow{\text{Enzyme}}$ _____ $\longrightarrow$ H^+ Binds to Hb + _____ Shifts to plasma in exchange for Cl^-

Figure 27-2.

D6. Define dyspnea.

_____

_____

_____

Describe several mechanisms that may explain dyspnea. _____

_____

_____

How can dyspnea be assessed?

_____

_____

_____

D7. Contrast *tachypnea* with *hyperventilation*.

_____

_____

_____

Alterations in Respiratory Function: Respiratory Tract Infections, Neoplasms, and Childhood Disorders

■ Review Questions

A. RESPIRATORY TRACT INFECTIONS
(pages 605–621)

A1. Circle the correct answers in this exercise.

(a) *(Bacteria? Viruses?)* are the most common cause of respiratory tract infections.

(b) *(The common cold? Influenza or "flu"?)* is the most common viral infection of the respiratory tract. Most adults have *(2-4? 8-10?)* colds per year.

(c) The common cold is known to be caused by *(one specific virus? more than 200 types of viruses?)*. In persons 5 to 40 years of age, the *(adeno? corona? rhino?)*virus most commonly causes colds.

(d) Cold viruses *(can? cannot?)* live on hard surfaces. Colds are spread primarily by *(coughing or sneezing? infected fingers?)*.

(e) Effective vaccines for the common cold *(have? have not?)* been developed. Explain.

_____

_____

A2. Explain the importance of hand washing in preventing colds in yourself.

_____

_____

_____

A3. Circle the single best treatment for the common cold.

(a) Antibiotics

(b) Antihistamines

(c) Vitamin C

(d) Decongestants

(e) Rest and drugs that reduce fever

A4. Mrs. Kelley has right maxillary sinusitis. Complete this exercise about her condition.

(a) Arrange sinuses according to location from most superior to most inferior:

Ethmoid and sphenoid Frontal Maxillary

_____, _____,

_____

(b) All of these sinuses are known as _____ sinuses; they drain into the _____. Explain how nasal polyps can interfere with drainage.

_____

_____

(c) These sinuses are lined with _____ membranes that *(do? do not?)* have cilia. Sinuses normally *(do? do not?)* have microbes present on the mucosa.

(d) Mrs. Kelley has had her sinusitis for 2 weeks; her condition is classified as *(acute? subacute? chronic?)* sinusitis. At this point, she *(is? is not?)* likely to experience irreversible changes of the lining of her sinuses.

(e) Circle the manifestations Mrs. Kelley is likely to exhibit.

(1) Pain in her right cheek

(2) Pain in her upper right teeth

(3) Pain in the right side of her forehead

(4) Increased headache when she bends forward

(5) A sense of fullness in the ears

(f) Circle the two most likely treatments for Mrs. Kelley at this point:

(1) Antibiotics

(2) Antihistamines

(3) Decongestants

(4) Surgery

A5. Ms. Drach, age 69 years, lives in her own home. She was infected with the flu on March 1 during a visit from her brother who had the flu. Complete this exercise about her.

(a) The virus is most likely to incubate until March ___ when symptoms begin *(rapidly? insidiously?)*. Ms. Drach probably will be contagious from about March ___ until March ___.

(b) List several symptoms of the flu.

_____

_____

(c) Ms. Drach's symptoms are likely to peak on about March ____ and disappear by about March ____.

(d) She is more likely to develop viral pneumonia if the infection begins by:

(1) Large droplet spray in the nose or throat or infection from fingers

(2) Small droplets that directly infect lungs before immune defenses can be built up

(e) Circle appropriate treatments for Ms. Drach beginning on March 4:

(1) Antibiotics

(2) Rest

(3) Cooling the body

(4) Drinking fluids

(f) It *(is? is not?)* advisable for Ms. Drach to get a flu shot. Once she does, she should get another flu shot *(each fall? in 5 years?)*.

A6. Choose the two true statements about influenza or "the flu."

(a) Almost all persons who die of influenza in the United States are **children**.

(b) Influenza is more commonly caused by the type B virus.

(c) The influenza vaccine **is** considered safe for pregnant women.

(d) The flu vaccine should **not** be taken by persons who are allergic to **eggs**.

A7. Complete this exercise about pneumonias.

(a) Circle the structures that are infected in pneumonia:

Alveoli   Bronchioles

Bronchi   Larynx

Pharynx (throat)

(b) Pneumonia *(is? is not?)* a common cause of death in the United States.

(c) List two causes of pneumonia other than infection.

_____

_____

(d) The presence of bacteria in lungs normally does not cause infection. State three reasons why such infection might occur.

_____

_____

(e) List examples of host defenses, which, if inadequate, can "invite" pneumonia.

_____

_____

A8. Ms. Drach (Question A5) developed a secondary bacterial infection superimposed on her flu. Answer these questions about her.

(a) She is admitted to the medical unit with pneumonia on March 9 because her brother is concerned that "she just isn't acting right—she seems a little incoherent and she hasn't had a thing to eat in 2 days." She has *(community? hospital?)*-acquired pneumonia that is classified as category *(2? 3? 4?)* pneumonia according to American Thoracic Society Guidelines.

(b) The most likely bacteria to cause her pneumonia are *(Streptococcus? Klebsiella?)* *pneumoniae*. These microbes also are known as _____cocci. These are gram-*(positive? negative?)* bacteria with virulence based largely on the presence of a polysaccharide _____.

(c) It is likely that her oxygen saturation of hemoglobin is *(increased? decreased?)* and her respiratory rate *(increased? decreased?)*. Lung consolidation *(is? is not?)* likely to occur. (See textbook Figure 28-2A.)

(d) Explain why sputum or bronchoscopy samples are likely to be obtained.

_____

_____

(e) To what does the "23-valent" pneumococcal vaccine refer?

_____

_____

Is Ms. Drach in a category of persons who should receive this vaccine?

_____

A9. Tabatha, age 4 years, has a diagnosis of sickle cell anemia. Explain why she is at increased risk for pneumococcal pneumonia.

_____

_____

_____

A10. Legionnaire's disease is a *(common? rare?)* community-acquired pneumonia. The gram-*(positive? negative?)* microbe can be found *(only in the human body? in warm, standing water?)*. Explain the derivation of the name "Legionnaire's disease."

_____

_____

_____

A11. Mr. Lungren, age 75 years, was admitted July 21 with dyspnea related to cancer of the pleura (mesothelioma). He has chest tubes draining excessive pleural fluid. On July 28, he received a diagnosis of pneumonia. Based on the timing of its onset, Mr. Lungren has *(community? hospital?)*-acquired pneumonia. It also is called _____. Almost all of such pneumonias are *(bacterial? viral?)*.

A12. Identify the type of immunodeficiency most likely in each of these cases.

Bacteria (B) *Staph aureus, Aspergillus, Candida,* or gram-negative bacilli (SACG) Viral, fungal, mycoplasmal, or protozoan (VFMP)

(a) Franklin has neutropenia: _____

(b) Grace's antibody production is deficient:

_____

(c) Erich has a T4 count of 148 as a result of his HIV infection: _____

A13. Choose the three true statements about *Pneumocystis carinii* pneumonia (PCP).

(a) PCP is caused by **bacteria.**

(b) PCP occurs at some time during the course of AIDS in **most** patients with AIDS.

(c) The onset of PCP is **gradual** with a **low fever, dyspnea,** and a **nonproductive cough.**

(d) Diagnosis involves microscopic identification of **boat-shaped cysts** from lungs.

(e) Children with HIV **rarely** contract PCP.

(f) Prophylactic treatment for PCP **is** recommended for many HIV-infected adults.

A14. Complete this exercise about tuberculosis (TB) infection.

(a) TB is a *(rare? common?)* disorder globally. Its incidence is greater in *(crowded? sparsely populated?)* communities because this *(is? is not?)* an airborne infection.

(b) TB bacteria are resistant largely because of the *(capsules? spores?)* that they form. This structure helps make these microbes identifiable by _____ staining.

(c) Which organs are most affected by *Mycobacterium tuberculosis hominis?* _____ TB in other organs is known as _____ TB. A form of TB known as MAC or *Mycobacterium* _____-*intracellulare* complex particularly affects lungs and the *(gastrointestinal? urinary?)* tract of persons living with HIV.

(d) TB bacteria harm lungs by:

(1) Direct destruction of lung tissue

(2) Initiating hypersensitivity responses that lead to chronic granulomatous lung inflammation

A15. Arrange in correct sequence the events in a primary TB infection.

(a) Engulfment of TB bacilli by macrophages in which the microbes slowly grow for up to 3 months

(b) Embedding of TB bacilli in the distal airways or alveoli

(c) Inhalation of droplet nuclei containing the TB bacillus

(d) Presentation of TB bacilli antigens to T cells as part of a cell-mediated response

(e) Lesions known as *Ghon's foci* form from TB bacilli, macrophages, and T cells

(f) Caseous necrosis of *Ghon's foci* and migration into lymph nodes leads to *Ghon's complexes.*

___ ___ ___ ___ ___ ___

A16. Complete the following exercise about TB.

(a) Explain why immunosuppressed persons such as those with AIDS are more likely to develop active cases of tuberculosis.

_____

_____

_____

_____

(b) Describe how chest x-rays can reveal a history of TB._____

_____

_____

(c) Contrast symptoms of primary TB to those of progressive primary or reactivated TB.

_____

_____

_____

(d) Describe the Mantoux (or ppd) test for TB.

_____

_____

_____

(e) What does a positive tuberculin test indicate? _____

_____

_____

_____

(f) Immunodeficient persons who have been exposed to TB are likely to have false-*(positive? negative?)* reactions known as anergy.

(g) How can results from (f) be verified?

_____

_____

(h) What is isoniazid (INH)? _____

_____

_____

TB drug therapy is typically *(long? short?)*-term. Explain why multidrug regimens are used. _____

_____

_____

A17. Select the fungal infection that fits each description.

Blastomycosis   Coccidioidomycosis
Histoplasmosis

(a) Distinctive among fungal infections by its productive cough and purulent sputum and by the fact that a skin test is not available; may spread to skin, bones, or prostate:

_____

(b) The most common fungal infection in the U.S., present in about 20% of the population; found especially in river valleys; the fungus grows well in soil:

_____

(c) About two of five infected persons have symptoms, and those resemble manifestations of TB; like TB, the infection

involves a delayed hypersensitivity response for which there is a skin test:

_____

(d) Present in soil and dust; most prevalent in the southwest and Texas; may affect lungs, skin ("desert bumps"), or joints ("desert arthritis"); rarely disseminates to other organs: _____

B. CANCER OF THE LUNG (pages 621–623)

B1. Complete the following exercise about Mr. Polk, age 62 years, who has lung cancer.

(a) He has the *(leading? fourth leading?)* cause of cancer deaths in the United States.

(b) Mr. Polk was an asbestos worker for 30 years; he smoked for 45 years and stopped smoking last year. About *(20%? 50%? 80%?)* of lung cancer causes are associated with smoking. Because of being a smoker in his profession, Mr. Polk's risk of having lung cancer develop was _____ to _____ times greater than that for nonsmoker asbestos workers.

(c) Mr. Polk has high levels of ADH and ACTH. Explain._____

_____

_____

(d) Sharp, severe chest pain *(is? is not?)* a typical early symptom of lung cancer. Write several early manifestations that Mr. Polk is likely to experience. _____

_____

_____

_____

(e) Mr. Polk's chart indicates that he exhibits these additional signs of lung cancer. Describe them.

(e1) Hemoptysis _____

(e2) Hoarseness _____

(f) Mr. Polk's presenting symptoms were pain in his right hip and thigh, which led to evidence of metastasis in these bones. Explain the clinical significance.

_____

_____

(g) High levels of CEA correlate to *(localized? metastasized?)* disease.

(h) Overall, the 5-year survival rate for individuals with lung cancer is about _____%.

B2. Match the types of lung cancer to the related descriptions.

Adenocarcinoma   Large cell carcinoma
Small cell carcinoma   Squamous cell carcinoma

(a) Mr. Polk's carcinoma is a type found commonly in male smokers; it started in his right bronchus, and carcinoma cells eventually were identified in his sputum:

_____

(b) Highly anaplastic (poorly differentiated); this type of lung cancer metastasizes early:

_____

(c) Mrs. Jordan has this type of cancer, which is common in women; she was never a smoker. The cancer started in her smallest airways (bronchioles) and her alveoli:

_____

(d) Which type of lung cancer is not staged by the TNM method? _____

(e) Which two types of lung cancer are associated with the best prognosis because they are less likely to spread?

_____ ,

_____

C. RESPIRATORY DISORDERS IN CHILDREN (pages 623–632)

C1. Choose the three true statements about lung development.

(a) Lungs mature **faster** than most other organs of the body.

(b) Lungs develop embryologically as outgrowths of the **esophagus**.

(c) Lungs typically **are** developed sufficiently so that they are capable of adequate respiration to permit survival by 25 to 28 weeks of gestation.

(d) **Type I** alveolar cells produce surfactant.

(e) The alveolar-capillary membrane normally grows **thinner** by the end of gestation.

(f) Normally all 300 million alveoli are present in lungs by **the time of birth**.

C2. Circle correct answers in each statement.

(a) Just before birth, an infant's lungs normally are filled with (air? fluid?).

(b) Fetal breathing movements begin (before? after?) birth.

(c) A newborn's chest wall and lungs normally are (compliant? stiff or rigid?). This factor typically makes the neonate's breathing (easier? more difficult?).

(d) Chest retractions are (normal? abnormal?) movements of the chest wall during (expiration? inspiration?).

(e) Adult arterial PO_2 is about _____ mm Hg. This value is _____ mm Hg in a fetus, and about _____ mm Hg in a neonate.

C3. Contrast respiratory disorders in three children, all 13 months old.

(a) Paulette's respirations are shallow and 38 breaths per minute. She emits audible grunts on expiration. It is likely that she has a(n) (obstructive? restrictive?) lung disorder because she cannot adequately inflate her lungs. How does the grunting help her?

_____

_____

(b) Paul has bronchial asthma, which is an (extra? intra?)thoracic disorder characterized by (crowing or stridor? wheezing or whistling?) as airways collapse during ____spiration.

(c) Patrice has croup, which is a(n) (obstructive? restrictive?) lung disorder that is (extra? intra?)thoracic. Her respiratory rate is likely to be (faster? slower?) than normal because her ____spirations are prolonged. Sounds she makes during inspiration are known as _____.

C4. Zachariah is born by cesarean section at 26 weeks of gestation. He is African American, and his mother has Type I diabetes mellitus.

(a) Circle the factors above that make Zachariah at high risk for respiratory distress syndrome (RDS).

(b) Surfactant (increases? decreases?) lung compliance, (increasing? decreasing?) the work of breathing. With surfactant deficiency, Zachariah is at (higher? lower?) risk for atelectasis.

(c) Explain why RDS is also called hyaline membrane disease._____

_____

_____

(d) Neonates with RDS typically (do? do not?) exhibit cyanosis and retractions. Grunting and _____pnea are likely to be present as indicators of (obstructive? restrictive?)

lung disorders. *Hint*: see Paulette in Question C3(a).

(e) Describe possible treatments for Zachariah's RDS.

———————————————————————

———————————————————————

C5. BPD refers to _____ dysplasia. What factor causes infants to be at high risk for BPD? _____ Explain why these infants typically develop signs of right-sided heart failure (cor pulmonale).

———————————————————————

———————————————————————

———————————————————————

C6. Respiratory infections are *(common? rare?)* in young children. List two reasons why.

———————————————————————

———————————————————————

———————————————————————

C7. Complete this exercise about croup.

(a) Croup most often occurs in children *(younger? older?)* than 5 years, and it is likely to be *(bacterial? viral?)*.

(b) Which form of croup is related to allergy and does not involve a fever?

(1) Spasmodic

(2) Viral

(c) Circle the interventions most likely to help a child with croup:

(1) Antibiotics

(2) Bronchodilators

(3) Exposure to cold air

(4) Being placed in a bathroom with the shower running

(5) Being placed in a supine position

C8. Distinguish characteristics of these three respiratory conditions in small children.

Bronchiolitis   Croup   Epiglottitis

(a) Caused by the bacterium *Hemophilus influenzae*: _____

(b) Most likely of these conditions to be fatal within hours of onset: _____

(c) The child has dysphagia and tends to assume a position sitting up with mouth open and chin thrust forward:
_____

(d) Most likely to occur in the trachea:
_____

(e) Prolonged expiration with wheezing is a typical sign: _____

(f) Breathlessness, rapid breathing, and retractions of lower ribs and sternum occur in young infants with the disorder:
_____

(g) A barking cough and hoarseness are typical signs: _____

C9. Signs of impending respiratory failure can include:

(a) Very *(rapid? slow?)* respirations

(b) Very *(rapid? slow?)* heart rate

(c) *(Extreme agitation? Decreased level of consciousness?)*

CHAPTER 29

Alterations in Respiration: Alterations in Ventilation and Gas Exchange

■ Review Questions

A. DISORDERS OF LUNG INFLATION (pages 633-638)

A1. Review the pleural coverings over lungs, pleural cavity, and intrapleural pressure in Chapter 27, Questions A12 and B2(b).

A2. Mr. Martini has chest pain in the lower left region of the chest. His breathing is shallow, and he splints the left side of his chest while he breathes. He states that it hurts to take a deep breath or to cough. Based on this information, circle the most likely cause of his pain.

   (a) Bronchial irritation

   (b) Myocardial infection

   (c) Musculoskeletal pain

   (d) Pleural pain

A3. The pleura normally secretes a small amount (10 to 20 mL = _____ tsp) of *(mucous? serous?)* fluid into the pleural cavity. Pleural _____ is a term that means abnormal fluid in the pleural cavity. Identify four factors that cause edema that can also cause pleural effusions. (*Hint:* See Study Guide Chapter 21, Questions E3, E4, and E6.)

   _____

   _____

   _____

A4. Use the term that best fits the description below. One answer will be used twice.

   Chylothorax   Empyema
   Exudate   Hemothorax
   Hydrothorax   Pneumothorax

   (a) Conrad has three ribs fractured in a motorcycle accident. Three of his intercostal arteries bleed into the thoracic cavity (or pleural space): _____

   (b) Ms. Blanchard has a streptococcal infection of the lungs with rupture into the pleural space: _____

   (c) Lymph has accumulated in Mrs. Ivey's chest cavity because her lymph nodes are blocked by metastases: _____

   (d) Hospitalized for congestive heart failure, Mr. Schefflein has serous transudate in his pleural cavity: _____

   (e) Fibrothorax—with fusion of pleural layers—is a serious consequence of: _____

   _____

   (f) Air in the pleural cavity: _____

   _____

A5. Complete this exercise about pleural effusions.

   (a) The most common sign is _____. Other signs include _____ noted on percussion and *(normal? diminished?)* breath sounds.

   (b) Define thoracentesis. _____

   _____

A6. Contrast types of pneumothorax in this exercise.

   Spontaneous   Tension   Traumatic

   (a) Conrad's three fractured ribs (see Question A4[a]) have caused _____ pneumothorax; treatment involves insertion of a large-bore needle into the chest to allow lung reexpansion.

   (b) Mr. DePalma has a life-threatening condition in which air can enter but not leave the right side of his thorax; his trachea has shifted to the left, and his left lung has collapsed: _____

   (c) Mick, age 19, is 6′ 2″ tall and weighs 150 pounds. He has a ruptured air-filled bleb on the surface of his left lung:

   _____

A7. Circle all signs of tension pneumothorax.

(a) Decreased respiratory rate

(b) Decreased heart rate

(c) Diminished breath sounds

(d) Dyspnea

(e) Hypoxemia followed by vasoconstriction in the affected lung

A8. Identify the type of atelectasis in each case by writing "C" for compression or "O" for obstructive.

(a) Caused by mucus plug: ____

(b) Coughing and deep-breathing postsurgery are designed to prevent this type of atelectasis: ____

(c) Pleural effusions, hemothorax, pneumothorax, and tumor all lead to: ____

A9. Signs of atelectasis are typically *(similar to? different from?)* those of pneumothorax (see Question A7).

A10. Treatment for both atelectasis and pneumothorax are aimed at: _____

_____

.

B. OBSTRUCTIVE AIRWAY DISORDERS (pages 638-653)

B1. Choose the two true statements.

(a) People with obstructive airway disorders are likely to have more difficulty in **expiration** than with **inspiration**.

(b) Sympathetic stimulation tends to cause airways to **constrict**.

(c) Histamine causes airways to **constrict**.

(d) Incidence of bronchial asthma in the United States is **decreasing**.

B2. Describe bronchial asthma in this exercise.

(a) Asthma is a chronic *(inflammatory? noninflammatory?)* condition. Cough with asthma is typically worse *(in the afternoon? during the night?)*.

(b) The acute or early response typically occurs within ____ minutes of exposure to an allergen. Airborne antigens bind to *(epithelial? mast?)* cells coated with Ig __ antibodies lining airways. Chemical mediators are then released and cause the three major characteristics of bronchial asthma:

(1) Broncho-_____

(2) Mucosal edema related to increased _____ of mucosal blood vessels

(3) *(Increased? Decreased?)* mucus secretions. All of these effects lead to a(an) *(increase? decrease?)* in the diameter of airways.

(c) The late-phase response recruits more cells such as _____. Resulting chronic inflammation leads to changes that *(are always? may not be?)* reversible.

B3. Complete this exercise about triggers of asthma attacks.

(a) Asthma caused by inhaled allergens typically begins in *(younger? older?)* persons who *(do? do not?)* have a family history. List several common household allergens. _____

_____

_____

_____

(b) Exercise-induced asthma (EIA) is a *(rare? common?)* form of asthma and is more likely to occur when people exercise in a *(cold? warm?)* environment.

(c) Respiratory infections, especially those caused by *(bacteria? viruses?)* can lead to asthma attacks.

(d) List several examples of inhaled irritants that can cause such attacks. _____

_____

_____

(e) Emotional upsets *(do sometimes? are not known to?)* precipitate asthma attacks.

(f) List medications that can lead to these attacks. _____

`_____

B4. Besides those listed in Question B2(b), circle signs of asthma in the following list:

(a) Increased $FEV_{1.0}$

(b) Shortened expiration period

(c) Hyperinflation of lungs as more air is retained in lungs (FRC increases)

(d) Wheezing as air is exhaled through narrowed airways

(e) Increased forced vital capacity (FVC)

(f) Contraction of sternocleidomastoid muscles during ventilation

(g) Cough due to extra mucus production and irritated mucosa

(h) Dyspnea and fatigue

B5. Explain why chronic asthma increases the risk of right-sided congestive heart failure.

_____

_____

_____

B6. Jodi, age 14, has asthmatic symptoms about every other day with episodes at night about once a week. She has had to curtail participation in physical education classes. Her forced expiratory volume in 1 second is about 75% of normal levels.

(a) Jodi's asthma is classified as:

(1) Mild intermittent

(2) Mild persistent

(3) Moderate persistent

(4) Severe persistent

(b) Her PEF is currently about 75% of her "personal best." She is in the *(green? yellow? red?)* zone.

B7. Describe categories of treatments for asthma in this exercise.

(a) List several examples of how contributing factors may be controlled. _____

_____

(b) Medications for asthma include the following, many of which are administered by MDI or_____:

(1) Broncho-*(constrictors? dilators?)* that mimic *(sympathetic or adrenergic? parasympathetic or cholinergic?)* neurotransmitters or block _____ pathways. These drugs *(constrict? relax?)* smooth muscle of airways. To prevent toxic levels of these drugs (e.g., theophylline), _____ levels are checked regularly.

(2) Anti-_____ such as corticosteroids

(3) Another category of drugs known as _____ modifiers that inhibit synthesis or action of bronchoconstrictor chemicals released from the asthmatic person's own mast cells.

B8. Circle the risk factors for death from asthma listed in the following paragraph. Marisol has had four visits to the ER over the past year, one 3 weeks ago. She has been hospitalized once in the past year and that stay required intubation. Marisol uses one β_2-stimulator inhaler about every 3 weeks and she knows how to use a peak flow meter. From an upper-middle-class family with good health insurance, Marisol is a happy, sociable adolescent who does not smoke, drink alcohol, or use other illegal drugs.

B9. Circle the two true statements about asthma.

(a) Status asthmaticus refers to a **mild, chronic** form of asthma.

(b) Most asthma deaths have occurred **outside** the hospital.

(c) Asthma is a **rare** cause for admission to children's hospitals.

(d) Most children who develop asthma have symptoms **before** they reach school age.

B10. What signs might suggest onset of bronchial asthma in an 18-month-old child?

_____

_____

_____

B11. Discuss special delivery systems of asthma medications for young children.

_____

_____

_____

B12. Fill in the blanks or circle the correct answers in these statements about COPD.

(a) An estimated _____ million Americans have asthma, and _____ million have COPD.

(b) The largest single cause of COPD is _____.

(c) Signs or symptoms *(are? are not?)* typically present in early stages of COPD.

(d) Circle the characteristics that are true of both COPD and asthma.

(1) Inflammation occurs

(2) Bronchoconstriction

(3) Excessive secretion of mucus

(4) Loss of elastic fibers in alveolar walls

(5) Difficult expiration

B13. Complete this exercise about emphysema.

    (a) Emphysema involves (*thickening? breakdown?*) of alveolar walls causing a(n) (*increased? decreased?*) surface for gas exchange.

    (b) Most people with emphysema develop it as a result of (*smoking? a genetic disorder?*). Cigarette smoke stimulates movement of _____ cells into lungs, and these cells release the enzyme _____, which digests the (*fat? protein?*) elastin in alveolar walls. Loss of elasticity in alveolar walls causes the characteristic barrel-chested appearance in which lungs are (*hypo? hyper?*)inflated (textbook Figure 29-12).

B14. Refer to Table 29-2 in the textbook and write "CB" (chronic bronchitis) or "Emph" (emphysema) next to descriptions that fit each disorder.

    (a) Clients have a productive cough of more than 3 months' duration for at least 2 consecutive years, and possibly for many years: ____

    (b) In the simple form, airflow is not affected; in the chronic obstructive form, airflow is blocked: ____

    (c) Called "blue bloaters": cyanosis results from CO_2 retention, and bloating derives from cor pulmonale. (See Question D8): ____

    (d) Hypoxemia also results in polycythemia and sluggish blood, with possible clot formation: ____

    (e) Called "pink puffers" because they respond to hypoxia by working extra hard to breathe and they do maintain quite normal blood gas values: ____

    (f) More likely to experience major weight loss related to the extra work of breathing: ____

    (g) Before age 40, the major cause is deficiency of the enzyme α_1-antitrypsin that normally protects alveolar walls from destruction: ____

B15. Mr. Eggers, age 48, complains of shortness of breath (dyspnea) and a productive cough early in the morning. He does not have an infection.

    (a) List the components of a work up for Mr. Eggers that ultimately reveals the diagnosis of COPD. _____
_____

    (b) Circle the results likely to be found in his diagnostic work up:

        (1) Prolonged (*in? ex?*)piration

        (2) Forced vital capacity (FVC) of (*4 to 5? 7 to 8?*) sec.

        (3) The volume of air that can be forcibly exhaled in 1 sec ($FEV_{1.0}$) is (*greater? less?*) than normal.

        (4) The total lung capacity (TLC) is (*greater? less?*) than normal.

B16. Mrs. Rice, age 68, has advanced emphysema. The home health nurse is assessing Mrs. Rice's management of her emphysema. Circle Mrs. Rice's statements that indicate good management of COPD.

    (a) "I got my flu shot this fall."

    (b) "My friend Sadie always seems to have a cold. I ask her if we can talk on the phone then—instead of her visiting me here."

    (c) "My sister still smokes two packs a day, and I just can't ask her to not smoke when she's here."

    (d) "I wear that face mask thing you got me when I go outside and it's freezing."

    (e) "No, I don't look at the stuff I cough up— I just can't deal with checking the color."

    (f) "I eat a little something every 2 or 3 hours; I get too tired if I eat big meals."

    (g) "I tried doing those breathing exercises— it's too much for me, so I stopped."

B17. Circle the interventions that are typically used to treat COPD.

    (a) Adrenergic bronchodilators

    (b) Anticholinergic bronchodilators

    (c) Oral corticosteroids

    (d) Oral theophylline

    (e) Oxygen by nasal cannula to maintain PO_2 at 90 mm Hg

B18. Circle the correct answers or fill in blanks about bronchiectasis.

    (a) This condition involves broncho- (*constriction? dilatation?*) associated with _____. Since the introduction of vaccinations and the use of antibiotics, the incidence of bronchiectasis is (*increasing? decreasing?*).

    (b) Causes of obstructive bronchiectasis include _____

(c) Causes of nonobstructive, generalized bronchitis include _____

_____

(d) This is a *(reversible? permanent?)* condition that may lead to *(thickening? destruction?)* of bronchial walls, usually *(bi? uni?)*laterally.

(e) Describe the "vicious cycle" that is likely to occur in bronchiectasis.

(f) Signs and symptoms include *(low body temperature? fever?)*; coughing up *(small? large?)* amounts of sputum that contains _____ and *(is? is not?)* foul smelling; weight *(gain? loss?)*; and changes in fingers known as _____ that may occur with cardiac or pulmonary disease.

B19. Complete this exercise about Brent, age 8, who has cystic fibrosis (CF).

(a) CF is a *(rare? common?)* fatal hereditary disorder. Both of Brent's parents must have the CF gene because this is a(n) *(autosomal dominant? autosomal recessive? sex-linked?)* disorder. It is likely that Brent's parents have *(no? some?)* symptoms of CF.

(b) Mapped to chromosome ___, the defective gene known as _____ fails to code for a protein needed for *(Ca^{++}? Cl$^-$? Mg^{++}?)* transport. As a result *(endocrine? exocrine?)* secretions are affected. Sweat has *(high? low?)* salt content, which can lead to salt depletion. Mucus becomes extremely *(thin? thick?)* and blocks ducts.

(c) The most serious effects of CF are on these major organs: _____ and the _____. Initial respiratory signs are _____ of airways, including those caused by *Staphylococcus aureus* and _____. Repeated infections lead to _____ and related destruction.

(d) Blockage of ducts of the _____ prevents enzymes from this organ from breaking down foods, especially fats. Brent experiences fatty stool, known as _____-orrhea, as well as diarrhea, and abdominal pain. As a result, Brent's weight, as in most CF clients, tends to be *(higher? lower?)* than normal.

(e) Brent is at high risk for infertility because bilateral failure of _____ development accompanies CF in most males.

B20. Explain why early diagnosis of cystic fibrosis (CF) is important.

_____

_____

_____

Describe diagnostic tests for CF in this exercise.

(a) The standard test for CF is analysis of _____ collected from skin.

(b) Newborn screening tests for blood levels of _____, which is produced in the *(lungs? pancreas?)*. Obstruction of ducts prevents passage of the chemical out of the organ, so that blood levels *(drop? elevate?)*. This test is ____% accurate for diagnosis of CF.

(c) Genetic tests check for mutations in the _____ gene. This test *(is? is not?)* conclusive without a family history of CF or clinical signs of CF. The genetic test *(can? cannot?)* detect carriers of CF which provides information for genetic counseling.

B21. Currently, about *(3? 13? 33?)*% of persons living with CF have reached adulthood. Treatment of CF focuses on replacement of _____ enzymes and methods of keeping _____ clear. Describe several treatments for airways.

_____

_____

_____

C. INTERSTITIAL LUNG DISEASES (pages 653-656)

C1. Choose the three true statements about interstitial lung diseases.

(a) These conditions are classified as **restrictive** rather than **obstructive**.

(b) They have their primary effects on **airways** of lungs.

(c) Interstitial diseases **do** involve injury, inflammation and formation of scar tissue.

(d) These conditions **are all** rapidly progressive.

(e) Interstitial lung diseases are **rarely** caused by occupational and environmental inhalants.

(f) Such diseases **decrease** lung compliance.

C2. Circle the signs or symptoms typical of interstitial lung diseases.

(a) Rapid, shallow breathing

(b) Bradypnea

(c) Decreased $FEV_{1.0}$ (as in COPD)

(d) Dyspnea with wheezing (as in COPD)

(e) Dyspnea without wheezing

(f) Clubbing of fingers

(g) Increase in total lung capacity with hyperinflated lungs (as in COPD)

C3. List several examples of occupational lung diseases in each category.

(a) Pneumoconioses: caused by inhalation of *(organic? inorganic?)* matter such as

_____

_____

(b) Hypersensitivity: caused by inhalation of *(organic? inorganic?)* matter such as

_____

_____

_____

C4. Explain the increased incidence of:

(a) Lung disease among asbestos workers who also smoke _____

_____

_____

(b) Tuberculosis among persons with silicosis

_____

_____

_____

C5. Sarcoidosis involves granular lesions that are most likely to affect three areas of the body, namely: *(brain? ears? eyes? lungs? skin? spleen? teeth?)*. The cause of this condition is _____. How is it diagnosed?

_____

D. PULMONARY VASCULAR DISORDERS (pages 656-660)

D1. Discuss pulmonary emboli (PEs) in this exercise.

(a) Most PEs are composed of blood clots (or thrombi). List three other types of substances that can form emboli.

_____

_____

_____

(b) Almost all PEs originate as _____ (DVTs) in *(upper? lower?)* extremities.

(c) Write examples of each of the three major factors that lead to DVTs (and therefore to PEs):

(1) Venous stasis due to: _____

_____

(2) Injury to the inner lining of veins as occurs in: _____

(3) Hypercoagulability related to:

_____

(d) PEs affect blood flow through lungs by two mechanisms. Briefly describe these.

_____

_____

(e) List the three most common signs or symptoms of PEs. _____

_____

_____

(Hypoxemia? Carbon dioxide retention?) is more likely to occur. *(Small? Medium-sized? Large?)* emboli are most likely to result in collapse, shock, loss of consciousness, and possibly death.

D2. Match diagnostic techniques for pulmonary emboli with descriptions below.

D-dimer testing
Lower-limb compression ultrasonography
Pulmonary angiogram
Ventilation-perfusion scan

(a) Measures products of coagulation factors activated when clots form:

_____

(b) An invasive technique that involves placement of a catheter through a vein into the right side of heart and pulmonary artery: _____

(c) A noninvasive means for detecting DVT that is 97% specific: _____

(d) Involves inhalation of a radiolabeled gas:

_____

D3. Match purposes (I-III) of interventions for PEs with their descriptions.

I. Prevention of clot formation
II. Prevention of movement of clots to lungs
III. Sustaining of life when PEs are already present by clot dissolution

(a) Administration of a plasminogen activator:

_____

(b) Insertion of a filter into the inferior vena cava: _____

(c) Use of compression stockings or IPC boots: _____

D4. Write a typical pulmonary artery (PA) blood pressure: ____/____ mm Hg with a mean PA pressure of ____ mm Hg. Compared with systemic circulation, pulmonary circulation is a *(low? high?)* pressure system with *(thin and compliant? thick and stiff?)* vessels.

D5. Most cases of pulmonary hypertension are *(primary? secondary?)*. Select the category of cause of pulmonary hypertension that fits the related description.

EPPV. Elevation of pressure in pulmonary veins

IPBV. Increased pulmonary blood flow

PHPV. Pulmonary hypoxemia leading to reflex pulmonary vasoconstriction

(a) COPDs such as chronic bronchitis or emphysema: _____

(b) Mitral valve stenosis or left-sided heart failure: _____

(c) Living in a town at an elevation of 12,000 feet: _____

(d) Congenital heart defects (VSD, ASD, or PDA) with left-to-right shunting that overloads and stimulates structural damage to the pulmonary artery: _____

D6. List major signs and symptoms of secondary pulmonary hypertension.

_____

_____

_____

D7. Complete this exercise about Mrs. Budd, who has a diagnosis of primary pulmonary hypertension.

(a) Her mean pulmonary artery blood pressure is most likely to be *(14? 26? 94?)* mm Hg.

(b) This is a relatively *(common? rare?)* condition, occurring in about one person in a *(thousand? million?)*. The 5-year survival rate is about ____ %.

(c) What signs or symptoms is Mrs. Budd likely to manifest? _____

_____

(d) What treatments may help? _____

_____

D8. Cor pulmonale refers to a heart ("cor") problem resulting from a _____ problem. Arrange in the correct sequence the events in development of cor pulmonale.

(a) Retrograde blood flow from lungs to right ventricle

(b) Pulmonary hypoxemia that causes reflex pulmonary vasoconstriction

(c) Some chronic lung problem such as chronic bronchitis

(d) Right ventricular hypertrophy that soon "outgrows" coronary blood supply

(e) Right ventricular failure with back flow into systemic veins

(f) Increased resistance to flow through pulmonary vessels

(g) Jugular vein distension, ankle edema, hepatomegaly, and ascites

____ → ____ → ____ → ____ → ____ →

____ → ____

D9. Mr. Sokolski has chronic bronchitis and cor pulmonale. Blood work reveals a hematocrit of 56; physical exam indicates presence of "plethora." Explain.

_____

_____

_____

D10. Mr. Ellison suffered severe burns and multiple fractures in the collapse of a burning building. He experienced significant bleeding and has now been diagnosed with ARDS. Complete this exercise about ARDS.

(a) ARDS is an acronym for a_____ r_____ d_____ syndrome. Refer to textbook Chart 29-2 and list possible causes of ARDS in Mr. Ellison.

_____

_____

_____

(b) Lung changes resulting from ARDS involve injury to alveoli that cause a(an) *(increase? decrease?)* in permeability of the alveolar-capillary membrane, *(increase? decrease?)* in surfactant production, and *(increase? decrease?)* in gas exchange. Resulting pulmonary edema, alveolar collapse, and fibrosis *(increase? decrease?)* Mr. Ellison's work of breathing.

(c) His treatment involves administration of _____ needed by vital organs and multiple interventions to address the other pathologies associated with his injuries.

E. RESPIRATORY FAILURE (pages 660-666)

E1. _____ is a term that means low level of O_2 in blood, whereas _____ means excess CO_2 in blood.

E2. Complete Table 29-1 below on blood gas values (all in mm Hg); one is done for you. Recall that in "PaO_2," "P" stands for _____ pressure of the gas, "a" stands for (alveolar? arterial?) blood. Capital letters A through F refer to letters in Study Guide Figure 27-1 (page 128); these values would differ for persons with chronic lung disease. Letters G and H are not shown on the figure, but would replace E and F in respiratory failure.

Now fill in values on any blank lines in the figure.

E3. Choose the two true statements about hypoventilation.

(a) **Hypoventilation** refers to a significant reduction of pure oxygen moving into or out of the lung.

(b) If hypoventilation decreases PaO_2 by 40% (from 100 to 60 mm Hg), $PaCO_2$ is likely to increase 100% (from 40-80 mm Hg).

(c) In clients who are hypoventilating, administration of oxygen can bring PaO_2 **back to normal**, but $PaCO_2$ will remain **high**.

(d) Hypoventilation is commonly caused by **lung disorders**.

E4. Match each condition in the list that follows with the related description below. Use each answer only once.

Cyanosis   Hypercapnia
Hypoxemia   Impaired diffusion
Shunt

(a) Occurs with atelectasis of a portion of a lung or a congenital heart defect such as tetralogy of Fallot: _____

(b) Pneumonia, pulmonary edema, interstitial disease, and ARDS all increase the thickness of the alveolar-capillary membrane: _____

(c) Bluish discoloration of skin (more readily detected in light skin) and mucosa due to reduction of at least 5g/dL of hemoglobin (Hb); can be central (as in tongue and lips) or peripheral (as in extremities); can occur in polycythemia without hypoxia because too many Hb molecules are present to bind with a normal level of O_2 molecules: _____

(d) Indicated by a $PaCO_2$ level greater than 50 mm Hg and a low arterial pH. Occurs with hypoventilation sufficient to cause hypoxia, such as COPD, Guillain-Barré syndrome, or severe scoliosis: _____

(e) If mild, produces few signs or symptoms. Can lead to impairment of vital centers (such as brain with visual effects) and activation of compensatory mechanisms (such as tachycardia, hyperventilation, cool skin, sweating, erythropoiesis). If not reversed, will lead to bradycardia, hypotension and death: _____

E5. Describe two noninvasive methods for oxygen assessment.

_____
_____
_____

E6. Complete this exercise about Mrs. McLaughlin, who has advanced COPD.

(a) Before developing COPD, Mrs. McLaughlin's respiratory center would have been stimulated by (central? peripheral?) chemoreceptors that sense an increase in (H^+? HCO_3^-?) ions directly related to (low blood levels of O_2? high blood levels of CO_2?).

Table 29-1. Blood and Alveolar Gas Valves

	Venous Blood: Normal	Alveolar Air: Normal	Arterial Blood: Normal	Arterial Blood: Respiratory Failure
PO₂	(A) PvO_2:	(C) PaO_2:	(E) PaO_2: **80-100**	(G) PaO_2:
PCO₂	(B) $PvCO_2$:	(D) $PaCO_2$:	(F) $PaCO_2$:	(H) $PaCO_2$:

(b) However, because persons with COPD have chronic hypercapnia, buffering occurs which *(increases? reduces?)* reactivity of those chemoreceptors. People with COPD must turn to another mechanism for control of ventilation: that involving *(central? peripheral?)* receptors located in the aorta and in _____ arteries.

(c) Mrs. McLaughlin normally inspires 1 to 2 L/min of by nasal cannula. If she were to breathe higher concentrations of oxygen, her $PaCO_2$ would *(increase? decrease?)*. Explain.

_____

_____

_____

_____

E7. Address mechanisms that can lead to hypercapnia by completing this exercise.

(a) Respiratory muscles cannot produce normal CO_2 exhalation if they:

(1) Require more energy for breathing than normal, for example: _____

(2) Lack normal energy resources or muscle strength, for example: _____

(b) Excessive CO_2 is produced:

(1) When activity level or body temperature *(increases? decreases?)*, for example:

_____

(2) When dietary intake of *(carbohydrates? fats?)* is increased as in TPN (or total _____ nutrition). Carbohydrates have a respiratory quotient (RC) of *(1.0? 0.7?)*. meaning that they lead to a greater level of *(CO_2 production? O_2 consumption?)*.

E8. June has a $PaCO_2$ level of 58 mm Hg and a PaO_2 level of 62 mm Hg. Describe her state of hypercapnia.

(a) She is likely to be in respiratory *(acidosis? alkalosis?)* as indicated by an arterial blood pH of *(7.25? 7.45?)*. Write the chemical reaction that shows the mechanism.

_____

(b) June is likely to manifest signs and symptoms of hypercapnia when $PaCO_2$ is *(slightly? markedly?)* elevated above the normal level of about _____mm Hg. One effect is *(increase? decrease?)* of central nervous system activity. Manifestations such as skin flushing and headache are related to hypercapnic effects of vaso*(constriction? dilatation?)*.

(c) Treatments for June are likely to focus on:

_____

_____

_____

F. HYPERVENTILATION SYNDROME (pages 667-669)

F1. Mr. Tomlinson is admitted to the emergency department after his involvement in a four-vehicle accident. He is highly anxious and fearful about his son who is in critical condition. He is sweating, breathing rapidly, and has heart palpitations.

(a) Circle the signs or symptoms likely to be present in his hyperventilating state.

(1) Blood pH of 7.5

(2) Blood level of $PaCO_2$ of 30 mm Hg

(3) Numbness and tingling in his arms and hands

(4) Headache

(5) Shortness of breath

(b) How can rebreathing into a paper bag help Mr. Tomlinson?

_____

_____

(c) How can adrenergic blocking drugs help?

_____

_____

_____

CHAPTER 30

Control of Renal Function

■ Review Questions

A. KIDNEY STRUCTURE AND FUNCTION
(pages 673–686)

A1. Complete this exercise about kidney structure.

(a) Kidneys are normally situated (*at waist level? in the pelvis?*). They are located (*in the anterior of the abdomen? retroperitoneally?*). State the significance of this location: _____

_____.

(b) Arrange in correct sequence from outermost to innermost: Renal

Medulla   Capsule   Cortex

_____ → _____ →

_____

(c) Urine formed in the cortex and medulla flows into the renal _____ from which urine enters the (*ureters? urethra?*) and passes to the urinary bladder.

(d) Refer to textbook Figures 30-3 and 30-4 and arrange blood vessels in correct sequence from first to and through kidneys:

Afferent arteriole   Efferent arteriole
Glomerular capillary   Intralobular artery
Intralobular vein   Peritubular capillary
Renal artery   Renal vein

_____ → _____ →
_____ → _____ →
_____ → _____ →
_____ → _____

A2. Describe the structure of a nephron in this exercise.

(a) Fill in the blanks or circle the correct answers to show that a nephron consists of:

(1) A cluster of capillaries known as a _____ in which blood is filtered and collected into _____'s capsule. Taken together, the glomerulus and capsule are known as a renal _____.

(2) A _____, which transports the filtrate (or "forming urine") and allows reabsorption of much of the filtrate into _____ capillaries.

(b) Glomeruli consist of three layers. The middle layer, which is the (*basement membrane? endothelium? epithelium?*), determines the permeability of the glomerulus. Normally, this membrane (*allows? prevents?*) passage of red blood cells and plasma protein from blood into filtrate. It is responsible for leakage in many glomerular diseases.

(c) _____ cells cover areas of glomeruli lacking a basement membrane. State two functions of these cells.

_____

_____

(d) Refer to textbook Figure 30-4 and arrange the following portions of the renal tubule in correct sequence from first to last:

Ascending limb of the loop of Henle (ALLH)
Collecting duct (CD)
Distal convoluted tubule (DCT)
Descending limb of the loop of Henle (DLLH)
Proximal convoluted tubule (PCT)

_____ → _____ →
_____ → _____ →
_____

A3. Refer to Figure 30-1 and identify the three steps in urine formation. Note the direction of movement of substances in each step. (Note that glomerular filtrate and tubular fluid are different stages of "forming urine.")

highly stressed, his sympathetic nerves will cause constriction of his ___ferent arterioles. This leads to *(increased? decreased?)* GFR and *(increased? decreased?)* urine production, as well as *(increased? decreased?)* blood volume and BP.

A5. Describe Steps II and III (from Question A3) of urine formation in this exercise.

   (a) Refer to textbook Figure 30-8 and trace the path of Na^+ from right to left in the figure. This process depends on the "sucking" of Na^+ from renal tubule cells into the *(lumen of the tubule? interstitial fluid and blood?)*, a process driven by the _____ pump (shown on the left side of the figure). In fact, most ATP used by kidneys is devoted to the *(filtration? reabsorption? secretion?)* of Na^+ from tubular fluid via tubule cells to blood. Simultaneously, glucose and amino acids are *(co? counter?)*transported in the same direction. The latter is also known as *(primary? secondary?)* active transport.

   (b) H^+ ions move the *(same? opposite?)* direction to Na^+, and therefore undergo ATP-dependent *(co? counter?)*-transport. This results in *(reabsorption? secretion?)* of H^+ into urine, a mechanism that reduces acidity of blood. Name three buffers that assist in secretion of H^+ ions: _____, _____, and _____. (Hint: see text page 679.)

   (c) Movement of H_2O in the same direction as Na^+ occurs during the *(active? passive?)* process of osmosis. Most such resorption of H_2O and Na^+, as well as that of glucose and amino acids, normally occurs in the *(PCT? DCT?)*. This process helps to prevent dehydration and loss of nutrients in urine.

   (d) In uncontrolled diabetes, blood levels of glucose are *(higher? lower?)* than normal, so *(more? less?)* glucose than normal is filtered in glomeruli. If the amount of glucose in tubular fluid surpasses the _____ (reabsorption) maximum for glucose as shown in textbook Figure 30-9, then glucose *(does? does not?)* appear in urine.

A6. Philippe runs 10 miles on a sweltering day. As a cooling mechanism, his sweat glands become *(more? less?)* active. How do his kidneys respond to help to prevent dehydration?

   (a) His kidneys produce a *(larger? smaller?)* amount of *(concentrated? dilute?)* urine.

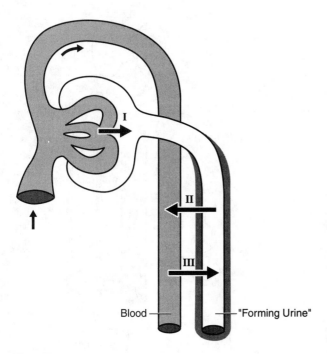

Figure 30-1.

   (a) Step I: _____ is the movement of substances out of blood into filtrate ("forming urine").

   (b) Step II: _____ is the return of substances from filtrate ("forming urine") now present in tubular fluid back into blood (in peritubular capillaries).

   (c) Step III: _____ is the movement of substances out of peritubular blood via kidney tubule cells into tubular fluid ("forming urine").

A4. Answer these questions about urine formation in Julian, age 46, whose kidneys and blood pressure are normal.

   (a) Julian's kidneys are likely to move about ____mL/min of substances from blood to filtrate (forming urine). This is known as his _____ rate (GFR). The filtrate formed is similar to his blood plasma except that filtrate lacks _____.

   (b) His kidneys are likely to reabsorb about ____ mL/min back into his blood. In other words, Julian's urinary output will be about ____ mL/min (or ____ mL/hour or ____ mL/day).

   (c) Normal glomerular capillary blood pressure (BP) is about ____ mm Hg; this is considerably *(higher? lower?)* than BP in all other capillaries of the body. When Julian is

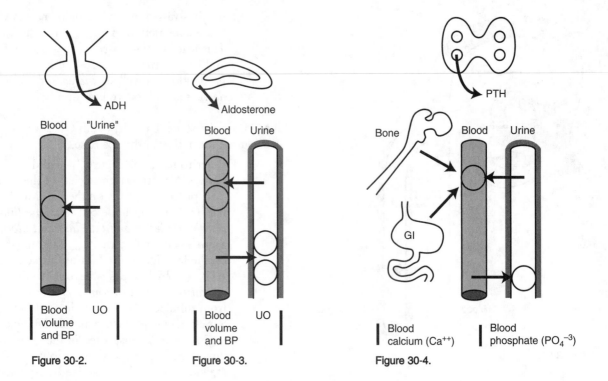

Figure 30-2.

Figure 30-3.

Figure 30-4.

(b) The mechanism involved is known as the _____ mechanism, which is based on the flow of fluids in *(the same? opposite?)* direction(s) within the two limbs of the loop of Henle and also in the parallel capillaries known as _____. This arrangement causes the renal medulla to become *(hyper? hypo?)* tonic (comparable to a desert) so it draws water out of urine.

A7. Refer to Figures 30-2 through 30-4 above and describe effects of hormones on kidneys. Fill in lines to show where hormones are produced; complete arrows to show their impact on urinary output (UO) as well as blood volume and blood pressure (BP); and fill in names of electrolytes (Na^+, K^+, H^+, or Ca^{++}) or H_2O in circles.

(a) ADH (Figure 30-2) causes insertion of water channels into membranes of renal tubules. The result is a(an) *(increase? decrease?)* in permeability of the collecting tubules and reabsorption of water.

(b) Cells in the *(PCT? DCT?)* and collecting tubules are sensitive to aldosterone (Figure 30-3), which causes resorption of *(Na+? K+?)* and water, and secretion of ____ and ____ into urine.

(c) Although aldosterone and ADH work by different mechanisms, they both *(increase? decrease?)* urinary output and *(lower? raise?)* BP. The hormone ANP, produced by the _____, *(mimics? opposes?)* release and action of ADH and aldosterone.

(d) Parathyroid hormone (Figure 30-4) acts on the *(PCT? DCT?)* to increase reabsorption of ____ ions. Vitamin D *(mimics? opposes?)* effects of PTH as they "pull" from several sources to *(increase? decrease?)* blood levels of Ca^{++}.

A8. Normally about *(2.5%? 25%?)* of cardiac output flows into kidneys each minute. Discuss variations in blood flow through kidneys (with direct effects on GFR and urinary output) in this exercise.

(a) Indicate effects of each of the following neural or chemical factors on kidneys.

Antidiuretic hormone (vasopressin)
Angiotensin II
Dopamine
Nitric oxide
Sympathetic nerve activity

(1) Cause renal vasoconstriction, decreased GFR, and decreased urinary output:

_____, _____,

_____

(2) Cause renal vasodilation, increased GFR, and increased urinary output: _____, _____

(b) When renal blood pressure increases, for example when blood pressure is high, the process of _____ causes renal vessels to dilate, increasing GFR and urinary output, and (increasing? decreasing?) blood pressure.

(c) The juxtaglomerular (JG) complex (textbook Figure 30-14) consists of two types of cells:

(1) _____ cells in the distal tubule that monitor NaCl levels.

(2) JG cells in the walls of _____ and _____ arterioles that respond to stretching of these vessels. JG cells then release renin which leads to the production of _____, a vasoconstrictor that regulates glomerular flow. Angiotensin II also stimulates release of the hormone _____. See also Question A7(b).

(d) Increase in dietary intake of protein and increased blood glucose levels (as associated with uncontrolled diabetes), both (increase? decrease?) renal blood flow and urinary output.

A9. "Renal clearance" means the volume of plasma that is "cleared" (or cleaned) of a given chemical each minute. Renal clearance is greatest for substances that are (well? poorly?) filtered from blood and (well? poorly?) reabsorbed back into blood. An example is (inulin? insulin? glucose?); its clearance is directly related to the person's GFR because this chemical is (highly? slightly? not at all?) reabsorbed.

A10. Mr. Charles has gouty arthritis. This is related to increased blood levels of _____ acid. Name two types of medications that Mr. Charles should avoid because they lead to hyperuricemia and exacerbate gout:

_____

_____

_____

A11. Complete this exercise about Ms. Jensen, age 55, who has a history of rheumatoid arthritis and diabetes mellitus. Her BUN level is 67 mg/dL, and her GFR is 24 mL/min. Ms. Jensen's blood calcium level is low.

(a) BUN refers to blood _____ nitrogen. Normal values range from ____ to ____ mg/dL; Ms. Jensen's BUN is (low? normal? high?).

(b) High levels of BUN can result from increased breakdown of (fats? proteins?), which contain about 16% nitrogen (N), (increased? decreased?) ability of kidneys to clear nitrogen-containing wastes, or (de? over?)hydration.

(c) Breakdown of protein leads to production of ammonia in the (intestine? kidney? liver?) which is converted to urea in the _____, which is then eliminated by _____.

(d) State several reasons why Ms. Jensen's BUN levels may be high.

_____

_____

(e) If the cause of Ms. Jensen's high BUN is related to renal failure, blood levels of some of her medications may (increase? decrease?). Explain the clinical significance.

_____

_____

(f) Ms. Jensen's hematocrit level is 18. Her physician prescribes "epoetin-a." Explain why. _____

_____

(g) What might explain Ms. Jensen's hypocalcemia? _____

_____

_____

B. TESTS OF RENAL FUNCTION (pages 686-689)

B1. Conrad has a urinalysis performed. Circle those findings that are abnormal.

Casts	Cloudy (high turbidity)
A small number	Glucose
of epithelial	Pink color
cells	Specific gravity of 1.015

90-mg protein in a 24-hour urine sample
400-mL total volume in a 24-hour urine sample

B2. Complete this exercise about renal function tests involving urine.

(a) On a day when a person produces a large amount of sweat, specific gravity is likely to be (1.010? 1.025?). Urine with a specific gravity of 1.003 is likely to appear (yellow-amber? colorless?).

(b) Explain why a specific gravity 1.060 may be found in a person with diminished renal function. _____

_____

(c) Casts are more likely to be found in urine that has a *(high? low?)* concentration of proteins, as in nephrotic syndrome, and is *(acid? alkaline?)*.

B3. Creatinine is a(n) *(abnormal? normal?)* product of muscle metabolism. Describe its role in renal function testing in this exercise.

(a) Because it is filtered out of blood and *(is? is not?)* reabsorbed, creatinine clearance directly reflects GFR levels. Normal creatinine clearance is about *(120? 90? 60?)* mL/minute. In other words, a high level of creatinine clearance indicates *(good? poor?)* kidney function.

(b) As kidneys fail, *(more? less?)* creatinine will end up in ("be cleared into") urine, so blood levels of creatinine *(increase? decrease?)*. Therefore, a high serum creatinine level indicates *(good? poor?)* kidney function.

(c) Circle the normal serum creatinine level (See Table 30-2): *(1.0? 5.0?)* mg/dL of blood. If the serum creatinine level is three times normal (such as 3.0 mg/dL), then GFR is *(three times? one third of?)* normal. Serum creatinine level tends to be *(higher? lower?)* among elderly persons.

(d) The normal BUN:creatinine ratio is about *(10:1? 1:1? 1:10?)*, such as 12 mg/dL of BUN to ___ mg/dL of creatinine.

B4. Which is the most specific indicator of renal failure? High blood levels of *(BUN? creatinine? K^+? H^+?)*. Explain.

_____

_____

_____

B5. Circle the two true statements.

(a) Cystoscopy is a technique that involves direct observation of the inside of the **bladder.**

(b) Ultrasonography is an **invasive** procedure that is used diagnostically.

(c) In an intravenous pyelogram (IVP), dye is injected **directly into kidneys.**

(d) Renal angiography involves introduction of a catheter into the **femoral** artery.

C. PHYSIOLOGIC ACTION OF DIURETICS (pages 689–691)

C1. Diuretics cause diuresis, which is the *(increase? decrease?)* of urinary output. List several categories of persons who are likely to be helped by diuretics.

_____

_____

_____

C2. Mrs. Johansen has just started on a diuretic. She is advised to eat a banana every day. Explain.

_____

_____

_____

C3. Select the diuretic that best fits each description below.

Aldosterone-antagonists   Loop diuretics
Osmotic diuretics   Thiazide diuretics

(a) The most effective diuretics, they work by inhibiting Na^+ resorption in the thicker portion of the loop of Henle; as a result, the extra Na^+ within urine takes water with it; furosamide (Lasix) is an example:

_____

(b) The least effective diuretics, but they offer the advantage of being "potassium sparing":

_____

(c) Used to reduce intracranial pressure (ICP); must be given IV because of their poor absorption; mannitol is an example:

_____

(d) They interfere with sodium reabsorption, but cause potassium loss and may lead to hyperglycemia: _____ and

_____

CHAPTER 31

Alterations in Fluid and Electrolyte Balance

■ Review Questions

A. COMPOSITION AND COMPARTMENTAL DISTRIBUTION OF BODY FLUIDS (pages 693-700)

A1. Identify the body fluids that fit the following descriptions.

Intracellular fluid   Interstitial fluid
Plasma or serum

(a) Fluid within cells; comprises about two thirds of body fluids: _____

(b) Contains a high level of potassium, and small amounts of sodium and chloride:

_____

(c) Fluid that is measured clinically (because of its accessibility): _____

(d) Extracellular fluids (ECF): _____
and _____

A2. Complete this exercise about body fluids and electrolytes.

(a) Circle the anion(s) in this list:

Bicarbonate   Chloride   Glucose
Potassium   Protein

(b) Which of the answers in A2(a) is/are nonelectrolyte(s)? _____

_____

(c) *(Diffusion? Dissociation? Osmosis?)* is the movement of water across a semipermeable membrane.

(d) Almost all of the osmotic pressure in extracellular fluids (ECF) is due to:

(1) Na^+, Cl^-, and HCO_3^-

(2) BUN and glucose

(e) A 0.9% NaCl solution is *(hyper? iso? hypo?)*tonic to human cells.

(f) Human cells placed in hypotonic solutions are likely to *(shrink? swell?)*.

(g) Name two or more "transcellular spaces":
_____, _____.
Accumulation of fluids here is known as
_____-spacing.

A3. Timothy, a healthy 12-year-old, weighs 100 pounds. His body weight contains about ___ pounds of fluid. This fluid includes ___ pounds of fluid within cells (ICF) and ___ pounds of ECF. Most of his ECF is likely to be *(blood plasma? interstitial fluid?)*.

A4. Refer to Figure 31-6 and Chart 31-1 in the textbook. Edema is most likely to result from any of the following factors. Give examples of causes in each case.

(a) An increase in *(capillary? tissue?)* hydrostatic pressure that is a force that *(pushes out of? pulls into?)* blood vessels.

_____

(b) Decrease in *(capillary? tissue?)* colloidal osmotic pressure (COP), a force that normally *(pushes out of? pulls into)* vessels. _____

(c) *(Increase? Decrease?)* in capillary permeability. _____

(d) Blockage of _____ flow.

_____

A5. Complete this exercise about edema.

(a) Mrs. Sella has dependent edema. This is more likely to be cased by:

(1) Hypoalbuminemia

(2) Congestive heart failure

(b) Renal failure is more likely to lead to large amounts of _____ in urine.

(1) Albumin

(2) Fibrinogen

(c) Which edema is typically life threatening? Edema of:

(1) Larynx or lungs

(2) Ankles and feet

(d) Edema increases risk of tissue breakdown (as in pressure ulcers) because edema _____ the distance between blood vessels and cells.

   (1) Increases

   (2) Deceases

(e) Mrs. Kuczkowski has +3 pitting edema that indicates that blood proteins such as fibrinogen _____ accumulated in tissues.

   (1) Have

   (2) Have not

(f) A weight gain of 9 pounds associated with edema indicates a water gain of about ___ liters.

   (1) 2

   (2) 4

   (3) 9

(g) Ascites refers to "third-spacing" of fluid in the _____ cavity.

   (1) Pleural

   (2) Pericardial

   (3) Peritoneal

B. SODIUM AND WATER BALANCE (pages 700-714)

B1. Refer to Figure 21-1 and identify major mechanisms that help to increase fluid volume and blood pressure.

(a) Sympathetic nerve activity *(increases? decreases?)* heart rate and causes blood vessels to vaso*(constrict? dilate?)*.

(b) *(Elimination? Retention?)* of sodium and water occurs by several mechanisms.

(c) Which of the above effects does angiotensin facilitate? _____
_____

B2. List three important functions of sodium in the body.

_____

_____

_____

B3. Jack, age 19, has no known health problems. He is sedentary, and he consumes about 10 g/d of sodium in his foods. This amount is about *(20 times? 10 times? 2 times? one-tenth of?)* the amount of sodium required by his body. List two other possible sources of sodium

besides dietary intake: _____, _____. Most of Jack's loss of sodium will typically be through his *(kidneys? skin? GI tract?)*.

B4. Indicate whether each of the following factors will cause the body to save or lose sodium by circling the correct answer.

(a) Vasoconstriction of renal arteries with decreased GFR:
Save Na+   *Lose Na+*

(b) The renin-angiotensin mechanism:
Save Na+   *Lose Na+*

(c) ANP (atrial natriuretic peptide):
Save Na+   *Lose Na+*

(d) Vomiting or diarrhea:
Save Na+   *Lose Na+*

(e) ACE-I:
Save Na+   *Lose Na+*

(f) Aldosterone:
Save Na+   *Lose Na+*

B5. Identify the major site where each of these chemicals is produced.

Adrenal cortex   Hypothalamus   Kidneys
Liver   Lungs

(a) Renin: _____

(b) Angiotensin converting enzyme (ACE):
_____

(c) Aldosterone: _____

(d) ADH: _____

B6. In healthy adults, total body water (TBW) normally ranges from about ___% to ___ % of body weight. Circle the persons more likely to have a higher proportion of total body water (TBW).

60-year-old woman   20-year-old woman
Lean person   Obese person
Person with body temperature of 104°F
Person with body temperature of 99.0°F
2-month-old infant   2-year-old child

List several reasons why. _____
_____

B7. Refer to Table 31-2 in the text and answer these questions about fluid exchange.

(a) The body typically gains about 90% of its body fluids through _____. The reminder comes from the _____ of foods.

Table 31-1. Alterations in Fluid Volume and Sodium Concentration: Causes and Manifestations

Disorder	Causes	Manifestations

Fluid volume deficit (FVD) or isotonic fluid volume loss	↑ Na^+ and H_2O loss
	  Addison's (↓ aldosterone)
	  GI loss (vomiting, diarrhea)
	  Skin loss (fever, burns)
	↓ Na^+ and H_2O intake
	  Third-spacing (burns, ascites)
		Serum Na^+ normal, thirst, ↑ pulse, ↓ BP
		↑ UO
		↓ UO
		↓ UO
		↓ UO
		↓ UO

Fluid volume excess (FVE) or isotonic fluid volume gain	↓ Na^+ and H_2O loss
	  Renal failure
	  Primary aldosteronism (↑ aldosterone)
	↑ Na^+ and H_2O intake
		Serum Na^+ normal, edema, weight gain
		↓ UO
		↓ UO
		↓ UO
		↑ UO

Hyponatremia	↑ Na^+ loss and replacement with tap H_2O (exercise)
	↑ H_2O intake compared with output
	  SIADH (↑ ADH)
	  Psychogenic polydipsia
		Serum Na^+ <135 mEq/L, fingerprint edema, personality change, stupor, coma
		
		↓ UO
		↑ UO

Hypernatremia	↑ H_2O loss Diabetes insipidus (↓ ADH) ↓ H_2O intake	Serum Na^+ >145 mEq/L, thirst, ↑ pulse, ↓ BP ↑ UO ↓ UO

BP, blood pressure; UO, urine output. Refer to text Figures 31-4 through 31-7 and add other manifestations of the four disorders as desired.

(b) Normally, kidneys eliminate about _____ mL of urine per day (or ____ mL/minute).

(c) In association with GI infections, more fluid is likely to be lost through *(exhalations? GI tract? kidneys? skin?)*. During vigorous exercise, more fluid is likely to be lost through _____.

B8. Thirst is a(n) *(early? late?)* sign of hemorrhage or other fluid volume deficits. Explain how thirst helps to maintain fluid volume in this exercise. (*Hint*: refer to Figure 31-10.)

(a) The "thirst center" is located in the _____, which is located just *(inf? sup?)*erior to the pituitary gland. Cells here shrink when the body is *(de? over?)*hydrated and send the message to drink water. List several other locations of thirst receptors. _____

_____

_____

(b) Hypothalamic cells also contribute to the maintenance of fluid level by secreting

(ADH? aldosterone? renin?) which is stored and released from the ___terior pituitary (see question B10).

B9. Complete this exercise about alterations in thirst.

(a) Mrs. Litwin, age 89, states "I don't drink much water; I just don't feel thirsty anymore." She is likely to have *(hypo? poly?)*dipsia.

(b) Mr. Le Sourd, age 38, is an inpatient in a psychiatric unit. He had been drinking 2 to 3 gallons of water a day. He is a 2-pack-a-day cigarette smoker. Name his thirst disorder: _____

(c) Mrs. San Domenico, age 70, is a person with diabetes whose blood glucose was 420 mg/dL. She produced more urine and was thirsty. Her thirst disorder is classified as _____ thirst.

(1) False

(2) Inappropriate

(3) True or symptomatic

B10. Visualize the hypothalamus when blood passing through it is slightly "thicker" or more concentrated than normal. These cells secrete ADH, which has the following effects.

(a) ADH stimulates kidney tubule cells to become *(more? less?)* permeable to water. In other words, ADH tells kidneys to "save the water!" See Study Guide Figure 30-2 (page 152). ADH *(increases? decreases?)* blood volume (blood becomes "less thick") as urine output is *(increased? decreased?)*. The name antidiuretic hormone (ADH) indicates that its effects are *(similar to? opposite of?)* those of diuretics.

(b) ADH is also known as vaso_____ because it can vaso*(constrict? dilate?)* blood vessels to raise blood volume and blood pressure.

B11. Urinary output is likely to increase considerably after Ray drinks large quantities of beer. One reason is that beer contains a high percentage of water; the other is that alcohol *(increases? decreases?)* ADH production. (See textbook Table 31-3.)

B12. Discuss two disorders of ADH in this exercise. Refer to Study Guide Table 31-1 (page 157).

(a) Dr. Tony has diabetes insipidus (DI).

(1) Her body produces too *(much? little?)* ADH. Without treatment she is more likely to produce *(15? 0.5?)* L of urine each day, causing her thirst to *(increase? decrease?)* as her blood is *(concentrated? dilute?)*. Treatment typically involves administration of a form of ADH in a *(skin ointment? nasal spray?)*.

(2) In DI, the large urine output is *(sugary? nonsugary?)*, which accounts for the term "insipidus." In diabetes mellitus, a person produces a *(large? small?)* amount of urine that is *(sugary? nonsugary?)* because of a decrease in effective _____.

(3) Dr. Tony's DI is *(central or neurogenic? nephrogenic?)*. In nephrogenic DI, a person produces *(adequate? inadequate?)* ADH, and kidneys *(do? do not?)* respond to it.

(b) Marc has SIADH.

(1) His condition involves *(over? under?)*production of ADH. Fluid *(retention? deficit?)* occurs leading to *(dehydration? edema?)*, dilution of solutes such as sodium, which causes _____natremia, and dilution of red blood cells (_____).

(2) List several factors that can lead to SIADH._____

Refer to Study Guide Table 31-1 (page 157) and textbook Tables 31-4 to 31-7 as you complete Questions B13 through B16.

B13. Alterations in fluids and electrolytes are closely linked because body fluids contain electrolytes. The major electrolyte in plasma (or serum) is *(K⁺? Na⁺?)*. Two major categories of fluid and sodium disorders include:

(a) Gains or losses of water. Some of these disorders were discussed in Question B12 because they may involve imbalances in *(ADH? aldosterone?)*. For example, as much water is lost in diabetes insipidus (DI), serum sodium concentration *(increases? decreases?)* above the normal range of _____ mEq/L. See also Question B14.

(b) Excess or deficit in *both* sodium and water (isotonic fluids). The hormone most likely to be involved in these imbalances is *(ADH? aldosterone?)*. See Question B14.

B14. Identify the disorder that fits each description. See Study Guide Table 31-1 (page 157).

Fluid volume   Fluid volume
  deficit (FVD)   excess (FVE)
Hyponatremia   Hypernatremia

(a) Serum sodium level is 152 mEq/L; hematocrit is 52; thirst: _____

(b) Caused by increase in aldosterone. Hint: refer to textbook Figure 30-3:

_____

(c) Caused by increase in ADH (SIADH):

_____

(d) Caused by chronic renal failure (CRF):

_____

(e) Manifestations of FVD most resemble those of: _____

(f) Hypotension and tachycardia are most likely to accompany: _____,

_____

(g) Most likely to affect brain cells and cause altered personality and behavior:

_____, _____

B15. Identify the disorder described in each case. Use the answers listed in Question B14.

(a) Mr. Evanston has congestive heart failure, both pulmonary and generalized edema, and venous distension; a sodium-restricted diet is prescribed for him: _____

_____

(b) Ms. Annenburg has been diagnosed with adrenal insufficiency (Addison's disease): _____

_____

(c) Mr. Leon, age 55, has severely limited mobility related to his Huntington's disease, but he still lives in his own house. In July, he fell and was unable to get up from the floor for 40 hours while temperatures in his house reached 105°F. His eyes were sunken; his skin turgor and capillary refill were both diminished: _____

_____

(d) Dr. Tony, who has diabetes insipidus, who was discussed in Question B12(a), is injured in a fall; she becomes unconscious and does not get her medication. Her pulse is 120 beats/minute, her skin and mucous membranes are dry, and her reflexes are decreased. She produces copious amounts of urine: _____

(e) Kathryn has been exercising and sweating on a hot, humid day. She has drunk over 1.5 liters of water. She begins to feel weak, becomes nauseated, vomits, and faints: _____

_____

(f) Todd, age 5 months, is in the children's burns unit with extensive second- and third-degree burns acquired in an automobile accident. His anterior fontanel is depressed: _____

(g) Sammy, age 2 months, has had diarrhea for 3 days. His weight has decreased from 14 pounds to 13 pounds. He is at greatest risk for (two answers): _____,

_____

(h) Mr. Le Sourd, mentioned in Question B9(b), has added tap-water enemas to his psychogenic polydipsia in attempts to "cleanse his body of demons." The resulting "water intoxication" adds to his personality changes. Fingerprint edema is manifested over his sternum: _____

B16. Circle the correct answers. (*Hint:* refer to Study Guide Table 31-1, page 157.)

(a) Which one cause of FVD will result in an increased urine output?

    (1) Addison's disease

    (2) Burns

    (3) Inability to access fluids

    (4) Diarrhea

    (5) Fever

(b) Which one cause of hypernatremia will manifest an increase in urine output (polyuria)?

    (1) Addison's disease

    (2) Diabetes insipidus

    (3) Fever

    (4) Watery diarrhea

    (5) Excessive sweating

C. POTASSIUM BALANCE (pages 714-721)

C1. Refer to Study Guide Figure 31-1 on the next page and complete this exercise about potassium in the body.

(a) Almost all potassium ions (K^+) are located within *(ICF? ECF?).* Show this by writing (K^+) within the cell on Figure 31-1A. Circle the normal range for serum K^+: *(134 to 145 mEq/L? 22 to 27 mEq/L? 3.5 to 5.0 mEq/L?).* Write this value on the leader line drawn to the blood vessel on Figure 31-1A.

(b) The main source of potassium each day is typically through diet. List several good sources of this electrolyte.

_____

_____

(c) Figure 31-1B shows that the hormones insulin and epinephrine facilitate movement of K^+ *(into? out of?)* cells. Severe exercise and cell trauma (including burns or excessive GI activity) move K^+ *(into? out of?)* blood.

(d) The major route by which healthy persons lose potassium each day is through the *(GI tract? kidneys? skin?).* Aldosterone *(increases? decreases?)* tubular secretion of K^+ into urine. On Figure 31-1C, identify other actions of this hormone.

(e) Hyperkalemia tends to cause acidosis and vice versa, as a result of K^+-H^+ exchange mechanisms demonstrated in Figures 31-1 D and E. High blood levels of K^+ cause kidney

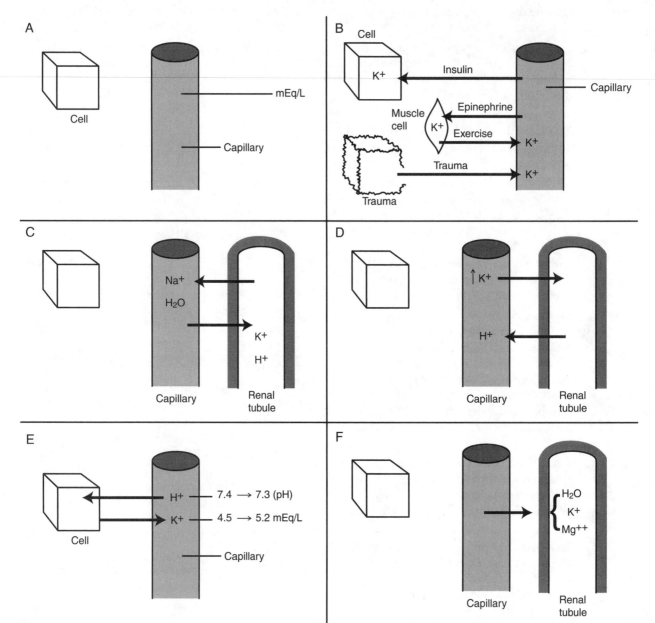

Figure 31-1.

tubules to secrete K^+ into urine and reabsorb another cation (___) back into blood (Figure 31-1D). During acidosis (Figure 31-1E), cells buffer H^+ and then give up K^+ to blood in exchange. An acidosis that lowers serum pH from 7.4 to 7.3 will typically raise serum K^+ by ____ mEq/L.

(f) The most common cause of excessive K^+ loss occurs by use of _____ shown in Figure 31-1F. Such medications also cause loss of ____.

C2. Consult Tables 31-8 and 31-9 in the textbook as well as alterations in K^+ regulation just discussed in Question C1. Apply this information to these cases of hypokalemia or

hyperkalemia by circling the correct answers or filling in the blanks.

(a) Ms. Annenburg (Question B15[b]) with Addison's disease has *(deficient? excessive?)* production of aldosterone. She is more likely to develop *(hypo? hyper?)*kalemia.

(b) Sammy (Question B15[g]) has lost much fluid during his prolonged diarrhea. He is at risk for _____kalemia.

(c) Todd (Question B15[f]) has extensive burns and other tissue trauma resulting from his accident. His damaged cells are likely to release K^+ initially causing _____ kalemia. Over time the K^+ in his ECF may leak out of his burned skin or exit in urine, leading to _____kalemia.

C3. Mr. Evanston (Question B15[a]) takes a thiazide diuretic and also digoxin for his CHF. Answer these questions about him.

(a) He is at increased risk for _____kalemia because of the diuretic. The most serious effects of hypokalemia are those affecting the _____ system, particularly if serum K^+ drops below ____ mEq/L.

(b) The drug digitalis is likely to (ameliorate = make better? exacerbate = make worse?) the situation. Both hypokalemia and digoxin tend to cause (brady? tachy?)cardia.

(c) Hypokalemia (increases? decreases?) resting cell membrane potential, leading to (increase? decrease?) in muscle and nerve activity. Write examples of such manifestations. _____
_____
_____

(d) List several approaches to increasing Mr. Evanston's serum K^+ level. _____
_____

If he does require IV , what assessment should be made first? Explain. _____
_____
_____

C4. Hye-Sun, age 35, (Chapter 34, Question B11) has end-stage renal disease (ESRD) with her glomerular filtration rate (GFR) currently less than 5 mL/min. Complete this exercise.

(a) Her serum K^+ is 7.2 mEq/L, indicating (hyper? hypo?)-kalemia. Decreased renal function is a (rare? common?) cause of hyperkalemia. Hyperkalemia is (common? rare?) among healthy persons.

(b) Hye-Sun (is? is not?) likely to manifest neuromuscular changes related to her hyperkalemia. Explain. _____
_____
_____

(c) Many manifestations of hyperkalemia are similar to those of hypokalemia (compare textbook Tables 31-9 and 31-8). Write two distinguishing manifestations of hyperkalemia._____
_____
_____

(d) The fact that her blood pH level is currently 7.1 is likely to (ameliorate? exacerbate?) her electrolyte disorder. Explain. _____
_____
_____

(e) Interventions for Hye-Sun (should? should not?) include use of salt substitutes.

D. CALCIUM, PHOSPHATE, AND MAGNESIUM BALANCE (pages 721-734)

D1. Virtually all of the body's calcium ions (Ca^{+2}) are located within (bones? blood?) (see textbook Figure 31-15). Two other major electrolytes that are concentrated in bone are ____ and ____. However, other tissues require these ions also. Discuss how the body controls locations of these three electrolytes in this exercise.

(a) Two major factors that regulate these ions are vitamin ___ and the hormone ____.

(b) Vitamin D is activated by several organs, namely _____, _____, and _____ under the influence of the hormone _____. The active form of vitamin D is known as _____.

(c) PTH is produced by the four parathyroid glands. What is their normal location? _____ What factor serves as the major stimulus for secretion of PTH? (Hyper? Hypo?)-calcemia. Name an electrolyte also needed for normal PTH function. _____

D2. Refer to Study Guide Figure 30-4 (page 152) and consider effects of PTH.

(a) An increase in PTH leads to a(n) (increase? decrease?) in serum Ca^{+2}. PTH either directly or indirectly "pulls" from three sources. Name them: _____,
_____, _____

(b) PTH also influences PO_4^{-3} levels of blood. The hormone (increases? decreases?) blood PO_4^{-3} levels by pulling the ion from bones, but (increases? decreases?) blood PO_4^- by triggering _____ excretion of this ion. The latter effect is greater so PTH tends to (increase? decrease?) serum PO_4^{-3}.

(c) PTH also increases blood _____ levels by pulling the ion from bones. Add a labeled arrow on Figure 30-4 to show movement of PO_4^{-3} and Mg^{+2} from bone to blood.

D3. List several causes of hypoparathyroidism.

_____

_____

Diagnosis of the condition is indicated by low levels of ____ and ____, and high levels of ____. Treatment involves supplements of ____, ___, and ____.

D4. Explain how renal failure can lead to the following conditions. (See Chapter 34, Questions B5[d] to [f], B6[c], and B8[e].)

(a) Hyperparathyroidism

_____

_____

_____

(b) Renal osteodystrophy

_____

_____

_____

D5. List several functions of calcium in the body.

_____

_____

_____

D6. Circle the correct answers about calcium.

(a) A serum level of 10.9 mg/dL is _(high? normal? low?)_.

(b) List several calcium-rich foods:

_____,

_____,

_____.

(c) Dietary deficiency of calcium exerts more effects on Ca^{+2} levels in _(blood? bone?)_. Hypocalcemia due to inadequate dietary Ca^{+2} or vitamin D is _(common? rare?)_ in the United States.

(d) The main route by which the body normally loses Ca^{+2} is _(feces? skin? urine?)_.

(e) The form of Ca^{+2} that is free to leave blood and take part in cell functions is the form that is _(complexed or chelated? ionized? protein-bound?)_.

D7. Write _hyper_ or _hypo_ next to factors that are likely to cause hypercalcemia or hypocalcemia.

(a) Failure to activate vitamin D due to liver or kidney disease: _____

(b) Leg immobilization for 2 months following a tibial fracture: _____

(c) Production of high levels of osteoclastic chemicals from tumor cells:_____

(d) Hyperphosphatemia and hypomagnesemia:

_____

(e) Renal failure: _____

D8. _(Rapid? Slow?)_ blood transfusions are more likely to lead to hypocalcemia. Explain.

_____

_____

_____

D9. Complete this exercise about Hye-Sun, age 35, (question C4) who has end-stage renal disease (ESRD).

(a) Her failing kidneys eliminate _(more? less?)_ than normal PO_4^{-3} and _(more? less?)_ than normal Ca^{+2}. Hye-Sun's serum calcium is more likely to be _(7.0? 11.5?)_ mg/dL, indicating _____calcemia.

(b) Hye Sun's bones are soft and painful and prone to fracture. Explain. _____

_____

(c) The nurse practitioner performs a Chvostek's sign on Hye-Sun. This involves _(inflating a blood pressure cuff on the arm? tapping on the face?)_. Describe a positive Chvostek's sign._____

_____

_____

(d) Hye-Sun's personality and behavior exhibit signs of psychoses and dementia. Explain.

_____

_____

(e) She experiences tingling known as _____ around her mouth and in extremities, as well as spasms of wrists and ankles (_____ spasms). Spasms of the _____ would exert potentially fatal effects.

(f) What treatments may improve Hye-Sun's condition? _____

_____

D10. Write _hyper_ or _hypo_ next to signs or symptoms of hypercalcemia or hypocalcemia.

(a) Decreased neuromuscular activity as indicated by muscle weakness and atrophy, constipation, lethargy, stupor, and coma:

_____

(b) Inability of kidneys (damaged by calcium) to concentrate urine, which leads to production of copious amounts of urine and excessive thirst:_____

(c) Cardiovascular alterations: _____

D11. Complete this exercise about phosphate (PO_4^{-3}).

(a) Most phosphate is located in *(bones? serum?)*. Of the phosphate that is outside of bone, most is in *(ICF? ECF?)*, so injury to cells is likely to *(increase? decrease?)* serum levels of PO_4^{-3}.

(b) Normal serum phosphate levels are in the range of *(2.5 to 4.5? 8.5 to 10.5?)* mg/dL. Increasing serum levels by three or four times is likely to cause *(fatal? no immediate?)* effects on the body.

(c) Circle the chemicals that contain phosphorus (needed to form phosphate):

(1) ATP

(2) Some buffers

(3) Coenzymes for cell function

(4) DNA

(5) Glucose

(d) List dietary sources of phosphate that can help to prevent and also treat hypophosphatemia._____

_____

_____

(e) The overall effect of PTH is to *(raise? lower?)* serum phosphate (text Table 31-12).

(f) Most of the manifestations of hypophosphatemia such as muscle weakness are related to lack of the energy source ___ and changes in _____ blood cells.

D12. Write *hyper* or *hypo* next to causes of hyperphosphatemia or hypophosphatemia.

(a) Chronic use of antacids with aluminum or calcium that bind phosphate: _____

(b) Alcoholism (with associated malnutrition): _____

(c) Phosphate-containing enemas accompanied by hypovolemia: _____

(d) Massive trauma: _____ (*Hint*: see question D11[a].)

D13. Explain why adequate magnesium levels are critical to normal body function.

_____

_____

_____

D14. Compare calcium, phosphate, and magnesium by circling all correct answers in this exercise.

(a) Serum level of 2.5 mg/dL is most normal for: Ca^{+2} Mg^{+2} PO_4^{-3}

(b) Renal failure is likely to cause high serum levels of: Ca^{+2} Mg^{+2} PO_4^{-3}

(c) Malnutrition is likely to cause low levels of: Ca^{+2} Mg^{+2} PO_4^{-3}

(d) Tetany and muscle spasms with positive Trousseau's and Chvostek's signs typically accompany low levels of: Ca^{+2} Mg^{+2} PO_4^{-3}

(e) Lethargy or coma are likely to accompany high levels of: Ca^{+2} Mg^{+2} PO_4^{-3}

CHAPTER 32

Alterations in Acid-Base Balance

■ Review Questions

A. MECHANISMS OF ACID-BASE BALANCE (pages 735-742)

A1. Choose the two true statements.

(a) An acid is a molecule that can **accept** a hydrogen (H⁺) ion.

(b) Most of the body's acids, such as carbonic acid, are **weak** acids.

(c) A pH of 7.5 is **more** acidic than a pH of 7.4.

(d) **Carbonic** acid is classified as a volatile acid because exhalation can eliminate it.

(e) Almost all of the CO_2 in blood is transported **attached to hemoglobin.**

A2. Write the chemical reactions that show formation and dissociation of carbonic acid. Write CA (carbonic anhydrase) above the reaction that is accelerated 5,000 times by this enzyme.

_____

_____

_____

Note that if bicarbonate (HCO_3^-) combines with H⁺, carbonic acid (H_2CO_3) results. But bicarbonate can also combine with another cation (Na⁺ in ECF or K⁺ in ICF) to form sodium bicarbonate ($NaHCO_3$) or potassium bicarbonate ($KHCO_3$), respectively.

A3. Name two or more acids in each category that are produced by metabolism.

(a) Organic

_____

_____

_____

(b) Inorganic

_____

_____

_____

A4. Complete this exercise about maintaining blood pH.

(a) Arterial blood pH is normally maintained at about *(7.2? 7.3? 7.4?)*, or within a range of pH ____ to ____.

(b) Refer to the reactions in Question A2. To maintain a pH of 7.4 in the plasma (ECF) of arterial blood, a ratio of Na.HCO_3 to H.HCO_3 ($NaHCO_3$ to H_2CO_3) of ___ : ___ must be maintained. This is determined by the _____-_____ equation. *Note: if one of these values increases, then the other value must also increase to maintain the ratio.*

(c) The concentration of bicarbonate in plasma is within the range of ____ to ____ mEq/L, or a mean of about ____ mEq/L. (*Hint: see textbook Table 31-1.*)

(d) Because H_2CO_3 cannot be measured directly, it is determined by the amount of CO_2 dissolved in plasma. This is calculated by multiplying PCO_2 by 0.03 (the solubility coefficient of CO_2).

(1) Refer to Study Guide Figure 27-1 (page 128) and note the PCO_2 of blood in venous blood (____ mm Hg) and in arterial blood (____ mm Hg).

(2) Venous blood contains 45 × 0.03 = ____ mEq/L. Dissolved CO_2 and arterial blood contains ____ × 0.03 = ____ mEq/L. It is logical that arterial blood contains a little *(more? less?)* dissolved CO_2 than venous blood.

(e) Now calculate the normal ratios that must be maintained for acid-base balance:

(1) Ratio in venous blood
$$\frac{NaHCO_3}{H_2CO_3 = \text{dissolved } CO_2} = \_\_\_ \text{mEqL} = \frac{20}{1}$$

(2) Ratio in arterial blood
$$\frac{NaHCO_3}{H_2CO_3 = \text{dissolved } CO_2} = \_\_\_ \text{mEqL} = \frac{20}{1}$$

(f) Calculate an acid-base *imbalance* in which hypoventilation causes retention of CO_2 so that the level of dissolved CO_2 doubles from 1.2 to ____ mEq/L. $NaHCO_3$ will need to *(increase? decrease?)* to ____ mEq/L to maintain a 20:1 ratio. So, as one value increases, the body compensates by causing the other value to *(increase also? decrease?)*. (See A4[b].) Complete the new ratio.

$$\frac{NaHCO_3}{H_2CO_3 = dissolved\ CO_2} = \frac{24\ mEqL}{1.2} = \frac{\_\_\_}{2.4}$$

(g) Bicarbonate ($NaHCO_3$) levels fluctuate widely in the body because this chemical is expended in buffering acids produced by metabolism. For example, lactic acid released during vigorous muscle metabolism decreases plasma levels of bicarbonate as it is used as a buffer. Therefore *(metabolic? respiratory?)* acid-base imbalances are reflected by altered *($NaHCO_3$? H_2CO_3 = dissolved CO_2?)*. Respiratory acid-base imbalances result from some respiratory condition that alters *($NaHCO_3$? H_2CO_3 = dissolved CO_2?)*. The disorder in Question A4(f) is an example of a compensated *(metabolic? respiratory?)* acid-base imbalance.

A5. List the three major mechanisms that work to maintain acid-base balance.

_____

_____

_____

Arrange them in correct sequence from fastest-to slowest-acting in responding to acid-base imbalances. _____, _____,

_____

A6. Visualize buffers as tiny sponges floating around in plasma. This exercise focuses on the carbonic acid-bicarbonate buffer system.

(a) The buffer consists of an anion (in this case, _____)— the "sponge" that can either absorb or eject different cations such as Na^+ or H^+. Typically, there are ____ bicarbonates attached to Na^+ for every ___ bicarbonate attached to H^+ (the 20:1 ratio).

(b) When the body develops acidosis and needs to buffer a strong acid such as HCl, the Na^+ ions are "squeezed out" of the "sponge" (HCO_3^-) such that the H^+ ions can enter the sponge and form the weaker acid, _____. The remaining Na^+ ions combine with ____. Complete the reaction: $HCl + NaHCO_3 \rightarrow$ _____ + _____

A7. Identify the buffer system that fits each description below. Choose from these answers:

Ammonia buffer system
Bicarbonate-carbonic acid
Protein
Plasma potassium-hydrogen exchange
Phosphate

(a) The most common buffer system in cells (ICF); albumin is a major buffer of this type: _____

(b) Involves the most common acid in the body (formed from CO_2 + H_2O):

_____

(c) This system allows kidneys to increase elimination of H^+: _____

(d) Allows kidneys to eliminate ammonia, H^+ and Cl^-, in the form of ammonium chloride (NH_4Cl): _____

(e) The result of this system is that when plasma H^+ increases (acidosis), K^+ will increase, as will Ca^{+2}, and vice versa (see Chapter 31 question C1e and related Figure 31-1D and E about shifts of H^+ and K^+): _____

A8. Complete this exercise about respiratory and renal mechanisms that regulate acid-base balance.

(a) Slight acidosis stimulates hyperventilation that will tend to *(raise? lower?)* blood pH because, as the person exhales, less CO_2 is available for formation of _____ acid and free hydrogen ion.

(b) Kidneys regulate acid-base balance by altering their tubular secretion of _____ or elimination of _____ ion over several days (see Chapter 30, Questions A5[a] and [b]). Several mechanisms are employed.

(1) H^+s are removed in urine by the carbonic anhydrase–mediated system that causes kidneys to retain _____ and _____ (see textbook Figure 32-5).

(2) H^+s are removed in urine by the _____ buffer system that again involves kidney retention of _____ and _____ (see textbook Figure 32-6).

(3) H^+s are removed in urine by the _____ buffer system. In this

system, ammonia (_____) combines with H+ to form ammonium (_____) that is excreted as NH_4Cl while again kidneys retain _____ and _____ (see textbook Figure 32-7).

    (4) All these systems allow acid to be eliminated and alkaline $Na^+HCO_3^-$ to be retained. How else are the different buffers helpful? _____

A9. Discuss other mechanisms that help to regulate pH.

    (a) Hyperkalemia (high levels of ____) tends to cause acidosis (high levels of ____) and vice versa (see Figure 31-1D and E). Conversely, hypokalemia leads to _____osis.

    (b) High aldosterone levels cause kidneys to retain ____ and ____ and to secrete ____ and ____. Thus, primary aldosteronism tends to lead to _____osis (and hypokalemia), whereas Addison's disease leads to _____osis (and hyperkalemia).

    (c) During a meal, the stomach secretes gastric juices including the acid _____. In response, the body will retain another anion (_____) to maintain electrochemical balance. Then, after a meal (postprandially), _____osis occurs briefly.

A10. Teri, age 42 and a life-long smoker, is in early stages of emphysema. Blood is removed from her left radial artery for testing of arterial blood gases (ABGs). Circle "yes" or "no" to indicate whether each result is normal. (*Hint*: refer to Study Guide Figure 27-1, page 128.)

    (a) Her arterial pO_2 is 88 mm Hg.   Yes   No

    (b) Her arterial PCO_2 is 48 mm Hg.   Yes   No

    (c) Her arterial pH is 7.30.   Yes   No

    (d) Her arterial HCO_3^- is 36 mm mEq/L.   Yes   No

    (e) Her arterial base excess is 3.3 mm Hg.   Yes   No

A11. Larry completed a 15-mile run 2 hours ago. Look at his arterial blood gases (ABGs) and serum electrolyte values and determine his anion gap. Is this high, low, or normal?

Na^+: 136 mEq/L   Arterial PCO_2: 44 mm Hg

Cl^-: 86 mEq/L   Arterial PO_2: 86 mm Hg

HCO_3^-: 34 mEq/L   Arterial pH: 7.35

Explain your answer. _____
_____
_____
_____

B. ALTERATIONS IN ACID-BASE BALANCE (pages 742-752)

B1. Identify whether a correction or a compensation is taking place in each case.

    (a) Tyler, age 5, overdosed on children's aspirin. He is lethargic but hyperventilating:

    _____

    (b) Mr. Hershey has increased blood levels of BUN, creatinine, K^+ and H^+ as a result of acute renal failure caused by nephrotoxic drugs. ECG changes, abdominal cramping, and diarrhea result from his hyperkalemia. His doctor changes his prescription to one that is not toxic to kidneys: _____

    (c) Mrs. Litzinger is hyperventilating during labor and delivery. Her kidneys start producing more highly alkaline urine. She begins involuntary wrist and ankle movements (carpopedal spasms): _____

    _____

B2. Describe effects of altered pH on the central nervous system (CNS).

    (a) In acidosis, H^+ *(increases? decreases?)*, pH *(increases? decreases?)*, and CNS activity *(increases? decreases?)*. (*Hint*: as pH goes down, so does CNS activity.) Write typical signs and symptoms: _____
    _____
    _____
    _____

    (b) In alkalosis, H^+ *(increases? decreases?)*, pH *(increases? decreases?)*, and CNS activity *(increases? decreases?)*. Write typical signs and symptoms: _____
    _____
    _____
    _____

B3. Identify the source of the signs or symptoms in question B1.

    (a) Signs of the primary disorder:

    _____
    _____

(b) Signs of altered pH:

_____

_____

_____

(c) Signs of a compensatory mechanism:

_____

_____

_____

B4. Indicate which of the four categories of acid-base imbalances is most likely to occur as a result of each condition.

Metabolic acidosis   Metabolic alkalosis
Respiratory acidosis   Respiratory alkalosis

(a) Tyler (Question B1[a]) who overdosed on children's aspirin: _____

(b) Mr. Hershey (Question B1[b]) during his acute renal failure: _____

(c) Teri (question A10) with emphysema:

_____

(d) Myocardial infarction: _____

(e) Suzanne who is on a ketogenic 400 cal/day diet for weight reduction: _____

_____

(f) Lisa, age 4, who ingests about 2 tablespoons (30 mL) of the "pretty yellow stuff that's sweet" (antifreeze): _____

(g) Severe diarrhea with loss of pancreatic secretions (high in HCO_3^-): _____

_____ `

(h) Hyperalimentation with liquids high in Cl-:

_____

(i) Diuretics that cause potassium loss:

_____

(j) Primary aldosteronism:
_____ (See Question
A9[b].)

(k) Loss of gastric juices (with hypochloremia) by nasogastric suction:
_____ (See Question A9[c].)

B5. Complete this exercise about acid-base imbalances.

(a) Mary Emma, age 11, has diabetes and is currently in ketoacidosis. She is breathing as if she just finished running hard. This is known as _____'s breathing and is a classic compensatory sign of *(metabolic? respiratory?)* acidosis. The pH of her urine is likely to be *(5.0? 7.0?)*. Acidosis *(can? does not?)* affect Mary Emma's skeletal growth.

(b) Emily has purging bulimia. Her plasma pH is 7.54, PCO_2 is 48 mm Hg, and HCO_3^- is 36 mEq/L. Her breathing is slow and shallow. Explain why KCl is administered.

_____

_____

_____

(c) Mr. Feinberg cannot breathing deeply after fracturing a rib 3 days ago. His blood pH is 7.33, PCO_2 is 48 mm Hg, and HCO_3^- is 36 mEq/L. His bicarbonate has *(increased? decreased?)* as a compensatory mechanism because PCO_2 is increased; this is an attempt to maintain the 20:1 ratio between these two chemicals (See Questions A4[b] and [f]). The change in bicarbonate level happens *(quickly? slowly?)*. State the clinical significance. _____

_____

_____

_____

(d) Julia has a panic attack and is in the psychiatric emergency department. Her hyperventilation is likely to lead to an arterial pH of *(7.3? 7.5?)* with *(hyper? hypo?)*excitability of her nervous system. Describe one simple method that can help to reverse her acid-base imbalance.

_____

_____

_____

_____

B6. How can you determine the type of acid-base imbalance when values for PCO_2 and HCO_3^- are similar, as for Emily and Mr. Feinberg in Questions B5(b) and (c)?

_____

_____

_____

_____

CHAPTER 33

Alterations in Renal Function

■ Review Questions

A. CONGENITAL DISORDERS OF THE KIDNEYS (pages 753-756)

A1. Choose the two true statements.

(a) Fetal kidneys **can** be detected by ultrasound by about 12 weeks' gestation.

(b) If fetal kidney function is less than normal, the volume of amniotic fluid is likely to be **greater** than normal.

(c) Renal hypoplasia is considered **more** serious than renal agenesis.

(d) **Potter's syndrome** refers to facial features that accompany renal agenesis.

A2. Jenny Rose was born with her kidneys located within her bony pelvis. Explain the clinical significance.

_____

_____

_____

A3. Complete this exercise about renal cysts.

(a) Renal cysts typically form from dilatation of *(glomeruli? renal tubules or collecting ducts?)*. They are *(solid? fluid-filled?)*.

(b) Cysts may range in size from 1 or 2 mm to 5 cm (about ___ inch[es]). Signs and symptoms range from none to fatality. What are typical effects of larger cysts? _____

_____

(c) Simple renal cysts are *(rare? common?)* and are typically *(benign? malignant?)*; most *(do? do not?)* alter kidney function. They occur more often in *(children? the elderly?)*.

A4. Match the type of renal cyst with the correct description.
Autosomal dominant polycystic kidney disease
Acquired renal cystic disease
Nephrophthisis-medullary cystic disease complex

(a) Almost always hereditary; accounts for 10% to 20% of renal failure in children; polyuria with bed-wetting are early indicators:

_____

(b) Disorder transmitted by PKD genes; systemic effects are common and often serious, as in liver, colon, mitral valve, and blood vessels; treatment is mostly supportive: _____

_____

(c) Typically occur in patients with renal failure who are receiving long-term dialysis:

_____

A5. Explain why each of the following signs or symptoms may accompany adult polycystic disease that is associated with long-term dialysis.

(a) Hypertension

_____

_____

_____

(b) Hematuria

_____

_____

_____

(c) Flank pain

_____

_____

_____

(d) Infected kidneys

_____

_____

_____

B. OBSTRUCTIVE DISORDERS (pages 756-761)

B1. Refer to Figure 33-4 and Table 33-1 in the textbook and identify possible causes of obstructions to urine flow.

_____

_____

_____

B2. Describe the major problems that arise from urinary tract obstructions leading to stasis of urine.

(a) Urine in a warm and moist environment predisposes to urinary tract _____ (UTIs). Repeated infection can lead to scar tissue in urine pathways that causes

_____.

(b) Urinary stasis concentrates urine which increases risk of formation of renal calculi (or _____), especially if urine is _(acid? alkaline?)_.

(c) The most serious consequence of obstructions arises from backflow of urine which can dilate ureters (_____ureter) and dilate and damage kidneys (_____). Irreversible kidney damage can begin as early as 7 _(days? months? years?)_ from the onset of obstruction.

(d) All these previously listed conditions may lead to pain. _(Acute? Gradual?)_ obstruction in kidneys or the upper ureter leads to stabbing flank pain, whereas _(acute? gradual?)_ obstruction, for example by prostate enlargement, leads to vague pelvic discomfort.

B3. The term nephro_____ refers to the condition of having kidney stones. Select the type of kidney stone that fits each description.

Calcium oxalate or calcium phosphate
Cystine   Struvite   Uric acid

(a) Occur in patients with gout when urine is abnormally acidic: _____

(b) Known as "staghorn stones" because they conform to the shape of the renal pelvis (much like a stag's horns); almost always occur in the presence of UTIs and alkaline urine: _____

(c) About three quarters of all kidney stones are of this type: _____

B4. Circle the answers that are predisposing factors to nephrolithiasis.

(a) Female gender

(b) Drinking 10 glasses of water a day

(c) High citrate level in urine

(d) Deficiency of stone formation inhibitors such as nephrocalcin or uropontin

(e) Urinary tract infections (UTIs)

(f) Hypercalcemia

B5. Mr. Laredo, age 68, has recently recovered from a fractured tibia that required immobilization for 2 months. He has benign prostatic hyperplasia (BPH) and a history of kidney stones. He is transported to the emergency room with excruciating pain in his left flank. Describe his condition by circling the correct answers or filling in the blanks.

(a) Mr. Laredo says his pain "comes and goes" and it intensifies. This is _(colicky? noncolicky?)_ pain that suggests _(left? bilateral?)_ kidney stones. Kidney stones are typically _(bi? uni?)_lateral.

(b) Mr. Laredo reports: "I tried drinking about a quart of water an hour ago—thought it might help this stone pass. But the pain just got worse." Explain. _____

_____

(c) Radiographs and an IVP _(are? are not?)_ likely to help to diagnose kidney stones. Mr. Laredo's stone is 1.2 cm and lodged in the left ureter. Because of its size, his stone _(is? is not?)_ likely to "pass" on its own. The treatment of choice is:

(1) Extracorporeal shock wave lithotripsy

(2) Percutaneous nephrolithotomy

(d) A ureteral stent is inserted and Mr. Laredo is instructed to "strain his urine." Explain.

_____

_____

(e) How may Mr. Laredo's stone be related to his BPH? _____

_____

(f) How may his stone be related to his fracture? _____

_____

(g) His stones are calcium oxalate. Which foods should he avoid because of their high oxalate content?_____

_____

C. URINARY TRACT INFECTIONS (pages 762-766)

C1. Choose the two true statements.

(a) Urinary tract infections (UTIs) are the **most** common type of bacterial infection in the body.

(b) Infections of the bladder (cystitis) are considered **more** serious than renal pelvis (pyelonephritis) infections.

(c) Most UTIs are caused by the gram-negative bacterium *E. coli*.

(d) Most UTIs occur from spread of infections from the **bloodstream.**

(e) Urine specimens **should** be refrigerated if they will be kept for longer than an hour.

C2. Circle the person who is at greater risk of UTIs in each case, then write a brief rationale.

(a)
   (1) A 12-year-old girl
   (2) An 82-year-old woman

_____

_____

(b)
   (1) A sexually active 21-year-old woman
   (2) A sexually active 21-year-old man

_____

_____

(c)
   (1) A 60-year-old man with BPH
   (2) A 60-year-old woman

_____

_____

(d)
   (1) A healthy 40-year-old woman
   (2) A 40-year-old woman with multiple sclerosis who is regularly catheterized

_____

_____

C3. Explain how the following factors contribute to risk of UTIs:

(a) Bacterial fimbriae or pili

_____

_____

_____

(b) Vesicoureteral reflux (backflow from bladder and ureter)

_____

_____

_____

C4. Use the following information to complete this exercise. Rochelle, age 20, reports that she "has been urinating two or three times an hour, and it burns and itches and smells something awful. And my belly feels yucky." When the nurse asks more about pain, Rochelle states: "It's not sharp pain, my belly just feels really bad." She denies any pain "at the back of my waist." Her temperature is 99.8°F. A clean-voided urine sample is positive for leukocytes (pyuria) and the bacterium, *E. coli*.

(a) Rochelle's UTI is most likely to be a(n):
   (1) Lower UTI: cystitis (bladder infection) and possibly lower ureters
   (2) Upper UTI (pyelonephritis)

(b) About *(2%? 20%?)* of all adult women develop at least one UTI during their lifetime. UTIs are more common in women between ages *(15 and 24? 45 and 54?)* years.

(c) Because Rochelle's diagnosis is an acute UTI involving the urethra and bladder, treatment is likely to include a *(3 to 7? 14 to 28?)*-day course of antifungal drug and of "forcing fluids." How does the latter help?

_____

_____

C5. Write a rationale to explain why UTIs are more common among each of these populations.

(a) Pregnant women

_____

_____

_____

(b) Elderly persons in nursing homes

_____

_____

_____

C6. Contrast signs and symptoms of UTIs that are likely to occur in these males:

(a) A 1-year-old

_____

_____

(b) An 80-year-old

_____

_____

_____

D. DISORDERS OF GLOMERULAR FUNCTION (pages 766-771)

D1. Refer to Chapter 30, questions A2(b) and (c), to review glomerular structure. Name the three layers: _____, _____, _____. In addition, mesangial cells cover areas of the glomerulus that *(have? lack?)* a basement membrane.

D2. Circle correct answers in this overview of glomerular disorders and use the list of terms to complete sentences about major signs and symptoms; one term will be used twice.

Azotemia	Coagulation disorders
Edema	Infections
Oliguria	Hematuria
Hypertension	Hypoalbuminemia
Proteinuria	Pyuria

(a) Glomerulonephritis is a *(nephritic? nephrotic?)* condition that is a *(rare? common?)* cause of chronic renal failure (CRF) in the United States. The suffix "-itis" indicates that this *(is? is not?)* an inflammatory disorder that reduces GFR. The inflamed membrane allows blood cells into urine.

   (1) Because of decreased GFR, BUN, and serum creatinine levels increase: _____

   (2) Decreased GFR tends to decrease urinary output (_____) with fluid retention that leads to _____ and _____.

   (3) Imagine gaping holes in inflamed glomerular membranes; these allow red blood cells to pass into urine, leading to the classic sign of cola-colored urine (_____). Presence of white blood cells in urine (_____) also occurs.

(b) *(Nephritic? Nephrotic?)* syndromes (or nephroses) involve damage to the glomerular membrane that allows protein and possibly lipids to escape into urine.

   (1) The passage of proteins from blood to urine results in _____ and _____.

   (2) Because depleted plasma proteins are not sufficient to create the osmotic "pull" of water into vessels, _____ occurs.

   (3) Loss of immunoglobulin proteins into urine increases risk for _____, and loss of fibrinogen can cause _____.

D3. Ms. Gowland has a form of glomerulonephritis. Her urinary output is higher than normal with a specific gravity of 1.005. Explain.

_____

_____

_____

D4. Discuss causes and categories of glomerulonephritis in this exercise.

(a) Most of these conditions *(are? are not?)* immune-related. Glomerular damage results from anti_____ that react with anti_____ on glomerular membranes (or from antigen-antibody complexes). These cause inflammatory changes in the membranes. List two or more examples of sources of such antigens. _____

_____

_____

(b) Glomerular disease that is widespread throughout kidneys is called *(diffuse? focal?)*. If it affects only certain segments of the glomerulus, it is called _____.

(c) Identify the type of damage to the glomerular wall that occurs in each of these categories of glomerulonephritis.

   Membranous   Proliferative   Sclerotic

   (1) Increased collagen between cells: _____

   (2) Increased number of cells in the glomerular wall: _____

   (3) Increased thickness by deposits of antigen-antibody complexes: _____

D5. Identify selected types of glomerular disease by their descriptions.

   Acute proliferative glomerulonephritis (APGN)
   Chronic glomerulonephrosis
   Focal segmental glomerulosclerosis (FSGS)
   IgA nephropathy
   Membranous glomerulonephritis (MGN)
   Nephrotic syndrome

(a) Dramatically increased permeability of glomeruli to proteins leads to the hallmark sign of this disorder: proteinuria more than 3.5 g/day causing systemic and pulmonary edema; altered lipid metabolism also occurs; usually primary in children; in adults may occur as MGN or FSGS, or secondary to diabetes or lupus: _____

(b) Involves increased collagen laid down in some but not all glomeruli; occurs in sickle cell disease, some congenital heart defects, with drug use or HIV; usually does lead to renal failure: _____

(c) Most commonly occurs one or two weeks post-strep infection as antigen-antibody complexes build up; occurs mainly in children, and has a 95% survival rate; cola-colored urine is a typical first sign: _____

(d) The most common cause of glomerular nephritis in Asian young adults; elevated serum IgA helps with diagnosis; currently no satisfactory treatment: _____

(e) May occur as a primary disorder affecting only kidneys, from lack of resolution of acute glomerular disease (such as APGN), or secondary to systemic disorders like diabetes or hypertension; gradual progression to end-stage renal disease: _____

D6. André, age 17, was diagnosed with diabetes mellitus at age 12. Complete this exercise about him.

(a) About 1 in *(3? 6? 10?)* people with type 1 diabetes develops diabetic nephropathy. Diabetes more commonly damages the *(glomerulus? renal tubule?)*.

(b) It is likely that André's glomerular membrane is becoming *(thinner? thicker?)* or sclerosing (See question D4c1). At least part of this change results from incorporation of excessive blood _____ into the glomerular wall.

(c) At this early stage of glomerulosclerosis, André's GFR is likely to be abnormally *(high? low?)*, enlarging glomerular pores. Protein in his urine then becomes *(dramatically? slightly?)* elevated, a predictor of future nephropathy. Such changes *(are? are not?)* likely to be minimized by control of blood sugar and blood pressure.

(d) André has taken up smoking. Smoking cessation *(is? is not?)* likely to reduce his degree of diabetic nephropathy.

D7. Is glomerular disease a cause or effect of chronic hypertension?

_____

_____

_____

E. TUBULOINTERSTITIAL DISORDERS (pages 771-773)

E1. Describe acidosis caused by renal tubule disorders by circling the correct answers or filling in the blanks.

(a) Proximal tubule injury causes *(more? less?)* than normal sodium bicarbonate (HCO_3^-) to pass into urine.

(b) In distal tubular disorders, *(more? less?)* than normal number of hydrogen ions (H^+) move into urine. Buffering of excessive blood acid leads to release of ____ from bone, which causes bone pain, decreased bone growth in children, and possible kidney stones. In addition, *(more? fewer?)* than normal sodium ions (Na^+) are reabsorbed by active countertransport.

(c) As a result of sodium loss by either route, secretion of aldosterone *(increases? decreases?)* in an attempt to *(reabsorb? secrete?)* more Na^+. But aldosterone causes *(loss? retention?)* of K^+, leading to _____kalemia. *Hint*: refer to Chapter 30, Questions A5(b), A7(b), and Figure 30-3.

E2. Pyelonephritis is typically more damaging to *(glomeruli? tubules and surrounding interstitium?)*. Identify whether the following descriptions indicate acute or chronic pyelonephritis.

(a) Infection leads to significant scar formation within kidneys; accounts for up to 20% of end-stage renal failure: _____

(b) Caused by bacterial infection with abrupt onset of fever, chills, back pain, and typical signs and symptoms of UTIs; likely to be short term: _____

E3. Explain why kidneys are at right risk for damage by toxic drugs.

_____

_____

_____

E4. Mrs. Stein, age 75, has rheumatoid arthritis and hypertension. Explain why she may be at increased risk for drug-related nephropathy.

_____

_____

_____

F. NEOPLASMS (pages 773-775)

F1. Wilms' tumor is a kidney tumor of *(young children? adults?)*. Incidence is *(higher? no greater?)* in children with congenital genitourinary anomalies. Almost all cases are *(bi? uni?)*lateral. Most common presenting symptoms are abdominal mass and *(hyper? hypo?)*tension. With aggressive treatment, survival is about ___%.

F2. Adult renal carcinoma (kidney cancer) is most likely to affect persons who are *(20? 40? 60?)* years old. The most common presenting sign is *(an abdominal mass? hematuria?)*. It is most commonly detected in *(early? late?)* stages. The treatment of choice is _____ectomy. Persons in stage *(I? IV?)* of the disease are likely to have a 5-year survival rate of 65% to 85%.

CHAPTER 34

Renal Failure

■ Review Questions

A. ACUTE RENAL FAILURE (pages 777-781)

A1. Choose the two true statements.

(a) Acute renal failure (ARF) is potentially reversible, whereas chronic renal failure (CRF) **is not.**

(b) The mortality rate of patients with ARF in intensive care units is about 4% to 8%.

(c) The most common sign of ARF is increase in blood levels of BUN and **creatinine.**

(d) ARF is most likely to be caused by **postrenal** causes.

A2. Identify the category or cause of acute renal failure in each case.

Intrarenal (or intrinsic)   Postrenal   Prerenal

(a) Decreased renal perfusion as by hemorrhage, shock, or renal vasoconstriction: _____

(b) Prostatic hyperplasia or bladder cancer: _____

(c) Long term use of NSAIDs for control of arthritis pain: _____

(d) Most commonly caused by acute tubular necrosis (ATN): _____

A3. Complete this exercise about acute renal failure (ARF).

(a) In ARF, both GRF and urinary output *(increase? decrease?)*. The ratio of BUN to creatinine is more likely to be *(10:1? 20:1?)* because the small amount of creatinine that is filtered is *(largely? not?)* reabsorbed.

(b) Signs and symptoms of renal failure do not typically occur until renal perfusion falls to about _____ % of normal. Ischemia is more likely to destroy cells of *(glomeruli? tubules?)* because of their greater oxygen demands. Toxins are also more damaging to *(glomeruli? tubules?)*. An early sign of tubular damage is inability of kidneys to

_____ urine, a condition that may mask a decrease in GFR.

A4. Identify the most likely cause of acute tubular necrosis (ATN) in each case.

Ischemia   Intratubular obstruction
Nephrotoxic

(a) Mr. Barkley is undergoing cisplatin chemotherapy for his cancer: _____

(b) Elena's urinary output decreases while she is taking the aminoglycoside kanamycin to treat her infection: _____

(c) Nate completes his first marathon but is hospitalized shortly after this extreme exertion with severely reduced urinary output and tea-colored urine: _____

(d) Allesandra has been in the children's burn unit for 2 weeks following severe burns and multiple fractures: _____

A5. Mr. Yoho's 24-hour urine output is 640 mL; his BUN is 32 g/dL, and his creatinine level is 1.7 g/dL. His potassium level is 6.2 mEq/L. Mr. Yoho is likely to be in the _____ of acute tubular necrosis (ATN).

(a) Initial phase

(b) Maintenance phase

(c) Recovery or repair phase

A6. Explain why early diagnosis of acute renal failure is critical, especially for elderly persons.

_____

_____

_____

B. CHRONIC RENAL FAILURE (pages 781-790)

B1. Choose the correct answers in this exercise about kidneys.

(a) Kidneys have *(a high level of? very limited?)* compensatory abilities.

(b) In chronic renal failure (CRF), which functions decrease?

(1) Glomerular filtration

(2) Reabsorption

(3) Renal endocrine function

(c) The outlook for chronic renal failure (CRF) patients has (*improved? gotten much worse?*) over the past three decades.

B2. Identify the phase of chronic renal failure demonstrated in each patient.

Diminished renal reserve   End-stage renal disease
Renal failure   Renal insufficiency

(a) Mr. Ash, aged 49, has type 2 diabetes. His blood pressure is 148/92 even when taking antihypertensive medication; his GFR is 32% of normal and he has signs of azotemia: _____

(b) Mrs. LaRocca, aged 61, has only one kidney following nephrectomy for renal carcinoma 5 years earlier. Her blood pressure is 136/82, GFR is 60%, BUN is 21 mg/dL, and her creatinine level is 1.1 mg/dL: _____

(c) Mrs. Rodriguez-Rivera's GFR is 18% of normal. Her feet and ankles are so swollen that she can wear only large slippers on her feet. Her hematocrit is 27, arterial pH is about 7.25 and she is lethargic: _____

B3. Contrast azotemia with uremia.

_____
_____
_____

B4. Explain why clients with CRF may become overhydrated and edematous, or may become dehydrated.

_____
_____
_____

B5. Insert arrows to indicate how blood levels, chemicals, or other factors change with chronic renal failure (↑ = increase; ↓ = decrease).

Blood:

(a) Na^+: ____

(b) K^+: ____ when in severe CRF (GFR <5 mL/min

(c) H^+: ____ (so pH ____) with buffering by bone leading to ____ in bone density

(d) PO_4^{-3} ____ which may be treated by (*increasing? decreasing?*) intake (especially in dairy products)

(e) Active vitamin D levels ____ which causes ____ in blood levels of Ca^{+2}

(f) Ca^{+2}: ____, which causes ____ secretion of PTH, which causes ____ in bone density

(g) Red blood cell count and hematocrit: ____

B6. Circle the correct answer or fill in the blanks in each statement about CRF.

(a) Blood levels of PO_4^{-3} and Ca^{+2} are (*directly? inversely?*) related. Because kidneys fail to excrete ____, they excrete excessive amounts of ____.

(b) Most people with end-stage renal disease (ESRD) tend to develop (*hyper? hypo?*)-parathyroidism.

(c) Osteodystrophy derives from electrolyte changes shown in Question B5d through f and involves (*increased? decreased?*) bone mineralization. One form of this bone disorder, osteitis fibrosa cystica, involves (*over? under?*)active osteoblasts; cysts may form in porous spaces.

(d) Osteomalacia is another form of renal osteodystrophy, in which bones are (*softer? more brittle?*) than normal, which is related to a (*high? low?*) turnover of bone, as osteoblast activity (*increases? decreases?*). Two factors that cause this condition are _____ deficiency and high blood _____ that occur with CRF. Until recently, osteomalacia was common among CRF patients on _____ who developed high blood levels of _____ from the procedure.

B7. After you review textbook Table 34-1 write the name of the system that involves signs and symptoms below. Choose from these answers.

Cardiovascular   Gastrointestinal
Hematologic   Immune
Integumentary   Neurologic
Reproductive

(a) Uremic encephalopathy due to toxic substances in blood: _____

(b) Restless legs syndrome and asterixis:
_____

(c) Pruritus resulting from presence of phosphate or urea crystals; Terry's nails:
_____

(d) Impotence (in more than half of men on dialysis) and amenorrhea:

_____

(e) Failure to develop a fever in the presence of infection: _____

(f) Metallic taste in the mouth that may lead to anorexia: _____

(g) The system most responsible for death in end-stage renal disease: _____

(h) Decreased erythropoietin production by kidneys: _____ and

_____

B8. Write rationales for the following interventions for chronic renal failure.

(a) rhEPO and iron supplements

_____

_____

_____

(b) Salt and water restriction

_____

_____

_____

(c) Adjustment (often lowering) of medication dosages and caution taking over-the-counter (OTC) drugs

_____

_____

_____

(d) Restriction of dairy products

_____

_____

_____

(e) Caution about types of antacids used

_____

_____

_____

B9. Explain why the outlook for chronic renal failure (CRF) patients has improved in recent years.

_____

_____

_____

B10. Contrast forms of dialysis for end-stage renal failure patients by writing "H" for hemodialysis or "P" for peritoneal dialysis.

(a) A cellophane membrane is involved in the dialysis: ___

(b) CAPD involves continuous dialysis for 4 to 6 hours four times a day: ____

(c) Usually requires an arteriovenous fistula and heparin: ____

(d) Dialysis is usually performed three times a week: ____

B11. Complete this exercise about Hye-Sun, age 35, who has ESRD that was caused by IgA glomerulonephropathy (See Chapter 33, Question D5[d]). She is receiving hemodialysis.

(a) Hye-Sun weighs 132 pounds (60 kg). How much protein intake per day is likely to be recommended for this patient? _____

_____

_____

(b) Why should Hye-Sun avoid taking penicillin for infections and consuming foods such as orange juice and chocolate?

_____

_____

(c) She experiences nausea and vomiting as well as muscle cramps during the dialysis. Are these normal side effects of the procedure? _____

_____

_____

(d) Hye-Sun is constantly thirsty. Explain.

_____

_____

(e) The fact that she has gained 13 pounds since her last dialysis treatment 3 days ago suggests edema involving retention (possibly from drinking) of ___ liters of fluid.

B12. Choose the two true statements about treatments for CRF.

(a) Recent 1-year graft survival rates for patients who have received kidney transplants are about 30%.

(b) Acute rejection of a transplanted kidney is **more** likely to respond to immunosuppressants than chronic rejection is.

(c) The dialysates used for continuous ambulatory peritoneal dialysis (CAPD) **do** contain nutrients.

(d) Eggs and lean meat are **contraindicated** in the diet of dialysis patients.

C. RENAL FAILURE IN CHILDREN AND ELDERLY PERSONS (pages 790-793)

C1. Billy, age 17 months, has chronic renal failure from a congenital kidney disorder. He is currently on dialysis therapy as he awaits a transplant.

(a) Renal osteodystrophy is *(more? less?)* likely to exert damaging effects in a child than in an adult. Explain. _____

_____

_____

(b) *(Nutrition? Gonadotropic hormone?)* is the key factor in bone maturation during infancy.

(c) Billy has CCPD dialysis. This is a form of *(hemo-? peritoneal?)* dialysis administered *(all day? at night?)*.

(d) After Billy does receive a transplant, he is likely to be at increased risk for infections. Explain why._____

_____

_____

C2. Circle correct answers in these statements.

(a) GFR *(does? does not?)* tend to decrease with normal aging; as a result, nephrotoxic drugs are likely to exert *(greater? fewer?)* effects on older adults.

(b) In an 80-year-old, a decreased GFR *(is? is not?)* as likely to increase blood creatinine to high levels as in a 30-year-old. Explain.

_____

_____

(c) Oliguria and cola-colored urine are more likely the first signs of renal failure in *(elderly? younger?)* persons.

(d) State one factor that may increase survival rate from kidney transplant in elderly persons. _____

_____

CHAPTER 35

Alterations in Urine Elimination

■ Review Questions

A. CONTROL OF URINE ELIMINATION (pages 795–801)

A1. The elimination of urine from the bladder is a process known as _____. In the following exercise, discuss the structures involved in this process. (*Hint*: refer to textbook Figure 35-1).

(a) The floor of the bladder is composed of the triangular muscle known as the (*detrusor? trigone?*) with its three corners marked by openings. Two corners have openings from (*ureters? urethra?*), structures about 30 cm (___ inches) long, that carry urine from kidneys to bladder. These openings (*do? do not?*) have valves. Explain. _____

_____

_____

_____

(b) The other opening empties into the (*ureter? urethra?*) and is surrounded by the internal sphincter, and is longer in (*females? males?*).

(c) The bladder is lined with _____ epithelium. Explain how it is unique.

_____

(d) The empty bladder (*is smooth? has folds known as rugae?*).

(e) Arrange the layers of the bladder wall in correct sequence from outside to inside.

Mucosa (transitional epithelium)
Submucosa   Muscle
Serous membrane (continuous with
   peritoneum)

_____, _____, _____,

_____

(f) Most of the bladder wall consists of the _____ muscle, which has (*great? little?*) distensibility. When it does contract, micturition is (*stimulated? inhibited?*). The detrusor muscle can be thought of as the (*"stop"? "go"?*) muscle. Simultaneously, the (*internal? external?*) sphincter is pulled open, causing urine to (*flow out of? stay within?*) the bladder.

(g) Contraction of the (*internal? external?*) sphincter at the base of the bladder causes urine to (*flow out of? stay within?*) the bladder. It helps to maintain (*continence? incontinence?*), which is the ability to

_____.

A2. Refer to Table 35-1 in the Study Guide as well as Figure 35-2 and Table 35-1 in the text. Complete this exercise about regulation of micturition.

(a) The (*parasympathetic? sympathetic?*) division of the autonomic nervous system inhibits ("stops") micturition. These nerves stimulate contraction of the trigone and the ___ternal sphincter, and relax the _____. In other words, during stress, when the sympathetic nerves predominate, the focus (*is? is not?*) on urinating, and urine is allowed to distend the bladder. _____ drugs mimic sympathetic nerves.

(b) Parasympathetic nerves arise from levels (*T11 to L2? S2? to S4?*) of the cord and pass to the detrusor through (*pelvic? pudendal?*) nerves (on the left side of Fig. 35-2). These cause the flow of urine to (*"stop"? "go"?*). These nerves are (*adrenergic? cholinergic?*). Medications that relax detrusor muscles (to slow down "hyperactive bladder") and therefore "stop" micturition are (*cholinergic? anticholinergic?*).

(c) External sphincter control is (*involuntary? voluntary?*) or somatic and carried by (*pelvic? pudendal?*) nerves shown on the right side of Figure 35-2. External sphincter action is (*increased? decreased?*) by skeletal muscle relaxants.

(d) All the nerves discussed in A2(a) through A2(c) are (*motor? sensory?*). Afferent (sensory) nerves accompany (*sympathetic? parasympathetic? voluntary?*) nerves. They alert the CNS (including the micturition

Table 35-1. Innervation of Urinary Structures Regulating Micturition

Type of Nerves (Motor)	Source of Nerves	Voluntary or Involuntary	Structure Innervated	Effect on Micturition (Stop/Go)
Parasympathetic (pelvic nerves) (cholinergic)	S2-S4	Involuntary	Detrusor	Stimulates ("go")
Sympathetic (sympathetic nerves) (adrenergic)	T11-L2	Involuntary	Trigone and internal sphincter	Inhibits ("stop")
Lower motoneurons (pelvic nerves)	S2-S4	Voluntary (somatic)	Detrusor	Stimulates ("go")
Lower motoneurons (pudendal nerves)	S2-S4	Voluntary (somatic)	External sphincter	Inhibits ("stop")

center in the _____) of bladder distention. In infants, reflex contraction of the *(detrusor? external sphincter?)* and relaxation of the _____ results. After further growth of sphincters and bladder training, overriding nerve impulses initiated from the _____ can inhibit micturition until the appropriate time and setting are reached.

A3. Explain why a man is not likely to expel semen and urine at the same time. During ejaculation, *(sympathetic? parasympathetic?)* nerves contract the *(detrusor? trigone and internal sphincter?)* so that urination *(does? does not?)* accompany ejaculation.

A4. Normal capacity of the bladder is about _____ mL. The sensation of fullness is normally first perceived at about _____ mL. When the bladder is emptied adequately, less than _____ mL should remain (PVR).

A5. Select the method for evaluating bladder function that fits each description.

Cystometry   Cystoscopy
Postvoid residual   Sphincter
  volume (PVR)   electromyography
Uroflowmetry   Urethral pressure profile

(a) Measures the muscle strength of the voluntary perineal muscles, including that of the external urethral sphincter:

_____

(b) Measures the volume of urine left in the bladder after urination: _____

(c) A urodynamic study that measures bladder pressure during filling and voiding, as well as the ability to sense fullness and to inhibit urination: _____

(d) Direct visualization of the inside of the bladder: _____

B. ALTERATIONS IN BLADDER FUNCTION (pages 801-809)

B1. Explain how each of the following factors can obstruct urine outflow through the urethra. List examples of causes of narrowing of the urethral passageway.

(a) Myelomeningocele

_____
_____
_____

(b) Gonorrhea

_____
_____
_____

(c) Fecal impaction

_____
_____
_____

B2. In response to urinary obstruction, two major compensatory mechanisms are both designed to relieve distention of the bladder. Complete this exercise about them.

(a) Bladder wall *(a? hyper?)*trophy occurs. Ultimately, the thickened wall becomes ischemic and _____ sets in before the bladder is emptied. *(Frequent? Infrequent?)*

attempts at urination result. The bladder wall may form pockets known as diverticulas that increase risk for _____. Hypertrophy may also cause back pressure against ureters, leading to _____.

(b) *(Hypo? Hyper?)*sensitivity of the bladder to filling and stretching occurs. This leads to _____ and _____.

B3. Complete this exercise about bladder disorders resulting from neural dysfunction.

(a) Name two cerebral disorders that can cause neurogenic bladder. _____

_____

(b) Neurogenic bladder can produce two opposite effects. One is failure to *(store? empty?)* urine; this is a *(spastic? flaccid?)* bladder dysfunction that is likely to accompany spinal cord injury (SCI) *(above? at?)* S2-S4 levels of the cord. This condition, called bladder *(a? hyper?)*reflexia, also occurs during the first few months immediately after SCI, regardless of level of injury.

(c) Another form of neurogenic bladder, failure to store urine, is more likely to occur with *(higher? lower?)* SCI, such as at level *(T6-T7? S2-S4?)* of the cord. In such cases, the bladder is being controlled by *(spinal cord? brainstem?)* reflexes, and is *(a? hyper?)*reflexic.

(d) Decreased perception of bladder filling can lead to bladder overfilling. Name two disorders that cause such afferent nerve neuropathies and also affect motor neurons leading to flaccid bladder. _____,

_____

(e) In detrusor-sphincter dyssynergia, when the bladder wall contracts, the external sphincter *(constricts? dilates?)*, causing intravesicular pressure to *(increase? decrease?)*.

(f) List several interventions for flaccid bladder.

_____

_____

B4. Complete Table 35-2.

Table 35-2. Medications to Treat Neurogenic Bladder Incontinence

Type of Medication	Mimics (P?S?)	Effect on Detrusor	Useful to Treat
(a) Cholinergic	—	Stimulates	_____
(b) Anticholinergic	—	_____	Spastic bladder
(c) Adrenergic	—	Relaxes	_____

B5. Select the category of urinary incontinence that fits each case by filling in the blanks.

Overflow   Urge (overactive bladder)
Stress   Other cause

(a) Mr. Laredo, age 68, has benign prostatic hyperplasia (BPH): _____

(b) Ms. Patterson, age 56, has given birth to six children; she states that urine "leaks a little" when she coughs or laughs: _____

_____

(c) Mrs. Winston, age 93 and a resident of a skilled nursing facility, has recurrent fecal impaction: _____

(d) Mr. Aguilar has been diagnosed with Alzheimer's disease. He was transferred to an Alzheimer's unit yesterday: _____

_____

(e) Ms. Marshall-Petersen, age 61, has osteoarthritis and early stages of Parkinson's disease. She is aware of the urge to urinate, but she cannot get to the toilet in time; her physician has just prescribed an anti-cholinergic medication (oxybutynin or Ditropan XL): _____

(f) Mrs. Aufman takes a diuretic for her heart failure; she also takes a "sleeping pill":

_____

B6. Describe the following interventions for incontinence.

(a) Kegel's exercises

_____

_____

(b) Habit training (voiding on a regular schedule)

_____

_____

_____

(c) Surgically implanted inflatable cuff

_____
_____
_____

B7. Urinary incontinence occurs more often in *(elderly? younger?)* persons. Explain.

_____
_____

Most individuals with incontinence *(do? do not?)* seek help for it.

C. CANCER OF THE BLADDER (pages 809-812)

C1. Choose the two true statements.

(a) Bladder cancer is a **rare** form of urinary tract cancer.

(b) Almost all bladder cancers derive from the **epithelial** lining of the bladder.

(c) The 5-year survival rate for noninvasive cancer is 24%.

(d) Cigarette smoking **is** associated with bladder cancer.

C2. Complete this exercise on bladder cancer.

(a) State the most common sign of bladder cancer. _____

List other signs. _____
_____
_____
_____

(b) Tumors that express the A, B, or H antigens have a *(better? worse?)* prognosis than those that do not express these antigens.

(c) State possible complications of bladder cancer other than metastases.

_____
_____
_____
_____

(d) Treatment with diathermy involves *(electrocautery? external beam radiation? intravesicular chemotherapy?)*. If the bladder is removed, urinary diversion is typically effected by creating an alternative urine reservoir from the part of the small intestine known as the _____.

CHAPTER 36

Control of Gastrointestinal Function

■ Review Questions

A. STRUCTURE AND ORGANIZATION OF THE GASTROINTESTINAL TRACT (pages 815–819)

A1. Complete this overview of the digestive system.

(a) Write a brief description of functions of the digestive system.

_____

_____

(b) Contrast the gastrointestinal (GI) tract with accessory organs.

_____

_____

(c) What is the lumen of the GI tract?

_____

_____

A2. Refer to text Figure 36-1 and complete this exercise about parts of the GI tract.

(a) Name the organs of the upper GI tract.

_____

The *(pharynx? esophagus?)* is the throat.

(b) The esophagus is about *(10? 25?)* inches long. Its *(upper? lower?)* sphincter normally prevents gastric reflux. The esophagus empties into the *(cardiac? fundic? pyloric?)* portion of the stomach.

(c) The wall of the stomach normally offers *(minimal? great?)* distensibility. The _____ portion of the stomach is attached to the small intestine.

(d) Arrange the parts of the small intestine from first to last in the pathway of food.

Duodenum   Ileum   Jejunum

_____ → _____ → _____

(e) Arrange these parts of the large intestine from first to last in the route of wastes.

Ascending colon   Anus
Cecum   Descending colon
Rectum   Sigmoid colon
Transverse colon

_____ → _____ → _____
_____ → _____ → _____
_____ → _____ → _____
_____

(f) The appendix normally arises from the

_____.

(Select an answer from A2[e].)

A3. Refer to text Figure 36-3 and describe the GI wall.

(a) Arrange the layers of the wall from the deepest to the most superficial.

Mucosa   Muscularis
Peritoneum   Submucosa

_____ → _____ →
_____ → _____ →

(b) Match layers of the GI wall (from A3[a]) with the following descriptions:

(b1) The largest serous membrane in the body; adhesions can occur here:

_____

(b2) Epithelial cells in this layer are replaced every 4 to 5 days: _____

(b3) Composed largely of blood vessels, nerves, and glands: _____

(b4) The myenteric (Auerbach's) nerve plexus is located here: _____

A4. Describe the peritoneum and its extensions in this exercise.

(a) The *(parietal? visceral?)* layer of peritoneum adheres to the outside of organs of the abdomen and pelvis, whereas the _____ layer lines the abdominopelvic cavity. The accumulation of abnormally large volumes of fluid between these membranes is a condition known as

_____.

(b) The *(greater omentum? lesser omentum? mesentery?)* supports loops of small intestine and provides routes for blood and lymph vessels and nerves. The *(greater? lesser?)* omentum anchors the stomach to the liver.

B. MOTILITY (pages 819–824)

B1. Describe control of movement of the GI tract wall in this exercise.

(a) Most of the wall of the GI tract contains *(skeletal? smooth?)* muscle. Peristalsis is an example of *(rhythmic? tonic?)* movement of this muscle.

(b) Of the two plexuses that control the GI tract, the *(myenteric? submucosal?)* regulates both motility and secretion.

(c) The *(parasympathetic? sympathetic?)* division of the autonomic nervous system (ANS) stimulates motility and secretion of most of the GI tract. The _____ nerves transmit such impulses to the stomach, small intestine, cecum, and the first half of the colon. The _____ nerves carry parasympathetic fibers to the last portions of the colon. Excessive vagal or other parasympathetic nerve impulses *(overexcite? inhibit?)* GI activity.

(d) Sympathetic nerves *(decrease? increase?)* blood flow to the GI tract, *(stimulate? inhibit?)* contractions of the GI wall, and *(stimulate? inhibit?)* contractions of the GI sphincters. The overall effect of the sympathetic nerves is to *(decrease? increase?)* GI activity.

(e) Enteric nerves exert local control as they *(are located within? extend outside of?)* the GI wall. Afferent nerves carry *(sensory? motor?)* impulses.

B2. Choose the two true statements about swallowing.

(a) The three phrases of the swallowing process are **oral, pharyngeal**, and **esophageal**.

(b) During swallowing, the **soft palate** normally prevents the bolus of food from entering the nasopharynx.

(c) The control center for swallowing is located in the **cerebral cortex**.

(d) Cranial nerve X (the vagus) regulates the **oral** and **pharyngeal** phases of swallowing.

B3. Describe the major factor that normally prevents esophageal reflux.

_____

_____

B4. Complete this exercise about gastric and intestinal motility.

(a) Typically, gastric peristaltic contractions are initiated by a "pacemaker" in the stomach wall at a rate of _____ contractions per minute; each contraction lasts up to _____ seconds.

(b) List several factors that normally prevent premature emptying of chyme from the stomach. _____

_____

_____

(c) Diabetic neuropathy is more likely to lead to gastric *(atony and retention? dumping?)*.

(d) *(Propulsive movements? Segmentation waves?)* move chyme alternately forward and backward. Explain how these movements help digestion. _____

_____

_____

_____

_____

(e) Propulsive movements ultimately convey chyme through the *(pyloric? ileocecal?)* sphincter into the large intestine.

(f) Explain how motility of the small and large bowel can be easily assessed. _____

_____

_____

_____

(g) Where do haustration movements occur?

_____

_____

(h) Mass movements of the colon involve propulsion of *(small? large?)* amounts of wastes. How often do these typically occur?

_____

_____

_____

B5. Discuss defecation in this exercise.

(a) Defecation is initiated by movement of feces into the *(rectum? anus?)*. Afferent impulses travel into the _____ segments of the spinal cord. Reflex *(sympathetic? parasympathetic?)* impulses then travel to relax the *(external? internal?)* sphincter to allow feces to be expelled.

(b) Simultaneously sacral impulses pass to the cerebral cortex, which can send impulses to the *(external? internal?)* sphincter to override the process and stop defecation if the timing is not appropriate.

C. SECRETORY FUNCTIONS (pages 824–827)

C1. A total of approximately ___ liters (quarts) of fluid is secreted into the GI tract each day. List the three major mechanisms that regulate GI secretion.

_____

_____

_____

As described earlier, the *(sympathetic? parasympathetic?)* division of the ANS plays the major role in stimulating motility and secretion.

C2. Select the hormone that fits each description.

Cholecystokinin   Gastrin
Gastric inhibitory peptide   Motilin
Secretin

(a) Stimulates production of alkaline pancreatic secretions that neutralize acids from the stomach: _____

(b) Stimulates production of pancreatic secretions rich in digestive enzymes; also stimulates contraction of the gallbladder:

_____

(c) Stimulates gastric secretion and motility; enhances blood flow to the stomach:

_____

(d) Two hormones that inhibit gastric secretions and emptying: _____ and

_____

(e) All of these hormones are produced by the intestine except: _____

C3. Describe two peptides produced by neurons of the gut.

(a) _____ act through opioid receptors to inhibit GI motility, which helps to explain how certain opioid drugs (such as Paregoric or Lomotil) act in the treatment of diarrhea.

(b) Because _____ stimulates production of gastric acid, H_2-antagonists block related receptors and reduce gastric acid production.

C4. Match the correct organ with the chemicals it produces.

Large intestine   Small intestine
Salivary glands   Stomach

(a) Enzymes that complete digestion by breakdown of dipeptides, disaccharides, and fats: _____

(b) Mucus and a starch-digesting enzyme:

_____

(c) Enzymes that produce pepsinogen and HCl, which initiate protein digestion: _____

_____

(d) Mucus but no digestive enzymes:

_____

C5. Choose the two true statements.

(a) Sympathetic activity, for example, during stressful times, **decreases** salivary flow and duodenal mucus production.

(b) The **sublingual** glands are the largest of the salivary glands.

(c) Brunner's glands are **gastric** cells that produce **mucus**.

(d) Most of the GI secretions produced each day are made by combined efforts of the **stomach** and the **small intestine**.

C6. Select the gastric secretion that fits each description.

Gastrin   Hydrochloric acid
Intrinsic factor   Mucus
Pepsinogen

(a) The only chemical listed that is a hormone; secreted by cells lining the pylorus:

_____

(b) Produced by chief cells within gastric pits, this is the inactive form of the protease pepsin: _____

(c) Deficiency causes a type of anemia resulting from lack of vitamin B_{12}:

_____

(d) Cells that produce this chemical are harmed by chronic use of "barrier breakers," such as aspirin or nonsteroidal anti-inflammatory drugs (NSAIDs): _____

(e) Two secretions produced by parietal cells in gastric pits: _____ and

_____

D. DIGESTION AND ABSORPTION (pages 827–830)

D1. Discuss digestion in this exercise.

(a) Explain why foods must be digested.

_____

_____

_____

_____

(b) Almost all digestion occurs in the *(stomach? small intestine? colon?)*. List three structural features of the small intestine that enhance its ability to carry out digestion.

_____

_____

_____

(c) Distinguish functions of these cells on villi:

(c1) Goblet cells _____

_____

(c2) Enterocytes and brush border enzymes

_____

_____

(d) Describe the roles of lacteals

_____

_____

D2. Refer to Table 36-3 in your text and Study Guide Table 36-1 and complete the following exercise.

(a) Digestion of starch begins in the _____. Name two organs that produce amylase to digest starch into disaccharides.

_____ , _____

(b) The disaccharide lactase normally breaks down lactose into _____ and _____.

Describe the effects of lactase deficiency.

_____

_____

(c) Name the products of the disaccharidase sucrose. _____ , _____ Which of these simple sugars does not require

adenosine triphosphate (ATP) for absorption? _____

Which requires ATP and a sodium-dependent carrier for absorption? _____

(d) Which organ secretes virtually all of the enzymes that digest fats? _____

Which chemical is needed for absorption of fat-soluble vitamins and products of fat digestion? _____ Circle the fat-soluble vitamins:

A   B   C   D   E   K

(e) Steatorrhea refers to _____ in the stool. What does this condition indicate?

_____

_____

(f) Most proteases are produced in *(active? inactive?)* form. Explain.

_____

_____

_____

(g) Name two inactive precursors of proteases and their active counterparts.

_____

_____

_____

(h) Which two types of products of digestion are absorbed into blood capillaries within villi?

(1) Amino acids from protein digestion

(2) Monosaccharides from carbohydrate digestion

(3) Fatty acids from fat digestion

Table 36-1. Roles of Digestive Organs in Secreting Enzymes and Other Chemicals*

Organ	Carbohydrates	Proteins	Lipids	Other Functions
Salivary glands	Amylase	—	—	Mucus
Stomach	—	Pepsinogen	—	HCl, intrinsic factor
Pancreas	Amylase	Trypsinogen, chymo-trypsinogen, carboxypeptidase	Lipase	Bicarbonate
Liver	—	—	—	Bile
Small intestine	Brush border enzymes: disaccharidases (lactase, maltase, sucrase)	Brush border enzymes: dipeptidases	—	Mucus
Large intestine	—	—	—	Mucus

*Note: Hormones are not included.

CHAPTER 37

Alterations in Gastrointestinal Function

■ Review Questions

A. MANIFESTATIONS OF GASTROINTESTINAL DISORDERS (pages 831–833)

A1. Explain links among nausea, vomiting, and anorexia.

_____

_____

Now describe these conditions further in this exercise.

(a) Describe the "good news and bad news" of vomiting._____

_____

_____

(b) Control centers for appetite are located in the *(hypothalamus? medulla? thalamus?)*, whereas centers for nausea and vomiting are present in the _____.

(c) Mary Lizbeth is feeling nauseous. What signs is she likely to manifest?

_____

_____

(d) Emesis is a term that means _____. As Mary Lizbeth vomits, how are her heart rate and blood pressure likely to change?

_____

_____

(e) Use key words provided below to help you describe triggers for vomiting.

(e1) Vestibular apparatus

_____

_____

(e2) Hypoxia

_____

_____

(e3) Inflammation or distention

_____

_____

_____

(e4) The neurotransmitter dopamine

_____

_____

_____

A2. Contrast signs of gastrointestinal (GI) bleeding disorders in this exercise. Select from these answers.

Bright red blood   Blood urea nitrogen
Hematemesis   Melena
Occult blood

(a) "Tarry stool" that is malodorous; it often indicates bleeding in the upper bowel:

_____

(b) "Coffee grounds" appearance of vomitus shows evidence of digestive action upon blood in the upper GI tract: _____

(c) Elevated nitrogen in blood indicates absorption of products of digestive blood into vessels of the GI wall: _____

(d) Bleeding in the lower bowel (as from hemorrhoids) coats the stool; also may be attributable to upper GI bleeding with GI hypermotility: _____

(e) Blood hidden in the stool that can be detected by a guaiac test; may point to peptic ulcer or GI cancer: _____

A3. Paul has obtained a kit for a guaiac test on his stool. The directions inform him to avoid vitamin C or red meats before the test. Explain.

_____

_____

_____

B. DISORDERS OF THE ESOPHAGUS (pages 833–836)

B1. Match the esophageal disorder with the correct description.

Achalasia   Aspiration
Diverticulum   Dysphagia
Odynophagia

(a) Outpouching of the esophagus (or other organ) caused by muscle weakness of the wall: _____

(b) Failure of the lower esophageal sphincter to relax; an entire meal or two may lodge in the esophagus: _____

(c) Movement of esophageal contents into the lung, potentially leading to infection there: _____

(d) Painful swallowing: _____

(e) Difficulty in swallowing, possibly caused by stroke, esophageal cancer, or scarring: _____

B2. Choose the two true statements about gastroesophageal reflux.

(a) **Most** people **do** occasionally experience this condition.

(b) Even small hiatal hernias **are** considered causes of this disorder.

(c) The most frequently occurring symptom of this condition is **heartburn** within an **hour** after eating.

(d) Sitting up and antacids typically **do not** relieve symptoms of this condition.

B3. Describe these two complications of gastroesophageal reflux.

(a) Esophageal strictures _____

(b) Barrett's esophagus _____

B4. Describe treatments for gastroesophageal reflux.

(a) Prevention methods _____

(b) Medications _____

B5. Gastroesophageal reflux is *(common? rare?)* in infants. State your rationale.

_____
_____
_____
_____

B6. Circle risk factors for esophageal cancer:

(a) Alcohol

(b) Barrett's esophagus

(c) Age younger than 30 years

(d) Female gender

(e) Smoking

B7. State the most common sign of esophageal cancer. _____ This type of cancer typically is diagnosed *(early? late?)* in the course of the disease and is associated with a *(good? poor?)* prognosis.

C. DISORDERS OF THE STOMACH (pages 836–842)

C1. List major factors that contribute to the "gastric mucosal barrier."

_____
_____
_____

C2. Mrs. Snyder, age 54 years, has "been plagued with arthritis for years." Describe mechanisms by which the following practices have contributed to her current diagnosis of "stomach ulcers."

(a) "I've taken aspirin and ibuprofen for as long as they've made them."_____
_____
_____

(b) "I know my drinking and smoking don't help, but they get me through the day with all my pain." _____
_____
_____

C3. Stephen ate *Staphylococcus*-contaminated food at a picnic about 4 PM today. He is likely to experience an abrupt onset of vomiting at about *(6 PM? 9 PM? 1 AM?)*. His gastritis is *(acute? chronic?)*.

C4. Explain why the following two conditions may be linked in patients with chronic gastritis: achlorhydria and pernicious anemia.

_____

_____

_____

C5. State the "claim to fame" of *Helicobacter pylori*. _____

Explain how each of the following factors contributes to the "success" of *H. pylori*.

(a) Flagella _____

_____

(b) Mucin-degrading enzyme _____

_____

(c) Urease _____

_____

C6. Choose the two true statements.

(a) Peptic ulcers can affect **either** the stomach or the duodenum.

(b) The incidence of peptic ulcer in the United States is 1 in 10,000 adults.

(c) Duodenal ulcers are **much more common** than gastric ulcers.

(d) The incidence of peptic ulcer is about four times higher in **women than in men**.

(e) There **is** evidence that special diets are beneficial in treating peptic ulcers.

C7. Complete this exercise about peptic ulcers.

(a) List the two most common causes of peptic ulcer. _____, _____

About ____% of people with gastric ulcer have *H. pylori* infection, and ____ % of people using nonsteroidal anti-inflammatory drugs (NSAIDs, such as Mrs. Snyder in Question C2) have these ulcers develop.

(b) List three methods for identifying *H. pylori* infection._____

_____

_____

(c) Circle the times when burning or gnawing pain is likely to be experienced by patients with peptic ulcer.

(1) 8 AM

(2) 3 PM

(3) 6 PM

(4) 1 AM

(d) Mrs. Snyder (Question C2) passed loose, tarry stools in the past 24 hours and has felt dizzy, weak, thirsty, and cold. What do these symptoms suggest? _____

_____

_____

(e) What symptoms signal possible perforated ulcer? _____

_____

_____

(f) Match the peptic ulcer medication with its correct description.

Antacid   Antibiotic
Bismuth subsalicylate (Pepto-Bismol)
Histamine (H_2) blocker

(f1) Neutralizes gastric acids; examples: calcium carbonate (Tums), aluminum or magnesium hydroxide (Gaviscon, Maalox, Mylanta): _____

(f2) Decreases secretion of gastric acid:

_____

(f3) Raises pH within the stomach, which inhibits bacterial growth; darkens stool:

_____

(f4) Destroys *H. pylori* directly; examples: amoxicillin, tetracycline: _____

_____

C8. Identify the gastric condition most likely in each client described.

Curling's ulcer   Cushing ulcer
Zollinger-Ellison syndrome

(a) Ms. Innes has second- and third-degree burns over 50% of her body. _____

(b) Mr. Edwards has a gastrin-secreting tumor of his stomach (gastrinoma). _____

(c) Timothy was admitted with severe head trauma and elevated intracranial pressure after he was hit by a car. _____

C9. Circle the correct answers about stomach cancer.

(a) The incidence of cancer is *(decreasing? increasing?)* in the United States. Worldwide, stomach cancer is *(common? rare?)*.

(b) Like esophageal cancer, stomach cancer typically is diagnosed *(early? late?)* in the course of the disease.

(c) The treatment of choice for stomach cancer is *(chemotherapy? subtotal gastrectomy?)*.

D. DISORDERS OF THE SMALL AND LARGE INTESTINE: INFLAMMATIONS AND INFECTIONS (pages 842–848)

D1. Circle statements that are true of irritable bowel syndrome (IBS).

(a) In Western countries, approximately 1 person in 1000 has the disorder.

(b) This disorder **is** explained by structural abnormalities (such as inflammation) of the wall of the intestine.

(c) IBS involves abdominal pain that **is not** relieved by defecation.

(d) Manifestations include gas production, bloating, nausea, and anorexia.

(e) Patients with IBS experience a change in consistency (hard, loose, or watery) or frequency of stools.

(f) IBS is associated with **stress.**

D2. Identify which of the two major forms of inflammatory bowel disease fits each description below. Mark CD for Crohn's disease and UC for ulcerative colitis. In some cases, both CD and UC will apply or neither may apply.

(a) A familial predisposition is present: Susan is at increased risk because both her mother and aunt have this disorder. _____

(b) Leonard states that he has been in "a vicious cycle for weeks" of diarrhea and fecal urgency that subsides, then recurs; he also has a "stiff, sore back," with fatigue (showing anemia) and recurrent eye inflammation (uveitis). _____

(c) Rhoda has two fistulas connecting portions of her jejunum and ileum and strictures in several areas of the small bowel. _____

(d) Polly received a diagnosis of this inflammatory bowel disease when she was 14 years old; the surface of her ileum resembles cobblestones and exhibits "skip lesions" with thickened areas that resemble lead pipes. _____

(e) Charles averages 30 to 40 bowel movements a day; his stools are bloody (derived from mucosal inflammation). _____

(f) A stool culture demonstrates that Mr. Okerson has a parasitic infection. _____

(g) Faith, age 8 years, is small for her age, and she eliminates fatty stools (steatorrhea) (both indicators of malabsorption); she requires a high-calorie, high-protein diet.

_____

(h) J. T.'s diagnosis is proctosigmoiditis with confluent, necrotic lesions and pseudopolyps; his disorder is classified as acute, fulminating with increased risk for toxic megacolon. _____

D3. Choose the two true statements.

(a) Ulcerative colitis **does significantly** increase risk for colon cancer.

(b) Smokers and people who use nicotine patches are **more** likely to have ulcerative colitis develop.

(c) Fiber supplements are likely to **decrease** the diarrhea of ulcerative colitis.

(d) Toxic megacolon refers to abnormal **strictures** that **narrow** the colon.

D4. List several types of medications used to treat ulcerative colitis.

_____

_____

_____

D5. Define each of these terms.

(a) Nosocomial _____

_____

_____

_____

(b) Broad-spectrum _____

_____

(c) Rebound tenderness _____

_____

_____

D6. Identify the large bowel condition most likely to occur in each case.

C. difficile colitis   Diverticulosis
E. coli 0157:87 infection

(a) Melinda has eaten a hamburger that was not fully cooked. _____

(b) Monique has just completed a course of broad-spectrum antibiotics. _____

(c) Bryan eats a low-fiber diet and often "fails to respond to nature's call" to defecate.

_____

D7. Describe *C. difficile* colitis in this exercise.

(a) What characteristics of *C. difficile* warrant its name ("difficult")? _____

(b) The pseudomembranous form of this colitis is typically *(more? less?)* severe. Explain.

_____

_____

(c) Patients with *C. difficile* colitis should *(continue? discontinue?)* the broad-spectrum antibiotic that leads to this infection. (See Question D6[b])

D8. Circle the correct answers and explain where indicated.

(a) Diverticular disease is *(more? less?)* common in the United States than in developing countries. Explain._____

_____

_____

(b) *(Diverticulitis? Diverticulosis?)* is an inflammatory disease. A common complaint of this condition is pain in the:

(1) Lower left quadrant (LLQ)

(2) Lower right quadrant (LRQ)

(3) Upper left quadrant (ULQ)

(4) Upper right quadrant (URQ)

(c) What condition is indicated by air in the urine (pneumaturia)?

_____

(d) Barium enema *(is? is not?)* recommended for diagnosing diverticular disease. Explain.

_____

_____

D9. Complete this exercise about appendicitis.

(a) Appendicitis is *(common? rare?)* in the United States with greater incidence among *(young? elderly?)* persons.

(b) Pain within 12 hours of onset is likely to be *(colicky? steady?)* and located in the *(LLQ? LRQ? ULQ? URQ?)*. Temperature and white blood cell count both typically *(decrease? increase?)*.

(c) State the usual treatment of appendicitis.

_____

_____

E. DISORDERS OF THE SMALL AND LARGE INTESTINE INVOLVING MOTILITY, ABSORPTION, AND NEOPLASMS (PAGES 848–856)

E1. Circle correct answers about changes in intestinal motility.

(a) Intestinal motility increases as a result of enteric nerve action (meaning nerves located within the _____), as well as from *(sympathetic? parasympathetic?)* stimulation.

(b) Typically, the colon eliminates about _____ g (or mL) of stool each day. Increased frequency of stool passage is known as *(constipation? diarrhea?)*. Increased volume of feces is known as _____ diarrhea.

(c) Diarrhea is *(sometimes? always?)* pathological. Diarrhea of 3 days' duration is considered *(acute? chronic?)*.

(d) Refer to Chart 37-1 and classify each of the following cases of diarrhea according to categories of cause.

Large volume: osmotic
Large volume: secretory
Small volume: inflammatory
Small volume: infectious

(d1) Chad has a case of *Staphylococcus* food poisoning after eating potato salad that sat on the picnic table for 4 hours.

_____

(d2) Rebecca has been diagnosed with *Salmonella* food poisoning after eating infected chicken. _____

(d3) Polly (Question D2[d]) has Crohn's disease with colicky diarrhea, urgency, and straining upon defecation (tenesmus). _____

(d4) Luther has lactose intolerance, in which indigestible lactose attracts water to the intestinal lumen. _____

(e) Most acute diarrhea *(is? is not?)* serious. Explain when diarrhea may become serious and even lethal. _____

_____

(f) Feeding *(should? should not?)* be continued during diarrhea. Describe the traditional BRAT diet. _____

_____

(g) Explain how medications such as Lomotil and Imodium are effective against diarrhea.

_____

_____

E2. Complete this exercise about constipation and fecal impaction.

(a) What is considered "normal" for frequency of bowel movements?

_____

_____

(b) State several examples of causes of constipation in each category.

(b1) Drugs _____

_____

_____

(b2) Disease _____

_____

_____

(b3) Aging _____

_____

_____

(c) List several health behaviors designed to prevent constipation. _____

_____

_____

_____

(d) Mrs. Jones, age 92 years, is confined to bed after a stroke. She has incontinence of bowel and bladder, but her stools have been watery. State a possible diagnosis.

_____

_____

E3. Match the terms related to intestinal obstruction with the descriptions provided.

Borborygmus   Intussusception
Paralytic ileus   Strangulation
Volvulus

(a) Complete twisting of the bowel:

_____

(b) Seen most often after surgery; indicated by absence of bowel sounds in all four quadrants: _____

(c) Mechanical obstruction complicated by ischemia, necrosis, and possibly gangrenous bowel: _____

(d) Telescoping of the bowel into an adjacent segment; most common in infants:

_____

(e) Rumbling sounds related to intestinal gas propulsion: _____

E4. *(Mechanical? Paralytic?)* intestinal obstruction is more likely to involve severe, colicky pain. List two treatments for intestinal obstruction.

_____

E5. Identify the cause of intestinal malabsorption in each case provided.

Lymphatic obstruction   Digestive disorder
Mucosal malabsorption

(a) Deficiency of pancreatic enzymes, as in cystic fibrosis: _____

(b) Metastasis that blocks the thoracic duct or periaortic nodes; interferes with fat absorption: _____

(c) Celiac disease or sprue: _____

E6. Discuss these two cases of intestinal malabsorption.

(a) Kara, age 7 years, has received a diagnosis of celiac disease (sprue). Circle the dietary restrictions likely for Kara.

Barley   Corn   Oat   Rice   Wheat

(b) Adam, age 4 years, has steatorrhea.

(b1) What color are his stools likely to be?

_____

(b2) Explain why Adam's stools float in the toilet. _____

_____

(b3) Explain the possible connection between his steatorrhea and his tendency to bleed and bruise excessively. _____

_____

E7. Discuss intestinal neoplasms in this exercise.

(a) Adenomatous polyps of the intestine are *(common? rare?)*. These are *(benign? cancerous?)* and may be pedunculated, meaning _____.

(b) These polyps consist of excessive growth of *(mucosa? submucosa?)*. There also may be *(excessive? deficient?)* apoptosis (normal cell death). *(Tubular? Villous?)* forms of these growths are much more likely to develop into invasive carcinoma (colorectal cancer). Removal of suspect polyps *(does? does not?)* reduce the incidence of colorectal cancer.

E8. Mildred is undergoing tests to rule out colorectal cancer.

(a) This form of cancer is *(common? rare?)* in the United States

(b) Circle the factors in Mildred's personal and family history that increase her risk for colorectal cancer.

(1) She is 58 years old.

(2) Her mother died of breast cancer.

(3) Her younger brother has had a total colectomy for familial adenomatous polyps of the colon.

(4) Her husband has kidney cancer.

(5) Mildred has ulcerative colitis.

(6) She regularly takes aspirin or ibuprofen for her "stiffness."

(7) Her favorite snack foods (which she says she "eats too much") are ice cream, chocolate, and chips.

(c) List signs related to Mildred's bowel movements that would suggest colorectal cancer. _____

_____

(d) Signs such as those just listed typically appear *(early? later?)* in the course of the cancer. Mildred's tumor has spread through the entire wall of her colon and it has metastasized to abdominal lymph nodes. Her tumor is likely to be a Duke stage *(A? B? C?),* which is associated with a 5-year survival rate of approximately _____%.

E9. Indicate whether each of the following is a primary (1°), secondary (2°), or tertiary (3°) form of prevention or treatment for colorectal cancer.

(a) Radiation therapy to shrink the tumor, followed by surgical removal of the malignant segment: ___

(b) Annual guaiac test for occult blood and digital rectal examination: ___

(c) Flexible sigmoidoscopy or colonoscopy: ___

(d) Low-fat, high-fiber diet: ___

F. DISORDERS OF THE PERITONEUM (pages 856–857)

F1. Describe the location of the peritoneum.

_____
_____
_____
_____

What makes infection of this membrane (peritonitis) potentially serious?

_____
_____
_____
_____

F2. List four or more causes of peritonitis.

_____
_____
_____
_____
_____
_____

F3. Circle typical early manifestations of peritonitis.

(a) Pain that is:

(1) Diffuse

(2) Localized over the inflamed area

(b) The person is likely to appear:

(1) Highly restless and active

(2) Subdued

(c) The abdominal wall becomes:

(1) Rigid

(2) Soft

(d) Blood work indicates:

(1) Leukocytosis

(2) Leukocytopenia

F4. Write a rationale for each of the following treatments of peritonitis.

(a) Intravenous fluids and electrolytes

_____
_____

(b) "Holding fluids" (n.p.o. = nothing by mouth) and nasogastric suctioning

_____
_____

CHAPTER 38

Alterations in Hepatobiliary Function

■ Review Questions

A. THE LIVER AND THE HEPATOBILIARY SYSTEM (pages 859–867)

A1. Choose the two true statements about the liver.

(a) In healthy persons, the liver **can** be palpated inferior to the rib cage.

(b) The bulk of the liver lies in the **upper right quadrant**.

(c) The liver receives blood from the **portal artery** and the **portal vein**.

(d) Bile is formed in the **liver** and is emptied into the **small intestine**.

A2. The portal vein transports blood from _____ into the liver. This vein *(has? lacks?)* valves. Explain the significance.

_____

_____

A3. Identify the term that fits the related description.

Bile canaliculi   Hepatocytes
Kupffer's cells   Lobules
Sinusoids

(a) Phagocytic cells that remove bacteria, old blood cells, and other debris from blood that enters the liver: _____

(b) Functional units of the liver; up to 100,000 per liver: _____

(c) Liver cells that perform the many roles of the liver listed in text Table 38-1: _____

(d) Wide channels between hepatocytes that contain blood supplied by hepatic artery and portal vein; lined with Kupffer's cells:

_____

A4. Arrange in correct sequence (from first to last) the structures that carry bile.

Ampulla of Vater   Bile canaliculi
Common hepatic duct   Sphincter of Oddi
Right and left hepatic ducts

_____ → _____ →
_____ → _____ →
_____

A5. Identify the chemical that fits the related description below.

Amino acid   Albumin   Bile
Fibrinogen   Glycogen   Ketone
Urea

(a) Clotting protein synthesized in the liver:

_____

(b) Acetoacetic acid produced when fat breakdown is excessive: _____

(c) The type of chemical used for protein synthesis: _____

(d) Most is formed in the liver and later excreted by kidneys or converted to ammonia within the intestine: _____

(e) Yellow-green secretion produced by the liver and required for digestion and absorption of fats and fat-soluble vitamins: _____

(f) Carbohydrate formed when blood glucose levels rise: _____

(g) Contributes greatly to colloidal osmotic pressure; if inadequate, leads to edema:

_____

A6. Mr. Newman's liver has been seriously damaged by cirrhosis. Explain how these signs or symptoms are related.

(a) Sensitivity to medications requiring that Mr. Newman receive small dosages

_____

_____

(b) Gynecomastia_____

_____

_____

(c) Bleeding disorder with a high prothrombin time _____

_____

_____

A7. Identify each process performed by the liver.

Beta oxidation   Deamination
Gluconeogenesis   Glycogenolysis
Transamination

(a) Breakdown of glycogen to release glucose when blood glucose level is low:

_____

(b) Conversion of amino acids or portions of fats into glucose when blood glucose is low:

_____

(c) A vital step in fat breakdown and energy release in which fatty acids are converted into two carbon acetyl groups that will enter the citric acid cycle: _____

(d) Processes in which amino groups are removed when amino acids are converted into other chemicals: _____ and

_____

A8. Mrs. Lennon takes a "statin" drug (Lipitor) to lower her blood cholesterol. Explain how this medication works.

_____

_____

_____

A9. Complete this exercise about bile pathways and blockage.

(a) Once bile reaches the duodenum (Question A4), where does it go next?

_____

_____

_____

This is known as _____ circulation.

(b) Define cholestasis and state two causes.

_____

_____

_____

(c) List common manifestations of cholestasis.

_____

_____

_____

_____

_____

A10. Arrange in correct sequence the chemicals formed in the "life cycle" of bilirubin.

Biliverdin   Conjugated bilirubin
Free bilirubin   Hemoglobin
Urobilinogen

Red blood cells → _____ →

_____ → _____ →

_____ → _____

Write * next to the chemical form that is present in bile.

Write ** next to the form that is reabsorbed into portal circulation or is excreted in feces.

A11. Jaundice refers to an abnormally high serum level of _____. Complete this exercise about jaundice.

(a) Circle serum levels of bilirubin that are higher than normal: ____ mg/dL

(1) 0.2

(2) 1.0

(3) 1.8

(4) 2.5

(b) At which blood levels of bilirubin will sclerae (and also white skin) appear yellow? _____

(c) Categorize types of jaundice that fit descriptions below:
Intrahepatic   Posthepatic   Prehepatic

(c1) Gallstones or tumors block bile ducts; cholestatic jaundice with pruritus; stools are clay colored because of lack of bilirubin in bile: _____

(c2) Cirrhosis, hepatitis, the anesthetic halothane, or liver cancer impairs liver function, preventing removal of bilirubin from blood as quickly as it is formed: _____

(c3) Excessive destruction of red blood cells in sickle cell anemia or in an "Rh disorder" (hemolytic disease of the newborn): _____

_____

(c4) Serum bilirubin is elevated; stools appear normal in color: _____

(c5) Urine may appear dark, indicating high levels of bilirubin: _____
or _____

A12. Explain why "serum levels of liver enzymes" increase with liver damage.

_____

_____

_____

Which enzyme level is specific for hepatic injury? _____

B. ALTERATIONS IN HEPATIC AND BILIARY FUNCTION (pages 867–882)

B1. List six or more causes of liver disease.

_____

_____

_____

_____

_____

B2. Discuss drug-induced liver disease in this exercise.

(a) Explain how chemicals that enter the body, including drugs and alcohol, can injure the liver. _____

_____

_____

(b) Drugs should be altered or detoxified by bio_____; this occurs in two phases:

(b1) Phase 1: the drugs are chemically modified or _____. These "detox" reactions take place in parts of cells known as _____; many are performed by enzymes that make up the cytochrome _____ system. This system can be activated to (decrease? increase?) breakdown of drugs, thereby leaving (more? fewer?) active drugs circulating in blood. Inactivation of cytochrome P450 has the opposite effect.

(b2) Phase 2: additional reactions convert _____-soluble drugs to _____-soluble ones that can be eliminated by _____. Explain why nutritional deficiency interferes with Phase 2 liver functions.

_____

_____

(c) The pain reliever acetaminophen (Tylenol) normally is metabolized by the _____.

(c1) One in (5? 50? 500?) cases of acutely painful liver failure is caused by acetaminophen overdose.

(c2) How does an overdose of this over-the-counter drug affect the liver?

_____

_____

(c3) Does withdrawal of acetaminophen lead to complete recovery of the liver?

_____

_____

(d) Many hormones produced by the body also are normally metabolized by the liver. Name several.

_____

_____

Liver damage is likely to (decrease? increase?) circulating levels of hormones. Describe effects.

_____

_____

(e) Explain how polypharmacy in an 84-year-old woman can affect her liver.

_____

_____

_____

(f) Drugs with cholestatic reactions cause decreased flow of _____, with manifestations of jaundice and

_____.

How does withdrawal of the drug affect the liver? _____

_____

(g) Idiosyncratic drug reactions refer to those that (are? are not?) predictable. Explain what causes these.

_____

_____

B3. Hepatitis refers to _____ of the liver. Complete this exercise about hepatitis.

(a) Circle possible causes of hepatitis.

Bacteria   Drugs   Protozoans
Toxins   Viruses

(b) One major mechanism of liver injury in hepatitis is direct cellular injury. State the other. _____
Contrast two types of these responses:

(b1) A prompt and intense immune response during acute injury (does? does not?) cause cellular injury (and possible liver necrosis), while it (does? does not?) eliminate the virus.

(b2) A more moderate immune response produces (more? fewer?) immediate symptoms and (eliminates the virus? leads to a chronic or carrier state?). Carriers (always? sometimes?) have symptoms. Circle the types of hepatitis that can produce carriers.
Hepatitis A   B   C   D

(c) The three phases of hepatitis are characterized partially by whether icterus (or _____) is present. Identify manifestations of the phases. _____

_____

    (c1) The prodromal phase or *(icterus? preicterus?)* phase occurs first. Circle typical manifestations.

        Sense of well being   Hearty appetite
        Jaundice   High blood
        Malaise   bilirubin
        Myalgia   Severe anorexia
        Nausea, vomiting, diarrhea
        High serum levels of liver enzymes
          (AST and ALT)   Severe pruritus

    (c2) Identify signs or symptoms of the icterus phase; choose from the answers above. _____

    _____

    (c3) Choose from answers above to identify signs of the convalescence phase.

    _____

    _____

(d) Complete clinical recovery is likely for hepatitis A within ___ months and for hepatitis B within ___ months.

B4. Refer to Table 38-1 (page 197) and contrast the five major types of viral hepatitis in this exercise.

(a) Hepatitis *(A? B?)* typically is a more serious health problem with longer duration.

(b) Relatively rare in the U.S., hepatitis ___ has the highest mortality in infected pregnant women.

(c) Hepatitis ___ occurs only when it accompanies hepatitis ___.

(d) Hepatitis ___ typically has mild signs or symptoms; however, it is the most common cause of chronic hepatitis, cirrhosis, and primary liver cancer worldwide.

(e) Most likely to be transmitted by improper hand washing techniques: ___ ___

(f) Health care workers are at greatest risk for these three types of hepatitis via accidental needle sticks: ___, ___, ___

(g) Three forms of hepatitis that are known to become chronic: ___, ___, ___; more than three fourths of chronic viral hepatitis is of type ___.

(h) Janelle is born of an HBV-infected mother. Janelle's risk of being a chronic carrier is approximately *(10%? 50%? 90%?)*. Her risk of dying of chronic liver disease as an adult is ___ %. The presence of *(anti-HBs? HBV DNA?)* in serum is the most certain indicator of HBV infection.

(i) It *(is? is not?)* recommended that Janelle receive hepatitis B vaccine. List six or more other categories of candidates for HBV vaccine. _____

_____

_____

_____

_____

_____

B5. Describe two possible types of treatments for chronic viral hepatitis.

    _____

    _____

B6. Contrast primary biliary cirrhosis (PBC) with primary sclerosing cholangitis (PSC).

(a) Inflammation and obstruction of large bile ducts either inside or outside of the liver; retention of bile leads to hepatic necrosis with potential liver failure; occurs more in males: _____

(b) Incidence is greater in persons with autoimmune disease; scarring of the liver leads to accumulated bile with green hue to the liver: _____

(c) Liver transplantation is the only treatment of advanced disease: _____

B7. Describe the effects of chronic alcoholism in this exercise.

(a) Alcohol *(is? is not?)* readily absorbed into the stomach lining. Digestion of alcohol yields about *(4? 7? 9?)* kcal, which is *(more? fewer?)* calories than carbohydrates.

(b) About *(10% to 20%? 80% to 90%?)* of alcohol is metabolized by the liver. All metabolic pathways of alcohol lead to production of _____. As a result of increased alcohol metabolism, the alcoholic liver cannot perform many of its normal functions and is *(more? less?)* susceptible to the toxic effects of industrial toxins, anesthetics, carcinogens, and acetaminophen.

Table 38-1. Types of Hepatitis

Type: Virus	Distinguishing Characteristic; Incidence	Mode of Transmission; Risk Factors	Manifestations	Serological Markers; Vaccine
A: HAV (RNA virus)	Formerly known as infectious hepatitis	Fecal–oral route via contaminated water or shellfish (not by blood). At risk: pre-schoolers; food handlers with poor hand washing; those practicing rectoanal sex; travelers to regions with poor sanitation	A benign, self-limited (acute, not chronic) disease with duration <2 months. Virus replicates in the liver, is excreted into bile and then into stool. 90% of adults develop jaundice. Children <2 years often have no symptoms	IgM anti-HAV indicates acute hepatitis; IgG anti-HAV documents past exposure. Vaccine: HAV is available for prevention; little help for persons with known HAV exposure
B: HBV (DNA virus): in blood	Formerly called serum hepatitis. As many as 300,000 new cases/year in the U.S. with >1 million carriers; epidemic in parts of Africa and Asia	Through blood, but also by other body secretions via oral or sexual contact. At risk: infants of HBV-infected mothers, persons with multiple sex partners or those who have recto-anal sex, IV drug users, and health care workers with accidental needle injuries	Can be acute, fulminant with massive liver necrosis; can be chronic, carrier state, and develop into cirrhosis	Anti-HBs signal recovery from HBV infection or successful immunization. HBV vaccine is effective long term; immune globulin helps if given within a week of HBV exposure
C: HCV (RNA virus with >50 subtypes)	Greatest concern is high risk for chronic hepatitis and cirrhosis. Formerly known as non-A, non-B hepatitis	By blood transfusions before HCV testing started in 1990. Now injected drug use is most common source; may be transmitted by tattoos, acupuncture or body piercing, or accidental needle sticks	Most infected persons do not know they are ill: symptoms are absent or mild, such as malaise or weight loss. May have long incubation period (5 months). Rarely fulmin-ant but commonly chronic	Test for HCV in serum is the most accurate, but costly. Anti-HCV antibody test has lower cost but is less accurate. No vaccine related to diverse subtypes
D: HDV (RNA virus)	Coinfection with hepatitis B	Routes of transmission similar to those of HBV. Mostly seen in drug users and those receiving clotting factors	HDV can exacerbate HBV infection and cause it to become chronic or progress to cirrhosis	Detected by anti-HDV or HDV RNA in serum
E: HEV (RNA virus)	High mortality rate (20%) if occurs in pregnant women. Seen mostly in developing countries	Fecal–oral route	Fulminating manifestations similar to those of HBA. Does not lead to chronic or carrier state	

(c) The U.S. has an estimated _____ alcoholics. *(Women? Men?)* are more vulnerable to the effects of alcohol because estrogen *(decreases? increases?)* the toxic effects of alcohol, whereas testosterone *(decreases? increases?)* acetaldehyde production.

(d) Liver disease is more common in women who drink more than 40 g/day of alcohol (or men who drink twice that). This is equivalent to ___ 8-oz (250-mL) glasses of beer per day for women (or twice that for men).

(e) List several effects of acetaldehyde that alter hepatic lobules. _____

_____

_____

_____

(f) Are these effects reversible if alcohol consumption is discontinued?

_____

B8. List the three major disorders of the liver associated with chronic alcoholism in the sequence in which they are likely to appear: _____ → _____ → _____.

Complete this exercise about these disorders.

(a) A fatty liver appears _____ in color. Explain how fatty liver is related to alcohol:

(a1) When alcohol is present, *(alcohol? fatty acids?)* become(s) the preferred fuel for the liver.

(a2) Alcohol *(stimulates? inhibits?)* fatty acid and triglyceride synthesis by the liver, and *(decreases? increases?)* fatty acid breakdown.

(b) List triggers for alcoholic hepatitis.

_____

_____

Circle signs typical of this alcoholic hepatitis:

(1) Anorexia and nausea

(2) Inflammation of hepatocytes in the central zone of the liver

(3) Necrosis of peripheral liver cells

(4) Upper right quadrant (URQ) tenderness

(5) Accumulation of fluid within the peritoneal cavity (ascites)

(c) Early stages of alcoholic cirrhosis involve *(small? large?)* nodules. How do these nodules injure the liver?

_____

_____

Is cirrhosis considered a serious disorder?

_____

B9. Mr. Nardella has received a diagnosis of hepatic failure. About *(10% to 15%? 45% to 50%? 85% to 90%?)* of liver function must be lost before liver failure occurs. Discuss his case in this exercise.

(a) Mr. Nardella states: "I've never taken a drink in my life." List several factors other than alcohol that can lead to liver failure.

_____

_____

_____

(b) Mr. Nardella's liver is palpable and tender. He is weak and has no appetite; he speaks about having a "belly for the first time in my life," yet he has not gained weight; his ankles are swollen. Explain.

_____

_____

_____

_____

_____

_____

_____

B10. Mr. Maloney has advanced-stage hepatic failure related to chronic alcoholism. Explain his manifestations.

(a) Mr. Maloney has a balloon tamponade to compress his bleeding esophageal veins.

_____

_____

(b) He cannot breathe well when he lies down; he is taking diuretics and has had a number of paracentesis treatments.

_____

_____

(c) His prothrombin time has doubled, indicating decreased ability to clot blood, and his hemoglobin level is 7 g/100 mL.

_____

_____

(d) Mr. Maloney also has hemorrhoids.

_____

_____

B11. Describe possible treatments for Mr. Maloney (Question B10). _____

_____

_____

_____

B12. Match the condition associated with portal hypertension and liver failure with the correct description.

Asterixis   Azotemia
Caput medusae   Esophageal varices
Fetor hepaticus

(a) Large, red veins in the skin around the umbilicus related to backup of portal vein blood into collateral vessels: _____

(b) Sweet, musty breath resulting from bacterial degradation of toxins within the intestine: _____

(c) Flapping of wrists related to the effects of hepatic encephalopathy; exacerbated by high-protein meals that increase production of ammonia: _____

(d) Highly elevated blood urea nitrogen (BUN) and serum creatinine levels, indicating renal failure: _____

(e) Occur in about two thirds of persons with advanced cirrhosis; in 50% of cases, lead to rupture, hypovolemic shock and death; may be treated by the TIP (transjugular intrahepatic portosystemic shunt) surgery:

_____

B13. Describe liver cancer in this exercise.

(a) Primary liver cancer accounts for approximately ___ % of all cancers. It is more common in *(the U. S.? developing countries?)*.

(b) Which type of primary liver cancer is more common: cancer of *(bile ducts? hepatocytes?)*. Almost all hepatocellular carcinoma in the U.S. is associated with _____. Which forms of chronic hepatitis are associated with this type of cancer? _____

(c) Primary liver cancers typically are diagnosed in *(early? late?)* stages. The 5-year survival rate is approximately ___ %.

(d) Most liver cancers are *(primary? metastatic?)*. In which organs are metastatic cancers likely to originate?

_____

_____

C. DISORDERS OF THE GALLBLADDER AND EXOCRINE PANCREAS (pages 882–887)

C1. Circle correct answers about the gallbladder.

(a) The major function of the gallbladder is to *(produce? concentrate?)* bile.

(b) The hormone *(cholecystokinin? secretin?)* stimulates contractions of the gallbladder.

(c) Bile exits from the gallbladder directly into the *(cystic? common bile?)* duct.

(d) After surgical removal of the gallbladder, the common bile duct *(constricts? dilates?)*.

C2. Complete this exercise about gallstones.

(a) Name the two main chemical components of gallstones: _____, _____

(b) List the three major factors that contribute to formation of gallstones.

_____

_____

(c) Circle factors that increase risk for formation of gallstones.

(1) Male

(2) Lean body

(3) Multiparous women

(4) Women taking oral contraceptives

(5) Native American heritage

(d) At what point is pain likely to accompany gallstones? _____

_____

Name two areas to which gallstone pain is likely to refer: _____, _____

C3. Match the term with the related description.

Cholangitis   Cholecystitis
Cholelithiasis   Choledocholithiasis

(a) Gallstones: _____

(b) Stones in the common bile duct:

_____

(c) Inflammation of the common bile duct:

_____

(d) Inflammation of the gallbladder:

_____

C4. Mrs. Jorgenson, age 52 years, has a history of cholelithiasis and now has cholecystitis.

(a) A history of gallstones *(is? is not?)* associated with both acute and chronic cholecystitis.

(b) What types of foods should Mrs. Jorgenson avoid in attempts to reduce acute attacks of cholecystitis?

_____

_____

(c) Pain that accompanies inflammation of the gallbladder is likely to begin as *(steady? colicky?)* pain. Potent analgesics such as meperidine (Demerol) typically *(do? do not?)* eliminate pain of attacks.

(d) The most widely used tool for diagnosing cholecystitis and cholelithiasis is:

(1) Cholescintigraphy scan

(2) Oral cholecystography

(3) Ultrasonography

(e) One of Mrs. Jorgenson's gallstones blocks her common bile duct; the purulent infection she now has is acute _____. Explain why this condition may lead to emergency surgery. _____

_____

_____

C5. Contrast the advantages and disadvantages of cholecystectomy performed by the traditional open surgical method versus the laparoscopic method. _____

_____

C6. Cancer of the gallbladder is *(common? rare?)*, typically with *(acute? insidious?)* onset. The 5-year survival rate is approximately ___ %.

C7. Complete this exercise about the pancreas and its disorders.

(a) The "head" of this fish-shaped organ rests against the *(duodenum? liver? spleen?)*, whereas the "tail" rests against the _____. Symptoms of pancreatic disorders are notable *(when changes are small? only when changes are great?)*. Explain._____

_____

(b) The pancreas produces *(many? few? no?)* digestive enzymes. Pancreatic amylases digest _____, whereas lipases digest _____.

(c) Explain why the pancreas does not normally digest itself by the protease trypsin produced by the pancreas. _____

_____

C8. Mr. Lowheide, age 61 years, has a history of alcoholism. He is being examined for a possible diagnosis of acute pancreatitis.

(a) List the two major causes of acute pancreatitis: _____, _____.

(b) Mr. Lowheide states that he "knocked off just a few beers last night with my buddies." Explain how alcohol triggers pancreatitis.

_____

_____

(c) Acute pancreatitis is likely to be *(mild? life threatening?)*. Explain. _____

_____

_____

(d) Explain why Mr. Lowheide has a rapid heart rate, low blood pressure, and cool and clammy skin. _____

_____

_____

(e) Mr. Lowheide's wife is informed that her husband's "blood levels of pancreatic enzymes" are high. Which two enzymes are likely to be high? _____, _____. How do these test results point to pancreatic damage?

_____

_____

(f) Explain why each of these treatments is ordered for Mr. Lowheide.

(f1) Intravenous fluid and electrolytes

_____

_____

_____

(f2) Nothing by mouth and nasogastric suction _____

_____

_____

(f3) Antibiotics _____

_____

_____

(f4) Percutaneous peritoneal lavage

_____

_____

C9. Brad, age 13 years, received a diagnosis of cystic fibrosis (CF) as an infant.

(a) Explain how CF can lead to chronic pancreatitis in the head of the pancreas.

_____

_____

(b) Describe signs and symptoms that Brad is likely to manifest.

_____

_____

(c) Explain why Brad is placed on a low-fat diet.

_____

_____

(d) Why does Brad receive pancreatic enzymes orally?

_____

_____

C10. Complete this exercise on pancreatic cancer.

(a) The 5-year survival rate associated with pancreatic cancer is approximately *(1%? 10%? 50%? 90%?)*. Incidence is especially high in *(young adult? elderly?)* persons. Pancreatic cancer typically is identified *(before? after?)* metastases have occurred.

(b) List dietary factors that appear to increase the risk for pancreatic cancer.

_____

_____

(c) What other factors are associated with the increased risk of pancreatic cancer?

_____

_____

(d) Onset typically is *(acute? insidious?)*. List typical manifestations.

_____

_____

(e) What health practices might help to prevent pancreatic cancer?

_____

_____

CHAPTER 39

Mechanisms of Endocrine Control

■ Review Questions

A. THE ENDOCRINE SYSTEM (pages 891–900)

A1. Describe the chemical links among these three systems: endocrine, nervous, and immune.

_____

_____

_____

A2. State one example of each of the following.

(a) A single hormone can affect several different organs._____

_____

_____

(b) A single function can be regulated by several different hormones. _____

_____

_____

A3. *(Auto? Juxta? Para?)*crine chemicals exert effects on the same cell that made the chemical, whereas _____crine chemicals act on cells adjacent to those that produce the chemical. Many hormones exert effects on distant organs; these hormones travel through *(blood plasma? ducts?)*.

A4. Classify the following hormones according to categories of chemical structure.

Amines or amino acids
Fatty acid derivatives
Peptides, polypeptides, and proteins
Steroids

(a) Eicosanoids including prostaglandins (involved with inflammation) and thromboxanes (active in hemostasis):

_____

(b) The smallest of all of these molecules; include epinephrine, norepinephrine, and dopamine: _____

(c) Derived from cholesterol; include sex hormones, cortisone, and aldosterone:

_____

(d) Comprise the largest category of hormones; include follicle-stimulating hormone (FSH), luteinizing hormone (LH), adrenocorticotropic hormone (ACTH), thyroid-stimulating hormone (TSH), antidiuretic hormone (ADH), oxytocin, releasing hormones, and insulin:

_____

(e) Thyroid hormone: _____

A5. Describe the synthesis and transport of hormones in this exercise.

(a) Steroids are synthesized in *(rough? smooth?)* endoplasmic reticulum (ER), whereas _____ hormones are formed on ribosomes located on *(rough? smooth?)* ER.

(b) Insulin is an example of a *(steroid? protein?)* hormone that is formed as a prohormone in rough ER. Then this chemical is converted to active insulin in *(Golgi? mitochondria?)*.

(c) Carrier-bound hormones are *(active? inactive?)* in that state. Circle hormones normally carried in blood bound to carriers.

Aldosterone   Cortisone
Estrogen   Growth hormone
Insulin   Parathyroid hormone
Thyroid hormone (thyroxine)

(d) About _____ % of thyroxine in blood is bound to protein carriers. What effect does aspirin exert on the effectiveness of thyroxine.

A6. Discuss metabolism of hormones in this exercise.

(a) How does metabolism of hormones affect hormone activity?

_____

_____

(b) Where does metabolism of hormones normally occur?_____

_____

(c) Name an enzyme that degrades and destroys catecholamines such as epinephrine or norepinephrine. _____

_____

(d) How are steroid hormones inactivated?

_____

_____

A7. Explain how a specific hormone "knows" which cells to affect.

_____

_____

_____

Describe receptors in this exercise.

(a) How many receptor molecules are present on (or in) one cell? _____

(b) Joyce has a decreased blood level of a particular hormone. As a result, her cells are likely to *(decrease? increase?)* the number of receptors for that hormone by *(induction? repression?)* of transcription of receptor genes. This mechanism is known as *(downregulation? upregulation?)*.

(c) Refer to Table 39-2 in the text. The hormones in the left two columns are likely to be more *(water? lipid?)* soluble. As a result, these *(can? cannot?)* penetrate the highly lipid cell membrane. As these hormones attach to *(surface? intracellular?)* receptors, they serve as *(first? second?)* messengers that trigger production of _____ (or a similar chemical) known as the *(first? second?)* messenger. The _____ messenger then triggers events within the cell that cause effects of the specific hormone.

(d) Steroid hormones *(can? cannot?)* penetrate the cell membrane. These hormones attach to *(surface? intracellular?)* receptors that initiate effects of the steroid hormone.

A8. Refer to Table 39-1 in the text and identify the organ that releases each hormone listed.

Adrenal cortex	Adrenal medulla
Anterior pituitary	Gastrointestinal tract
Hypothalamu	Kidney
Ovaries	Posterior pituitary
Testes	

(a) Releasing hormones such as corticotropin-releasing hormone (CRH), gonadotropin-releasing hormone (GnRH), or thyrotropin-releasing hormone (TRH): _____

(b) Tropic hormones such as ACTH, FSH, LH, or TSH: _____

(c) Growth hormone (GH): _____

(d) Cortisol and aldosterone: _____

(e) ADH and oxytocin: _____

(f) Erythropoietin: _____

(g) Androgens such as testosterone and related chemicals: _____ and _____

A9. Select the hormone(s) listed in Table 39-1 that fit(s) each description.

(a) Lowers blood calcium: _____

(b) Lowers blood glucose: _____

(c) Stimulate release of hormones from the anterior pituitary: _____

(d) Mimic effects of the sympathetic nervous system: _____

(e) Promotes protein synthesis in bones and muscles: _____

(f) Stimulates secretion of HCl by the stomach: _____

A10. Describe regulation of hormone levels in this exercise.

(a) The hypophyseal portal system is a system of _____ that transport hormones from the _____ to the _____. (Select from answers in Question A8). These hormones are known as *(releasing? tropic?)* hormones. (See Figure 39-5.)

(b) Tropic hormones are produced by the *(anterior? posterior?)* pituitary. For example, the tropic hormone TSH stimulates its target gland (_____) to release the target hormone _____. Increasing levels of thyroxine have a *(positive? negative or opposite?)* feedback effect, causing a(n) *(decrease? increase?)* in TRH and TSH.

(c) ACTH is the tropic hormone that stimulates adrenal *(cortex? medulla?)* production of the hormone *(cortisol? epinephrine?)*. Cortisol is known as a glucocorticoid because one of its functions is to regulate levels of _____ in blood. Cortisone injections are *(endo? exo?)*genous forms of cortisol, which will cause a(n) *(decrease? increase?)* in production of CRH and ACTH and *(stimulation? suppression?)* of adrenocortical function.

(d) Name two or more hormones that are regulated by blood levels of the chemicals that these hormones control.

_____

_____

A11. Describe tests of hormone levels in this exercise.

(a) Circle tests that require use of radiolabeled forms of the hormone being tested:

Enzyme-linked immunosorbent assay (ELISA)
Immunoradiometric assay (IRMA)
Magnetic resonance imaging (MRI)
Radioimmunoassay (RIA)

(b) Describe advantages and disadvantages of assessing endocrine function by urine testing. _____

_____

B. GENERAL ASPECTS OF ALTERED ENDOCRINE FUNCTION (pages 900–902)

B1. *(Hyper? Hypo?)*function refers to a decrease in function of an endocrine gland. List six or more possible causes of such an alteration.

_____

_____

_____

_____

_____

_____

B2. Identify the category of endocrine hypofunction in the following cases.

1° = Primary   2° = Secondary   3° = Tertiary

(a) Mr. Bagley's radiation treatments for brain cancer have led to his adrenal cortex hypofunction: ____

(b) Marguerite has a bilateral oophorectomy related to her ovarian cancer: ____

(c) Seth's low thyroid hormone is linked to a defect in his TSH production: ____

B3. Choose the two true statements about hypopituitarism.

(a) Manifestations of this condition are apparent by the time 25% of the pituitary is destroyed.

(b) This condition is **always** acquired (not congenital).

(c) **Adrenal cortex** hypofunction is the most serious endocrine deficiency secondary to hypopituitarism.

(d) Cortisol and thyroid hormone replacement therapy **can** help clients with this condition.

B4. List the anterior pituitary hormones in correct sequence as they are lost with hypopituitarism.

ACTH   FSH   GH   LH   TSH

_____ → _____ → _____ → _____ →

_____

CHAPTER 40

Alterations in Endocrine Control of Growth and Metabolism

■ Review Questions

A. GROWTH DISORDERS (pages 903–909)

A1. Complete this exercise about factors that regulate growth and maturation.

(a) List four hormones required for normal growth and maturation.

_____

_____

_____

(b) Circle functions of growth hormone (GH).

(1) Increases protein in body cells

(2) Increases blood glucose levels

(3) Acts directly on bones and muscles to increase growth of these tissues

(4) Decreases use of fats and increases use of carbohydrates as major fuel sources

A2. Circle the two true statements related to growth factors.

(a) Growth hormone normally is produced **only during childhood.**

(b) Insulin-like growth factors are also known as **somatomedins.**

(c) Somatomedins normally are produced by the **hypothalamus** and the **pancreas.**

(d) Hypoglycemia, starvation, stress, and the amino acid arginine all **decrease** production of GH.

A3. Complete this exercise about stature (height).

(a) Determine the "midparental height" for children of Cindy (5'7") and Alex (6'2").
Male children: _____
Female children: _____

(b) List the three factors that can most accurately diagnose short stature.

_____

_____

_____

(c) Children with congenital GH deficiency typically have *(short? tall?)* stature with *(normal? abnormal?)* intelligence. Growth hormone deficiency typically is treated with GH replacement therapy derived from *(cadaver pituitary? recombinant DNA?).*

A4. Select the term that best fits each description.

Constitutional short stature
Catch-up growth
Genetically short stature
Laron-type dwarfism
Psychosocial dwarfism
Panpituitarism
Somatotrope

(a) Caused by hereditary deficiency in insulin-like growth factor (IGF) production with normal GH production: _____

(b) Most likely to occur in severely neglected or abused children: _____

(c) Well-proportioned child who has short parents: _____

(d) Condition in which all pituitary hormones are deficient, including GH: _____

(e) Anterior pituitary cell that produces GH:

_____

A5. Match the condition to the related description.

Acromegaly   Gigantism   Somatopause

(a) Mr. Gordon, age 67 years, is the same height that he attained by age 20 years. He has gained weight, and he comments, "I have a belly that I never had before." He is fatigued and his blood GH levels are subnormal for a person of his age.

_____

(b) During the past 3 years, Mr. George's shoe size has increased, and his ring finger has outgrown his wedding ring. His lower jaw protrudes, and his voice has deepened. George is 46 years old and 6'1".

_____

(c) Billy, age 8 years, is in the 99th percentile for his age and parental height; his serum GH levels are extremely high. _____

A6. Complete this exercise about Mr. George (Question A5[b]).

(a) Mr. George's height (*is? is not?*) likely to increase. Explain._____

_____

(b) His condition is a quite (*common? rare?*) disorder with an (*acute? insidious?*) onset. Almost all cases of acromegaly are caused by (*benign? malignant?*) tumors of the pituitary that increase GH production.

(c) Mr. George has increased risk of heart failure. Explain. _____

_____

(d) Headaches and visual defects also have plagued Mr. George recently. Explain how these are related to his acromegaly.

_____

_____

(e) Mr. George will have his pituitary tumor removed. The nurse tells Mr. George that his sense of smell may be diminished after the surgery. Explain. _____

_____

_____

A7. Roberta, age 8 years, is diagnosed with a tumor of her hypothalamus. Identify each condition that relates to this tumor.

Isosexual precocious puberty
Menarche
Thelarche

(a) She began to develop breasts at age 6 years:

_____

(b) Her first menstrual period took place at age 7 years: _____

(c) Her sexual development has occurred much earlier than normal: _____

B. THYROID DISORDERS (pages 909–915)

B1. Use terms from the following list to fill in blanks about the thyroid gland and its hormone. (Not all terms will be used.)

De-Iodide	Four Isthmus	Free Lobules	In-Protein
TBG	Three	Thyroglobulin	
Thyroxine (T_4)		Triiodothyronine (T_3)	
Tyrosine			

(a) The thyroid consists of two lobes connected by the _____. Lobes consist of tiny, saclike _____ filled with _____.

(b) Thyroglobulin consists of long chains of the amino acid _____, to which the ion _____ is attached. The most active form of thyroid hormone appears to be _____, in which _____ iodides are attached to tyrosine.

(c) Almost all thyroid hormone exists bound to _____, primarily the binding protein named _____. Only the _____ form of thyroid hormone can enter cells and affect their metabolism.

(d) Corticosteroids, protein malnutrition, kidney disorders such as nephrosis (in which protein is lost in the urine), and aspirin, all ___crease T_3T_4 binding to TBG, causing a(n) ___crease in active thyroid hormone.

B2. Review negative feedback mechanisms that regulate thyroid hormone in Chapter 39, Question A10(b), Study Guide page 203. High thyroid hormone levels are likely to (*stimulate? inhibit?*) production of TRH and TSH. Cold temperature (*triggers? inhibits?*) thyroid production by stimulating TRH release from the (*anterior pituitary? hypothalamus? thyroid gland?*).

B3. Thyroid hormone exerts effects on (*all major? only a few specific?*) organs of the body. In general, it (*decreases? increases?*) metabolism. Write "IN" (for increase) or "DE" (for decrease) to indicate specific effects of thyroid hormone.

(a) ____ creased blood levels of cholesterol as fats are used for fuel.

(b) Gastrointestinal absorption of glucose from food is ____ creased, providing more fuel for metabolism.

(c) Muscle mass is ____ creased as muscle proteins are used for fuel. However, if thyroid hormone is excessive, muscle action ____ creases leading to tremor.

(d) Gastrointestinal tract motility and secretion ____ crease, providing more nutrients for metabolism. Risk for diarrhea ____ creases related to intestinal motility.

(e) Weight ____ creases and body temperature ____ creases as calories are "burned" for metabolism. Blood vessels of skin dilate in attempts to ____ crease body temperature associated with increased metabolism.

(f) Heart rate, cardiac output, and ventilation ____ crease, providing oxygen for metabolism.

(g) Nerve activity ____ creases, leading to anxiety and restlessness if thyroid hormone is excessive. Infants with thyroid deficiency are likely to experience ____ creased brain development.

B4. Consider the normal functions of thyroid hormone (Question B3) and also refer to Table 40-3. Now determine whether each of the following descriptions better applies to hypothyroidism (hypo) or hyperthyroidism (hyper).

(a) Neonatal retardation and developmental delay in infants: _____

(b) Sluggishness, sleeping more than normal:

_____

(c) Bradycardia and low cardiac output: _____

(d) Blood cholesterol is high: _____

(e) Weight gain related to accumulation of a mucopolysaccharide that presents as edema; may lead to life-threatening coma: _____

B5. Identify the thyroid condition that fits each description.

Cretinism	Goiter
Graves' disease	Hashimoto's disease
Myxedema	Thyroid storm

(a) Mrs. Ruiz has an enlargement in her neck in the area of her "Adam's apple." The growth is pressing against her trachea, esophagus, and veins of her neck causing difficulty breathing and eating and facial edema. Mrs. Ruiz lives in a region where iodized salt is not readily available: _____

(b) Screening of Antonio, born this week, indicates subnormal levels of T_4 and TSH. Additional tests indicate that he has congenital absence of a thyroid gland. Antonio is treated with T_4 to prevent mental retardation and short stature: _____

(c) Mrs. Jones has a history of thyroid cancer with radiation therapy 15 years ago. She has a "puffy" appearance with nonpitting edema: _____

(d) Nan has begun taking lithium carbonate for her bipolar disorder, diagnosed 2 months ago; she is weak and fatigued and is depressed about her recent weight gain:

_____

(e) Ms. Mason initially presents with a goiter; with time her T_4 levels decrease as a result of her antithyroid antibody production. Her skin is dry and rough; her hair is coarse and brittle. Ms. Mason is treated with T_4:

_____

(f) Mrs. Yokum has undiagnosed hyperthyroidism that is exacerbated as she experiences diabetic ketoacidosis. Her high fever, congestive heart failure, and delirium require rapid treatment to prevent death:

_____

(g) Dr. Oxford, age 37 years, has lost 30 pounds during the past month. Her eyes bulge so much that her eyelids barely close over her eyes. Her partner has noted that Dr. Oxford seems "anxious and restless." Dr. Oxford has experienced episodes of palpitations, dyspnea, and irritability that she attributes to her insomnia.

_____

B6. Choose the two true statements about the thyroid gland.

(a) Radiation of the neck is more likely to cause **primary** (rather than secondary) hypothyroidism.

(b) Graves' disease is **a rare** form of hyperthyroidism.

(c) Thyroid storm is **a mild** form of hyperthyroidism.

(d) Because manifestations of hyperthyroidism mimic the effects of **sympathetic** nerves, beta-blocker drugs (propranolol) can reduce symptoms.

C. DISORDERS OF ADRENAL CORTICAL FUNCTION (pages 915–922)

C1. Complete this exercise about the adrenal glands.

(a) Where are these glands located?

_____

(b) Contrast the adrenal cortex (C) and medulla (M).

(b1) Produces the hormones epinephrine and norepinephrine that both mimic sympathetic nerves: _____

(b2) Forms most of each adrenal gland; consists of zona glomerulosa, fasciculata, and reticularis: _____

(b3) Critical for stress responses needed for survival: _____

(b4) Its hormones are steroids (derived from cholesterol): _____

C2. Identify the adrenocorticoid hormone that fits each description.

Aldosterone   Cortisol
Dehydroepiandrosterone sulfate

(a) The chief mineralocorticoid; causes kidneys to retain Na^+ and H_2O and to eliminate K^+ into urine (see Study Guide Figure 30-1C):

_____

(b) Regulated by the renin-angiotensin mechanism and blood levels of K^+:

_____

(c) The primary sex hormone made by the adrenal cortex; levels decrease with aging (adrenopause): _____

(d) The major glucocorticoid; controlled by corticotropin-releasing hormone (CRH) and adrenocorticotropic hormone (ACTH) (see Chapter 39, Question A10[c]):

_____

C3. Circle the effects of cortisol.

(a) *(Decreases? Increases?)* blood glucose levels (See Study Guide Figure 41-1B, page 211.)

(b) Causes *(synthesis? breakdown?)* of muscle proteins, which can lead to striae (lines) in skin

(c) Enhances conversion of amino acids into glucose, a process known as *(glycogenesis? gluconeogenesis?)* (See Study Guide Figure 41-1B.)

(d) *(Decreases? Increases?)* capillary permeability and action of B- and T-cells

(e) *(Decreases? Increases?)* fever

(f) *(Decreases? Increases?)* formation of scar tissue

(g) The effects described just above (in C3[d], [e], and [f]) are all examples of cortisol's function as an *(anti-inflammatory? inflammation-enhancing?)* hormone.

C4. Describe diurnal variations in cortisol production. _____

_____

_____

_____

C5. Vanessa has been taking steroid medications for a year. Explain the following effects.

(a) She has become emotionally labile (has dramatic mood swings).

_____

_____

(b) Her own production of adrenal hormones is diminished. _____

_____

_____

(c) Vanessa suddenly decides to stop taking her steroid medications. _____

_____

_____

C6. Describe the following tests related to the adrenal cortex.

(a) Screening test for Cushing's syndrome

_____

_____

(b) Testing the CRH-ACTH-glucocorticoid axis

_____

_____

C7. Sophie is born with congenital adrenal hyperplasia.

(a) Congenital adrenal hyperplasia *(is? is not?)* a genetic disorder. Sophie lacks the enzymes necessary to synthesize *(ACTH? aldosterone? cortisol? sex hormones?)*.

(b) Decreased cortisol activates the negative feedback mechanism that *(decreases? increases?)* blood levels of ACTH. As a result, Sophie's adrenal cortex *(decreases? increases?)* in size (hyperplasia). In addition, her adrenal cortex *(decreases? increases?)* production of androgen. Describe the effects. _____

_____

C8. Contrast disorders of the adrenal cortex in this exercise. Select the correct name of the disorder (which may be used more than once).

Addison's disease
Cushing's disease
Cushing's syndrome
Incidental adrenal mass
Secondary adrenal cortical insufficiency

(a) Mrs. Tappin's deficiency of adrenocortical hormones is precipitated by removal of her pituitary gland: _____

(b) Vanessa's adrenal insufficiency (Question C5) caused by cessation of exogenous cortisol is an example of this type of disorder:

_____

(c) Mr. Joliet has had an adrenal mass found unexpectedly during a CAT scan of his abdomen related to his primary colon cancer: _____

(d) Mr. Fitzgerald is a 41-year-old white man whose adrenal cortex was destroyed by autoimmune mechanisms. His blood levels of cortisol are deficient, causing increased ACTH levels: _____

(e) Lieutenant Jackson has a pituitary tumor with excessive ACTH production that stimulates adrenal production of cortisol:

_____

(f) Mrs. Reed has a small cell lung carcinoma that is producing ectopic ACTH; adrenocorticoid replacement is required:

_____

C9. Describe Mr. Fitzgerald's condition (Question C8[d]) in further detail in this exercise.

(a) His disorder is a (*primary? secondary?*) adrenal insufficiency. He is likely to manifest signs of adrenal insufficiency once these hormones drop to approximately (*10%? 90%?*) of normal.

(b) Circle the typical manifestations of Addison's disease.

(1) Increased urinary output with low cardiac output and low blood pressure

(2) Decreased urinary output with high cardiac output and high blood pressure

(3) Excessive loss of salt in urine with abnormal craving for salt

(4) Hyperglycemia with high energy level

(5) Pale skin

(c) Mr. Fitzgerald (*will? will not?*) require lifetime replacement of adrenocortical hormones.

C10. Signs and symptoms of Cushing's syndrome are related to (*deficient? excessive?*) cortisol production. Circle common manifestations of this disorder.

(a) Lean trunk with obesity in extremities

(b) Excessive distribution of fat in the face and back

(c) Stretch marks in skin

(d) Osteosclerosis

(e) Hypotension

CHAPTER 41

Diabetes Mellitus

■ Review Questions

A. HORMONAL CONTROL OF BLOOD GLUCOSE (pages 925–930)

A1. Explain why diabetes mellitus (DM) is a major health problem in the United States.

_____

_____

_____

_____

A2. Pancreatic hormones are produced by *(acinar cells? islets of Langerhans?)*. List three hormones synthesized by the islet cells and summarize their functions.

(a) Alpha cells produce _____, which *(decreases? increases?)* blood glucose.

(b) Beta cells produce _____, which *(decreases? increases?)* blood glucose.

(c) Delta cells produce _____, which inhibits release of both _____ and _____ and *(decreases? increases?)* gastrointestinal activity.

A3. Refer to Study Guide Figure 41-1 and textbook Table 41-1. Complete this exercise about blood glucose regulation in Simon, who is a healthy 30-year-old man (without diabetes mellitus).

(a) It is 7 AM and Simon has not eaten for 12 hours. Which blood glucose level(s) would be considered normal at this time? _____ mg/dL.

36   76   136   780

Which value would indicate hypoglycemia?

_____

(b) How is Simon's blood glucose level being maintained to prevent hypoglycemia? Circle the processes that increase his blood glucose level between meals:

(1) Glycogenolysis

(2) Glycogenesis

(3) Gluconeogenesis

(c) Which one of these processes (in A3[b]) involves conversion of amino acids or parts of fats into glucose? _____ Where does this process occur? _____

(d) Which process (in A3[b]) releases glucose by breakdown of glycogen? ___

(e) Identify hormones that promote glycogenesis or gluconeogenesis to help maintain Simon's blood glucose throughout the night (Figure 41-1B).

Cortisol   Epinephrine
Glucagon   Insulin

(f) Which of Simon's tissues relies on glucose as its fuel source and depends on a constant blood supply of glucose because this tissue can neither synthesize nor store much glucose?

(1) Adipose tissue

(2) Brain

(3) Skeletal muscle

(4) Liver

(g) When Simon eats a hearty breakfast, his blood glucose level *(decreases? increases?)*. High blood glucose stimulates the pancreas to release *(glucagon? insulin?)*. This hormone promotes movement of glucose from *(blood into cells? cells into blood?)* and also *(stimulates? inhibits?)* liver storage of glucose as _____. In other words, insulin *(raises? lowers?)* blood glucose. (See Figure 41-1C.)

A4. Further describe insulin and its functions in this exercise.

(a) Insulin is a *(carbohydrate? lipid? protein?)* composed of two peptide chains. Which chain is removed when active insulin is formed in the pancreas? *(A? B? C?)* chain

(b) Pancreatic release of insulin is signaled by entrance of _____ into beta cells.

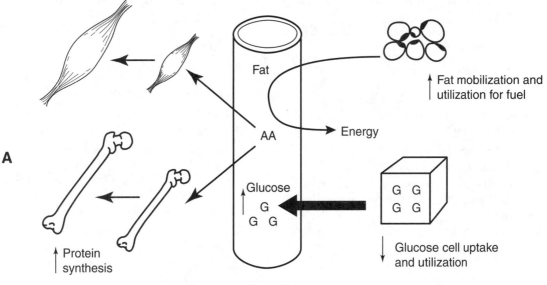

Functions of growth hormone

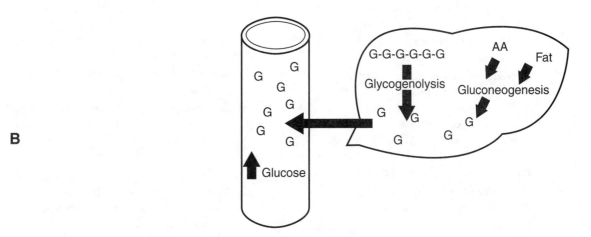

Functions of glucagon, epinephrine, and cortisol

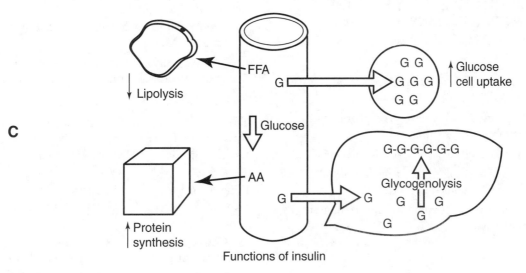

Functions of insulin

Figure 41-1.

Glucose enters cells by means of the glucose transporter named _____. Within minutes, (pre-formed? newly synthesized?) insulin is released.

(c) Insulin released from the pancreas passes into the (inferior vena cava? portal vein?) and travels to the liver. Once in general circulation, insulin has a half-life (T$_{1/2}$) of approximately ____ minutes.

(d) GLUT-4 is the glucose transporter for glucose entrance into (Hint: circle two answers) (adipose? brain? liver? skeletal muscle?) cells; this transporter requires the presence of _____. GLUT-___ is the transporter for glucose available in all body cells, including neurons; this transporter (does? does not?) require insulin.

(e) Insulin also promotes transport of _____ into cells, which facilitates _____ synthesis. Insulin also stimulates movement of _____ into cells and inhibits fat breakdown known as lipo-_____. (See Figure 41-1C.)

(f) Catecholamines such as epinephrine (stimulate? inhibit?) insulin release, and growth hormone (GH) (antagonizes? mimics?) the effects of insulin. As a result (and because of other actions shown in Figure 41-1A and B), these hormones (decrease? increase?) blood glucose.

(g) Explain why acromegaly and chronic stress can lead to hyperglycemia and DM.

_____

_____

B. DIABETES MELLITUS: CLASSIFICATION, ETIOLOGY, MANIFESTATIONS, DIAGNOSIS, AND MANAGEMENT (pages 930–942)

B1. Choose the two true statements about diabetes mellitus (DM).

(a) Diabetes mellitus primarily is a problem of **unavailability of insulin.**

(b) The term "mellitus" in DM refers to **urine.**

(c) A value of 108 mg/dL on a fasting blood glucose test is considered **normal.**

(d) Type 1 diabetes accounts for approximately 90% of DM.

B2. Complete this exercise about DM.

(a) A blood glucose level of 170 mg/dL on a 2-hour postload glucose test indicates (see textbook Table 41-3):

(1) Diabetes mellitus

(2) Impaired glucose tolerance

(3) Normal value

(b) Most type 1 DM is type (1A? 1B?), which is (idiopathic? immune-mediated?). This form of DM formerly was known as (insulin? noninsulin?) dependent because patients with type 1 diabetes (do? do not?) require exogenous insulin replacement.

(c) After diagnosis of type 1 DM, a _____ period may occur in which manifestations disappear and insulin replacement is not required. Explain.

_____

(d) Insulin normally (stimulates? inhibits?) lipolysis (Study Guide Figure 41-1C). With absolute absence of insulin, as in type (1? 2?) DM, formation of _____ is more likely to occur as a result of excessive fat breakdown.

(e) Four of five persons with type 2 diabetes are (obese? underweight?), especially if waist:hip ratio is (high? low?). Explain how obesity contributes to this form of DM._____

(f) How do high levels of free fatty acids contribute to DM? Free fatty acids (stimulate? inhibit?) insulin secretion and (stimulate? inhibit?) glucose uptake by cells. Free fatty acids also (decrease? increase?) release of glucose from the liver.

(g) Weight loss and exercise in obese persons (can? cannot?) help to prevent and manage type 2 DM.

(h) Women with gestational DM (are? are not?) at increased risk of having diabetes develop within the next 10 years.

B3. The many types of DM are classified by (cause? treatment?). Refer to textbook Table 41-2 and identify the class of DM present in each client.

Type 1   Type 2
Drug disorder   Endocrine disorder
Exocrine pancreas   Gestational diabetes
  disorder   mellitus

(a) Clarissa, age 34 years, is pregnant. At 25 weeks of pregnancy, her screening load glucose tolerance test reveals a blood glucose of 202 mg/dL: _____

(b) Timmy received a diagnosis of DM at age 8 years; his beta cells were destroyed by his own autoantibodies, so his pancreas produces no insulin: _____

(c) Annette has pheochromocytoma, and Allison has Cushing's syndrome, both of which cause hyperglycemia: _____

(d) Harry is taking steroids for a severe case of pneumonia and also is taking Lasix (a loop diuretic) to reduce fluid in his lungs: _____

B4. Circle risk factors for gestational DM.

(a) African American

(b) Native American

(c) 23 years old

(d) Previously delivered a healthy 10-pound baby

(e) Third pregnancy

(f) Family history of DM

(g) Weight of 105 pounds

(h) Absence of glucose in urine

(i) History of two miscarriages

B5. Explain why early diagnosis and management of gestational DM are essential.

_____
_____
_____
_____

B6. Discuss signs and symptoms of DM in this exercise.

(a) Type *(1? 2?)* DM typically has a more insidious onset.

(b) One sign of diabetes is *(decreased? increased?)* urinary output. Explain the mechanism._____
_____
_____

How does polyuria contribute to fatigue of DM?

_____
_____

(c) Which of the three "poly's" of DM refers to excessive thirst and drinking?

Polydipsia   Polyphagia   Polyuria

(d) Polyphagia is more likely to accompany type *(1? 2?)* DM. Explain. _____
_____
_____

(e) Weight loss is more likely to be a sign of type *(1? 2?)* DM. List three factors that may account for weight loss. _____
_____
_____

(f) Infections are *(more? less?)* common in people with diabetes. Explain.

_____
_____

(g) How is hyperglycemia related to blurred vision? _____
_____
_____

B7. Identify each blood test designed for diagnosing or monitoring diabetes.

Fasting blood glucose test
Glycosylated hemoglobin (HbA$_{IC}$ test)
Glucose tolerance test
Random blood glucose test
Self-monitoring test

(a) After a "load" (such as 100 g of glucose) is given, blood samples are drawn; individuals without diabetes exhibit normal blood glucose levels within 2 to 3 hours:

_____

(b) The preferred diagnostic test: easily administered and low cost: _____

(c) Administered at any time regardless of last meal; glucose >200 mg/dL is considered an unequivocal elevation: _____

(d) Measures percentage of hemoglobin that has combined permanently with glucose during the past 3 months since those red blood cells were formed; a measure of diabetes control (and patient compliance): _____

(e) Involves placing a drop of blood on a strip then read by a glucometer; allows rapid, low-cost testing several times a day:

_____

B8. Discuss nonpharmacologic management of diabetes in this exercise.

(a) Which type of testing for glucose is considered more accurate? *(Blood? Urine?)*

(b) List three mechanisms for control of type 2 diabetes other than by insulin.

_____
_____
_____

(c) The American Diabetic Association (ADA) *(does? does not?)* recommend a specific diet for individuals with diabetes.

However, eating foods at (consistent? varied?) times is recommended.

(d) Counting grams of carbohydrates on food labels is recommended for individuals with diabetes. A food serving with 25 g of carbohydrate contains approximately ____ Cal.

(e) Mr. Jensen has type 2 DM with high low-density lipoproteins (LDLs) and diabetic nephropathy. Of his daily intake of 2000 Cal, no more than approximately ____ Cal should come from saturated fats. Because of his renal impairment, his daily intake of _____ may be restricted.

(f) Describe the benefits and risks of exercise for individuals with diabetes, including the potential problem of delayed hypoglycemia for those with type 1 diabetes.

_____

_____

B9. Oral hypoglycemic drugs can be effective for individuals with type (1? 2?) diabetes. Identify mechanisms of action of these drugs.

IHC = Inhibits hepatic glucose production (by glycogenolysis or gluconeogenesis)

ISC = Increases sensitivity of cells of liver, skeletal muscle, and fat to insulin; thus, enhances uptake of glucose

SBC = Stimulates beta cells to release insulin (which works only for patients with some functional beta cells); can lead to hypoglycemia

RFFA = Reduce free fatty acids (thus, may prevent beta cell exhaustion)

(a) Thiazolidinediones: ____, ____, and ____

(b) Biguanides: ____ and ____

(c) Sulfonylureas: ____ and ____

B10. Complete this exercise about Melissa, age 19 years, who has type 1 diabetes.

(a) The medication she takes is more likely to be (insulin? an oral hypoglycemic?). She takes her medication by injection, not by mouth. Explain. _____

_____

(b) Her insulin is U-100 strength. What does this mean? _____

_____

_____

(c) Melissa's insulin is Humalog injections three times a day. What advantage does this regimen offer over once-a-day dosing with Ultralente? _____

_____

(d) Her insulin is human insulin made by recombinant DNA methods. How is this insulin preferable to porcine insulin?

_____

_____

_____

(e) Melissa is being considered for an insulin pump (CSII). Describe this method of treatment and explain why Melissa must be highly motivated to qualify as a candidate for CSII. _____

_____

_____

C. DIABETES MELLITUS: COMPLICATIONS (pages 943–951)

C1. Identify correct descriptions of the three major acute complications of DM. More than one answer will be appropriate in some cases.

Diabetic ketoacidosis (DKA)
Hyperglycemic hyperosmolar nonketotic syndrome (HHNK)
Hypoglycemia

(a) An insulin reaction caused by an insulin level in excess of the body's current needs:

_____

(b) Most associated with excessive fat breakdown (lipolysis) when insulin is lacking: _____

(c) Associated with high blood glucose levels:

_____

(d) Condition with the most rapid onset:

_____

(e) Precipitated by stress: _____

(f) Involves movement of water out of brain cells as extremely high blood glucose exerts an osmotic effect; may involve severe neurological alterations: _____

(g) Involves dehydration of mucosa (leading to extreme thirst) and dry skin: _____

(h) Seen most often in association with type 2 DM: _____

C2. Melissa (Question B10) is more likely to have diabetic ketoacidosis (DKA) develop when her blood glucose level is *(35? 100? 260?)* mg/dL. Complete this exercise about her episode of DKA.

(a) Circle the factors that increase Melissa's risk for DKA. She:

   (1) Has type 1 diabetes

   (2) Is 7 months pregnant

   (3) Is a college student and approaching midterm examinations

   (4) Has had a respiratory infection this week

   (5) Self-monitors her blood glucose three or four times a day

(b) In DKA, excessive fat breakdown leads to formation of _____ in the liver. These chemicals are *(acids? bases?)*, so they *(decrease? increase?)* blood pH. Blood levels of bicarbonate *(decrease? increase?)* as bicarbonate buffers acids.

(c) How can Melissa's ketonemia be readily detected?

   _____

(d) Melissa's blood pressure is likely to *(decrease? increase?)* in DKA; *(brady? tachy?)*cardia also may occur. Explain.

   _____

   _____

(e) Melissa is admitted to the hospital. List three major goals of her treatment.

   _____

   _____

C3. Nick, age 17 years, has type 1 DM and is a football player. He self-monitors to carefully balance his insulin doses with his meals and football practice. Today he had an insulin reaction.

(a) Circle factors most likely to trigger such a reaction:

   (1) Skipping an insulin injection

   (2) Taking too large a dose of insulin

   (3) Working harder than usual at practice

   (4) Skipping a meal

(b) Circle signs of hypoglycemic effects on his cerebrum:

   (1) Making a mistake on a play at practice

   (2) Headache

   (3) Hunger

   (4) Rapid heart rate and cool, clammy skin

   (5) Starting a fight with another player

(c) Which sign (in C3[b]) indicates sympathetic response to the hypoglycemia? ____

(d) Nick is unconscious and lying on the field. Which treatments for his insulin reaction are most helpful right now?

   (1) Insulin injection

   (2) Glucagon injection

   (3) Hard candy

   (4) Orange juice

   (5) Glucose gel placed in the side of his mouth

C4. Colleen, a 50-year-old woman with type 2 DM, recently has increased carbohydrates and calories in her diet. Describe her experience.

(a) Her recent changes in diet are likely to *(decrease? increase?)* her blood glucose level.

(b) Colleen notices this change as she self-monitors. She decides to increase her insulin dosage to "cover" the extra blood glucose. The extra insulin puts her into a mild *(hyper? hypo?)*glycemia.

(c) As a result, four counterregulatory hormones are released; all of these will *(decrease? increase?)* her blood glucose. Name these four hormones. (See Study Guide Figures 41-1A and B.)

   _____

   _____

   _____

(d) Colleen then may increase her insulin dosage further, creating a vicious cycle. This cycle is known as the *(dawn? Somogyi?)* phenomenon, in which "_____glycemia begets _____glycemia."

(e) If Colleen also exhibits the "dawn phenomenon," her blood glucose level will increase in early *(morning? evening?)*; this can *(exacerbate? reduce the effects of?)* her Somogyi phenomenon.

C5. Describe three mechanisms that lead to chronic complications of DM.

(a) Excessive blood glucose causes accumulation of *(fructose? sorbitol?)*, which can lead to damage of blood vessels, eyes, and kidneys. Excesses of this chemical also can damage the Schwann cells of _____.

(b) Extra glucose combines with protein to alter _____ membranes of small blood vessels, *(decreasing? increasing?)* blood supply to tissues.

(c) In DM, glucose attached to hemoglobin (HbA$_{1c}$) has a *(higher? lower?)* affinity for oxygen, and thus *(decreases? increases?)* oxygen supply to tissues.

C6. Choose the two true statements about chronic complications of DM.

(a) Research indicates that intensive treatment for type 1 DM **can** reduce chronic complications.

(b) Nephropathies refer to alterations in **nerves**.

(c) Kidney damage is a **rare** complication of DM.

(d) Most diabetic kidney damage involves **renal tubules**.

(e) **Elevated protein in urine** is an early sign of diabetic nephropathy.

C7. Further describe chronic complications of DM in these cases.

(a) Colleen (Question C4) is showing signs of peripheral neuropathies. These are most likely to start in her *(hips and shoulders? feet and hands?)* and progress *(proximally? distally?)*. This is known as the _____ pattern and is likely to be *(bilateral? unilateral?)*.

(b) Explain why Colleen's peripheral neuropathies can lead to further complications. _____
_____
_____
_____

(c) Daniel, age 65 years, received a diagnosis of type 2 DM 9 years ago. Circle the manifestations associated with autonomic nerve damage:

(1) Pain in his hands

(2) Burning pain in his legs

(3) Urinary tract infections

(4) Constipation

(5) Erectile dysfunction

(6) Feeling dizzy when he stands up quickly

(d) Circle factors that increase Daniel's risk for diabetic nephropathy and end-stage renal disease (ESRD).

(1) Daniel is Native American

(2) His father had diabetic nephropathy

(3) Daniel smokes a pack of cigarettes a day

(4) His blood pressure typically is approximately 150/92 mm Hg

(5) His HbA$_{1c}$ usually is 6% to 7%

(6) His total cholesterol is 246 mg/dL

(e) List three regions of Daniel's body particularly at risk for macrovascular disease. _____
_____
_____

(f) Daniel is tested with a Semmes-Weinstein monofilament. What is being tested?
_____
_____

In addition to decreased circulation, what factors might contribute to foot ulcers in Daniel? _____
_____
_____

(g) Blindness in individuals with diabetes most commonly results from:

Cataracts   Glaucoma
Retinopathy

Which factors listed in Question C2(a) increase Melissa's risk for diabetic retinopathy? _____
_____
_____

C8. Summarize measures that can best prevent chronic complications of DM. _____
_____
_____
_____

CHAPTER 42

Structure and Function of the Male Reproductive System

■ Review Questions

A. STRUCTURE OF THE MALE REPRODUCTIVE SYSTEM (pages 955–959)

A1. List two functions of the male reproductive system.

_____

_____

A2. Choose the two true statements about the male reproductive system.

(a) Males have XX (rather than XY) chromosomes.

(b) At 6 weeks of gestation, the gender of an embryo **is** evident anatomically.

(c) Male reproductive tracts develop from **wolffian** (not müllerian) ducts.

(d) Development of testes requires genes in the short arm of the Y chromosome.

A3. Match each male reproductive hormone with its function.

Anti-müllerian hormone   Dihydrotestosterone
Testosterone

(a) Stimulates wolffian ducts to develop male reproductive ducts (epididymis and vas deferens); without this hormone, XY embryos will develop female genitalia:

_____

(b) Formed from testosterone, it stimulates development of the male urethra, prostate, penis, and scrotum: _____

(c) Inhibits males from developing female organs from müllerian ducts:

_____

A4. Discuss these clinical applications of male reproductive anatomy in the following exercise.

(a) Dennis is born at 29 weeks of gestation. Palpation of his scrotum indicates absence of testes. What is the likely explanation?

_____

_____

Explain why eventual descent of testes is important. _____

_____

(b) Mr. Jamison, age 66, has testicular cancer that has metastasized to lymph nodes surrounding his abdominal aorta. Explain.

_____

_____

Where do testes develop during embryologic life? _____ At what point do they typically descend into the scrotum?

_____

(c) Patrick and Jane both lift heavy machinery as part of their jobs. Patrick has had bilateral inguinal hernias develop; Jane has not. Explain. _____

_____

_____

_____

(d) Sean has a vasectomy on March 1. He is advised to "use protection" to prevent pregnancy until April 15. Explain.

_____

_____

A5. Circle or fill in correct answers about structures associated with the testes or scrotum.

(a) The tunica (*albuginea? vaginalis?*) is derived from abdominal peritoneum and immediately surrounds testes, whereas the tunica _____ is tougher and more external and protects testes.

(b) Name the two sets of muscles that contract to pull the testes and scrotum closer to the body during cold temperatures: _____ muscles and _____ muscles

(c) The pampiniform plexus consists of (*arteries? veins?*) that supply testes.

A6. Arrange from first to last the structures in the pathway of sperm from their formation to the point at which they exit from the body:

Efferent ductules	Ejaculatory duct
Epididymis	Rete testis
Seminiferous tubules	Urethra
Vas (ductus) deferens	

_____ → _____ →

_____ → _____ →

_____ → _____ →

_____

Which of these structures is/are unpaired?

_____

A7. Circle or fill in the correct answers about glands and the seminal fluid they produce.

(a) There is/are *(one? two?)* seminal vesicle(s) located just *(inferior? posterior?)* to the urinary bladder. *(Fructose? Prostaglandins?)* in seminal vesicle secretions provide energy for sperm, whereas _____ cause cervical mucus to be ideal for sperm passage.

(b) The *(seminal vesicles? prostate?)* is/are responsible for forming about 70% of semen.

(c) The prostate surrounds the urethra just *(inferior? posterior?)* to the urinary bladder. Explain the significance of this location.

_____

_____

(d) One function of the prostate is production of secretions. The *(mucosal? submucosal? main?)* prostatic glands are enlarged in benign prostatic hyperplasia (BPH). The _____ prostatic glands secrete the fluid that contributes to semen. This *(acid? alkaline?)* secretion neutralizes fluid from the vas deferens that is strongly acidic. The pH of semen must be about _____ for sperm to be motile.

(e) A second function of the prostate is based on its _____ tissue, which helps in the process of _____. State one other function of the muscle of the prostate.

_____

_____

A8. Complete this exercise about the penis.

(a) The enlarged end of the penis is known as the *(glans? prepuce? shaft?)*; the foreskin is known as the _____. The foreskin is removed in the surgery known as a

_____.

(b) Bodies composed of erectile tissue are known as _____. The urethra passes through the corpus *(cavernosa? spongiosum?)*.

B. SPERMATOGENESIS AND HORMONAL CONTROL OF MALE REPRODUCTIVE FUNCTION (pages 959–961)

B1. Refer to Figure 42-6 in the textbook and describe hormones that regulate male reproduction.

Anti-müllerian hormone
Estradiol
Follicle-stimulating hormone
Gonadotropin releasing hormone (GnRH)
Inhibin
Luteinizing hormone (LH)
Testosterone

(a) Hormone produced by the hypothalamus that stimulates production of gonadotropins; boys begin making this hormone at about age 10 to 11 years: _____

(b) Gonadotropins made by the anterior pituitary: _____,

_____

(c) Stimulates testes to produce sperm; the same hormone in females stimulates follicle cells to produce eggs: _____

(d) Hormones made by Sertoli cells of testes:

_____, _____,

_____

(e) Also known as interstitial cell-stimulating hormone (ICSH) because it triggers production of testosterone by these cells:

_____

(f) A female reproductive hormone that is required in males for sperm production.

(g) Inhibits production of FSH, which then inhibits spermatogenesis: _____

(h) The major androgen produced in testes; small amounts also produced in the adrenal cortex; can be converted to dihydrotestosterone (DHT) or to estradiol:

_____

(i) Inhibits production of GnRH and LH by a negative feedback effect: _____

B2. Choose the two true statements about sperm production.

(a) Sperm production typically begins at about age 13 years.

(b) Sperm are made by Sertoli cells.

(c) Each human cell that begins the process of spermatogenesis produces **four** cells that each contain 46 chromosomes.

(d) The process of sperm production requires about 6 to 7 days.

B3. Arrange in correct order in the process of sperm formation:

Spermatogonia   Spermatids
Primary   Secondary
   spermatocytes   spermatocytes

_____   _____

_____   _____

(a) Which of these cells are involved in meiosis?

_____, _____

(b) Which cells contain 23 chromosomes?

_____, _____

B4. Describe the function of each of these parts of a sperm.

(a) Acrosome

_____

_____

_____

(b) Tail

_____

_____

_____

(c) Mitochondria

_____

_____

_____

B5. The number of sperm in a normal ejaculate is about *(1 to 4? 100 to 400?)* million. Sperm can live in the female reproductive tract for about 1 to 2 *(hours? days? weeks?)*.

B6. Describe the effects of testosterone at different stages of life:

(a) In embryo

_____

_____

_____

(b) At puberty

_____

_____

_____

(c) Throughout the life of the male

_____

_____

_____

B7. List potentially harmful effects of use of anabolic steroids on skin, reproductive organs, vital organs, blood cholesterol, and personality.

_____

_____

_____

C. NEURAL CONTROL OF SEXUAL FUNCTION AND AGING CHANGES (pages 962–964)

C1. Complete this exercise about male sexual response.

(a) The major source of sexual stimulation for males is:
(1) Psychic stimuli
(2) Sensory stimuli to the glans penis

(b) Erection is due primarily to:
(1) Filling of the penis with blood
(2) Contractions of ischiocavernosus and bulbocavernosus muscles of the penis

In which areas of the penis does blood accumulate during erection? _____

(c) The *(sympathetic? parasympathetic?)* division of the autonomic nervous system is responsible for erection. These nerves travel though *(L1-L2? S2-S4?)* spinal nerves.

(d) The *(sympathetic? parasympathetic?)* division of the autonomic nervous system is responsible for emission and ejaculation. These nerves travel though *(L1-L2? S2-S4?)* spinal nerves.

(e) Nitric oxide released within the penis causes *(contraction? relaxation?)* of smooth muscles in blood vessels, contributing to the *(erect? flaccid?)* state of the penis.

(f) Ischiocavernosus and bulbocavernosus muscles are located *(in the glans? at the base?)* of the penis. What is their function?

_____

_____

C2. Match the correct term to the related description.

Detumescence   Ejaculation   Emission

(a) The state in which the penis attains or maintains a flaccid state: _____

(b) Passage of semen from the epididymides into the urethra: _____

(c) Ejection of semen from the urethra to the outside of the body: _____

C3. Circle the correct answers in statements about male sexual response.

(a) Psychic stimulation such as sexual thoughts *(is? is not?)* required for erection or ejaculation.

(b) The total volume of ejaculate typically is *(2-5? 12-15?)* mL of semen. (Note: 4-5 mL = 1 teaspoon.)

C4. Describe aging changes related to male sexual response.

(a) Define the term andropause.

_____

_____

_____

(b) Contrast the effects of normal aging with those caused by cardiovascular disease or diabetes on the male reproductive system.

_____

_____

_____

(c) Explain the role of self-esteem as it relates to sexual function in older men.

_____

_____

_____

C5. Describe the effects and contraindications of testosterone administration in older men.

_____

_____

_____

CHAPTER 43

Alterations in Structure and Function of the Male Genitourinary System

■ Review Questions

A. DISORDERS OF THE PENIS (pages 965–970)

A1. Circle the correct answers in each statement about disorders of the penis.

(a) In *(epi? hypo?)*spadias, the urethral opening lies on the under (ventral) surface of the penis. This disorder occurs in about 1 in *(300? 30,000? 3 million?)* male infants born each year. Hypospadias is much *(more? less?)* common than epispadias. Surgery for one of these conditions is more likely to be performed at age *(9 months? 5 years?)*.

(b) In phimosis, the foreskin of the penis is so tight that it cannot *(cover? be retracted over?)* the glans? What is paraphimosis?

_____

_____

(c) Which condition is inflammation of the glans and the foreskin? *(Balanitis? Balanoposthitis?)*

A2. Select the name of the disorder that best fits each description.

Balanitis xerotica obliterans   Chordee
Cryptorchidism   Paraphimosis
Peyronie's disease   Phimosis

(a) Undescended testes; more common in infant boys with hypospadias and chordee:

_____

(b) Ventral bowing of the penis:

_____

(c) Stiffening of the fibrous covering around the corpora cavernosa; may cause upward bowing of the penis and pain during intercourse: _____

(d) This condition increases the risk of inflammation of the glans and foreskin:

_____

(e) Atrophy and sclerosis of the glans penis in uncircumcised males; leads to white, patchy areas on the glans and thickened, unretractable foreskin: _____

A3. Choose the two true statements about disorders of the penis.

(a) Most newborns **do not** have a fully retractable foreskin.

(b) The foreskin of all 2-year-old boys **should** be forcibly retracted for thorough cleaning of the area.

(c) Smegma is accumulated mucus from the male urethra.

(d) Balanitis is inflammation of the **glans** of the penis.

A4. Review the autonomic and chemical factors that regulate male sexual response in Chapter 42, Question C1. Now identify the correct summary of factors leading to:

Detumescence   Erection

(a) Parasympathetic nerve impulses that cause release of nitric oxide and the enzyme guanyl cyclase, forming GMP and causing smooth muscle relaxation in cavernous sinuses; compression of veins restricts outflow of blood from the penis:

_____

(b) Sympathetic nerve response causing contraction of cavernous smooth muscle that expels blood from the penis:

_____

A5. Mr. Rathwell is 62 years old, divorced, and has erectile dysfunction (ED) He has been a smoker for 48 years and recently celebrated 4 years of sobriety. His type 1 diabetes mellitus is under poor control. In addition to his oral hypoglycemic, he also takes medications for hypertension, a cholesterol-lowering agent, and an antidepressant.

(a) In which category of ED is Mr. Rathwell's condition classified?

Mixed   Organic   Psychogenic

(b) What factor included in his patient history indicates a neurogenic origin of his disorder? _____

_____

(c) Which factors contribute to decreased vascular flow to his external genitalia?

_____

_____

(d) List any other factors in Mr. Rathwell's history that may contribute to his ED.

_____

_____

(e) Mr. Rathwell has his blood levels of hormones evaluated. Which of his hormone levels are likely to be decreased? _____ and _____

(f) He begins taking Viagra. How does this help patients with ED? _____

_____

A6. Define priapism. _____

_____

(a) State the major concern about the long-term effects of priapism. _____

_____

_____

(*High-flow? Low-flow [stasis]?*) priapism is more likely to lead to ischemia with permanent damage.

(b) Write two or more causes of priapism in each category:
(b1) Primary _____

_____

(b2) Secondary _____

_____

(c) Explain how sickle cell disease can lead to priapism. _____

_____

A7. Complete this exercise about penile cancer by circling or filling in the correct answer.

(a) This condition is most common among (*young? middle-aged?*) men. It is (*highly? rarely?*) curable if diagnosed early. What factor do you think is most likely to hinder early diagnosis? _____

_____

_____

(b) List four risk factors for cancer of the penis.

_____

_____

_____

_____

(c) Penile cancer is more common in (*the United States? other countries?*). It occurs more in men who (*have? have not?*) been circumcised.

(d) The most definitive prognostic indicator for penile cancer is _____.
For men with metastasis to inguinal and iliac nodes, the 5-year survival rate is (*60%–90%? 20%–50%?*).

B. DISORDERS OF THE SCROTUM AND TESTES (pages 970–975)

B1. Zachariah (see Chapter 28, Question C4) was born at 26 weeks of gestation. In addition to his respiratory distress syndrome, he has cryptorchidism of the left testis.

(a) Define this condition.

_____

_____

(b) Cryptorchidism is (*common? rare?*) among premature boys, and relatively (*common? rare?*) in full-term infants. It is typically (*uni? bi?*)lateral.

(c) Spontaneous descent of the testis is more likely to occur in months (*0 to 3? 6 to 9?*) of Zachariah's life.

(d) Contrast a retractable testis with one that is undescended. _____

_____

(e) State three reasons why early diagnosis and treatment of Zachariah's condition are important. _____

_____

_____

(f) Surgical placement and fixation of Zachariah's undescended testis into his scrotal sac is a procedure known as

_____.

B2. Match the condition with the correct description.

Hematocele   Hydrocele
Spermatocele   Varicocele

(a) Accumulation of blood around the testes:

_____

(b) Accumulation of fluid within the tunica vaginalis around the testes:

_____

(c) Varicose veins of the testes:

_____

(d) Sperm-containing cyst at the end of the epididymis; rarely causes problems:

_____

B3. Choose the three true statements.

(a) Most hydroceles of infancy **do** resolve spontaneously before the age of 1 year.

(b) A dense hydrocele that does not transilluminate is **more** likely to be cancerous than a soft mass that does illuminate.

(c) In adults, hydroceles typically **do** require treatment.

(d) Incidence of varicoceles is greatest **after** age 60 years.

(e) Varicocele is more likely to occur on the **right** side than on the **left**.

(f) "Heaviness" of the scrotum is a sign of **both** hydrocele and varicocele.

B4. List four or more causes of hydrocele.

_____

_____

_____

_____

B5. Discuss each of these phrases related to hydrocele.

(a) "Bag of worms"

_____

_____

(b) Valsalva's maneuver with a Doppler stethoscope placed over the scrotum

_____

_____

(c) Examination in standing and recumbent positions _____

_____

B6. Describe testicular torsion in this exercise by circling or filling in the correct answers.

(a) This condition involves twisting of the spermatic cord; this structure includes

_____

_____

(b) Extravaginal testicular torsion occurs more often in _(neonates? boys 8 to 18 years?)._

(c) _(Extra? Intra?)_vaginal testicular torsion is a true surgical emergency in which patients are in acute distress; the condition _(can? does not?)_ lead to destruction of the involved testis.

B7. Claude, age 20 years, has epididymitis. Discuss his condition in this exercise.

(a) Describe the location and functions of the two epididymides. _____

_____

(b) Claude's epididymitis is caused by _Chlamydia trachomatis._ Name another sexually transmitted disease (STD) that commonly leads to epididymitis: _____. Identify the population most likely to experience this form of epididymitis. _____

(c) Explain how urethritis or prostatitis could spread to cause epididymitis.

_____

_____

(d) State two other sources of infection that can cause epididymitis._____

_____

(e) Claude's infection was typical in that it led to pain and swelling by 1 or 2 _(hours? days? weeks?)_ after onset of epididymitis. His fever and painful urination are _(common? rare?)_ signs. Is he likely to have a urethral discharge? _____

(f) _(Bed rest? Exercise?)_ is likely to be recommended for Claude. Explain why his scrotum is elevated on a pillow or rolled towel as he rests. _____

_____

Name three "A" types of medications that he will receive: _____, _____, _____. During this recovery period, sexual activity is _(encouraged? discouraged?)._

(g) Claude's condition spreads to cause orchitis, which is an infection of _____.

B8. What childhood infection is most likely to lead to orchitis? _____

(a) Compare and contrast signs and symptoms of orchitis with those of epididymitis.

_____

_____

(b) What percentage of bilateral orchitis cases caused by mumps result in sterility? _____

B9. Discuss neoplasms of the scrotum or testes in this exercise by circling or filling in the correct answers.

(a) *(Scrotal? Testicular?)* carcinoma is more common.

(b) Explain what is distinctive about scrotal cancer in the history of medicine.

_____

_____

In addition to exposure to these occupational carcinogens, what other factors can lead to scrotal cancer? _____

_____

(c) Testicular cancer is the leading cause of cancer in males ages *(15 to 34? 35 to 55?)* years old. If diagnosed early, it *(is? is not?)* highly curable.

(d) Name the disorder that has the strongest association with cancer of the testes: _____. Seminomas are testicular tumors that develop from _____ tubules, and these develop most commonly in *(children? men in their 20s? men in their 30s?)*. Seminomas are *(highly? rarely?)* curable tumors.

(e) Which is the most common first sign of testicular cancer?

   (1) Slight enlargement of the testis with feeling of heaviness with or without pain

   (2) Swelling of legs and back pain

   (3) Cough and blood in sputum (hemoptysis)

(f) To detect testicular cancer early, how often is testicular self-examination recommended? _____. This self-exam should take place while *(in a warm shower? lying in bed?)*.

(g) Stage I and II testicular tumors are associated with a ____ % survival rate. A stage *(I? II? III?)* testicular cancer involves metastasis above the diaphragm, for example, to lungs. Circle the tumor markers used to evaluate testicular cancer.

Alpha-fetoprotein   Alkaline phosphatase
Human chorionic   Lactic dehydrogenase
   gonadotropin   Prostate serum antigen

(h) Treatment of *(some? all?)* testicular cancers involves surgical removal of the affected testis, a procedure known as an _____. Such surgery *(is? is not?)* likely to affect fertility and sexual function.

C. DISORDERS OF THE PROSTATE (pages 976–981)

C1. Contrast types of prostatitis in this exercise.

Acute bacterial prostatitis
Chronic bacterial prostatitis
Chronic prostatitis/chronic pelvic pain syndrome

(a) Mr. Harrell has a prostate condition that is not contagious; urine cultures reveal no bacteria in urine; he has the form in which prostatic fluid shows evidence of leukocytes, a sign of inflammation: _____

(b) Mr. Tomlinson presents with dull, aching pain in the perineal area, frequent and urgent urination of cloudy and malodorous urine, fever and chills; most commonly caused by *E. coli*; treatment includes antibiotic therapy for up to 4 weeks:

_____

(c) Rev. Peter has recurrent urinary tract infections (UTIs) with *Pseudomonas*. Like Mr. Tomlinson, he has frequent and urgent urination and perineal discomfort; his condition is more difficult to treat than acute bacterial prostatitis because antibiotics do not readily penetrate his chronically inflamed prostate: _____

_____

C2. Circle the two urine specimens that are most likely to identify chronic bacterial prostatitis.

(a) First part of the voided stream

(b) Midstream specimen

(c) Specimen obtained by prostatic massage

(d) Specimen obtained after prostatic massage

C3. Choose the two true statements related to benign prostatic hyperplasia (BPH).

(a) The prostate gland lies **posterior** to the urinary bladder.

(b) BPH typically affects the **outer** regions of the prostate gland.

(c) This condition affects at least **half** of men older than 75 years of age.

(d) In the prostate gland, almost all testosterone is normally converted to dihydroxytestosterone.

(e) The enzyme *5a*-reductase is likely to **improve** BPH.

C4. Circle risk factors for BPH.

African American descent
High levels of dihydroxytestosterone
Family history of BPH
Japanese descent
Older men

C5. Discuss manifestations and diagnoses of BPH in this exercise.

(a) State the major clinically significant effect of BPH. _____
_____

(b) Now list three or more significant sequelae of BPH. _____
_____
_____

(c) Explain the diagnostic information indicated by these clinical findings:

(c1) Presence of bacteria and leukocytes in urine _____

(c2) Smooth, rubbery, enlarged prostate palpated by digital rectal examination
_____

(c3) Normal PSA _____

(c4) Residual urine volume of 180 mL detected by postvoiding catheterization_____

(c5) Flow rate of 8 mL/second indicated by uroflowmetry_____

(c6) Serum creatinine level of 2.5 mg/100 mL _____

C6. American Urological Survey Symptom Index scores in the range of 12 to 18 indicate *(mild? moderate? severe?)* BPH.

C7. Discuss treatments for BPH in this exercise.

(a) Prostatectomy surgery *(is? is not?)* currently the primary treatment for BPH. What is the meaning of the acronym TURP?
T _____
U _____
R _____
of the P_____.

List several possible complications of a TURP.
_____
_____
_____

(b) Describe the effect of a TURP.
_____
_____

(c) Mr. Davidson, age 89 years, has congestive heart failure (CHF) and advanced emphysema. How can a stent help his BPH?
_____
_____
_____

C8. Choose the two true statements about prostate cancer

(a) This form of cancer is **rare** in the United States.

(b) More than 80% of all prostate cancers are diagnosed in men **older than** 65 years.

(c) Incidence of prostate cancer is **greater** in men with a family history and also with high dietary fat content.

(d) Prostate cancer typically presents with symptoms **early** in the course of the disease.

C9. Explain what the following signs or symptoms suggest in patients with prostate cancer.

(a) Voiding pattern similar to that of BPH
_____
_____

(b) Dyspnea (shortness of breath)
_____
_____

(c) Low back pain and pathological fracture of a lumbar vertebra_____
_____

C10. List three methods of screening for prostate cancer.
_____
_____
_____

C11. Mr. van den Ende, age 51 years, has been in apparently good health but recently was diagnosed with prostate cancer that is Grade 4, and staged T3, N1 and M1. The grading indicates that his tumor is *(highly? poorly?)* differentiated. What do his TNM values indicate? _____ Given his age and otherwise good health, what treatment is likely? _____

CHAPTER 44

Structure and Function of the Female Reproductive System

■ Review Questions

A. STRUCTURE OF THE FEMALE REPRODUCTIVE SYSTEM (pages 983–987)

A1. Arrange these female external genitalia from anterior to posterior in location.

Anus   Clitoris
Perineal body   Urinary meatus
Vaginal orifice

_____, _____, _____,
_____, _____

A2. Match the structure to the related description.

Clitoris   Introitus
Labia majora   Labia minora
Mons pubis   Urinary meatus
Vaginal orifice   Vestibule

(a) Vaginal opening; may be surrounded by hymen: _____

(b) Prepuce is the "hood" of this structure:
_____

(c) Surrounded by Skene's glands: _____

(d) Most common site of pubic lice infestation in females: _____

(e) Located between labia minora; site of urethral and vaginal openings: _____
_____

(f) Structures that are developmentally analogous to the male scrotum:
_____ and _____

A3. Choose the two true statements about internal genitalia.

(a) The vaginal lining contains **no** sensory receptors.

(b) Fornices refer to the **uterine cervix.**

(c) Vascular tissue within labia minora becomes **engorged** during sexual excitement.

(d) An intact hymen **does** indicate virginity.

A4. Complete this exercise about vaginal pH.

(a) Vaginal pH is normally about *(4? 6? 8?).* Explain what accounts for this pH.
_____
_____

(b) How is this pH helpful? _____

(c) List three factors that can alter vaginal pH.
_____
_____
_____

A5. Describe the uterus in this exercise.

(a) Arrange parts of the uterus from most superior to most inferior in location:

Body   Cervix   Fundus
_____, _____, _____

(b) Arrange from most posterior to most anterior in location:

Bladder   Rectum   Uterus
_____, _____, _____

(c) Which is more anterior in location?
(1) Pouch of Douglas
(2) Vesicouterine pouch

(d) Which is a sheetlike ligament that attaches the uterus laterally to the sides of the pelvis?
(1) Broad
(2) Cardinal
(3) Round
(4) Uterosacral

(e) Arrange layers of the uterine wall from most deep to most superficial:

Endometrium   Myometrium
Perimetrium
_____, _____, _____

(f) Which layer of the uterus is the thickest? _____metrium. Explain the relationship between this layer and dysmenorrhea. _____
_____
_____

A6. Select the female reproductive organ that fits each description.

Fallopian tubes   Ovaries   Uterus

(a) Fingerlike fimbriae draw in ova:

_____

(b) Part of the lining is shed as menses:

_____

(c) Usual site where fertilization occurs:

_____

(d) Sites where ova and the hormones estrogens and progesterone are produced:

_____

B. THE MENSTRUAL CYCLE (pages 987–993)

B1. Choose the two true statements about the menstrual cycle.

(a) **Ovaries** are primarily responsible for changes within the menstrual cycle.

(b) Menarche refers to the **first** menstrual bleeding.

(c) For a woman to menstruate, it **is** necessary for her to ovulate.

(d) The average length of the female menstrual cycle is 38 days.

B2. Ability to maintain a regular menstrual cycle *(is? is not?)* related to body fat.
Explain._____

_____

Circle women who are likely to experience amenorrhea.

(a) Karen, age 20, who is 5′6″ tall, weighs 95 lbs, and has a diagnosis of anorexia

(b) Eileen, age 30, who weighs 340 lbs

(c) Sandra, who runs 70 miles a week

(d) Geraldine, age 38, with end-stage cancer

B3. Indicate where each hormone related to female reproduction is made.

Estrogen
Follicle-stimulating hormone
Gonadotropin-releasing hormone
Luteinizing hormone
Prolactin
Progesterone

(a) Hypothalamus: _____

(b) Anterior pituitary: _____,

_____, _____

(c) Ovaries: _____, _____

B4. Which hormones listed in Question B3 are gonadotropic?

_____

B5. Circle the two true statements about female reproductive hormones.

(a) During pregnancy, estrogens, progesterone, insulin, and cortisol **all** help to prepare breasts for lactation.

(b) Dopamine **inhibits** production of prolactin.

(c) ER_1 receptors **increase** the action of estrogens.

(d) The most abundant and potent form of estrogen is **estriol** (E3).

B6. Circle the actions of estrogens.

(a) Antioxidant effects

(b) Increase blood levels of the "good cholesterol" (HDLs)

(c) Increase risk of osteoporosis

(d) Help to maintain memory by promoting cerebral blood flow

(e) Cause retention of Na^+ and H_2O

(f) Stimulate development of reproductive organs in the developing embryo and fetus

(g) Stimulate glandular development of breasts at puberty

(h) Stimulate development of pubic hair and other secondary sexual characteristics

B7. Explain how progesterone is "pro gestation."

_____

B8. Women normally *(do? do not?)* produce androgens. Where are these made?

_____

B9. Arrange in correct sequence the events in the ovarian cycle.

Corpus albicans, a white scar on the ovary, formed postovulation (CA)
Corpus luteum formed postovulation (CL)
A surge of LH triggers ovulation of the oocyte with its corona radiata (LH)
One dominant follicle (ODF)
Primary follicle develops under FSH stimulation (PF)
Secondary follicles (6 to 12) develop (SF)

_____ → _____ → _____ → _____ →

_____ → _____

B10. Describe these terms related to the female reproductive cycle.

(a) "Mittelschmerz" refers to a pain that may accompany *(menstruation? ovulation?)*.

(b) HCG is a hormone that maintains the *(follicle? corpus luteum?)*. Presence of this hormone in a woman's blood or urine indicates that she is *(ovulating? pregnant?)*.

(c) During menstruation, part of the *(basal? functional?)* layer of the endometrium sloughs off.

(d) *(Estrogen? Progesterone?)* increases cervical mucus production and causes the mucus to be *(thin? viscous?)* and more conducive to passage of sperm.

(e) "Spinnbarkeit" refers to _____ of cervical mucus. "Ferning" refers to the pattern that this mucus takes when it *(is moist? dries?)*. The absence of ferning is an indicator of low *(estrogen? progesterone?)* levels.

B11. Complete this exercise about Ms. Grayling, who is age 51 years old.

(a) Ms. Grayling has experienced menstrual irregularity for 3 years; her last menstrual period was 4 months ago. She is said to be _____ menopausal.

(b) Her estrogen levels are likely to be *(zero? diminished?)*. Explain.

_____
_____

(c) Ms. Grayling experiences "vasomotor instability," commonly manifested as

_____.

(d) She has some sleep deprivation. Explain.

_____
_____

(e) She is at *(increased? decreased?)* risk for osteoporosis. Explain. _____

_____
_____

(f) Hormone replacement therapy (HRT) includes doses of *(estrogen only? progesterone only? both estrogen and progesterone?)*. Explain why the inclusion of progesterone is important.

_____
_____

(g) List several positive effects of HRT.

_____
_____

(h) Describe concerns about estrogen replacement. _____

_____
_____

C. BREASTS (pages 993–994)

C1. Select the term that fits the related description.

Alveoli   Areolar tissue
Cooper's ligaments   Lobules
Nipple

(a) Milk-producing glandular cells located in grapelike clusters within lobes of breast:

_____

(b) Fibrous tissue in spoke-like arrangement that supports breasts: _____

(c) Smooth area surrounding the nipple; darkens at puberty and during pregnancy; contains Montgomery's tubercles:

_____

C2. Identify the hormones involved in breast development and function.

Estrogen
Follicle-stimulating hormone (FSH)
Luteinizing hormone (LH)
Oxytocin
Prolactin
Progesterone

(a) Hormone most directly responsible for growth of alveolar epithelium at puberty and during pregnancy; may be protective against breast cancer: _____

(b) Ovarian hormone most directly responsible for growth of ducts of breasts: _____

(c) Pituitary hormones that stimulate release of estrogen from ovaries at puberty:

_____, _____, _____

(d) Released in response to suckling of an infant, causes ejection of milk from glands into ducts: _____

C3. Circle the tissue most involved in postmenopausal loss of breast size (atrophy).

Adipose (fat)   Alveolar (gland)
Connective   Ductile

CHAPTER 45

Alterations in Structure and Function of the Female Reproductive System

■ Review Questions

A. DISORDERS OF THE EXTERNAL GENITALIA AND VAGINA (pages 997–1001)

A1. The vulva consists of *(external? internal?)* female genitalia. Inflammation of the vulva *(does? does not?)* typically involve itching. The most common cause of vulvitis is infection with the microbe _____. List three or more other causes of vulvitis.

_____

_____

_____

A2. Select the condition that fits each description.

Bartholin's cyst   Cyclic vulvovaginitis
Nevi   Vulvodynia
Vulvar dystrophy

(a) Syndrome of vulvar pain sufficient to interfere with daily activities: _____

(b) Episodes of vulvodynia that coincide only with premenstrual phase or after sexual activity: _____

(c) Moles; should be observed for changes that could indicate carcinoma: _____

(d) Fluid-filled sac lateral to the vagina that can reach the size of an orange: _____

(e) Parchment-thin, white lesions of lichen sclerosus are examples of this disorder; treated by topical testosterone or corticosteroids: _____

A3. Choose the two true statements about vulvar lesions in this exercise.

(a) The risk for invasive vulvar carcinoma is **greater** in women in their 30s than for women in their 60s.

(b) Vulvar intraepithelial neoplasia (VIN) is a diagnosis that **means** vulvar cancer.

(c) Human papilloma virus (HPV) infection **increases** risk for VIN and cancer of the vulva.

(d) The 5-year survival rate for vulvar cancer lesions less than an inch in diameter is at least 90%.

A4. Complete this exercise about vaginal disorders.

(a) Doderlein's bacteria are *(pathogens? normal flora?)* of the vagina. They break down *(glycogen? proteins?)* in the lining of the vagina. Products of this breakdown normally cause the vaginal lining to have a pH of about *(4.5? 7.0? 9.5?)*.

(b) Postmenopausal women are likely to have a(n) *(decreased? increased?)* number of Doderlein's bacteria and a more *(acidic? alkaline?)* vaginal pH. This environment *(decreases? increases?)* risk of vaginal infections. Describe two primary preventions to help avoid vaginal infections.

_____

_____

A5. Sally, age 27 years, is recovering from 3 weeks of bronchitis for which she took antibiotics. She is highly stressed as semester exams approach. Answer these questions about her.

(a) Sally has been producing a malodorous vaginal discharge; her vagina is red, burning, and itching. Are these simply normal changes within the menstrual cycle?

_____

(b) The nurse practitioner places a sample of Sally's vaginal mucus on a slide, adds KOH, and identifies "hyphae and buds." Name the likely microbe causing Sally's infection.

_____

(c) How does this diagnosis relate to Sally's recent history?

_____

_____

A6. List several health practices that can reduce the incidence of vulvar and vaginal irritation or infection.

_____

_____

_____

A7. Complete this exercise about vaginal cancer.

(a) This form of cancer is *(common? rare?)*, and occurs mostly in women aged ___ years or older. Write two causes of vaginal cancer in women about 35 years of age.

_____

_____

(b) DES (diethylstilbestrol) was taken by women *(for nausea? to prevent miscarriage?)* primarily during the years *(1940–1971? 1972–2002?)*. Daughters of these women have a greatly increased risk for *(benign? malignant?)* extension of cervical tissue into the vagina, which predisposes to cancer.

(c) The most common sign of cancer of the vagina is _____.

(d) List four types of treatment that may be used depending on the nature of the malignancy._____

_____

_____

_____

(e) How can sexual intercourse be possible for a woman with surgical removal of vaginal cancer? _____

_____

_____

B. DISORDERS OF THE CERVIX AND UTERUS (pages 1002-1008)

B1. Refer to text Figure 45-2 and discuss disorders of the cervix of the uterus in this exercise.

(a) The cervix is normally lined with ___ epithelium, whereas the vagina is lined with ___ epithelium. Label these regions A and B on the left side of the text figure.

(1) Simple columnar

(2) Stratified squamous

(b) Which of these tissues undergoes a change to form the other? Some of *(A becomes B? B becomes A?)*. The region where such change occurs is known as the _____ zone.

(c) This change results in *(dysplasia? metaplasia?)*, which means growth of tissue that is *(abnormal? normal for the body but not for this region?)*. Such change *(can? cannot?)* lead to dysplasia and neoplasia (such as cancer).

(d) List factors that can increase such transformation. _____

_____

_____

(e) _____ cysts may develop in the transformed tissue. Are these malignant?

_____

B2. Contrast acute (A) and chronic (C) cervicitis.

(a) Often results from minute tears in the cervix that develop during childbirth: ____

(b) Most commonly caused by *Chlamydia trachomatis* infection: ____

(c) The cervix becomes red and edematous with large amounts of white mucopurulent discharge: _____

B3. Karla, age 30 years, has received a diagnosis of cervical intraepithelial neoplasia (CIN) grade II.

(a) It is likely this condition has been developing for *(days? weeks? years?)*. Explain._____

_____

_____

(b) Karla's cervical tissue is classified as *(mild? moderate? severe?)* dysplasia (see Table 45-1). Her epithelial cells are likely to be graded as *(ASCUS? HSIL? LSIL? SCC?)*, which means the tissue *(has? has not?)* progressed to cervical cancer by this time (see Table 45-3).

(c) Because the abnormal cells have not spread beyond her cervix, Karla's neoplasm is considered to be stage *(I? II? III?)*. The 5-year survival rate associated with Karla's cancer is likely to be approximately *(50%? 70%? 90%?)*.

(d) Defend or dispute this statement, "Cervical cancer is a sexually transmitted disease."

_____

_____

(e) List several other risk factors for cervical cancer. _____

_____

_____

(f) The incidence of cervical cancer has *(decreased? increased?)* in the last half century, largely related to early diagnosis. Explain._____

_____

_____

(g) Karla's gynecologist performs loop electrode excision procedure (LEEP) because Karla's lesions are of a "SIL grade." This procedure is *(more? less?)* invasive than cone biopsy.

B4. Emily, age 27 years, has received a diagnosis of endometriosis.

(a) Circle the factors that increased Emily's risk for this condition.

   (1) She started menstrual periods at age 16 years.

   (2) Her periods have been heavy with intense cramping.

   (3) Her mother and older sister both have endometriosis.

   (4) Her age

(b) Emily has "chocolate cysts." Describe these in terms of location, composition, and possible complications.

_____

_____

(c) List two possible mechanisms by which endometrial tissue reached Emily's ovaries.

_____

_____

(d) Why does this tissue continue to grow?

_____

_____

(e) In addition to her dysmenorrhea, what other symptoms are likely for Emily?

_____

_____

(f) The definitive diagnostic method for endometriosis is _____. The most definitive treatment is _____. Incidence of recurrence after surgery is *(high? low?)*.

B5. Match each uterine disorder with the correct description.

Adenomyosis   Endometritis
Endometriosis   Leiomyoma

(a) "Fibroids" that grow within the myometrium; the most common form of pelvic tumor; often asymptomatic; typically do not interfere with pregnancy:

_____

(b) Endometrial tissue is present within the myometrium; likely to occur in middle-aged, multiparous women and resolve with menopause: _____

(c) Infection of the endometrial lining with a variable clinical picture but often marked by a foul-smelling vaginal discharge:

_____

(d) Presence of endometrium in ectopic sites usually within the pelvic cavity; likely to occur in young women who are infertile or who have chronic pelvic pain:

_____

B6. Circle correct answers about endometrial cancer.

(a) Endometrial cancer is much *(more? less?)* common than cervical cancer. It almost always occurs in women *(younger than? older than?)* 40 years of age.

(b) Circle risk factors for endometrial cancer:

   (1) Obesity

   (2) Hormone replacement therapy that combines estrogen and progesterone

   (3) Tamoxifen therapy for breast cancer

   (4) Diabetes mellitus

   (5) Hypertension

(c) Circle typical early manifestations of endometrial cancer:

   (1) Vaginal bleeding between menstrual periods in a 40-year-old woman

   (2) Vaginal bleeding in a 65-year-old woman

   (3) Pain that accompanies abnormal bleeding

   (4) Enlarged inguinal lymph nodes

(d) Circle the most definitive tool for diagnosing this type of cancer:

   (1) Papanicolaou smear

   (2) Biopsy

   (3) Transvaginal ultrasonography

   (4) Dilation and curettage (D & C)

(e) With early diagnosis and treatment, the 5-year survival rate is *(20%? 50%? 90%?)*.

C. DISORDERS OF THE FALLOPIAN TUBES AND OVARIES (pages 1008–1013)

C1. Discuss pelvic inflammatory disease (PID) in this exercise.

(a) List the three major organs most involved in PID. Then add the names of inflammations of these organs. _____,

_____, _____

(b) Name the two microbes that most often cause PID. _____, _____ What is the origin of these microbes? _____

_____

(c) Circle risk factors for PID.

(1) Age 25 to 35 years

(2) Married, multiparous woman

(3) Previous history of PID

(4) History of multiple sex partners

(5) Use of an intrauterine device (IUD)

(d) What signs or symptoms of PID distinguish this condition from other pelvic disorders?

_____

_____

In addition, white blood cell count and erythrocyte sedimentation rate both *(decrease? increase?)*. Because this is a widespread infection, fever *(is? is not?)* likely to occur.

(e) Name two categories of medications typically administered to clients for pain associated with PID. _____

_____

C2. Elizabeth, age 40 years, is being examined for a possible ectopic pregnancy.

(a) Name the most common site of an ectopic pregnancy. _____

(b) Circle the factors in Elizabeth's history that increase her risk for ectopic pregnancy.

(1) She has been on infertility drugs during the course of 2 years.

(2) The lumen of her fallopian tubes is narrowed by PID.

(3) She had an ectopic pregnancy 14 months ago.

(c) Elizabeth reports "a little spotting for the last few days," and "a kind of uncomfortable belly for about the last week-but unbearable pain since last night." List several other disorders that would need to be ruled out in diagnosing ectopic

pregnancy. _____

_____

(d) A pregnancy test reveals that Elizabeth is pregnant. It is likely that her human chorionic gonadotropin (HCG) level (used in the home pregnancy test) will be *(higher? lower?)* than expected for her stage of pregnancy, which she thinks is almost 6 weeks.

(e) It is determined that Elizabeth's tubal pregnancy has ruptured. Explain why the tube is ruptured.

_____

_____

(f) A *(salpingectomy? salpingostomy?)* is likely to be performed. Elizabeth *(is? is not?)* likely to be prescribed a regimen of methotrexate for about a week. Explain. _____

_____

C3. Choose the three true statements.

(a) Cancer of the fallopian tube is a **common** malignancy of female reproductive organs.

(b) Polycystic ovarian cysts are **rare forms** of ovarian tumors.

(c) Women with polycystic ovary syndrome (PCOS) are likely to experience a **low** blood level of follicle-stimulating hormone (FSH) and **high** level of androgens.

(d) Weight loss in obese women has been found to **increase** ovulation in women with PCOS.

(e) Dermoid cysts are **malignant** ovarian tumors.

(f) Androgen-secreting ovarian cysts are likely to **increase** growth of **hair** in women.

C4. Complete this exercise about ovarian cancer.

(a) Circle women at increased risk for this type of cancer:

(1) Stacy is 27 years old.

(2) Tanya's mother died of ovarian cancer.

(3) Joan's father has colorectal cancer.

(4) Yvonne has given birth to five children.

(5) Patrice has used oral contraceptives for 8 years.

(6) Molly eats a low-fat diet.

(b) Ovarian cancer is *(frequently? rarely?)* fatal. It usually is diagnosed *(before? after?)* metastasis because early symptoms are *(severe? vague?)*. Which system most commonly manifests early symptoms?

_____

(c) There *(are? are no?)* definitive screening tests for ovarian cancer. Name a serum marker that can identify most women with stage II or higher ovarian cancer: _____. These women are more likely to have surgery followed by *(chemotherapy? radiation?)*. Overall, the 5-year survival rate is approximately *(50%? 90%?)* for ovarian cancer.

D. DISORDERS OF PELVIC SUPPORT AND UTERINE POSITION (pages 1013-1016)

D1. Describe supportive structures of the pelvis and uterus in this exercise.

(a) Which ligaments secure the cervix laterally to the pelvis to help prevent uterine prolapse?

(1) Round

(2) Broad

(3) Cardinal

(4) Uterosacral

(b) Which structure provides the most support for pelvic viscera?

(1) Pelvic diaphragm

(2) Bony pelvis

(3) Peritoneum

(c) List several factors that lead to relaxation of pelvic support structures.

_____

_____

(d) Which condition involves sagging of the urinary bladder into the anterior wall of the vagina?

(1) Rectocele

(2) Uterine prolapse

(3) Cystocele

(4) Enterocele

(e) Evelyn's cervix has prolapsed so that it protrudes outside of her vaginal opening. This is a _____-degree uterine prolapse.

(1) First

(2) Second

(3) Third

(f) The most common variation in uterine position is:

(1) Acute anteflexion

(2) Retroflexion

(3) Simple retroversion

D2. Describe treatments for pelvic support disorders.

(a) Nonsurgical _____

_____

(b) Surgical _____

_____

E. MENSTRUAL DISORDERS (pages 1016–1019)

E1. Identify the type of dysfunctional menstrual cycle in each case.

Amenorrhea   Hypomenorrhea
Menorrhagia   Metrorrhagia
Oligomenorrhea

(a) Bleeding between periods: _____

(b) Excessive menstruation: _____

(c) Absence of menstruation: _____

(d) Periods more than 35 days apart:

_____

E2. Complete this exercise about abnormal menstrual cycles.

(a) Estrogen inadequacy causes a *(thinner? thicker?)* than normal endometrium.

(b) Estrogen without progesterone leads to a *(thinner? thicker?)* than normal endometrium. Progesterone is reduced when a follicle *(does? fails to?)* mature, ovulate, and form a corpus luteum.

(c) *(High? Low?)* levels of both estrogen and progesterone lead to anovulatory bleeding with *(light? heavy?)* flow that *(is? is not?)* typically accompanied by cramps. List two populations of women likely to experience such cycles. _____

_____

(d) List two components of a minimal evaluation of menstrual cycle disorders.

_____

_____

(e) Indicate whether each of the following causes of amenorrhea is primary (P) or secondary (S).

(e1) Juliette, age 25 years, runs 6 to 10 miles a day and has a diagnosis of bulimia; she has not had a period since she was 21. ___

(e2) Roberta, age 18, has never menstruated. ___

E3. Menstruation with cramping and possibly diarrhea and headache is known as _____-menorrhea. Severe dysmenorrhea caused by endometriosis or pelvic adhesions is classified as primary (P) or secondary (S)?

E4. Choose the three true statements related to premenstrual syndrome (PMS).

(a) Premenstrual syndrome (PMS) **is** a psychosomatic disorder.

(b) The incidence of PMS is greatest among women in their **early 20s.**

(c) The cause of PMS is **estrogen deficiency.**

(d) Fluid retention, headache, and swollen breasts are **typical** manifestations of PMS.

(e) PMS usually is relieved by **menstruation.**

(f) Premenstrual dysphoric disorder is a **psychiatric** diagnosis in which symptoms are **not** relieved by onset of menses.

E5. Describe an integrated treatment approach for PMS.

_____

_____

_____

F. DISORDERS OF THE BREAST (pages 1019-1022)

F1. Match each breast disorder with the related description.

Ductal ectasia   Fibroadenoma
Fibrocystic disease   Galactorrhea
Mastitis

(a) Inflammation of the breast starting with nipple irritation, infection, or hormonal changes: _____

(b) Condition with gray-green discharge from nipples; occurs in older women:

_____

(c) Milk secretion in nonlactating breasts of women or men: _____

(d) Single, firm, movable breast mass that usually is painless; incidence greatest in premenopausal women: _____

(e) The most common breast lesion, in as many as four of five women, especially those 30 to 50 years: _____

F2. Describe fibrocystic disease in this exercise.

(a) Discomfort that accompanies fibrocystic disease typically occurs within the *(first? second?)* half of the menstrual cycle.

(b) A *(biopsy? mammogram?)* is more likely to provide information needed for diagnosis of fibrocystic disease.

(c) Coffee, tea, cola, and chocolate should be *(increased? avoided?)* by women with fibrocystic disease. Explain. _____

_____

_____

F3. Mrs. Cappel, age 34 years, with a history of normal menstrual cycles, has received a diagnosis of breast cancer. Complete this exercise about her.

(a) Mrs. Cappel's cancer is a *(common? rare?)* form of female cancer. One in *(8? 80? 800?)* women is likely to develop breast cancer in her lifetime. The incidence of breast cancer has *(decreased? increased?)* within the last 25 years. Explain. _____

_____

_____

(b) Circle Mrs. Cappel's risk factors for breast cancer:

(1) Her age

(2) Onset of menarche at age 11

(3) Mrs. Cappel gave birth to her first child 12 years ago.

(4) Both her mother and her older sister have breast cancer.

(5) She has the BRCA1 mutation on chromosome 17.

(c) Based on her BRCA1 gene, Mrs. Cappel's risk for breast cancer is increased by _____ percent.

(d) Which will serve as a better indicator of Mrs. Cappel's diagnosis of breast cancer?

(1) Size of her tumor

(2) Degree of metastasis to lymph nodes

F4. List the three diagnostic methods that can best diagnose breast cancer.

_____

_____

_____

(a) Mammography can identify lesions as small as _____, whereas palpation (breast self-examination [BSE]) can identify tumors as small as _____. Palpated malignancies typically are found to be *(painful? painless?)*.

(b) In what part of her monthly cycle should Mrs. Cappel perform BSE?

_____

_____

(c) List several other diagnostic methods for identifying and evaluating breast cancer tumors. _____

_____

_____

F5. Circle the true statements about treatment for breast cancer.

(a) Radical mastectomy is **no longer** used as surgical therapy for most breast cancers.

(b) Prognosis depends **more** on the size of the breast tumor than on nodal involvement.

(c) A sentinel node refers to the **farthest** node that cancer cells are likely to reach.

(d) Tamoxifen **blocks** estrogen receptors, so it is likely to **decrease** growth of breast cancers that are estrogen receptor-positive.

(e) The 5-year survival rate for localized cancers is 21%.

(f) Paget's disease, which usually affects **bone** tissue, is a **rare** form of breast cancer.

G. INFERTILITY (pages 1023–1027)

G1. Fill in the blanks in this exercise about infertility.

(a) Infertility is defined as the inability of a couple to conceive a child after _____ of unprotected sex. About ____% of U.S. couples are affected by infertility. About ____% of U.S. couples are sterile.

(b) _____ infertility occurs in couples who have difficulty conceiving another child after one or more previous pregnancies.

(c) Causes of infertility include about _____% related to male factors, _____% based on female factors, and _____ % related to combined factors.

G2. Mr. Peterson is being evaluated for infertility.

(a) Circle all values that indicate that Mr. Peterson is likely to be infertile.

(1) Sperm density: 5 million mL

(2) Sperm morphology: 75% normal

(3) Motility: 30%

(4) 5 mL semen per ejaculation

(b) Given Mr. Peterson's clinical values (in G2[a]), which conditions does he appear to have?

(1) Asthenospermia

(2) Azoospermia

(3) Oligospermia

(c) List several causes of male infertility.

_____

_____

G3. Circle the structures, chemicals, or other factors that are listed with correct descriptions.

(a) Dominant follicle: normally reaches a diameter of approximately 1.5 to 2 cm

(b) Estradiol: an estrogen that is responsible for the luteinizing hormone (LH) surge that triggers ovulation

(c) FSH: converts follicle into corpus luteum

(d) Corpus luteum: produces both progesterone and estradiol

(e) Estradiol: causes the endometrium to become secretory

(f) Progesterone: causes rise in basal body temperature (BBT)

(g) Rise in BBT: basis of a pregnancy test

(h) Luteal phase of the menstrual cycle: should be 7 days long

(i) HCG: supports corpus luteal production of hormones during early months of pregnancy and is the basis of home pregnancy tests

G4. Circle the chemicals that can help a woman develop cervical mucus that is ideal for sperm penetration.

(a) Clomiphene citrate

(b) Cough medicines that are mucolytic

(c) Estradiol

G5. Explain why the following factors may lead to the inability of a woman to carry a baby to term.

(a) PID_____

_____

_____

(b) Endometriosis_____

_____

G6. Match the procedure or chemical used to enhance fertility to the correct description:

Assisted hatching   Clomiphene citrate
Gamete intrafallopian   Human chorionic
  transfer   gonadotropin
Partial zona dissection   Tubal embryo
Zygote intrafallopian   transplant
  transfer

(a) Sperm and ovum are placed directly into a fallopian tube by laparoscopy:

_____

(b) The zygote is placed directly into a fallopian tube laparoscopically: _____

(c) An embryo is placed directly into a fallopian tube laparoscopically: _____

(d) Stimulates production of a large number of follicles: _____

(e) Stimulates an LH surge to cause ovulation of multiple ova from many mature follicles:

_____

(f) Creation of small opening in the layer around the egg so that sperm can penetrate:

_____

(g) A procedure that helps the fertilized ovum escape from the zona pellucida:

_____

CHAPTER 46

Sexually Transmitted Diseases

■ Review Questions

A. INFECTIONS OF THE EXTERNAL GENITALIA (pages 1029–1034)

A1. Choose the two true statements about sexually transmitted diseases (STDs).

(a) STDs are **more** common in persons who have more than one sexual partner.

(b) It **is** possible for a person to be infected with more than one STD at a time.

(c) Human papilloma virus infections are **decreasing** in numbers each year.

(d) Viral STDs are **more** easily eliminated than bacterial STDs.

A2. List five possible portals of entries for microbes that cause STDs.

_____

_____

_____

_____

_____

A3. Complete this exercise on human papilloma virus (HPV) infections.

(a) Circle the type of external genital warts most likely to infect moist surfaces such as the vulva.

(1) Flat warts

(2) Papular warts

(3) Keratotic warts

(4) Condyloma acuminata

(b) Approximately 99.7% of _____ cancers have been associated with HPV viruses. List several other factors that increase risk for these cancers.

_____

_____

_____

(c) There are approximately ____ different types of HPV viruses. Types ___ and ___ are the ones most correlated to invasive

carcinomas. Most reinfections involve *(the same? different?)* types of HPV viruses.

(d) Amelia is exposed to HPV on January 1. During what period of time is she likely to exhibit signs or symptoms? February 15 through _____. List typical manifestations that would lead to a diagnosis of HPV.

_____

_____

(e) Describe treatments that can eradicate HPV infections. _____

_____

_____

(f) Describe how HPV infections may be prevented. _____

_____

_____

A4. There are ____ known types of herpesviruses that cause infections in humans. Herpes (or varicella) zoster is known to cause _____ and _____. Genital herpes is caused by the herpes _____ virus (HSV). Describe genital herpes in this exercise.

(a) HSV-*(1? 2?)* is responsible for more than 90% of cases of genital herpes. HSV-1 typically causes "cold sores" or _____. HSV-I *(also can? does not?)* cause genital herpes by orogenital sex.

(b) In the United States, 1 of *(5? 50? 500?)* adolescents or adults is infected with HSV-2. The incidence of genital herpes is greater in *(men? women?)*. Explain why.

_____

_____

(c) HSV viruses on skin or mucosa travel to _____ of *(sacral? thoracic?)* spinal nerves, where they reside during a latent period of months or years. Antiviral medications *(are? are not?)* effective against these latent viruses.

(d) Most episodes of herpes *(do? do not?)* have recognizable manifestations, and most

Copyright © 2002. Lippincott Williams & Wilkins. *Study Guide to Accompany Porth: Pathophysiology: Concepts of Altered Health States, 6th edition*

spread of HSV-2 occurs from persons who *(do? do not?)* have symptoms, which explains the *(limited incidence? epidemic proportions?)* of herpes globally.

(e) List several areas where herpes lesions are likely to form in women, in men, or in either gender. _____

_____

_____

(f) List examples of systemic manifestations of HSV-2._____

_____

A5. Discuss these cases involving genital herpes.

(a) Philip states that he has a history of fever blisters but that this is the first episode of genital herpes of which he is aware.

(a1) Philip's genital herpes diagnosis is most likely to be classified as:
  A. Initial nonprimary infection
  B. Primary infection
  C. Recurrent infection

(a2) Signs or symptoms of *(primary? nonprimary?)* episodes of genital herpes typically are more acute. Explain.

_____

_____

(a3) Philip's symptoms are likely to last about *(2 to 4? 7 to 10? 12 to 14?)* days.

(a4) There *(is? is no known?)* cure for genital herpes. Why does Philip's physician prescribe antiviral drugs for Philip?

_____

_____

(a5) The clinic nurse advises Philip to be extremely careful to wash his hands well, especially before applying his contact lenses. Explain.

_____

_____

_____

(b) Mary Lee has a history of genital herpes outbreaks about once a month; she is 8 months pregnant.

(b1) She is experiencing prodromal manifestations of genital herpes. These include:
  A. Burning, tingling (paresthesia), or itching
  B. Painful vesicles that rupture, crust over, and heal

(b2) If Mary Lee continues to have active lesions at the time her baby is due, it is likely that she will be advised to have a *(cesarean? vaginal?)* delivery. About *(0.6%? 6%? 60%?)* of neonates infected with HSV die during the neonatal period.

A6. Identify the category that fits each microbe:

Bacteria   *Chlamydia*   Fungi
Parasites   Protozoa   Virus

(a) Genital warts (condyloma acuminata):

_____

(b) Granuloma inguinale: _____

(c) Lymphogranuloma venereum (LGV):

_____

(d) Molluscum contagiosum: _____

B. VAGINAL INFECTIONS (pages 1034–1036)

B1. Circle all terms that refer to *Candida* infections.

Bacterial vaginosis   Moniliasis   Thrush
Trichomoniasis   Yeast infection

B2. Circle the three true statements about *Candida* infections.

(a) **One** of four women in the United States is likely to experience candidiasis within a lifetime.

(b) Candidiasis is **always** transmitted through sexual contact.

(c) Pregnancy and use of oral contraceptives **increase** the risk of *Candida* infections.

(d) Healthy women **rarely** harbor the yeast in moist areas of skin or mucosa.

(e) Vulvar candidiasis typically is accompanied by **pruritus**.

(f) Candidiasis **can** be effectively treated by over-the-counter medications.

B3. Where else (other than external genitalia) can *Candida* infections occur?

_____

_____

B4. Mr. Emerus has a diagnosis of trichomoniasis. Complete this exercise about his condition.

(a) He has a copious discharge from his urethra that *(has an? has no?)* odor and has a pH *(under 4.5? over 6.0?)*.

(b) Mr. Emerus receives a prescription for Flagyl. The nurse advises him that he can expect a *(metallic? putrid? salty?)* taste in his mouth and that alcohol use while taking this drug is *(acceptable? contraindicated?)*. She also describes side effects to the _____ and _____ systems that also may accompany use of this drug.

(c) Trichomonas *(is? is not?)* transmitted through sexual contact. Cessation of sexual activity during the course of the infection *(is? is not?)* recommended for Mr. Emerus.

C. VAGINAL-UROGENITAL-SYSTEMIC INFECTIONS (pages 1036–1040)

C1. Which is the most prevalent STD in the United States: *(Chlamydia? gonorrhea? syphilis?)?*

Write one characteristic that distinguishes the effects of gonorrhea, syphilis, and *Chlamydia* from those of STDs discussed thus far in this chapter.

_____
_____
_____

C2. Discuss *Chlamydia* in this exercise.

(a) In the United States, *Chlamydia* transmission is *(primarily? rarely?)* by sexual contact.

(b) There *(is one type? are many types?)* of *Chlamydia*.

These microbes exist in two forms: _____ bodies and _____ bodies.

(c) Manifestations of *Chlamydia* and gonorrhea are *(quite similar? very dissimilar?)*, although *(Chlamydia? gonorrhea?)* is more likely to be asymptomatic. In fact, more than *(10%? 50%?)* of these patients have no symptoms. Explain why this lack of symptoms may be problematic.

_____
_____
_____

(d) In addition to infection of the urethra, list other parts of the body affected by Reiter's syndrome. _____
_____
_____

(e) Identify the most common organ affected by neonates who are infected by their mothers' chlamydial infections. _____ "
_____

(f) The diagnostic method of choice for *Chlamydia* is _____

C3. Discuss gonorrhea in this exercise.

(a) It is estimated that there are approximately *(6,500? 650,000?)* new cases of gonorrhea in the United States each year. Infection typically occurs 2 to 7 *(days? months? years?)* after exposure. In addition to the genitourinary tract or anorectum, what areas can serve as portals of entry?

_____
_____
_____

(b) Myra, age 22 years, has gonorrhea. Describe these symptoms that accompany her condition:

(b1) Dysuria_____
_____

(b2) Dyspareunia_____
_____

(b3) Salpingitis_____
_____

(c) Suzy, age 5 years, has gonorrhea in her throat. What is the likely cause?

_____
_____

C4. Contrast major STDs by completing Table 46-1.

Table 46-1. Comparison of Sexually Transmitted Diseases

Name of STD	Causative Microbe	Description
(a)		Genital warts, pruritis; increased risk of cervical cancer; rapidly growing STD in the U.S.
(b)	Protozoan: turnip-shaped with flagellae	
(c)		The most prevalent STD in the U.S.; often no symptoms, but women may have mucopurulent discharge and men, pruritis; may spread; causes blindness in 25%–50% of infected neonates
(d) Chanchroid		
(e)	Neisseria bacteria (gram-negative diplococci)	
(f)		Thin, gray-white discharge with foul, fishy odor; "clue cells" seen on slides; very common
(g)	Spirochete bacteria: Treponema pallidum	
(h) Genital herpes		
(i)		Most women have this infection at least once; thick, cheesy, odorless discharge; antifungals can cure

CHAPTER 47

Organization and Control of Neural Function

■ Review Questions

A. NERVOUS TISSUE CELLS (pages 1043-1049)

A1. Complete this exercise about structures that make up the nervous system.

(a) Circle structures that form the central nervous system (CNS):

Spinal cord   Brain

Cranial nerves   Spinal nerves

(b) *(Neurons? Glial cells? Satellite cells?)* conduct nerve impulses.

(c) Motor neurons are known as *(afferent? efferent?)* neurons.

A2. Describe neurons in this exercise.

(a) The nucleus of a neuron is located in the:

(1) Axon

(2) Dendrite

(3) Cell body

(b) Nissl bodies contain *(chromosomes? mitochondria? ribosomes?).*

(c) A(n) *(axon? dendrite?)* carries nerve impulses away from a cell body. Most neurons have *(one? many?)* axon(s) with *(no? some?)* branches.

A3. Schwann cells are found in the *(central? peripheral?)* nervous system. Complete this exercise about them.

(a) These cells wrap around axons ("jelly roll" fashion) to form _____ sheaths. Composed of lipid, myelin gives nerves their *(gray? red? white?)* color.

(b) Myelin functions as an _____ for axons. Myelin *(decreases? increases?)* velocity of nerve conduction as impulses are forced to "jump" between nodes of Ranvier, where myelin is *(extra thick? lacking?).* This type of conduction is known as _____.

(c) Myelin *(is? is not?)* required for survival of axons. Explain how this fact is related to multiple sclerosis (MS) and Guillain-Barré syndrome. _____

_____

(d) The endoneurial sheath (textbook Figure 47-5) around Schwann cells is required for the process of _____ of axons. This sheath is absent in the *(central? peripheral?)* nervous system. Explain the significance.

_____

_____

A4. Identify functions of supporting cells of the nervous system.

Astroglia   Ependymal cells   Microglia

Oligodendroglia Satellite cells   Schwann cells

(a) Together with endothelial cells, they form the blood-brain barrier: _____

(b) Link neurons to blood vessels, so critical for nourishing neurons; form scar tissue (gliosis) when CNS tissue is destroyed: _____

(c) Form cerebrospinal fluid (CSF): _____

(d) Phagocytic "clean-up" cells: _____

(e) Form myelin around axons of the brain and cord: _____

(f) Surround and protect cell bodies in ganglia of the peripheral nervous system (PNS): _____

(g) Supporting cells of the PNS: _____,

_____

A5. Mr. Jenkins, who has type 1 diabetes, has experienced a "small stroke," in which the blood supply to his brain was interrupted for approximately 90 seconds.

(a) The brain makes up approximately ___ % of body weight, yet uses approximately ___ % of the body's oxygen. Brain cells are *(hyper? hypo?)*metabolic.

(b) Neurons of the brain *(can? cannot?)* store glucose or glycogen. During the period when Mr. Jenkin's blood supply is interrupted, how can his brain receive nutrients?

_____

_____

(c) Is it likely that Mr. Jenkins has had brain cells die as a result of his episode?

_____

_____

(d) If Mr. Jenkins has an insulin reaction, how is this likely to affect his brain?

_____

_____

B. NERVE CELL COMMUNICATION (pages 1049–1053)

B1. A nerve impulse is also known as an _____. Refer to textbook Figure 47-7 and describe an action potential.

_____

(a) A "resting" neuron is polarized so that the inside of the membrane is more *(positive? negative?)* than the outside. A typical resting membrane potential for large neurons is approximately *(−70 to −90? −30 to −40?)* mV.

(b) A stimulus leads to entrance of *(sodium? potassium?)* into membrane channels. As a result, membrane potential on the inner side of the membrane becomes less *(positive? negative?)*. If threshold (approximately ___ mV) is reached, an action potential is initiated. As more sodium enters the neuron, the membrane potential approaches ___ mV, at which point this minute region of the membrane is completely depolarized. It may even become positive, described as _____.

(c) Repolarization takes place as sodium stops entering the neuron and *(sodium? potassium?)* exits through membrane channels; the membrane potential changes to approximately ___ mV before the resting potential is reinstated.

(d) An entire action potential lasts less than *(a millisecond? 0.1 second? 2 seconds?)*. During the *(early? late?)* portion of the action potential, the neuron is in an absolute refractory period. During this time, *(only large? no?)* stimuli can initiate an action potential.

B2. Choose the two true statements about synaptic transmission.

(a) Impulses **can** be transmitted between **axons** and **dendrites** and between **axons** and **cell bodies**.

(b) An excitatory postsynaptic potential (EPSP) is likely to **lower** the membrane potential (such as from −70 to −90 mV) so it is **farther** from threshold.

(c) Hyperpolarization (such as from −70 to −80 mV) accompanies an EPSP.

(d) **Spatial** summation involves additive effects of depolarization in at least several sites of the neuronal membrane.

B3. State an example of each of the following.

(a) A hormone that can function as a neurotransmitter.

_____

_____

(b) A neurotransmitter that can function as a hormone.

_____

_____

B4. Arrange in correct sequence the events in which the neurotransmitter acetylcholine (ACh) functions in synaptic transmission.

(a) Acetylcholine binds to a cholinergic receptor on the postsynaptic cell membrane.

(b) A presynaptic neuron synthesizes and stores ACh within the axon terminal.

(c) The presynaptic neuron is stimulated and releases ACh from vesicles into the synaptic cleft.

(d) Acetylcholine is broken down by acetylcholinesterase (ACh-ase), and choline is recycled into the presynaptic neuron.

(e) Excitation or inhibition of the postsynaptic neuron occurs (depending on the nature of the receptor and postsynaptic cell).

___ → ___ → ___ → ___ → ___

B5. Discuss the amazing complexity of neural networks in this exercise.

(a) Explain how neurons serve as integrators.

_____

_____

(b) Describe the numbers of neurons involved.

_____

_____

(c) Describe the "split-second timing" involved

_____

_____

(d) List examples of types of stimuli to neurons.

_____

_____

B6. Identify characteristics of these neurotransmitters.

Acetylcholine   Dopamine
Endorphins and enkephalins
Gamma-aminobutyric acid   Glycine
Norepinephrine   Serotonin

(a) Chemically classified as monoamines:

_____, _____, _____

(b) Peptides involved in pain
perception: _____

(c) Common inhibitory neurotransmitters:

_____, _____

(d) Excitatory to skeletal muscle but inhibitory
to cardiac muscle: _____

(e) Deficient in patients with Parkinson's
disease: _____

C. DEVELOPMENTAL ORGANIZATION OF THE NERVOUS SYSTEM (pages 1053–1061)

C1. Select the two true statements about
development of the nervous system.

(a) The mesoderm develops **after** the endoderm
and ectoderm, and it forms during the **third**
week of development.

(b) The neural plate develops **after** the neural
tube.

(c) The neural tube normally closes by the end
of the first **4 weeks** of development.

(d) The neural tube develops into the **PNS**.

C2. Circle correct answers about embryonic
development.

(a) The embryonic notochord is formed from
_(ecto? meso?)_derm, and it develops
primarily into the _(spinal cord? vertebral
column?)_.

(b) Neural crest cells are formed from _(ecto?
meso?)_derm. Circle structures derived from
neural crest cells.

(1) Autonomic ganglia

(2) Neuroglia

(3) Cranial nerve ganglia

(4) Dorsal root ganglia

(5) Meninges

(6) Many facial structures

(c) The brain is formed from the 10 segments of
the "rostral" _(front or cephalic? back or
caudal?)_ end of the neural tube. Two of
these segments form the prosencephalon (or
_____ brain); one forms the
_____ brain; and the next five form
the _____ brain. Basically, these 10
segments form the _(brain stem? cerebral
hemispheres?)_.

(d) Circle the other structures that derive later
from the prosencephalon (forebrain).

(1) Olfactory nerves

(2) Optic nerves and retina

(3) Cerebral hemispheres

(4) Oculomotor nerves

(5) Pons and medulla

(e) Circle structures derived from endoderm.

(1) Lining of the gastrointestinal tract

(2) Liver and pancreas

(3) Walls of major arteries and veins

(4) Lungs

C3. Circle the two true statements about
organization of the nervous system.

(a) **Each spinal nerve** and **cranial nerve** is
attached to the CNS by a dorsal root and a
ventral root.

(b) Dorsal roots of spinal nerves contain
sensory (afferent) neurons.

(c) Dorsal root ganglia contain **cell bodies** of
sensory neurons.

(d) The ventral horns of gray matter within the
spinal cord contain **sensory input
association neurons**.

(e) **Few** of the billions of neurons in gray matter
of the CNS are internuncial neurons.

C4. Identify the type of neuron that enables Jesse to
sense as he spends a hot summer day at a theme
park.

General somatic afferent
General somatic efferent
General visceral afferent
General visceral efferent
Special somatic afferent
Special visceral afferent

(a) Jesse is aware that he is moving in circles
and that his muscles are tense

(proprioception) as he spins on a ride at the park: _____

(b) Walking around the park involves Jesse's use of his lower motor neurons (LMNs), which are _____ pathways. As he walks around, Jesse feels the heat of the sun on his skin: _____

(c) Jesse smells and tastes the lunch that he buys: _____. Parasympathetic (vagus) nerves begin the process of digestion: _____. Soon Jesse becomes aware of a full stomach and bladder: _____ .

C5. Longitudinal tracts consist of *(gray? white?)* matter located in the *(inner or "butterfly-shaped"? outer?)* portion of the cord. Answer questions about these longitudinal pathways.

(a) The *(archi? paleo? neo?)* layer is considered the oldest layer in evolutionary development. This layer consists of the *(longest? shortest?)* pathways.

(b) Spinothalamic tracts (for pain and temperature) lie in the *(archi? paleo? neo?)* layer, which is the *(inner? middle? outer?)* layer of white tracts.

(c) The *(archi? paleo? neo?)* layer extends the entire length of the nervous system and is even "suprasegmental," meaning that it extends into the _____. Myelination of this part of the spinal cord usually is complete at *(birth? approximately 6 years of age?)*. State the significance of this fact._____

_____

C6. What is the function of the reticular activating system?

_____

_____

D. THE SPINAL CORD (pages 1061–1068)

D1. Circle correct answers in these statements about the spinal cord.

(a) The spinal cord is *(longer? shorter?)* than the vertebral column. The cord ends as the *(cauda equina? conus medullaris? filum terminale?)* at about level *(L1 or L2? L3 to L4?)*. The spinal nerve roots that extend below the inferior end of the spinal cord are known as the _____.

(b) At what level is a spinal tap typically performed? Between vertebrae ___ and ___. Explain. _____

_____

_____

(c) A cross section of the cord reveals an inner "H" or butterfly-shaped region of *(gray? white?)* matter. The *(dorsal? lateral? ventral?)* gray horns contain cell bodies of *(motor? sensory?)* neurons. These are known as *(lower? upper?)* motor neurons; they innervate *(skeletal? smooth?)* muscle.

(d) Which regions of the cord contain relatively great amounts of gray matter? (See Figure 47-18.) _____, _____ Explain.

_____

_____

(e) List three examples of anatomical structures that anchor the spinal cord in place.

_____

_____

D2. Complete this exercise about spinal nerves and spinal reflexes.

(a) The human body has a total of ___ pairs of spinal nerves. How many pairs in each location?

Cervical: ___   Thoracic: ___

Lumbar: ___   Sacral: ___

Coccygeal: ___

(b) Spinal nerves are attached by a *(motor? sensory?)* dorsal root and a *(motor? sensory?)* ventral root. Spinal nerves are *(mixed? motor? sensory?)*.

(c) What are "rami" of spinal nerves?

_____

_____

Which are larger *dorsal* or *ventral* rami? Explain._____

_____

(d) What do white "rami communicantes" supply? _____

_____

(e) List the three components of a spinal reflex.

_____

_____

(f) A stretch reflex is also known as a _____ reflex. Describe two functions of this type of reflex.

_____

_____

(g) Diminished capacity for stretch reflexes is likely to cause *(hyper? hypo?)* tonia with weakness or paralysis. Excessive stretch reflex responses can lead to _____.

(h) What type of stimulus triggers a withdrawal reflex? _____
_____
_____

E. THE BRAIN (pages 1068–1080)

E1. Identify components of the three major regions of the brain. Write one brain part on each line provided.

Cerebellum   Cerebrum   Hypothalamus
Medulla   Midbrain   Pons
Thalamus

(a) Forebrain: _____, _____,
_____

(b) Midbrain: _____

(c) Hindbrain: _____, _____,
_____

E2. Use answers from Question E1 to identify which brain part fits each description.

(a) The name means a "bridge" connecting midbrain with medulla as well as right to left cerebellar hemispheres: _____

(b) Inferiormost portion of the brain stem:
_____

(c) The cerebral aqueduct carries CSF through this brain part: _____

(d) The fourth ventricle lies anterior to the _____ and posterior to the _____ and _____.

(e) Contains the "pyramids": _____

(f) Coordinates and "dampens" movements, keeping them "smooth": _____

E3. Identify which cranial nerves (I-XII) are attached to each brain part.

(a) Medulla: _____

(b) Pons: _____

(c) Midbrain: _____

E4. Identify by name and number the cranial nerve that is likely to be impaired in each case. Where indicated, circle whether the right or left nerve is damaged.

(a) Gail has lost most movements of her left eye; she has ptosis (drooping) of her left eyelid: _____, _____ R L

(b) Sean cannot raise his right shoulder, and his head is turned toward the left: _____,
_____ R L

(c) Val's blindness in her right eye is related to cranial nerve damage: _____,
_____ R L

(d) Michael has difficulty swallowing, has developed a husky voice, and his uvula is deviated to the right side: _____,
_____ R L

(e) Phoebe's tongue muscles are weak:
_____, _____

(f) Joyce has a cranial nerve disorder that causes dry mouth and dry eyes: _____,
_____

(g) Gus lacks facial expression on one side of his face (Bell's palsy): _____,
_____

(h) Mark cannot feel touch, pain, or temperature on the right side of his lower jaw, including his lower right teeth; his chewing muscles also are affected:
_____, _____

E5. Name the cranial nerves that serve the following functions.

(a) Provide the brain with information about blood pressure originating from baroreceptors in major arteries: _____,
_____

(b) Carry impulses related to taste: _____,
_____, _____

(c) Hearing and balance are most related to:
_____

(d) Carries most parasympathetic efferent impulses and many visceral afferents:
_____

(e) Supplies the only extrinsic eye muscle that turns the eye outward (abduction):
_____

(f) Carries sensations of smell (but not pain, pressure, or temperature) from the nose:
_____

(g) Shining light in an eye to check a photopupil reflex is an assessment of:
_____

E6. Refer to textbook Table 47-2 and identify the spinal nerves with the following functions.

C1-C4: Cervical nerves no. 1-4
C5-C8: Cervical nerves no. 5-8
L2-S1: Lumbar-upper sacral nerves
S2-S4: Lower sacral nerves

(a) Supply most nerves to lower extremities:
_____

(b) Supply nerves to upper extremities:

_____

(c) Supply nerves to most neck and shoulder muscles: _____

E7. Identify functions of each major part of the diencephalon by writing H (hypothalamus) or T (thalamus) next to related descriptions.

(a) Major regulatory center for hormones and autonomic responses: ____

(b) Major relay center for sensations; also involved with selected motor activities: ____

(c) Two egg-shaped masses connected by a cross bar that passes through the third ventricle: ____

(d) The posterior pituitary is an extension of this brain part: ____

E8. Discuss the cerebrum in this exercise.

(a) Refer to textbook Figure 47-25 and identify the structures that fit descriptions below. Then circle G or W to indicate whether each structure consists of gray or white matter.

Basal ganglia   Corpus callosum
Internal capsule

(a1) A bridge of tracts connecting the two cerebral hemispheres; located immediately superior to lateral ventricles: _____ _(G? W?)_

(a2) The caudate and lentiform nuclei; regulate association movements, such as arm movements that accompany walking: _____ _(G? W?)_

(a3) Major site of tracts located between basal ganglia and thalamus: _____ _(G? W?)_

(b) Identify which cerebral lobes contain the following structures:

Frontal   Occipital
Parietal   Temporal

(b1) Primary reception areas for hearing (41): _____

(b2) Primary reception areas for vision (17):

_____

(b3) Primary sensory areas (3, 1, and 2) for the sense of touch on fingers or face; located in the postcentral gyrus:

_____

(b4) Primary motor cortex (area 4) located in the precentral gyrus: _____

(c) In most persons, the (_left? right?_) cerebral hemisphere is the dominant hemisphere. Cerebral dominance typically develops (_completely by birth? gradually throughout childhood?_).

E9. Identify the area most likely to be dysfunctional in each neural disorder.

Auditory association area (22)
Basal ganglia
Limbic system
Premotor area (6)
Primary auditory cortex (area 41)
Somesthetic association areas (5 and 7)

(a) Huntington's and Parkinson's disease:

_____

(b) Apraxia, such as ability to handle scissors but inability to use them to cut paper:

_____

(c) Inability to hear the sounds of music:

_____

(d) Inability to identify a musical sequence as a commonly recognizable song:

_____

(e) Astereognosis, such as inability to distinguish whether an object held in the hand is a key or a paperclip: _____

(f) Violent behavior with explosive speech:

_____

E10. Discuss meninges in this exercise.

(a) Arrange meninges from most external to most internal:

Arachnoid   Dura mater   Pia mater

_____, _____, _____

(b) Which is a delicate layer that encases blood vessels to the brain? _____

(c) Its name means "tough mother"; it forms the falx cerebri and tentorium cerebelli:

_____

(d) Circle brain structures that are infratentorial.

Cerebellum   Cerebrum   Medulla   Pons

E11. Jacob experiences a mild blow on the side of his head. List structures that protect his brain during the trauma.

_____

_____

E12. Complete this exercise about CSF.

(a) Where is CSF formed?

_____

_____

(b) A total of approximately *(3 to 4? 1.5 to 2.0? 0.5 to 0.75)* cup(s) of CSF are found within or around the CNS.

(c) Arrange structures in the pathway of CSF from first to last:
Arachnoid villi
Cerebral aqueduct
Cranial venous sinuses
Fourth ventricle
Lateral ventricles
Subarachnoid space
Third ventricle

_____ → _____ →

_____ → _____ →

_____ → _____ →

_____

E13. Discuss the "barriers" that protect the brain.

(a) List structures that form the blood-brain barrier.

_____

_____

(b) Circle all substances that can cross the blood-brain barrier.

Alcohol   Bilirubin in newborns
Epinephrine   Heroin   Nicotine

(c) The CSF-brain barrier is formed by tight junctions of _____ cells of choroid plexuses.

(d) Which chemicals readily diffuse or osmose across the membrane?

CO_2 H_2O O_2 Protein   Vitamins

F. THE AUTONOMIC NERVOUS SYSTEM (pages 1080–1088)

F1. Summarize functions of the autonomic nervous system (ANS) in several words.

_____

_____

F2. Write P (parasympathetic) or S (sympathetic) to indicate which division of the ANS better fits each description.

(a) Prepares the body for stress or "fight or flight": ____

(b) Functions when the body is "peaceful" (nonstressed) to help it conserve energy:

____

(c) Exerts a more widespread effect: ____

(d) Slows heart rate: ____

(e) Increases salivation and motility of the stomach: ____

(f) The vagus nerve makes up 75% of its efferent nerves: ____

F3. Choose the two true statements.

(a) Autonomic pathways from CNS to effector consist of **two** neurons, whereas somatic pathways consist of **only one**.

(b) In general, sympathetic and parasympathetic nerves have **similar** effects.

(c) Enteric plexuses in the wall of the gastrointestinal tract are **sympathetic** neurons.

(d) Visceral afferent neurons sensitive to changes in blood pressure (BP) pass from **carotid** arteries via **cranial nerve IX** to cardiovascular centers in the brainstem.

F4. Refer to Figure 47-35 and complete this exercise about ANS pathways.

(a) Parasympathetic nerves are found in cranial nerves ____, ____, ____, and ____.

(b) Axons of preganglionic neurons are shown by *(solid? broken?)* lines in this figure. Most *(P? S?)* preganglionic axons reach all the way to viscera.

(c) Known as the "thoracolumbar" outflow, preganglionic neurons of this division begin at levels T1 through L2 of the cord: ____

(d) The *(P? S?)* division has relatively short preganglionic neurons with branches that synapse with *(few? many?)* postganglionic neurons.

(e) The ganglia situated by major abdominal arteries (celiac, superior and inferior mesenteric) are sites where *(P? S?)* neurons synapse. The chains of ganglia that parallel vertebrae are sites where *(P? S?)* neurons synapse.

(f) White and gray rami both contain axons of *(P? S?)* neurons.

(g) Segments S2 through S4 of the spinal cord give rise to *(P? S?)* preganglionic neurons, which then travel in pelvic nerves.

(h) Circle the viscera that receive sympathetic but not parasympathetic innervation:

Adrenal medulla   Blood vessels of skin
Heart   Hair muscles of skin
Stomach   Sweat glands

F5. Describe roles of the following structures in mediating autonomic activities.

(a) Hypothalamus

_____

_____

(b) Visceral afferent neurons

_____

_____

F6. Refer to Figure 47-34 and write the correct neurotransmitter next to each type of cell that releases it.

Acetylcholine   Norepinephrine
                  (or other catecholamines)

(a) All postganglionic parasympathetic neurons:

_____

(b) All somatic neurons (for example, to the gastrocnemius muscle):

_____

(c) Most postganglionic sympathetic neurons:

_____

(d) A few postganglionic sympathetic neurons (to sweat glands and vasodilator neurons in skeletal muscles): _____

(e) Adrenal medulla cells: _____

F7. Describe ANS neurotransmitters and their receptors in this exercise.

(a) Write the two chemicals that combine to form the neurotransmitter ACh: _____ + _____ → ACh. Name the two types of receptors for ACh: _____, _____. On which of these receptors does the anticholinergic drug atropine exert its effect? _____

(b) Which enzyme destroys ACh?

ACh-ase   COMT   MAO

(c) List in correct sequence the chemicals involved in the formation of the catecholamine norepinephrine (NE):

Dopamine   L-DOPA
Tyrosine (an amino acid)

_____ → _____ → _____ → NE

(d) In the adrenal medulla, most NE is converted to epinephrine by the addition of a (*carboxyl? hydroxyl? methyl?*) group. Production of both of these hormones

(*does? does not?*) depend on the influence of adrenal cortical hormones such as cortisol.

(e) List three mechanisms by which catecholamines can be removed from synapses or neuromuscular junctions.

_____

_____

(f) Explain how the following medications work to allow NE to remain active in synapses:

(f1) MAO inhibitors

_____

_____

(f2) Tricyclic antidepressants, such as amitriptyline

_____

_____

(g) Receptors for NE are known as (*adrenergic? cholinergic?*). Describe roles of several of these receptors.

(g1) β_1-adrenergic receptors are located on ___ cells.

(1) Smooth muscle of blood vessels

(2) Smooth muscle of airways

(3) Cardiac muscle

(g2) When NE stimulates a β_1-adrenergic receptor, heart rate (*decreases? increases?*). A β_1-adrenergic-blocking drug such as propranolol (Inderal) will (*decrease? increase?*) heart rate.

(g3) When NE stimulates a β_2-adrenergic receptor, smooth muscle of airways will (*contract? relax?*) so that airways (*constrict? dilate?*).

(g4) When NE stimulates an α_1-adrenergic receptor, smooth muscle of blood vessels in skin and GI tract will (*contract? relax?*), causing vaso(*constriction? dilation?*) and a(n) (*decrease? increase?*) in BP.

(h) Sympathomimetic drugs act on (*adrenergic? cholinergic?*) receptors.

CHAPTER 48

Somatosensory Function and Pain

■ Review Questions

A. ORGANIZATION AND CONTROL OF SOMATOSENSORY FUNCTION (pages 1091–1100)

A1. With her right hand, April attempts to pick up an extremely hot cup of tea from the microwave. Describe the sensory pathway in this exercise.

(a) At least *(two? three?)* orders of neurons form the pathway for burning pain. The first-order neuron has its cell body in April's *(central? peripheral?)* nervous system, specifically in a _____ ganglion just lateral to the right side of her spinal cord. Refer to the dermatome map in Figure 48-2 of the text. At which level of the spinal cord do first-order neurons from April's hand enter her spinal cord? *(C6-8? T6-8?)*

(b) April's second-order neurons *(do? do not?)* cross to the left side of her spinal cord and ascend her spinal cord in *(anterolateral? posterior?)* pathways that reach to the *(right? left?)* side of her thalamus.

(c) The third-order neuron axons terminate in April's _____, specifically in the *(right? left?)* *(frontal? parietal?)* lobe. Refer to textbook Figure 48-7 and determine the exact location of the cortex that receives impulses from April's hand. The map of these sensory neurons is known as the _____ pattern because it roughly parallels a "little man" laid across a cerebral hemisphere. The exact parietal lobe location for reception of sensations from April's fingers is:

(1) Lateral

(2) Medial

(3) Between medial and lateral

(d) Figure 48-7 indicates that most of April's primary sensory cortex would be devoted to perception of sensations from ___ because

these areas have a high density of sensory receptors.

(1) Fingers and face

(2) Trunk, hips, and feet

A2. Contrast the two major somatosensory pathways in this exercise.

Anterolateral pathway   Discriminative pathway

(a) Includes tracts for pain, hot, cold, and "crude touch": _____

(b) Carries impulses that allow distinction between a paperclip and a key (stereognosis): _____

(c) Permits proprioception (awareness of body position and muscle tension) as well as two-point discriminative touch: _____

(d) The second-order neuron crosses to the opposite side of the cord to ascend in neospinothalamic or paleospinothalamic tracts: _____

(e) First-order neurons ascend in dorsal columns (or enter via cranial nerves) to the medulla where they synapse: _____

(f) Second-order neurons convey impulses through the medial lemniscus tract of the brain: _____

(g) Destruction of the left side of the spinal cord would result in loss of these pathways from the right arm and leg: _____

A3. Circle the two true statements.

(a) Type A nerve fibers convey impulses **more slowly** than do type C fibers.

(b) Burning pain (such as April's pain in Question A1) is transmitted along **both** A and C nerve fibers.

(c) Sensations of touch from the anterior thigh are located in dermatomes for spinal nerves S2 and S3 (see Figure 48-2).

(d) Somatosensory association areas apply **meaning** to sensations.

A4. Describe aspects of sensation in this exercise.

(a) List three or more *modalities* of sensation.

_____
_____

Explain what accounts for such modalities.

_____
_____

(b) Define *acuity* of sensation and describe what accounts for it.

_____
_____

(c) Define threshold for sensory stimuli.

_____
_____

A5. Identify the type of sensory receptor that fits each description.

Free nerve endings	Hair follicle end organs
Meissner's corpuscles	Merkel's disks
Pacinian corpuscles	Ruffini's end organs

(a) Abundant in your fingertips and lips where your sense of touch is well developed:

_____

(b) Deep to your skin, these receptors allow sensation for vibration and pressure:

_____

(c) Lacking a capsule, these account for sensitivity of your skin and the anterior of your eyes (corneas) to touch; they transmit their impulses along thin, slow fibers:

_____

(d) Very slow to adapt, these receptors make you aware of the lightest touch over your skin: _____

(e) Detect continuous pressure of a heavy weight on your skin or joints: _____

A6. Complete this exercise about other sensations.

(a) Which regions are more sensitive to cold? *(Lips? Fingers?)* Which are more sensitive to heat? *(Lips? Fingers?)*

(b) Cold and warmth receptors *(do? do not?)* completely adapt. Explain the clinical significance.

_____
_____

(c) Define *proprioception*.

_____
_____

(d) Kinesthesia refers to *(static? dynamic?)* position sense.

_____
_____

A7. Refer to textbook Figure 48-2 and explain what information is provided by pressing a pinpoint against the sole of a client's foot.

_____
_____

B. PAIN (pages 1100–1113)

B1. Describe the "good news" and "bad news" of pain.

_____
_____

B2. Circle the correct answers in these statements about pain.

(a) Suffering from pain is influenced more by *(intensity of? reaction to?)* pain.

(b) Approximately *(3.7? 13.7?)*% of people in the U.S. have their activities of daily living limited by pain.

(c) *(Nociceptive? Neuropathic?)* pain results from injury to nerves. Diabetic neuropathy is an example of *(analgesic? hyperalgesic?)* pain.

(d) Intense stimulation of *(only specific? virtually all?)* types of sensory receptors can lead to pain. This is a statement of the *(pattern? specificity?)* theory of pain.

B3. Describe theories of pain in this exercise.

(a) The "gate control theory" of pain states that tactile sensations that travel over *(fast? slow?)* fibers can block pain pathways that travel over *(fast? slow?)* pathways, thereby blocking pain. This theory was proposed by _____ and _____ in 1965. This theory *(does? does not?)* fully explain pain mechanisms. Describe how the gate control theory has been helpful.

_____
_____

(b) Describe Melzak's neuromatrix theory of pain (1999).

_____
_____

B4. Nociception means _____ sense. Describe nociceptive mechanisms in this exercise.

(a) List several sites in the body where nociceptors are located.

_____
_____

(b) List and give examples of three categories of stimuli that can be nociceptive.

(b1)_____
_____
_____

(b2)_____
_____
_____

(b3)_____
_____
_____

(c) Acute mechanical and thermal painful stimuli typically are transmitted along:
A δ: Fast, myelinated nerve fibers
C: Slow, unmyelinated nerve fibers

(d) Bright, sharp, or stabbing pain is more likely to be transmitted through *(neo? paleo?)*spinothalamic tracts, which are *(fast? slow?)* conduits to the brain. *(Neo? Paleo?)*spinothalamic tracts transmit dull, aching pain, such as chronic visceral pain.

B5. Choose the two true statements about pain.

(a) Prostaglandins tend to **cause** pain.

(b) Aspirin is an analgesic that **blocks** synthesis of prostaglandins.

(c) Glutamate and substance P both **inhibit** pain.

(d) The periaqueductal gray region is located in the **thalamus** and it **causes pain.**

(e) The antidepressant amitriptyline has the side effect of **causing pain.**

B6. Explain how a withdrawal reflex can be protective.

_____
_____

B7. Define and describe effects of endogenous opioids.

_____
_____

List three categories of such chemicals.

_____
_____

B8. Which refers to the "amount of pain a person is willing to endure before the person wants some relief"? Pain *(threshold? tolerance?)*. Which is more constant from person to person? Pain *(threshold? tolerance?)*.

B9. Contrast types of pain in this exercise.

(a) A sprained ankle is likely to cause *(cutaneous? deep somatic? visceral?)* pain. Cutaneous pain is considered *(diffuse? sharp, bright?)* pain.

(b) Appendicitis, gallstones, and kidney stones cause *(cutaneous? deep somatic? visceral?)* pain. This type of pain also is known as _____ pain. Explain why visceral pain is likely to be accompanied by sweating, pallor, nausea, and vomiting.

_____
_____

(c) Visceral pain is more likely to occur from:

(1) Abnormal contractions, distention, or ischemia of the intestinal wall

(2) Burning (cauterizing) or cutting the wall of the intestine

(d) Visceral pain *(is? is not?)* readily localized. Explain why. _____
_____

(e) Mr. Jefferson experiences pain of a heart attack in his left arm and the left side of the chest (see Figure 48-11). This phenomenon is known as *(phantom? referred?)* pain. Explain the mechanism. _____
_____
_____

(f) Liver and gallbladder pain "refer" to the *(right? left?)* side of the *(chest? neck?)*. Explain._____
_____
_____

(g) *(Acute? Chronic?)* pain is defined as pain caused by tissue damage (such as from surgery) that ends when tissues heal. This pain has a duration of less than ___ months. List three factors other than the actual pain stimuli that can exacerbate acute pain.

_____
_____

(h) *(Acute? Chronic?)* pain serves a useful function. Explain. _____
_____
_____

(i) *(Acute? Chronic?)* pain is more associated with depression, loss of appetite, and sleep disturbances.

B10. Ms. Templeton, age 42 years, has metastatic ovarian cancer; she is being evaluated for pain and possible treatment.

(a) The single most reliable indicator of the existence and intensity of acute pain is:

(1) The patient's self-report

(2) Patient blood pressure and heart rate

(3) Names of pain medications the patient is taking

(b) Describe methods that the nurse is likely to use to assess Ms. Templeton's pain.

_____

_____

B11. Choose the two true statements about treatment of pain.

(a) Treatment of acute pain is likely to be **more** complex than treatment of chronic pain.

(b) Pain management is considered to be **more** effective if it is initiated after pain becomes severe.

(c) Risk for addiction to opioid medications is considered **great** when drugs are prescribed for acute pain.

(d) It **is** recommended that a plan for control of postoperative pain be developed before surgery.

(e) Cancer **is** a common cause of chronic pain.

B12. Write examples of each of the following cognitive-behavioral methods that may be implemented for pain control for Ms. Templeton (Question B10).

(a) Relaxation

_____

_____

(b) Biofeedback

_____

_____

(c) Guided imagery

_____

_____

(d) Distraction

_____

_____

B13. Explain precautions that should be taken to reduce complications of these pain treatments.

(a) Cold packs for Janine, age 15 years, who has a sprained ankle and is sleeping much of the day.

_____

_____

(b) Heat treatments for Mrs. Snyder, age 73 years, who has disabling arthritis.

_____

_____

B14. TENS is a pain relief approach that refers to

T_____

E_____

N_____

S_____

across the skin. It is (*invasive? noninvasive?*) and (*can? cannot?*) be performed by the client. Describe several mechanisms by which TENS may work. _____

_____

B15. (*Acupressure? Acupuncture?*), which is a(n) (*ancient? recent?*) practice involves use of extremely fine needles introduced into specific sites to relieve pain. (*Acupressure? Acupuncture?*), also known as shiatsu, uses pressure exerted by _____.

B16. Analgesics are medications that decrease pain (*with? without?*) loss of consciousness. Describe analgesics in this exercise. Choose from these answers.

Acetaminophen   Aspirin   Codeine

Dynorphins   Endorphins

Nonsteroidal anti-inflammatory drugs

Morphine   Serotonin reuptake inhibitors

(a) Classified as opioid analgesics:

_____, _____,

_____, _____

(b) Non-narcotic analgesics that also are antipyretic and anti-inflammatory:

_____, _____

(c) A non-narcotic analgesic that is antipyretic but not anti-inflammatory: _____

(d) Adjuvant analgesics such as the tricyclic antidepressant amitriptyline: _____

B17. Choose the two true statements about pain treatments.

(a) Antiseizure medications (Dilantin or Tegretol) **are** examples of placebos.

(b) The World Health Organization (WHO) **does** recommend morphine use for persons with chronic cancer pain.

(c) Placebos **should** be used for clients with chronic cancer pain.

(d) Interdisciplinary approaches to pain management are **more** likely to be successful than are approaches with a single focus.

C. ALTERATIONS IN PAIN SENSITIVITY AND SPECIAL TYPES OF PAIN (pages 1113–1116)

C1. Select the term that fits each description.

Allodynia	Analgesia	Athermia
Hyperalgesia	Hyperpathia	Paresthesia

(a) Celia's foot "fell asleep" as her nerves were compressed by her crossed legs; now she feels "pins and needles" as her foot "wakes up": _____

(b) Anthony experiences increased sensitivity to pain: _____

(c) Joan has an "explosive" pain that radiates along the distribution of L1 spinal nerve: _____

(d) Elizabeth experiences intense pain initiated by light touch that should not normally induce pain: _____

(e) Dave has lost the ability to feel changes in temperature in his right leg: _____

C2. List several conditions that can cause neuropathy and neuropathic pain that is:

(a) Localized

_____

_____

(b) Widespread

_____

_____

C3. Describe two major categories of treatments for neuropathy by writing sentences using the following key words:

(a) Cause

_____

_____

(b) Palliative

_____

_____

C4. Hye-Sun experiences neuropathy based on her end-stage chronic renal failure (Chapter 34, Question B11). Explain why opioids, rather than acetaminophen, are selected for palliative pain control.

_____

_____

C5. Neuralgia refers to _____. Complete this exercise about neuralgias.

(a) Tic douloureux is another name for _____ neuralgia, which is pain along *(cranial nerve V? spinal nerve C5?)*. This condition typically is *(bilateral? unilateral?)* and involves *(mild, aching? severe, lightning-like?)* pain in the face. State one trigger for tic douloureux: _____. List several treatment approaches.

_____

_____

(b) Postherpetic neuralgia refers to pain more than 1 month after onset of herpes *(simplex? zoster?)*, also known as *(cold sores? shingles?)*. This condition is *(more? less?)* common among elderly persons. Explain.

_____

_____

(c) Explain why complex regional pain syndrome may be exacerbated by emotional upsets and possibly involve pallor, rubor, edema, sweating, or dryness.

_____

_____

C6. Phantom limb pain occurs in about *(17%? 70%?)* of clients who undergo amputation. Use key words listed below to possible causative mechanisms.

(a) Scar tissue

_____

_____

(b) Spinal cord

_____

_____

(c) Brain

_____

_____

D. HEADACHE AND ASSOCIATED PAIN (pages 1116-1119)

D1. Choose the two true statements about headaches.

(a) Approximately 75% of women experience at least one headache a month.

(b) **Most** headaches indicate serious intracranial disorders.

(c) Almost all migraines occur **with** an aura.

(d) Bruxism refers to **teeth grinding**, a condition that **is** associated with temporomandibular joint pain.

D2. List characteristics of headaches that should be investigated for possibly serious causes.

_____

_____

D3. Mari, age 16 years, has developed chronic headaches. What information should she include in her headache diary?

_____

_____

D4. Identify characteristics of major types of headaches in this exercise.

Cluster   Chronic daily
Migraine   Tension-type

(a) The most common type of headache; does not typically interfere with daily activities or involve nausea or vomiting: _____

(b) May be caused by caffeine withdrawal, temporomandibular joint pain, or prolonged neck muscle work such as computer activity: _____

(c) More common in women and may be associated with estrogen levels; tend to be familial: _____

(d) "One-handed" (unilateral) headaches that are pulsatile, throbbing, often accompanied by nausea and vomiting; may be disabling: _____

(e) Headaches that occur on more than half of the days in a month: _____

(f) Typically unilateral, radiating pain around eyes or in temples that may be mistaken for sinus infections; occur in clusters over weeks or months separated by headache-free intervals: _____

D5. Circle correct answers in these statements about migraines.

(a) What is the typical duration of the aura that occurs with some migraines? _____

(b) Describe the signs or symptoms that accompany these types of migraines:

_____

_____

(b1) Ophthalmoplegic migraine

_____

_____

(b2) Transformed migraine

_____

_____

(c) Migraines *(can? do not?)* occur in children. Circle all characteristics typical of childhood migraines:

(1) Continuous headaches without pain-free periods

(2) Bilateral head throbbing

(3) Intense nausea and vomiting

(4) Positive family history

(5) Seeking relief in dark environments

(d) Describe methods (nonpharmacologic and pharmacologic) of prevention of migraines.

_____

_____

_____

_____

E. PAIN IN CHILDREN AND OLDER ADULTS (pages 1119–1121)

E1. Defend or dispute this statement: "Young children and elderly persons do not feel pain."

_____

_____

E2. Describe tools for assessing pain in:

(a) Jewel, age 4 years

_____

_____

(b) Jade, age 12 years

_____

_____

E3. Jade (age 12 years) is scheduled for a painful surgery. It is preferable to teach pain interventions *(before? after?)* the surgery. List several such methods.

_____

_____

E4. Write one reason elderly persons may be reluctant to report pain.

_____

_____

E5. Describe important guidelines for pain interventions in elderly; use these key terms.

(a) Individualized_____

_____

_____

(b) Dosage _____

_____

_____

(c) Polypharmacy _____

_____

_____

CHAPTER 49

Motor Function

■ Review Questions

A. CONTROL OF MOTOR FUNCTION (pages 1123–1129)

A1. Explain the importance of inhibition of muscle activity.

_____

_____

A2. Define posture and summarize how it is maintained. _____

_____

_____

A3. Describe roles of each of the following in movements.

(a) Actin and myosin_____

_____

(b) Flexor _____

_____

_____

(c) A motor unit _____

_____

_____

A4. Circle correct answers in each statement.

(a) Large motor units may have *(several? thousands?)* of muscle cells innervated by a single lower motor neuron (LMN).

(b) Muscles that sustain contractions to maintain posture are more likely to incorporate high numbers of *(fast? slow?)*-twitch fibers. These depend on *(oxygen in blood? stored glycogen?)* for energy and are *(fast? slow?)* to fatigue.

(c) Muscles for jumping (such as the gastrocnemius) or for throwing a ball (triceps brachii) are composed largely of *(fast? slow?)*-twitch fibers.

A5. Refer to textbook Figures 49-2 and 49-3 and identify parts of the cerebrum with each function.

Prefrontal association cortex

Primary motor cortex

Supplementary motor cortex

(a) On medial aspects of area 6 and 8; involved with skillful movements on both sides of the body: _____

(b) Also called the "motor strip" or area 4; this thick area in the left side controls delicate movement sequences on the right side of the body: _____

(c) Programs complex activity patterns, such as picking up a spoon: _____

(d) Neurons are arranged in a person-shaped map known as the "motor homunculus":

_____

A6. Refer to textbook Figure 49-1 and arrange structures in pyramidal pathways from first to last.

(a) Tracts in the internal capsule

(b) Cell bodies of upper motoneurons (UMNs) in motor cortex in the posterior region of the frontal lobe

(c) Corticospinal tract in the spinal cord

(d) Decussation (crossing) of axons in pyramids of the medulla

(e) Ventral roots and then spinal nerves

(f) Cell bodies of LMNs in ventral horn of the spinal cord

____ → ____ → ____ → ____ → ____ → ____

A7. Choose the three true statements.

(a) The homunculus map demonstrates that about half of the primary motor cortex controls movements of **arms** and **legs**.

(b) Neurons on the lateral aspect of the primary motor cortex regulate **foot** movements.

(c) Most of the neurons in the right primary cortex control movements on the right side of the body.

(d) Axons of the lateral corticospinal tract are parts of UMNs.

(e) About half of the axons in the lateral corticospinal tract synapse with LMNs in **cervical** regions of the spinal cord and supply upper extremities.

(f) Extrapyramidal pathways do not cross in the medulla, and they provide supportive roles in movements.

A8. Describe roles of the cerebellum, basal ganglia, thalamus, and sensory cortex in corrections and adjustments that affect smooth movements._____

_____

_____

A9. Circle correct terms in this exercise about muscle disorders.

(a) Hypotonia refers to *(absent? less than normal? spastic?)* muscle tone.

(b) *(Paralysis? Paresis?)* refers to weakness of muscles. Paralysis of both legs is an example of *(mono? di? para? quadri?)*plegia.

(c) Injury to *(UMNs? LMNs?)* is more likely to lead to flaccid paralysis.

A10. Chad suffered a gunshot wound that severed his spinal cord at vertebra T6.

(a) From level T7 inferiorly, Chad has lost:

(1) Communication with the brain

(2) Spinal cord reflexes

(b) Chad's spinal cord injury (SCI) destroys pathways of *(UMNs? LMNs?)* *(above? below?)* his midthoracic area.

(c) He is likely to have *(complete use? spasticity? flaccidity?)* of his arms and *(complete use? spasticity? flaccidity?)* of his legs. Explain. _____

_____

_____

(d) When Chad shifts from his electric scooter to a chair, his thigh and leg muscles sometimes go into spastic movements. This is known as _____.

(e) Chad *(is? is not?)* likely to have bowel and bladder incontinence. He *(may? will not?)* have erections that could permit sexual intercourse. Explain._____

_____

_____

A11. Describe infections that can injure nerves.

(a) Dan steps on a rusty nail and develops tetanus in his right leg. *Clostridium tetani* toxin travels to Dan's spinal cord and irritates the cell bodies of *(UMNs? LMNs?)*. As a result, muscles innervated by these nerves become *(hyper? hypo?)*excited and develop sustained contractions known as _____.

(b) The polio virus is likely to attack *(UMNs? LMNs?)* such that muscles experience *(spastic? flaccid?)* paralysis and *(atrophy? hypertrophy?)*.

A12. Injury to Mr. Ross's right *(C7? T3? L4?)* spinal nerve by a herniated disk is most likely to lead to leg weakness and pain, specifically of his *(right? left?)* leg.

B. SKELETAL MUSCLE AND PERIPHERAL NERVE DISORDERS (pages 1129–1137)

B1. Identify the motor disorder of each client below.

Denervation atrophy	Disuse atrophy
Duchenne's muscular dystrophy	Myasthenia gravis
	Mononeuropathy
Polyneuropathy	

(a) Matt, age 10 years, is wheelchair-bound because of a progressive genetic disorder:

_____

(b) Mrs. Meyer, age 48 years, has been in a coma and has been paralyzed following traumatic brain injury in an automobile accident 10 years ago:_____

(c) Ms. Allen, age 27 years, has experienced muscle weakness and fatigue; tests indicate a diagnosis of an autoimmune disease that destroys acetylcholine (ACh) receptors at her neuromuscular junctions: _____

(d) Mrs. Schmidt has been wearing an immobilizer of her right leg since she fractured her tibia 2 months ago; as a result, she has lost 25% of her calf muscle tissue:

_____

(e) Lisette received a diagnosis of Guillain-Barré syndrome a short time after she recovered from a viral infection; she experienced paralysis in her legs that ascended to her upper body; her recovery is now complete:

_____

(f) Brandy, age 29 years, has worked an assembly line for 11 years; she has carpal tunnel syndrome of both wrists:

_____

B2. Discuss Matt's disorder (Question B1[a]) in this exercise.

(a) His condition occurs in (*females? males? both females and males?*). Explain.

_____

_____

(b) Matt's condition is a (*muscular? neural?*) disorder. Duchenne's muscular dystrophy (DMD) involves formation of a faulty protein, _____, which normally connects muscle cell membranes with actin and myosin filaments.

(c) Circle typical early manifestations of DMD:

(1) Hip muscle weakness, abnormal postures, and falls

(2) Inability to use utensils to eat

(3) Incontinence

(4) Weakness of thoracic muscles with respiratory infections and scoliosis

(d) Matt's serum levels of creatine kinase are likely to be (*high? normal? low?*). Explain.

_____

_____

(e) He (*is? is not?*) likely to have an emaciated appearance. Explain._____

_____

_____

(f) With early treatment, DMD (*is? is not?*) curable.

B3. Identify effects of the following chemicals at neuromuscular junctions or synapses.

Acetylcholinesterase
Clostridium botulinum toxin
Curare
Physostigmine and neostigmine

(a) Breaks down the neurotransmitter ACh (review Chapter 47, Question F7[b]):

_____

(b) Inhibits acetylcholinesterase (ACh-ase), causing ACh to linger longer in neuromuscular junctions: _____

(c) Acts as a muscle relaxant by blocking ACh action on muscles: _____

(d) Produced by microbes from soil, it can cause a serious food poisoning from improperly canned foods. Because it blocks release of ACh, it can be used clinically to reduce spasms of extrinsic eye muscles, eyelids,

neck, or larynx: _____

_____

B4. Discuss Ms. Allen's disorder (Question B1[c]) in this exercise.

(a) Myasthenia gravis is more common in (*women? men?*).

(b) Circle Ms. Allen's activities that are most likely to be affected by myasthenia gravis:

(1) Speaking

(2) Lifting her eyelids

(3) Chewing

(4) Writing

(5) Sensation in her feet

(c) Which type of drug listed in B3 is most likely to help Ms. Allen?_____

(d) Plasmapheresis is a treatment that removes _____ from Ms. Allen's blood.

(e) Identify the most serious problem associated with myasthenia crisis. _____

_____

B5. Identify events in peripheral nerve injury and repair.

Chromatolysis   Endoneurial tube
Schwann cells   Wallerian degeneration

(a) Destruction of myelin around injured peripheral nervous system (PNS) neurons:

_____

(b) Responsible for phagocytosis of injured tissue and production of new myelin:

_____

(c) Disappearance of Nissl granule (ribosomal) staining that indicates active protein synthesis is attempting repair of nerve fibers:

_____

(d) Structure that must be intact for growth of axonal tissue: _____

B6. Discuss Mr. Ross's "slipped disk" injury (Question A12) in this exercise.

(a) A "slipped disk" is technically known as a _____ intervertebral disk. The portion of the disk that protrudes out of position is the (*annulus fibrosus? nucleus pulposus?*). It is most likely to herniate (*anteriorly? posterolaterally?*). Explain why.

_____

_____

_____

(b) Herniation is most likely to occur at vertebrate level (*T6-T7? L1-L2? L4-L5?*). Trauma is a (*common? rare?*) cause of such herniations.

(c) Typically, the first sign of herniated disk is _____, and major muscle weakness is (*common? rare?*).

(d) When Mr. Ross lies supine and his leg is raised 50°, he feels pain in his hamstrings. This is a (*positive? negative?*) test for herniated disk.

(e) Circle conservative treatments for herniated disk:

    (1) Nonsteroidal anti-inflammatory drugs

    (2) Back surgery

    (3) Exercises to strengthen the back

    (4) Muscle relaxants

B7. Discuss Brandy's carpal tunnel syndrome (Question B1[f]) in this exercise.

(a) In addition to the repetitive wrist movements of her job, what other factors might contribute to Brandy's diagnosis? She:

    (1) Has diabetes

    (2) Takes oral contraceptives

    (3) Has hypothyroidism

(b) Circle typical manifestations of carpal tunnel syndrome:

    (1) Numbness of the little finger and ring finger in each hand

    (2) Difficulty gripping between thumb and index finger

    (3) Positive Tinel's sign (tingling sensation radiating into the palm when the anterior of the wrist is tapped)

(c) Wearing wrist splints (*can be? is not?*) helpful for Brandy.

B8. The effects of chronic alcoholism on nerves is an example of a (*mono? poly?*)neuropathy.

C. DISORDERS OF THE BASAL GANGLIA AND CEREBELLUM (pages 1137–1142)

C1. Describe functions of the basal ganglia.

(a) Basal ganglia are most involved with (circle two answers):

    (1) Initiating movements, so if basal ganglia are impaired, paralysis results

    (2) Adding gracefulness to highly learned, skilled movements

    (3) Regulating distal part of limbs (such as fingers) more than proximal parts

    (4) Preventing extra, involuntary movements

(b) Basal ganglia are (*excitatory? inhibitory?*). For example, they tend to inhibit the triceps brachii when the _____ brachii contracts. Impaired basal ganglia lead to:

    (1) Weakness and flaccidity

    (2) Stiffness, rigidity, and tremor

(c) Because basal ganglia are parts of (*pyramidal? extrapyramidal?*) pathways, the stiffness and rigidity that accompany impairment of basal ganglia are known as (*pyramidal? extrapyramidal?*) signs.

C2. Refer to textbook Figure 49-10, and describe components of the basal ganglia and associated structures.

(a) Basal ganglia are deep-lying regions of (*gray? white?*) matter known as "nuclei" within the (*cerebrum? cerebellum?*).

(b) The most lateral portion of the basal ganglia is the (*caudate? putamen?*). The white matter (axons) that lies between the caudate and the putamen is known as the _____. Collectively this gray-white-gray area is known as the "striped body" or the corpus (*nigra? striatum?*).

(c) The midbrain contains cells rich in the pigment melanin; this section of the midbrain is known as the substantia _____. These cells synthesize the neurotransmitter (*serotonin? dopamine?*) and supply it to the striatum.

(d) In (*Alzheimer's? Parkinson's?*) disease, substantia nigra production of dopamine is (*deficient? excessive?*). Inhibitory nerve impulses are reduced, leading to (*hyper? hypo?*)kinesis. Results are classic signs of Parkinson's (*hint:* see Question C1[b]): _____, _____, and _____. If only the right basal ganglia are involved, signs will be seen on the (*right? left? both right and left?*) side(s) of the body.

(e) Basal ganglia (*do? do not?*) form many connections with the cerebral cortex, cerebellum, brainstem, and thalamus in reciprocal circuits. State the significance.

_____

_____

(f) List five or more other neurotransmitters involved in complex pathways associated with basal ganglia.

_____

_____

_____

(g) Which neurotransmitter is deficient in the basal ganglia-related condition, Huntington's disease? _____

_____

_____

C3. Refer to textbook Table 49-1 and match involuntary movement disorders to each description.

Athetosis   Ballismus   Chorea

Dystonia   Tardive dyskinesia   Tic

(a) Brief, rapid, jerky and irregular movements of head and extremities; the term means "to dance"; may include piano-playing-type movement of fingers, curling and protrusion of tongue, raising eyebrows and shoulders:

_____

(b) Continuous, wormlike, twisting movements of extremities, trunk, or face: _____

(c) Violent, flinging movements of limbs; the term means "to jump around":

_____

(d) Repetitive, bizarre movements of face, including grimacing, protrusion of tongue, and deviations of the jaw; may occur as reaction to long-term use of antipsychotic drugs: _____

(e) Repetitive winking of eyelids, and brief abnormal movements of other parts of face, or shoulder: _____

(f) "Wry neck" or torticollis, affecting neck and shoulder, is the most common form of this disorder: _____

C4. Mr. Gustafson, age 68 years, has received a diagnosis of Parkinson's disease (PD). Review Question C2(d) and complete this exercise on Mr. Gustafson's condition.

(a) Parkinson's disease _(is? is not?)_ a progressive disorder. Symptoms begin once _(20%? 80%?)_ of dopamine production is lost from nigrostriatal pathways. List other possible causes of parkinsonism. _____

_____

_____

_____

(b) Identify the manifestations of PD exhibited by Mr. Gustafson:

Autonomic   Bradykinesia
manifestations   Cog-wheel movements
Dysphagia   Masklike face
Tremor

(b1) Slow, shuffling gait related to excessive inhibition of movement; difficulty initiating movements; most disabling of PD manifestations: _____

(b2) Ratchet-like movements of arms; a form of rigidity: _____

(b3) The most visible sign of PD in patients who are awake and at rest; present in 75% of patients with PD; includes "pill-rolling" movements of thumb and forefinger: _____

_____

(b4) Lack of facial expression: _____

(b5) Difficulty swallowing; one sign is drooling:

_____

(b6) Excessive sweating, salivation (with drooling), lacrimation, constipation, and impotence: _____

(b7) "Poverty of movement": _____

(c) Mr. Gustafson does not exhibit dementia. About one in _____ patients with PD will experience dementia.

(d) Explain how each type of drug might be helpful to Mr. Gustafson:

(d1) Levo-dopa

_____

_____

(d2) Carbidopa

_____

_____

(d3) Anticholinergic (anti-ACh) drugs such as Cogentin or Artane

_____

_____

C5. The cerebellum _(does? does not?)_ initiate movements. Briefly describe how the cerebellum contributes to skillful movements.

_____

_____

_____

C6. List possible causes of cerebellar impairment.

_____

_____

_____

C7. Mr. Daugherty is being assessed for possible cerebellar damage. Identify manifestations of cerebellar damage.

Nystagmus   Cerebellar dysarthria
Dysdiadochokinesia   Dysmetria
Dysphagia   Intention tremor
Truncal ataxia

(a) Mr. Daugherty is not able to stand with a steady posture: _____

(b) In a seated position, he has difficulty starting the movement of tracing the back of his left shin with the toes of his right foot: _____

(c) With hands on his knees, he cannot rapidly pronate and supinate his forearms: _____

(d) When he tries to touch his finger to his nose (with eyes closed), he repeatedly misses: _____

(e) His speech is slow and slurred: _____

(f) His eyes move rapidly from right to left, then slowly return to the right: _____

D. UPPER MOTONEURON DISORDERS (pages 1142-1156)

D1. Craig, age 40 years, received a diagnosis of amyotrophic lateral sclerosis (ALS) 2 years ago. Complete this exercise about his condition.

(a) Amyotrophic lateral sclerosis is commonly known as _____'s disease. Most cases of this disease *(are? are not?)* hereditary. The disease typically is diagnosed in men *(younger? older?)* than Craig. Survival usually is _____ years from onset of symptoms.

(b) What information does the name ALS provide about this condition?

(b1) Amyotrophic _____

(b2) Lateral_____

(b3) Sclerosis _____

(c) Circle manifestations likely to develop in Craig:

(1) Loss of sensation in hands and feet

(2) Paralysis of his hands and feet

(3) Dementia

(4) Difficulty swallowing, speaking, and making any sounds

(5) Loss of sexual sensation and ability to have an erection

(6) Weakness of respiratory muscles, leading to infections

(7) Elevated glutamine levels in his cerebrospinal fluid

(d) Name one type of drug approved for treatment of ALS. _____

(e) In final stages of ALS, how may Craig still be able to communicate? _____

D2. Therese, age 31 years, received a diagnosis of multiple sclerosis (MS) at the age of 25 years. Describe MS.

(a) This condition typically is diagnosed *(before? after?)* age 40 years and is more common in *(women? men?)*. There *(is? is not?)* a genetic predisposition.

(b) MS is a disorder of the *(CNS? PNS?)* in which axons lose their _____; as a result, velocity of nerve condition then *(decreases? increases?)*. MS is related to a decrease in _____ cells that normally produce myelin in the CNS. MS is likely to affect *(movements? sensations? both?)*.

(c) Explain the meaning of the term *multiple sclerosis.* _____

(d) This disorder *(is? is not?)* likely to be immune related. Explain. _____

(e) Circle two manifestations likely for initial presentation of MS.

(1) Forgetfulness

(2) Paralysis of one hand

(3) Numbness and tingling

(4) Double vision

(f) List other signs and symptoms of MS. _____

(g) Therese's MS has been characterized by remissions and exacerbations, as occurs in about *(one? four?)* of five cases of MS.

(h) List treatments that may help limit the progression of Therese's MS.

_____

_____

D3. Identify factors that increase the risk for SCI.

(a) Alcohol and other drugs

(b) Older than 30 years

(c) Female

(d) Motor vehicle accidents

D4. Refer to Figure 49-11 and complete this exercise about the vertebral column.

(a) Vertebral bodies are largest in *(cervical? lumbar? thoracic?)* vertebrae. Explain how this is helpful._____

_____

_____

(b) Circle structures that are located more anteriorly in each case:

(b1)

A. Vertebral bodies and intervertebral disks
B. Vertebral spines

(b2)

A. Laminae   B. Spinal cord

(c) Name structures that normally keep vertebrae in alignment. _____

_____

_____

_____

_____

D5. Contrast tetraplegia with paraplegia.

_____

_____

_____

D6. Identify which SCIs are complete (C) or incomplete (I).

(a) A digital examination of the anus produces a sphincter reflex: _____

(b) All sensory and motor function is lost below the injury, including the anal sphincter response: _____

(c) Cord hemisection: _____

(d) Has a better prognosis: _____

D7. Circle correct answers in each statement about SCIs.

(a) Anterior spinal artery infarction is more likely to result in loss of ability to sense:

A. Two-point discriminatory touch and proprioception
B. Pain and temperature

(b) Injury to the right spinothalamic tract is more likely to lead to loss of pain and temperature sensation in the *(right? left?)* side of the body. This is a(n) *(contralateral? ipsilateral?)* effect. Injury to a corticospinal (voluntary motor) tract has a(n) *(contralateral? ipsilateral?)* effect.

(c) With central cord syndrome, *(arms? legs?)* are likely to be affected to a greater degree. This condition occurs more commonly in *(children? the elderly?)*.

(d) Conus medullaris syndrome is least likely to affect *(arms? legs? bowel and bladder function?)*. Damage to nerve roots in the lumbosacral area is known as *(Brown Séquard? cauda equina?)* syndrome. It *(is? is not?)* likely to affect continence and sexual function.

(e) *(Primary? Secondary?)* SCI occurs at the time of the mechanical injury; such injury *(is? is not?)* reversible. Edema and vasospasm with ischemia are causes of *(primary? secondary?)* injury and may be reversible.

D8. State rationales for the following early treatments for SCIs.

(a) Immediate in-line immobilization and "log rolling" onto a rigid backboard

_____

_____

(b) Correcting hypotension and hypoxia

_____

_____

(c) Use of steroids _____

_____

(d) Use of the ganglioside GM-1 and calcium channel blockers _____

_____

_____

_____

D9. Ann experiences a complete C3 SCI during a traumatic fall from horseback. Circle true statements about her case.

(a) A complete SCI at C3 is likely to cause **less** loss of function than a complete SCI at T3.

(b) SCI injuries at C3 level or higher **do** require assistance with ventilation.

(c) Ann **is** at increased risk for serious respiratory infections.

(d) She **is** likely to be able to pick up items as a result of tenodesis.

(e) Ann **is** likely to be able to use an electric wheelchair.

D10. James has a T8 compression SCI resulting from a fall from the roof of a two-story house.

(a) Because his injury is at T12 or above, James *(is? is not?)* likely to have UMNs affected. UMN destruction with intact LMNs ultimately results in *(flaccid? spastic?)* paralysis.

(b) In the hours immediately after his fall, James goes into a period of spinal shock. This is a time of *(a? hyper?)*reflexia as his spinal reflexes below T12 are *(absent? exaggerated?)*. By the time he is airlifted to the hospital 90 minutes after his fall, spastic reflexes are observed. This fact is a *(positive? negative?)* sign regarding some recovery of function.

(c) James *(is? is not?)* likely to have impaired posture in a wheelchair.

D11. The diaphragm receives its innervation from spinal nerves that arise from levels *(C3 to C5? T3 to T5?)* of the cord. Mr. Tenley has a C7 SCI. Explain why his risk of respiratory infections (including pneumonia that may be fatal) is likely to be high. _____

_____

_____

D12. Both Ann (Question D9) and James (Question D10) are likely to experience *(high? normal? low?)* heart rate, blood pressure, and body temperature after their injuries.

(a) In both cases, vagus nerve function is likely to *(fail? persist?)* and contribute to bradycardia. Explain. _____

_____

_____

(b) *(Ann? James?)* is more likely to have these conditions persist. Explain. _____

_____

_____

(c) Ann's heart rate drops when she undergoes suctioning to remove mucus from airways. Explain. _____

_____

_____

(d) When Ann is raised from a supine to sitting position, she feels dizzy. This condition is known as _____ . What can prevent this disorder? _____

_____

D13. Autonomic dysreflexia leads to distinct contrasts in manifestations above and below the site of an SCI. Complete this exercise about this condition.

(a) Which two clients are most likely to experience episodes of autonomic dysreflexia? *(Ann? James? Mr. Tenley?)*. Explain why they are at risk for this disorder. _____

_____

(b) List common triggers for autonomic dysreflexia. _____

_____

(c) As a result of this trigger, unregulated sympathetic responses become *(absent? exaggerated?)* below the site of injury. Vasospasm leads to skin *(flushing? pallor?)*, goose bumps, and extremely *(high? low?)* blood pressure with headaches.

(d) Baroreceptor reflexes then call for decreased sympathetic activity above the injury site (where sympathetic structures still communicate with the brainstem). In the upper body, *(flushing? pallor?)* of skin is evident, along with nasal stuffiness (due to vaso-_____); _____cardia also develops.

(e) Summarizing: in autonomic dysreflexia, sympathetic signs are present in the *(upper? lower?)* body and are absent in the *(upper? lower?)* body. This condition *(is? is not?)* a clinical emergency.

D14. Briefly explain why each of the following conditions is likely to accompany SCIs.

(a) Poikilothermy_____

_____

_____

(b) Edema and deep venous thrombosis

_____

_____

_____

(c) Safety and skin integrity issues associated with spasticity (See James, Question D10[a]) and sensory loss_____

_____

_____

(d) Pain _____

_____

_____

(e) Bladder incontinence _____

_____

_____

(f) Bowel incontinence _____

_____

_____

(g) Sexual dysfunction _____

_____

_____

CHAPTER 50

Disorders of Brain Function

■ Review Questions

A. MECHANISMS AND MANIFESTATIONS OF BRAIN INJURY (pages 1159–1172)

A1. Complete this exercise about the brain and its blood supply.

(a) The brain makes up approximately ____ % of body weight, yet receives approximately ____% of the blood pumped out of the heart each minute.

(b) Cerebral *(hypoxia? ischemia?)* deprives the brain of blood flow, whereas ____ involves adequate blood flow but reduced oxygen level.

(c) Explain how hypoxic neurons can survive.

_____

_____

How can anaerobic metabolism be problematic?_____

_____

(d) A "stroke" (cerebrovascular accident [CVA]) is more likely to lead to *(focal? global?)* ischemia. List two causes of global ischemia.

_____

_____

(e) Global ischemia can lead to unconsciousness within 10 *(seconds? minutes?)*; the ATP resources of the brain are likely to be depleted within *(2? 5? 20?)* minutes.

(f) Most of the ATP used by brain cells goes toward maintenance of _____ within neurons. State two consequences of failure of these pumps. _____

_____

(g) Circle the two parts of the brain that are especially vulnerable to ischemia:

(1) Pons

(2) Midbrain

(3) Cerebellum

(4) Hippocampus

(h) "Watershed infarcts" most commonly develop at the *(proximal? distal?)* ends of the major cerebral arteries when perfusion is reduced.

A2. Explain how each of the following contributes to or counteracts ischemia.

(a) Sludging of blood _____

_____

(b) Hypermetabolism associated with increased catecholamines_____

_____

_____

(c) Hypothermia _____

_____

_____

A3. Describe glutamate toxicity in this exercise.

(a) List several neurological conditions that have pathogenesis related to overstimulation by amino acids such as glutamate or aspartate. _____

_____

_____

_____

(b) Describe an NMDA receptor.

_____

_____

_____

(c) List two specific types of neuronal injury caused by excessive exposure to glutamate.

_____

_____

(d) The concentration of glutamate normally is 16 times greater in *(ICF within? ECF around?)* neurons. Explain how prolonged ischemia affects this concentration.

_____

_____

_____

(e) Neurons of the _____ and the _____ have large numbers of NMDA receptors and thus are particularly sensitive to glutamate excitotoxicity. What functions do these neurons control? _____ and _____

(f) Explain how a neuroprotectant medication such as riluzole can help some persons with amyotropic lateral sclerosis (ALS). _____ _____ _____

A4. Mrs. Smith has been transported to a rural clinic. Her intracranial pressure (ICP) is increasing as a result of a severe head trauma in a domestic violence incident several hours ago. Her blood pressure is 200/110 mm Hg, and her pulse is 50 bpm. She appears lethargic and confused.

(a) List the three major components within Mrs. Smith's cranium and the percentage of intracranial volume that each is likely to form under normal conditions. Then state one or more mechanisms by which each of these might increase in volume, thereby elevating ICP.

(a1) _____ (___ %): _____

(a2) _____ (___ %): _____

(a3) _____ (___ %): _____

(b) Which of these volumes is likely to be increased in Mrs. Smith's cranium? _____ _____

(c) Mrs. Smith's ICP is likely to rise *(minimally? dramatically?)* when her intracranial volume increases significantly.

(d) List the manifestations that are reliable early indicators of increased ICP in Mrs. Smith. _____ _____

(e) If Mrs. Smith's ICP is 55 mm Hg, her cerebral perfusion pressure (CPP) is _____ mm Hg. This value is *(high? normal? low?)*.

(f) Mrs. Smith's blood pressure is significantly *(decreased? increased?)*, especially the *(systolic? diastolic?)* value. As a result, pulse pressure is *(widened? narrowed?)*. This "last ditch" effort to provide cerebral perfusion when ICP is high is known as _____'s reflex; it results from a *(tachycardic? vasoconstrictive?)* response to decreased cerebral perfusion. This reflex *(is? is not?)*

frequently observed clinically. Explain. _____ _____

(g) Mrs. Smith's reflex *(brady? tachy?)*cardia is likely to lead to *(high? low?)* pCO_2 levels in cerebral blood. Hypercarbia then stimulates vaso*(constriction? dilation?)*. How can this help Mrs. Smith's brain? _____ _____

A5. Describe factors that typically compartmentalize the brain and explain how these may be altered by increased ICP.

(a) The falx cerebri consists of tough *(dura? pia?)* mater that extends *(horizontally? vertically?)* to compartmentalize the *(two cerebral hemispheres? cerebrum from the cerebellum?)*. *(Cingulate? Uncal?)* herniations can pass under the falx cerebri and press on the *(anterior? middle? posterior?)* cerebral artery (Figure 50-8). Reduced flow through this vessel affects *(medial? lateral?)* aspects of a cerebral hemisphere that control *(arm? leg?)* muscles. (*Hint*: refer to the homunculus figure on text page 1126.)

(b) Describe normal functions of the following structures and name a type of herniation associated with each structure.

(b1) Tentorium cerebelli _____ _____

(b2) Incisura _____ _____

(c) Identify the manifestations associated with each type of herniation:

Arm weakness Respiratory arrest
Blindness   Leg weakness
"Clouding" of consciousness
Posturing (decorticate or decerebrate)
Death by compression of vital structures in the medulla
Dilated pupil (ipsilateral)

(c1) Uncal (lateral) herniation: _____ _____ _____

(c2) Transtentorial (central) herniation: _____

(d) Figure 50-4 indicates that elbows are flexed in *(decerebrate? decorticate?)* posturing.

(e) Contrast conditions related to increased ICP.

   (e1) Which type of herniation is more likely to compress the brainstem? *(Cingulate? Infratentorial?)*.

   (e2) Which condition is most life threatening: *(brainstem? cerebral? diencephalon?)* compression?

A6. Identify types of brain edema in each case.

   Cytotoxic   Interstitial   Vasogenic

   (a) Obstructions in cerebrospinal fluid (CSF) pathways press CSF from ventricles into adjacent white matter: _____

   (b) Caused by impaired blood-brain barrier function resulting from brain injury, infections, tumors, or ischemia; leads to increased extracellular fluid (ECF) between brain cells: _____

   (c) Neurons and neuroglia swell and may rupture as excessive fluid moves into them; causes include water intoxication (as in hyperglycemic hyperosmolar nonketotic syndrome [HHNK] with type 2 diabetes mellitus) or severe ischemia with adenosine triphosphate (ATP) depletion that disrupts the sodium pump; most likely to affect gray matter: _____

A7. List two categories of drugs that may be used to treat cerebral edema. _____

A8. Complete this exercise about hydrocephalus.

   (a) This condition involves an excessive volume of _____. Most cases of hydrocephalus are caused by *(overproduction? reduced reabsorption?)* of CSF.

   (b) Identify whether hydrocephalus caused by reduced reabsorption of CSF is communicating (C) or noncommunicating (NC):

   (b1) Narrowing of the (cerebral) aqueduct of Silvius connecting the third and fourth ventricles related to embryonic viral infection or midbrain tumor:

   _____

   (b2) Arachnoid villi are injured by scarring or infectious debris: _____

   (b3) Treatment includes surgical shunting:

   _____

(c) Enlargement of the head is likely to occur when hydrocephalus occurs in *(infants? older children or adults?)*. Explain.

   _____

   _____

(d) Circle the manifestations likely to be present in a 10-month-old infant with hydrocephalus.

   (1) Vomiting
   (2) Bulging fontanels
   (3) Signs of decreased intelligence
   (4) Weakness or seizures
   (5) Visual disorders
   (6) Ventricular enlargement observed by imaging

(e) Papilledema is a sign of high ICP and hydrocephalus. How is papilledema assessed? _____

   _____

   _____

A9. Complete this exercise about Missy's altered consciousness as her brother splashes her in the swimming pool.

   (a) Circle the structures that comprise Missy's reticular formation.

   Cerebral cortex   Medulla   Midbrain
   Hypothalamus   Pons   Thalamus

   (b) Arousal and wakefulness (for example, Missy's startle reaction as water splashes on her face) are functions most associated with the *(ascending reticular activating system [ARAS]? cerebral cortex?)*. The content and cognitive aspects of consciousness (for example, her awareness that it was water that was splashed on her face and that it was her brother who initiated that action) are regulated by the

   _____.

   (c) The ARAS relay to the *(hypothalamus? limbic system?)* is most likely to make Missy's heart race, whereas the ARAS relay to her _____ is most associated with Missy's determination to splash her brother in return.

A10. Circle the two true statements about levels of consciousness (LOC).

   (a) A CVA involving one cerebral hemisphere is likely to lead to altered level of consciousness (ALC).

(b) Shearing injury that traumatizes white matter of the RAS and cerebral hemispheres **can** lead to ALC.

(c) Hallucinations and delusions are most associated with a state of **confusion**.

(d) An obtunded person **may** respond to significant shaking.

(e) A state of stupor indicates a **higher** LOC than a state of obtundation.

(f) A client with doll's-head eye movements will have eyes **stay fixed** in the head (and **not** rotate) as the head is moved.

A11. Severity of altered LOC depends on the site of brain injury, progressing from most anterior/superior or *(caudal? rostral?)* to most posterior/inferior or *(caudal? rostral?)*. Determine which level of brain injury is indicated in each case.

Diencephalon   Medulla   Midbrain   Pons

(a) Mrs. Ellington lies rigid in full extension; her pupils are fixed and dilated (do not constrict to light); she exhibits doll's-head eye movements; her respirations are 42 per minute: _____

(b) Ms. Rutenschrorer is comatose with flaccidity; her sporadic respirations require ventilatory assistance: _____

(c) Mr. Lopez lies in full extension except for flexor posturing of elbows, wrists, and hands; his pupils react to light, and his gaze follows a moving finger; he exhibits Cheyne-Stokes breathing: _____

A12. Ms. Delgado scores a 14 on the Glasgow Coma Scale assessment. This is a relatively *(high? low?)* score. List the three aspects of neurological functioning measured by this scale: _____, _____, _____

A13. Explain why the definition of "brain death" has changed during the past several decades.

_____

_____

Circle criteria that indicate brain death.

(a) Absence of pupillary reactions to light and absent gag reflex

(b) Lack of electroencephalogram (EEG) activity for at least 15 minutes

(c) No effort to ventilate in response to arterial blood pCO_2 > 60 mm Hg

(d) Irreversibility of brain death

(e) Absence of perfusion of the circle of Willis

A14. Mrs. Meyer is in a persistent vegetative state (PVS). List six or more criteria used to determine PVS. _____

_____

_____

_____

B. CEREBROVASCULAR DISEASE (pages 1172–1182)

B1. Refer to Figures 50-7 and 50-8 and select the names of arteries listed below to fill in blanks in this exercise.

Anterior cerebral arteries
Basilar artery
Internal carotid arteries
Middle cerebral arteries
Posterior cerebral arteries
Posterior communicating arteries
Vertebral arteries

(a) Right and left _____ ascend in the posterior of the neck, enter the skull, and then form the _____ that lies at the base of the brain. These arteries are vital to survival because they perfuse the brainstem.

(b) The right and left _____ supply the anterior of the circle of Willis. Emboli from these arteries pass directly into the _____, which are the most common sites of embolic strokes.

(c) Located on the medial aspect of frontal and parietal lobes, the _____ supply motor neurons to lower extremities.

(d) Arteries that directly supply blood to deep-lying structures such as basal ganglia and thalamus include _____, _____, _____, _____, and _____.

(e) _____ connect middle cerebral arteries with _____ to complete the posterior portion of the circle of Willis.

B2. Describe the veins that drain the brain in this exercise.

(a) Which are more vulnerable: *(deep? superficial?)* veins? Explain.

_____

_____

_____

(b) Venous blood from the brain empties into venous sinuses composed of *(dura? pia?)* mater. These structures empty into

_____ veins that carry blood back toward the heart.

(c) Venous sinuses *(do? do not?)* have valves. State the significance.

_____

_____

B3. Discuss factors that regulate cerebral blood flow.

(a) Cerebral blood flow—especially *(deep? superficial?)* flow—normally is regulated by *(local? sympathetic nerve?)* control. These mechanisms are known as _____ regulation, and they work as long as mean arterial pressure (MAP) is maintained within a range of ____ to ____ mm Hg.

(b) Circle three local factors that dilate cerebral vessels.

(1) Acidosis

(2) Alkalosis

(3) Hypercarbia

(4) Hypocarbia

(5) Hypoxia

(c) Acidosis *(stimulates? depresses?)* CNS function. Explain how cerebral artery vasodilation helps to correct cerebral acidosis._____

_____

B4. Compare the terms in each pair.

(a) Heart attack (MI)–brain attack (CVA)

_____

_____

(b) Angina—transient ischemic attack (TIA)

_____

_____

B5. Circle the factors that increase risk of stroke.

(a) *(African American? White?)* race

(b) Age *(65 years? 75 years?)*

(c) Chronic *(hypotension? hypertension?)*

(d) *(History? No history?)* of previous stroke

B6. Write rationales for increased risk of stroke in the following clients.

(a) Angeline, age 8 years, has a sickle cell crisis.

_____

_____

(b) Mr. Polk, age 61 years, has atrial fibrillation. _____

_____

(c) Gustav has been "blood doping" and has a hematocrit of 64%._____

_____

B7. List five or more "lifestyle modifications" that can decrease the risk for stroke.

_____

_____

_____

_____

B8. Mrs. Everly, age 66 years, manifests early signs of a TIA.

(a) A TIA is best described as *(focal? global?)* ischemic cerebral defects with a duration of less than 24 *(hours? minutes?)*.

(b) Define "penumbra" as related to a CVA and a TIA. _____

_____

_____

B9. Circle the two true statements about strokes.

(a) Ischemic strokes are most often caused by **hemorrhage**.

(b) Strokes are **more** likely to occur at sites of bifurcation of arteries with atherosclerotic plaques.

(c) Thrombotic strokes **are** associated with increased activity in older adults.

(d) The name "lacunar infarcts" is based on the **small cavities** or **lacunae** in the brain that remain after such strokes.

(e) Lacunar infarcts cause **global cortical deficits,** such as the inability to **speak or to accomplish tasks performed before the stroke.**

B10. Which type of stroke is most frequently fatal?

(a) Cardiogenic embolic

(b) Hemorrhagic

(c) Lacunar

(d) Thrombotic
List several causes of this type of stroke.

_____

_____

B11. Review Question B1 and text Table 50-6, and then identify the cerebral artery involved in each case of stroke. Where possible, indicate whether the affected artery is on the right or left side of the brain.

Anterior cerebral artery
Middle cerebral artery
Posterior cerebral artery

(a) Ms. Weldon has paralysis and sensory loss of her right arm and the right side of her face; she cannot turn her eyes toward her right, and she is confused and sometimes appears delirious: *(L? R?)* _____

(b) Mr. Knowlton's left leg and foot are paralyzed with sensory loss resulting in impaired gait; his wife states that "his mind is slower, and he's distracted all the time": *(L? R?)* _____

(c) Mrs. Penn's daughter reports that her mother "just keeps repeating the same couple of phrases all day long, she's been having trouble remembering things, and her senses just aren't what they were—her vision, hearing, taste . . . .":

_____

B12. Ms. Weldon has been transported to the emergency department. A history and physical examination identify manifestations described in Question B11(a); onset was 2 hours ago and symptoms have persisted.

(a) The duration of her symptoms indicates that her condition *(is? is not?)* a TIA. Explain. _____

_____

(b) Ms. Weldon's symptoms of stroke are largely unilateral with sudden onset. This *(is? is not?)* a typical pattern for strokes. Her neurologic examination also reveals dysarthria, which means _____; ataxia, which means _____; and restlessness and some brief periods of delirium.

(c) Explain why it is critical to determine quickly the cause of her stroke.

_____

(d) *(Computed tomography? Magnetic resonance imaging?)* is the diagnostic imaging considered superior for differentiating ischemic from hemorrhagic lesions.

(e) Thrombolytic agents are most helpful for salvaging penumbral areas around _____ strokes. List several

thrombolytic agents.

_____
_____

(e) List five contraindications for taking thrombolytic medications. _____

_____
_____
_____

B13. Select the two true statements about aneurysmal subarachnoid hemorrhages.

(a) The incidence of this condition is greatest in **adolescents**.

(b) **Most** patients with this diagnosis **do** achieve complete recovery.

(c) Most aneurysms of the brain are **berry** aneurysms.

(d) The larger the aneurysm, the **more** likely it is that the aneurysm will rupture.

(e) There **is no** evidence of hereditary predisposition for these aneurysms.

B14. Circle manifestations of a ruptured subarachnoid aneurysm.

(a) Nuchal rigidity
(b) Mild headache
(c) Photophobia
(d) Altered extraocular muscle function
(e) Loss of consciousness

B15. Briefly describe three possible and serious complications of ruptured subarachnoid aneurysm.

(a) Vasospasm _____

_____
_____

(b) Rebleeding _____

_____
_____

(c) Hydrocephalus _____

_____
_____

B16. Discuss arteriovenous (A-V) malformations in this exercise.

(a) What is unique about blood flow through these vascular systems?

_____
_____
_____

(b) Arteriovenous malformations *(are? are not?)* thought to be congenital and *(do? do not?)* appear to increase risk for neurological deficits and learning disorders.

B17. Circle the two true statements about long-term disabilities associated with strokes.

(a) Motor and sensory deficits are likely to manifest **contralaterally.**

(b) Loss of **language** ability refers to loss of the motor act of verbal expression.

(c) A stroke affecting Broca's area is likely to result in some form of **aphasia.**

(d) A person with a right-sided stroke is more likely to exhibit hemineglect on the **right** side of the body than on the **left.**

B18. Match the following terms related to strokes with the correct meanings.

Anomic aphasia   Wernicke's aphasia
Apraxia   Dysarthria
Expressive aphasia   Fluent aphasia

(a) Inability to articulate words because of dysfunction of structures such as mouth, lips, or larynx: _____

(b) Inability to translate thoughts into meaningful speech: _____

(c) Loss of spontaneity of speech, including appropriate rate of speech: _____

(d) Inability to understand the speech of others, including written word: _____

(e) Loss of ability to correctly sequence motor acts to carry out an act such as speech: _____

(f) Nearly normal speech except inability to word-find: _____

C. TRAUMA, INFECTIONS, AND NEOPLASMS (pages 1182–1189)

C1. Discuss the "good news" and the "bad news" about the skull and CSF as protectors of the brain. _____
_____
_____

C2. Circle correct answers about head injuries.

(a) Most fatal head injuries result from *(falls? accidents involving vehicles and pedestrians?).*

(b) A skull fracture involving a multiple fracture line is known as a *(basilar? comminuted? laminar?)* fracture.

(c) Rhinorrhea refers to flow of CSF into the *(ear? eye? nose?),* suggesting a fracture of the ethmoid bone.

(d) Which of the following are primary head injuries?

Ischemia   Edema
Brain herniation   Subdural hematoma
Concussion   Infection
Contusion

(e) A *(concussion? contusion?)* involves a longer period of unconsciousness with bruising of the brain.

(f) When the skull is hit on the anterior, a contrecoup trauma involves injury to the *(anterior? posterior?)* of the brain.

C3. Refer to textbook Figure 50-12 and complete this exercise about hematomas.

(a) Alex was riding his bike without a helmet when his bike swerved and he fell on the right side of his head. He immediately became unconscious, then conscious and speaking for a brief period, then unconscious again.

(a1) This pattern suggests a(n) *(epidural? intracranial? subdural?)* hematoma. Tearing of Alex's right middle meningeal artery during the accident is likely to lead to *(rapid? slow?)* compression of his brain.

(a2) Neurological assessment of Alex is likely to reveal a fixed, dilated *(right? left?)* pupil and *(right? left?)*-sided hemiplegia of his arm and face.

(b) Miranda experienced jarring of her head as it snapped backward in an automobile accident on Saturday. At the accident site, Miranda stated that she felt "fine" and refused medical help. On Thursday, the onset of severe headache, lethargy, and confusion prompted her to see a physician.

(b1) Miranda receives a diagnosis of a subdural hematoma; its classification is *(acute? subacute? chronic?).*

(b2) A subdural hematoma is located between the dura mater and the *(arachnoid membrane? cranial bones?).* The torn vessels are likely to be *(arteries? veins?),* which bleed relatively *(rapidly? slowly?).*

C4. Discuss infections of the central nervous system (CNS) in this exercise.

(a) Infection of the brain is known as _____, whereas infection of the spinal cord is _____.

Encephalitis   Meningitis   Myelitis

(b) Circle the two major routes by which CNS infections occur:

(1) Via a lumbar puncture

(2) By spread of infection from vertebrae or skull bones

(3) Via a blood-borne infection that crosses the blood-brain barrier

(4) Through surgery

(c) Meningitis typically spreads *(rapidly? slowly?)*. Explain. _____

_____

_____

(d) Write B for bacterial or V for viral next to characteristics of each form of meningitis.

(d1) Likely to be more severe and possibly fatal: _____

(d2) A lumbar puncture will reveal presence of lymphocytes and normal glucose in CSF: _____

(d3) CSF is cloudy and contains enormous numbers of neutrophils, elevated protein, and low glucose: _____

(d4) Causes include the meningococcus and *Hemophilus influenzae*: _____

(e) Identify the following signs of acute bacterial meningitis:

Brudzinski's sign   Fever and chills
Kernig's sign   Nuchal rigidity
Petechiae

(e1) Neck stiffness: _____

(e2) Rash found on most persons with meningococcal meningitis: _____

_____

(e3) Hip and knee flexion when the neck is flexed: _____

(f) In addition to antibiotics, which other class of drugs is used to combat the effects of meningitis? _____ State a rationale for this treatment. _____

_____

_____

(g) Most cases of encephalitis are *(bacterial? viral?)*. Signs and symptoms typically *(do? do not?)* include fever and nuchal rigidity.

C5. Name the types of cells in each category that can develop into brain tumors.

Breast cancer cells   Meningeal cells
Neurons   Neuroglia: astrocytes
Neuroglia: ependymal   Pineal cells
  cells   Pituitary cells
Prostate cancer cells

(a) Primary tumors of CNS tissue:

_____, _____, _____

(b) Primary tumors of non-CNS tissue:

_____, _____, _____

(c) Secondary (metastatic) tumors:

_____, _____

C6. Choose the two true statements about brain tumors.

(a) Benign brain tumors **cannot** cause death.

(b) Most primary brain tumors in adults are **astrogliomas**.

(c) Many manifestations of brain tumors are **similar** to those of head injuries or infections.

(d) Meningiomas typically are **malignant** with **rapid** growth.

C7. Defend or dispute this statement: "Because the brain has no pain receptors, pain is not a symptom of a brain tumor." _____

_____

_____

_____

_____

_____

_____

C8. Choose the two true statements about diagnosis and treatment of brain tumors.

(a) A funduscopic examination checks for the presence of **papilledema**.

(b) Computed tomography scans are **more** sensitive in detecting brain tumors than are MRI scans.

(c) Most brain tumors **do** cause abnormal EEGs.

(d) Surgery is **rarely** a part of the initial management of brain tumors.

D. SEIZURE DISORDERS (pages 1189–1194)

D1. List several possible signs and symptoms of seizures. _____

_____

_____

Explain why manifestations vary from person to person.

_____

_____

D2. Circle the two true statements about seizures.

(a) Seizures are **rare** disorders.

(b) Seizures are **syndromes, not diseases.**

(c) Seizures may be caused by **decrease** of inhibitory neurotransmitters such as GABA.

(d) The **ictal** period is the time between seizures.

(e) A provoked seizure is also known as a **primary** fever.

D3. Complete this exercise about seizures.

(a) Kyle, age 18 months, has a seizure preceded by a fever. In children, fever *(is? is not?)* a common antecedent of seizure. Anticonvulsant drugs *(are? are not?)* likely to exert side effects on young children.

(b) List six systemic or metabolic disorders that can provoke seizure.

_____

_____

_____

_____

_____

_____

(c) A simple partial seizure *(does? does not?)* involve loss of consciousness, and it involves *(one? both?)* hemisphere(s).

(d) Generalized-onset seizures *(do? do not?)* involve unconsciousness with effects on *(one? both?)* hemisphere(s). This type of seizure is the most *(common? rare?)* type in children.

(e) Indicate whether the following manifestations of seizures are autonomic (A), motor (M), or sensory (S) alterations:

(e1) Flushing, excessive sweating, and change in blood pressure: ___

(e2) "Crawling" sensations: ___

(e3) "Jacksonian seizure": ___

(f) How does an aura or prodrome relate to seizures? _____

_____

During an aura or prodrome, the person *(is? is not?)* conscious.

(g) *(Clonic? Tonic?)* seizures involve alternating rhythmic contractions and relaxations of muscles.

D4. Identify the types of generalized-onset seizures.

Absence   Atonic
Myoclonic   Tonic-clonic

(a) Formerly called "grand mal" seizures; unconsciousness, incontinence, and impaired respirations may accompany dramatic muscle movements; phenobarbital is used for treatment: _____

(b) Called "drop attacks" related to loss of muscle tone; this type of seizure is highly resistant to therapy: _____

(c) Brief blank stare and unresponsiveness along with lip smacking are signs; may be treated with clonazepam:_____

D5. Complete this exercise on diagnosis and treatment of seizure disorders.

(a) Electroencephalograms *(are? are not?)* helpful in diagnosing seizures.

(b) State the first rule of treatment during a seizure. _____

_____

(c) Explain how monotherapy can help patients with seizures. _____

_____

_____

D6. Define *status epilepticus.* _____

_____

_____

E. DEMENTIAS (pages 1194–1197)

E1. Explain why depression must be ruled out in diagnosing dementia.

_____

_____

_____

_____

_____

E2. Select the term that fits the correct description related to Alzheimer's disease (AD).

Amyloid B-peptide   Acetylcholine
Amyloid precursor protein   Cortical atrophy
Neuritic plaques   Neurofibrillary
Sundown syndrome   tangles

(a) Indicated by narrowing of gyri and widening of sulci: _____

(b) Tendency of patients with stage 2 AD to wander, particularly in the early evening:

_____

(c) Fibrous proteins arranged in helical fashion within abnormal neurons of patients with AD: _____

(d) Patches of parts of degenerating neurons wrapped around amyloid; found in the hippocampus and other brain areas of patients with AD: _____

(e) A neurotransmitter required for memory; decreased in AD: _____

(f) A large protein that appears to be required for normal cytoskeleton; mutation of the gene for this chemical is associated with a hereditary form of early-onset AD:

_____

E3. The incidence of Alzheimer's disease is *(high? low?)* in people with Down syndrome. Explain.

_____
_____
_____

E4. Identify whether the following descriptions are characteristics of stage 1, 2, or 3 Alzheimer's disease.

(a) Confusional stage likely to last for several years; client may become hostile and abusive: ___

(b) Short-term memory loss with anomia; mild changes in personality: ___

(c) Inability to communicate; incontinence of bowel and bladder: ___

E5. Briefly describe diagnosis of Alzheimer's disease.

_____
_____
_____

E6. Identify each type of dementia according to its major characteristics.

Creutzfeldt-Jakob disease
Multi-infarct dementia
Pick's disease
Huntington's disease
Wernicke-Korsakoff syndrome

(a) Related to atrophy of frontal and temporal lobes; may involve echolalia, apathy, and hypotonia: _____

(b) Associated with vitamin B deficiency in alcoholics; severely affects recent memory and eye muscles: _____

(c) A rare autosomal dominant disorder that causes movement disorders (chorea and later rigidity), personality changes, and dementia:

_____

(d) A rare dementia transmitted by infective proteins known as prions; has a rapid progression; affects personality and motor coordination: _____

(e) Vascular dementia; incidence is greater in persons with hypertension: _____

CHAPTER 51

Sleep and Sleep Disorders

■ Review Questions

A. NEUROBIOLOGY OF SLEEP (pages 1201–1206)

A1. Describe several functions accomplished by sleep.

_____

_____

_____

A2. Explain roles of the following structures in the sleep-wake cycle.

(a) Reticular formation _____

_____

_____

(b) Thalamocortical loop _____

_____

_____

A3. Circle correct answers in each statement about brain waves.

(a) Amplitude of brain waves refers to the *(height? width?)* of waves.

(b) Brain waves at 10 Hz/sec have a *(higher? lower?)* frequency than do waves at 1 Hz/sec.

(c) Marty's brain waves are more likely to be of *(lower? higher?)* frequency when he is awake with his eyes closed (compared with when his eyes are open).

A4. Complete this exercise about types of brain waves seen in electroencephalograms (EEGs).

Alpha   Beta

Theta   Delta

(a) Arrange from highest to lowest frequency:

_____, _____, _____, _____

(b) Waves typical of a person who is awake with eyes open: _____

(c) Brain waves typical of deep sleep (stages 3 and 4): _____, _____

A5. Write *non-REM* or *REM* next to the descriptions of each of these types of sleep.

(a) Stages 1, 2, 3, and 4: _____

(b) Period of vivid, colorful, emotional dreaming: _____

(c) Heart rate, blood pressure, and respirations are relatively high; breathing is more irregular: _____

(d) Skeletal muscle movements are more active: _____

(e) Relatively short phase early in the night but increases in length as the night goes on: _____

A6. Refer to textbook Figure 51-3 (right side) and fill in the stages of sleep on blank lines to show the correct sequence in a normal sleep pattern. Choose from these answers.

1   2   3   4   REM

Stage 1 → 2 → 3 → ____ → ____ → ____

→ ____ → 2 → 3 → ____ → ____ → ____

→ ____ → ____

A7. Identify characteristics of stages 1, 2, 3, or 4 of non-REM sleep.

(a) Periods of deepest sleep: ___ and ___

(b) Longest stage of non-REM sleep: ___

(c) Person can be most easily awakened; this stage is commonly altered in sleep disorders: ___

A8. Explain why REM sleep is called *paradoxical sleep*.

_____

_____

_____

A9. Define these terms related to sleep.

(a) Circadian rhythms

_____

_____

(b) Entrainment

_____

_____

(c) Suprachiasmatic nucleus (SCN)

_____

_____

A10. Melatonin is released by the _____ gland during the *(day? night?)*. Describe its function.

_____

_____

B. SLEEP DISORDERS (pages 1206–1214)

B1. Mr. Strauss is visiting a sleep disorder clinic. Complete this exercise about the experience he is likely to have.

(a) Before his visit, Mr. Strauss is asked to fill out a sleep diary for 1 to 2 *(days? weeks?)*. List components of such a diary. _____

_____

(b) Define polysomnography and list four components of this study.

_____

_____

_____

_____

Which types of movements are reported by the electro-oculogram (EOG) during Mr. Strauss' overnight stay at the clinic? _____ What information does pulse oximetry provide? _____

(c) Mr. Strauss receives a multiple sleep latency test (MSLT) during the *(night of? day after?)* his night at the clinic. Sleep latency refers to the amount of time from the point at which lights are turned out until _____. This time normally is ___ minutes or more. What is indicated by Mr. Strauss' sleep latency period of 3 minutes? _____

_____

B2. Choose the two true statements about dyssomnias.

(a) Blind persons are **more** likely than sighted persons to experience sleep disorders.

(b) The effects of jet lag **increase** in proportion to the number of time zones crossed.

(c) Circadian rhythm is likely to take **longer** to resynchronize for a flight from New York to Los Angeles than for one from Los Angeles to New York.

(d) Insomnia is a **rare** sleep disorder among adults.

B3. Describe signs and symptoms of sleep disorders in night-shift workers. _____

_____

B4. Identify the sleep disorder that fits each person described below.

Acute insomnia	Advanced sleep phase
Chronic insomnia	syndrome
Delayed sleep phase	Narcolepsy
syndrome	

(a) Kay, age 56 years, falls asleep each night between 8:30 and 9 PM. She wakes up feeling refreshed each morning at approximately 5 AM: _____

(b) Elizabeth, age 15 years, is awake until 2 AM to 3 AM each night; she has difficulty getting up each morning for school, and she falls asleep in classes: _____

(c) Gladys, age 82 years, awakens frequently throughout the night because of arthritis pain and occasional bouts of angina:

_____

(d) Heidi, age 34 years, falls asleep during team meetings; often while she is speaking she lapses into unrelated verbiage; her daytime sleepiness occurs even if she has had a full night's sleep: _____

(e) Danielle, age 20 years, has been distraught by the breakup of a relationship last week; she "can't get to sleep at night" and has been "in a terrible mood and falling asleep at work every day": _____

B5. List several suggestions to help Danielle (Question B4[e]) achieve a more total state of wakefulness each morning. _____

_____

_____

_____

B6. Discuss Heidi's sleep disorder (Question B4[d]) in this exercise.

(a) Persons with narcolepsy are likely to have a *(faster? slower?)* than normal onset of REM sleep as well as a *(long? short?)* sleep latency.

(b) Episodes of cataplexy that Heidi experiences are periods of muscle *(spasms? weakness?)* similar to those of *(REM? non-REM?)* sleep.

(c) Describe a possible role of hypocretin in narcolepsy. _____

_____

_____

B7. Describe examples of sleep disorder treatment in each category.

(a) Behavioral therapies _____

_____

(b) Pharmacologic treatment

_____

_____

B8. Circle the correct term in each statement.

(a) Time asleep compared to time in bed is known as sleep (*efficiency? hygiene? latency?*).

(b) Establishing a regular wake-up time and a comfortable sleeping environment are examples of sleep (*efficiency? hygiene? latency?*).

(c) (*PLMD? RLS?*) involves movement of legs in response to a "creeping" or "crawling" sensation. First-line drugs for these patients are (*anticholinergic? dopaminergic?*) drugs.

B9. Circle the factors that are associated with obstructive sleep apnea.

(a) Alcohol use
(b) Middle-to-older age
(c) Obesity with thick neck
(d) Snoring
(e) Female
(f) Daytime sleepiness
(g) Male impotence
(h) Hypotension

B10. Select the parasomnia that fits each description.

Enuresis   Nightmares
Somnambulism   Sleep terrors

(a) Accompanied by sudden, loud, terrified screaming: _____

(b) Aimless wandering in sleep with possible furniture rearrangement activity:

_____

(c) Bed-wetting: _____

(d) May be early signs of brain tumor; increased incidents in elderly persons with cardiac problems: _____,

_____

(e) Common in children; these behaviors are typically outgrown: _____,

_____, _____

B11. Choose the two true statements about parasomnias.

(a) Most nightmares take place during non-REM sleep.

(b) The incidence of nightmares is **greater** among persons with post-traumatic stress disorder (PTSD).

(c) Sleepwalking and sleep terrors typically occur during stages 3 and 4 sleep within the **first third** of the night.

(d) Efforts **should** be made to interrupt sleepwalking episodes.

C. SLEEP AND SLEEP DISORDERS IN CHILDREN AND THE ELDERLY (pages 1214–1216)

C1. Annabelle, age 1 week, is likely to sleep about _____ hours a day. Typically, about (*one fourth? one half?*) of Annabelle's sleep is REM. By the age of 8 months, Annabelle is likely to sleep a total of ____ hours a night with a(n) (*increase? decrease?*) in REM sleep. By age ____ years, she is likely to sleep 8 hours a night.

C2. In both sleepwalking and sleep terrors, autonomic nerve activities such as tachycardia and sweating are likely to (*increase? decrease?*); children (*are? are not?*) likely to have memories of the events.

(a) The onset of sleep terrors typically is between ages _____ years; sleep terrors (*are? are not?*) likely to resolve by adolescence. Describe the appearance of a child in the midst of a sleep terror.

_____

_____

(b) Episodes of sleepwalking usually last approximately _____ minutes.

C3. Choose the two true statements about sleep disorders in elderly persons.

(a) Complaints of chronic sleep complaints among elderly are **common.**

(b) Older adults typically experience **more** deep sleep (stages 3 and 4) than younger persons.

(c) Older adults typically achieve **less** nighttime sleep than younger persons.

(d) The incidences of sleep apnea, RLS, and PLMD are **lower** in older adults than in younger persons.

C4. List several possible causes of sleep disorders in elderly persons. _____

_____

_____

_____

CHAPTER 52

Neurobiology of Thought, Mood, and Anxiety Disorders

■ Review Questions

A. EVOLUTION IN UNDERSTANDING OF MENTAL ILLNESS (pages 1219–1222)

A1. Psychiatric disorders include alterations in

_____, _____, or _____.

A2. Discuss "nature vs. nurture" theories in causation of mental illness.

_____

_____

_____

A3. Identify advances that have led to a better understanding of mental illness.

Diagnostic Statistical
   Manual of Mental
   Disorders (DSM-IV)

Genetic studies
Imaging studies
Psychotherapy

(a) Twin studies are examples: _____

(b) Lists criteria that can accurately predict whether a person has a particular mental illness _____

(c) Client-therapist relationship elucidates and treats mental disorders: _____

(d) Techniques such as magnetic resonance imaging or computed tomography scans that permit correlation of brain structures (including blood flow and metabolic rate) with symptomatic presentations: _____

_____

A4. Briefly trace the history of perspectives on mental illness. Include the relationship between deinstitutionalization and homelessness of the mentally ill, and the significance of chlorpromazine.

_____

_____

_____

A5. Choose the two true statements related to mental illness and its diagnosis.

(a) Magnetic resonance imaging is an imaging technique that **can** distinguish gray matter from white matter.

(b) Positive emission tomography (PET) is **less** expensive than single-photon emission computed tomography (SPECT).

(c) Concordance of mental disorders such as schizophrenia is **higher** for fraternal twins than for identical twins.

(d) Epidemiological studies have indicated that **both** genetic and environmental factors contribute to mental illness.

A6. Identify mechanisms of action of the following categories of antidepressants that permit neurotransmitters to linger longer in synapses.

Monoamine oxidase inhibitors (MAOIs)
Selective serotonin reuptake inhibitors (SSRIs)
Tricyclic antidepressants (TCAs)

(a) Inhibit reuptake of serotonin and norepinephrine into presynaptic neurons:

_____

(b) Block reuptake of serotonin into presynaptic neurons: _____

(c) Reduce destruction of norepinephrine and serotonin within synapses: _____

B. ANATOMIC AND NEUROCHEMICAL BASIS OF BEHAVIOR (pages 1222–1225)

B1. Identify functions of cerebral lobes in this exercise.

Frontal
Parietal

Occipital
Temporal

(a) Ability to integrate different types of sensory input and to filter out extraneous background stimuli: _____

(b) Ability to integrate auditory and spatial information required for recognizing the familiar: _____

(c) Reception and interpretation of visual experiences, including depth perception:

_____

(d) Abstract thinking, intellectual insights, judgment, problem solving: _____

(e) Language and speech: _____

(f) Control of impulses, aggression, and sexual expression: _____

(g) Aspects of emotional responses: _____ and _____

(h) Memory: _____ and _____

B2. Identify functions of the limbic system and related structures.

Amygdala   Hippocampus   Hypothalamus

(a) Involved with encoding, consolidating, and retrieving memories: _____

(b) Located deep within the temporal lobe; important in emotional function and for modulating affective responses, sexual arousal, and aggression: _____

(c) Not part of the limbic system but extensively connected to it; regulates autonomic functions, hunger, sleep-rest, sexual drives, and release of many hormones: _____

B3. Describe integrative processes in this exercise.

(a) Nick's perfecting of his fencing skills is an example of *(explicit? implicit?)* learning, whereas his acquiring an understanding of neurotransmitters is an example of *(explicit? implicit?)* learning.

(b) Review the steps in the transmission of an impulse across a synapse (Chapter 47, Question B4, page 242 of the Study Guide).

(c) Arrange in correct sequence the steps in the processing of information that begins as you observe an apple on the table:

Amyg = Amygdala receive information and may respond emotionally

Fro = Frontal lobe receives essential information about the apple

Hip = Hippocampus deposits information into short-term memory and groups input for memory encoding

Par = Parietal lobe filters out extraneous background information

Pre = Prefrontal association cortex integrates the new sensory input with long-term memories

Thal = Thalamus receives sensory information and determines if it is "safe" (nonthreatening)

_____ → _____ → _____ → _____
_____ → _____ → _____

B4. Relate the following neurotransmitters to mental illnesses.

Acetylcholine   Norepinephrine
Dopamine   and epinephrine
Gamma-aminobutyric acid   Serotonin

(a) Implicated in anxiety disorders:

_____

(b) Underactivity related to some depressions; antidepressants can increase activity of these chemicals: _____, _____

(c) Underactivity related to obsessive-compulsive disorder (OCD): _____

(d) Underactivity implicated in Alzheimer's disease: _____

(e) Overactivity related to schizophrenia:

_____

C. DISORDERS OF THOUGHT AND VOLITION: SCHIZOPHRENIA (pages 1225–1228)

C1. Describe the meaning and incidence of schizophrenia in this exercise.

(a) This disorder often is referred to as "split personality." What is the true meaning of schizophrenia? _____

_____

(b) Circle factors that increase the risk for schizophrenia:

(1) History of attention deficit disorder by age 4 years

(2) Having a mother who is schizophrenic

(3) Having a birth date in July

(4) Being male

(c) Circle the two phases of life when onset of schizophrenia is greatest:

(1) 5 to 15 years

(2) 20 to 35 years

(3) 43 to 53 years

(4) 66 to 76 years

(d) Currently, an estimated ____ % of homeless persons are schizophrenic. Write a rationale for this statistic. _____

_____

_____

_____

C2. What is the meaning of the terms *positive* or *negative* manifestations of schizophrenia?

_____

_____

Write *P* next to positive symptoms and *N* next to negative symptoms of schizophrenia.

(a) Apathy and flat affect: _____

(b) Hallucinations and delusions: _____

C3. Select the term that best fits each description of schizophrenic manifestations.

Alogia   Anhedonia
Delusions   Derailment and tangentiality
Echolalia   Echopraxia
Hallucinations Neologisms
Word salad

(a) Bridget states, "Kentucky shoe walks loud noise mushed leather tree far now":

_____

(b) When Bridget is asked to tell about her day, she changes the subject 15 times within 2 minutes: _____

(c) Yvonne sits rigidly and says nothing for hours: _____

(d) Yvonne no longer enjoys listening to her favorite classical music: _____

(e) Tom believes that he is an alien from the "flaming cauldron of fire deep within Mount St. Helen": _____

(f) Tom explains that he heard the "newsman on national TV" tell him that firebirds are rising from the cauldron and coming to destroy him: _____

C4. Identify the types of schizophrenia in each case.

Catatonic   Disorganized   Paranoid

(a) Yvonne's rigid posturing, alogia, and anhedonia are signs of _____ schizophrenia.

(b) Tom's belief that the firebirds are out to get him is a sign of _____ schizophrenia.

(c) Bridget appears unkempt, cannot dress herself appropriately, and spends her day wandering aimlessly picking food from trash barrels: _____ schizophrenia

C5. Circle the two true statements related to schizophrenia.

(a) To meet DSM-IV criteria for schizophrenia, symptoms such as those in Questions C3 and C4 must be present for at least 1 **year**.

(b) **Atrophy** of brain tissue and **increase** in the size of ventricles are found with this disorder.

(c) Schizophrenic brains are likely to have an **increase** in dopamine receptors.

(d) Dopamine **agonists** are likely to be effective antipsychotic drugs.

D. DISORDERS OF MOOD (pages 1228–1230)

D1. Complete this exercise about mood disorders.

(a) List two or more examples of mood disorders. _____

_____

_____

(b) Mood disorders are *(rare? common?)* conditions worldwide, and the incidence appears to be *(increasing? decreasing?).* Studies indicate that depression is *(more? less?)* likely in persons with a family history of depression and also in *(African Americans? whites and Hispanics?).*

(c) Dysthymia is a *(mild? severe?)* form of depression with a duration of at least 2 *(months? years?).*

(d) Persons with seasonal affective disorders (SAD) experience more depression in months when days are *(long? short?).*

(e) Episodes of depression and mania alternate in *(bipolar? unipolar?)* disorders. The onset of bipolar disorder is more likely to occur in people in their *(20s? 60s?).*

D2. List 10 or more signs or symptoms of depression. _____

_____

_____

_____

_____

For a diagnosis of a major depressive episode, at least ____ of these manifestations must be present for a period of at least ___ weeks.

D3. Contrast atypical (A) with melancholic (M) depression in this exercise.

  (a) Adrienne's depression is worse as the day goes on; she sleeps more than she ever has, and she is overeating and gaining weight:

  ___

  (b) Madeline's depression is worse in the morning; she wakes up "at the crack of dawn" and can't get back to sleep; she is agitated, cannot eat, is losing weight, and feels no joy in life: ___

D4. Draw arrows to indicate whether each factor increases ↑ or decreases ↓ with depression.

  (a) Volume and activity of gray matter in the prefrontal cerebral cortex: ____

  (b) Function in temporal lobes: ____

  (c) Brain levels of serotonin (5-HT) and norepinephrine: ____

  (d) During depressive episodes, thyroid hormone ($T_3 T_4$) levels: ____

  (e) During depressive episodes, cortisol levels erratically: ____

D5. In the manic state of bipolar disorder, the mood is *(depressed? elevated or expanded?)*. List seven or more specific manifestations of mania.

  _____

  _____

  _____

D6. Left untreated, bipolar episodes typically become *(more? less?)* severe with age.

D7. Describe the overall effect of the medications, such as SSRIs, TCAs, and MAOIs, that are used to treat mood disorders.

  _____

  _____

  _____

E. ANXIETY DISORDERS (pages 1230–1232)

E1. Complete this exercise about anxiety disorders.

  (a) Such disorders are very *(common? rare?)*, affecting approximately ____ % of the population. There *(is? is not?)* a known genetic defect related to anxiety disorders.

  (b) State the common features of all anxiety disorders. _____

  _____

  _____

E2. Identify the anxiety disorder in each case.

  Generalized anxiety disorder
  Obsessive-compulsive disorder
  Panic disorder
  Post-traumatic stress disorder
  Social anxiety disorder

  (a) Julia is unable to socialize at all; she fears that she will "do everything wrong, and everyone will just be watching me and laughing": _____

  (b) Jack must lock and unlock the door handle five times when he goes into his apartment; he meticulously opens a new bar of soap each time he washes his hands; he carefully walks around cracks on sidewalks:

  _____

  (c) Dale has worried incessantly for almost a year; his muscles are always tense; he continuously scans all around himself to check for attackers: _____

  (d) Katharine feels lightheaded as if she will faint; she is short of breath and her "heart is pounding"; she states, "I know I'll die if I can't get out of this place" (a grocery store):

  _____

E3. Answer questions about the cases in Question E2.

  (a) In Jack's OCD (Question E2[b]), his repeated acts are *(obsessions? compulsions?)*. There *(is? is not?)* evidence of anatomical brain change in persons with OCD. Circle the two treatments most likely to help Jack:

  (1) Electroconvulsant shock therapy

  (2) GABA inhibitors

  (3) Lithium

  (4) Selective serotonin reuptake inhibitors (SSRIs)

  (5) Tricyclic antidepressants (TCAs)

  (b) Most panic attacks, such as Katharine's, last *(15 to 30 minutes? 3 to 4 hours? 3 to 4 days?)*. She sees a therapist and begins psychotherapy and starts taking an SSRI medication. This drug is likely to be fully effective in approximately 3 to 4 *(days? weeks? months?)*.

CHAPTER 53

Control of Special Senses

■ Review Questions

A. THE EYE AND VISUAL FUNCTION
(pages 1237–1249)

A1. Arrange the following structures related to the eye in correct sequence.

(a) From outside to inside of the eyeball:

Retina   Sclera
Uveal tract (or vascular layer)

_____ → _____ → _____

(b) Bones of the orbit from superior to inferior:

Frontal   Maxillary   Sphenoid

_____ → _____ → _____

(c) From first to last in the pathway of tears:

Lacrimal glands and ducts
Medial canthus
Nasolacrimal duct

_____ → _____ →

_____

(d) From anterior to posterior:

Anterior cavity   Cornea
Lens   Posterior cavity

_____ → _____ →

_____ → _____

A2. Identify the answer that fits each description.

Aqueous humor   Canthus
Conjunctiva   Lysozyme
Meibomian glands   Optic foramen
Palpebrae   Pupil
Tarsal plate   Vitreous body

(a) Membrane covering the anterior of the eyes and lining the eyelids: _____

(b) Opening in the sphenoid bone for the optic nerve and ophthalmic artery: _____

(c) Eyelids: _____

(d) Antibacterial enzyme in tears: _____

(e) Points at medial and lateral corners of the eye where eyelids meet: _____

(f) Dense connective tissue that forms interior of eyelid: _____

(g) A hole surrounded by the iris: _____

(h) Gel-like substance that fills the posterior cavity and gives spherical structure to the eyeball: _____

A3. Complete this exercise about the middle layer (uveal tract) of the eye and related structures.

(a) All of the following are parts of the uveal tract except:

Choroid   Ciliary muscle   Ciliary
Iris   Lens   processes

(b) The part of the uveal tract that makes eyes brown, blue, or gray is the _____.

(c) State a function of the melanocytes present in the choroid layer._____
_____

(d) The choroid is *(highly? not?)* vascular. State the significance. _____
_____

(e) Contraction of the ciliary muscle changes the *(lens shape? pupil diameter?)*, whereas the iris regulates *(lens shape? pupil diameter?)*.

(f) *(Sympathetic? Parasympathetic?)* nerves carried in the *(oculomotor? optic?)* nerves stimulate constrictor (or sphincter) muscles of the iris. These nerves originate in the Edinger-Westphal nucleus located in the *(medulla? midbrain? pons?)*.

(g) Arrange in correct sequence the pathway of aqueous fluid:

Anterior chamber (of anterior cavity)
Ciliary processes
Trabeculae and canal of Schlemm
Posterior chamber (of anterior cavity)

_____ →

_____ →

_____ →

_____

(h) The lens is attached to the ciliary body by means of _____.

A4. Discuss processes involved as you look at a bird in a distant tree and then to the bird feeder just outside your window.

(a) Focusing images on the retina requires bending (or changing direction) of light rays, a process known as _____. Explain how light rays are refracted as they pass though the eye. _____
_____
_____

(b) As you focus from far to near, the anterior of your lens must be made more *(flat? rounded or convex?)*. *(Ciliary? Iris?)* muscles perform this process, which is known as
_____.

(c) If your eyeball is too long, the image of the bird (or feeder) will be focused *(anterior? posterior?)* to your retina. You would have the condition known as *(myopia? hyperopia?)*, also known as _____ sightedness because you can see near items but not those far away. *(Biconcave? Biconvex?)* lenses or radial keratotomy can correct this disorder.

(d) Other processes that increase your visual acuity as you focus on a nearby object are *(constriction or miosis? dilation or mydriasis?)* of the pupil (by contraction of _____ muscles) and *(widening? narrowing?)* of the palpebral slit to control light entering your eye.

(e) As you age, your lens will become *(thicker? thinner?)* and less able to accommodate; this condition is known as _____opia. Cycloplegia is a condition in which the ciliary muscle is *(hyperactive? paralyzed?)*. Identify one situation in which cycloplegia is induced purposely._____
_____

A5. Refer to textbook Figure 53-9 and complete this exercise about the retina.

(a) The top of the figure (labeled A) is most *(anterior? posterior?)* within the eye. Except for layer A (which is the choroid), all other parts of the figure form the *(retina? sclera?)*.

(b) State two reasons the proximity of the choroid to the retina is significant.
_____
_____

(c) Light passes from layer *(B to E? E to B?)* in the figure, whereas nerve impulses pass from *(B to E? E to B?)* and ultimately exit the eye in the _____ nerve.

(d) Arrange from first to last the neurons in the pathway of nerve impulses:

Bipolar layer   Ganglion layer
Photoreceptor layer

_____ →_____
→_____

(e) In which layer of retinal cells are rods and cones? _____ Which layer forms axons that become the optic nerve? _____ (Choose answers from A5[d].)

A6. Write C next to descriptions of cones and R next to descriptions of rods.

(a) Three types (for red, green, and blue) allow for color vision: ___

(b) Decomposition of the visual pigment rhodopsin occurs when light strikes these cells: ___

(c) Vitamin A deficiency impairs function of these cells: ___

(d) Involved with night (or low-illumination or scotopic) vision in black-gray-white: ___

A7. The fovea centralis is located in the *(anterior? posterior?)* of the eye near the origin of the optic nerve. The fovea is positioned in the center of the "yellow spot," known as the _____. This area *(does? does not?)* contain bipolar and ganglia cells and consists of *(cones? rods? both rods and cones?)*. The fovea is the *(blind spot? point of sharpest vision?)*.

A8. Most color blindness *(does? does not?)* involve defects in genes for all three types of cones. The genes for red-green color blindness are *(autosomal? sex linked?)*; thus, this disorder occurs *(more in females? more in males? equally in females and males?)*. How can a person with red-green color blindness "read" stoplights?
_____
_____
_____

A9. Imagine that the bird feeder (viewed in Question A4) is located slightly to the left of center of the field of view of your left eye. Draw the outline of a bird feeder just above the word "Temporal" on Figure 53-11. Now arrange in correct sequence the structures in the visual pathway that allow you to see that bird feeder.

Left optic nerve   Optic chiasma
Left eye: nasal retina   Right optic tract
Right lateral geniculate nucleus of thalamus
Right optic radiations and occipital cortex

_____	→	_____
→ _____	→	_____
→ _____	→	_____

A10. Refer to Figures 53-11 and 53-12 and determine visual losses in each case.

(a) Sister Martha has a pituitary tumor that has destroyed nasal portions of her optic nerves that cross just anterior to her pituitary. _____

_____

(b) Mr. Jarvi had a stroke that affects his left occipital cortex (areas 17-19). _____

_____

_____

(c) Mr. Frederick had a detachment of the superior portion of the retina of his left eye.

_____

_____

A11. Explain what information you gather when you shine a penlight into the right eye of a client.

_____

_____

_____

B. EYE MOVEMENTS AND CONJUGATE GAZE (pages 1249–1253)

B1. Binocular vision and depth perception require vision in (only one eye? both eyes?). Briefly describe how these processes are accomplished.

_____

_____

_____

B2. Select the extraocular eye muscles that fit these descriptions.

Inferior oblique   Inferior rectus
Levator palpebrae superioris Medial rectus
Lateral rectus   Superior rectus
Superior oblique

(a) Moves the eyeball so that you can look directly up to the sky: _____

(b) The only muscle that moves eyes directly medially (toward your nose = adduction):

_____

(c) When the lateral rectus of your right eye contracts (abducting your right eye), which muscle of your left eye is likely to contract (so that both eyes will be directed toward your right)? Your left _____

(d) Innervated by the right cranial nerve VI (abducens); damage to this nerve results in medial strabismus of the right eye:

_____

(e) Raises the upper eyelid; innervated by the oculomotor nerve: _____

(f) Innervated by cranial nerve III (oculomotor):

_____, _____,

_____, _____

B3. Define optokinetic eye movements.

_____

_____

_____

Complete this exercise about structures and mechanisms that allow your eyes to move in synchrony as they follow moving objects. Choose from these answers.

Conjugate   Convergence
Divergence   Nystagmus
Saccadic

(a) _____ gaze maintains your eyes in a parallel position so that you can steadily follow the path of your young niece as she toddles across the playground or climbs up and down the play equipment. As your niece walks closer to you, _____ movements allow you to continue your focus on her and facilitate depth perception.

(b) As you catch a ride home, you look out of the car. Your eyes attempt to follow what you see by making small, two or three jumping movements per second. These are known as _____ movements, and they continually focus on new scenes so that these scenes do not appear blurred to you. The combination of slow conjugate movements followed by rapid saccadic eye movements is known as _____.

B4. Identify locations of the centers (or nuclei) that control conjugate gaze movements.

Abducens nucleus   Oculomotor nucleus
Trochlear nucleus

(a) Control vertical gaze as you look up or down (involving cranial nerve III supplying superior and inferior rectus muscles):

_____

(b) Control lateral gaze as you look toward your right (involving cranial nerve VI innervating lateral rectus muscle of your right eye): _____

(c) Control torsional gaze as you rotate eyes (involving cranial nerve IV to superior oblique muscle): _____

B5. Explain how these centers (nuclei) work together to coordinate eye movements.

_____
_____
_____

B6. Explain the roles of the following structures in coordination of eye movements.

(a) Superior colliculi of the midbrain

_____
_____
_____

(b) Frontal eye fields of the frontal lobes

_____
_____
_____

C. THE EAR AND AUDITORY AND VESTIBULAR FUNCTION (pages 1253–1261)

C1. Distinguish different aspects of sound waves in this exercise.

(a) The frequency of sound waves is a measure of *(pitch? loudness?)*. The human ear is most sensitive to sound waves between *(20 to 30? 1000 to 3000? 20,000 to 30,000?)* cycles per second (cps) or hertz (Hz).

(b) Loudness of sounds is measured by the *(height? width?)* of sound waves, also known as *(amplitude? frequency?)*. Audible speech sounds fall in the range of *(1 to 5? 10 to 25? 42 to 70?)* decibels (dB).

C2. Select the part of the ear that fits each description.

External ear   Inner ear   Middle ear

(a) The eardrum (tympanic membrane) is located between the _____ and the _____.

(b) Includes the pinna and the external ear canal that is lined with ceruminous glands: _____

(c) Location of ossicles (ear bones), stapedius, and tensor tympani muscles: _____

(d) Site of entry of the eustachian (auditory) tube from the nasopharynx: _____

(e) Location of the cochlea, semicircular canals, and vestibular apparatus, which are collectively called the labyrinth: _____

(f) Location of perilymph, endolymph, and the organ of Corti: _____

C3. Explain the function or significance of each of the following.

(a) Mastoid air spaces_____
_____
_____

(b) The stapedius muscle and reflex _____
_____
_____

(c) Ossicles _____
_____
_____

(d) The difference in surface area of the eardrum compared to that of the oval window_____
_____
_____

C4. Circle the correct answers in these statements about the ear.

(a) The parts of the ear that are inside the skull are located within the *(parietal? temporal?)* bone.

(b) The stapes exerts a piston-like action against the *(oval? round?)* window.

(c) The *(cochlea? vestibule?)* is a snail shell-shaped structure that winds around the bony modiolus.

C5. Refer to Figures 53-16 through 53-19 and arrange structures in the correct sequence.

(a) From first to last in the pathway of sound waves and mechanical action:

External ear canal	Incus
Malleus	Oval window
Perilymph of the	Stapes
scala vestibuli	Tympanic membrane

_____ → _____ →
_____ → _____ →
_____ → _____ →
_____

(b) From superior to inferior within the cochlea:

Basilar membrane
Cochlear duct containing the organ of Corti
   and endolymph
Scala tympani containing perilymph
Scala vestibuli containing perilymph
Vestibular membrane

_____ → _____ →
_____ → _____ →
_____

(c) From superior to inferior within the organ of Corti:

Cochlear nerve fibers   Hair cells
Tectorial membrane

_____ → _____ →
_____

C6. Circle all answers that match a structure with its correct location.

(a) Helicotrema: at basal end of the cochlea

(b) Hair cells that detect high-pitch notes: at the basal end of the cochlea

(c) Cells that detect the loudness of sounds: the inner cells of the organ of Corti

(d) Medial geniculate nucleus: in the thalamus

(e) Primary and association auditory areas of the cortex: occipital lobe

C7. Choose the two true statements about the ear.

(a) Cranial nerve VII conducts impulses from the ear to the brainstem.

(b) Both sides of the brain receive nerve impulses from **both ears**.

(c) The superior olivary nuclei facilitate awareness of the **directions** from which sounds come.

(d) The auditory startle reflex activates **parasympathetic** responses.

C8. Describe two major functions of the vestibular system.

_____
_____
_____

C9. Identify characteristics of components of the vestibular system.

Saccule   Semicircular canals
Utricle

(a) Regulate responses to angular movement, such as riding around curves of a roller coaster: _____

(b) Facilitate awareness of body position, such as lying supine, sitting up, or tilting the head: _____, _____

(c) Function in "righting reflexes" and in reflex bracing of the neck, such as in response to rapid acceleration of a motor vehicle: _____, _____

(d) Located closest to (and continuous with) the cochlea: _____

(e) Contain calcium carbonate crystals (otoliths) that exert weight caused by gravity upon hair cells of the maculae:

_____, _____

(f) Consist of three canals each dilated into an ampulla with stereocilia extending from hair cells into a gelatinous cupula:

_____

C10. Briefly describe neural pathways that help to maintain posture and prevent falls as they extend from the vestibular system to the brain.

_____
_____
_____

C11. Defend or dispute this statement: "Nystagmus is always abnormal." _____

_____
_____

C12. When the head is moved from side to side, the eyes *(do? do not?)* normally move toward the opposite side of the orbit to maintain conjugate gaze on an original fixed point. This is known as the _____'s-head eye response; it demonstrates vestibular responses when brainstem function is *(damaged? intact?)*.

CHAPTER 54

Alterations in Vision

■ Review Questions

A. DISORDERS OF THE ORBIT AND SURROUNDING STRUCTURES (pages 1263–1267)

A1. Identify the disorders according to their descriptions.

Anophthalmos	Blepharitis
Chalazion	Dacryocystitis
Ectropion	Enophthalmos
Exophthalmos	Keratoconjunctivitis sicca
Proptosis	Ptosis
Sjögren's syndrome	Stye

(a) Mrs. Laufman has developed a staphylococcus infection of the upper eyelid:

_____

(b) Mr. Feinberg's left eye droops as a result of a weak levator palpebra muscle:

_____

(c) Mrs. St. George has deeply sunken eyes as a result of extreme weight loss during end-stage cancer: _____

(d) The right eye failed to form within baby Danamarie's right orbit: _____

(e) Newborn Ximena's right nasolacrimal duct has failed to open; tears well up and lead to infection of her lacrimal sac in the medial orbit of her right eye: _____

(f) Mr. Sanchez has an inflammation of eyelid sebaceous glands with swelling, pain, and redness; he is using warm compresses and topical antibiotics on his eyelids:

_____

(g) Professor Sears is having a nontender nodule on his upper lid excised because it is pressing on his eyeball; he has a history of an internal hordeolum at this site:

_____

(h) Ms. Sonnie has been diagnosed with Graves' disease; her eyeballs bulge forward excessively: _____

(i) Ms. Casteneda applies "artificial tears" solutions frequently to treat her "dry eyes":

_____

(j) Mrs. Vigna, age 57 years, has decreased production of tears and saliva, as well as rheumatoid arthritis: _____

A2. Complete this exercise about disorders of protective structures of the eyes.

(a) Damage to cranial nerve *(III? V? VII?)*, such as in _____'s palsy, is most likely to cause paralysis of orbicularis oculi muscle and lead to difficulty closing the eye; tears and saliva production also are reduced.

(b) Injury to cranial nerve *(III? VII?)* is more common. Explain. _____

_____

(c) Explain how tears are protective.

_____

_____

(d) List several conditions that can lead to "dry eyes." _____

_____

_____

B. DISORDERS OF THE CONJUNCTIVA, CORNEA, AND UVEAL TRACT (pages 1267–1270)

B1. Choose the two true statements about conjunctivitis.

(a) Conjunctivitis is a **common** condition and is known as **pink eye.**

(b) Severe eye pain suggests **conjunctivitis** rather than **corneal disease.**

(c) Conjunctivitis involves **enlargement** of blood vessels within the conjunctiva.

(d) Typically, conjunctivitis **does** affect vision.

B2. On Monday evening, Leslea's eyes feel irritated and appear red. By Tuesday morning, Leslea has a yellow-green discharge from both eyes. Complete this exercise about her case.

(a) Leslea sees her physician on Tuesday and reports that (to her knowledge) she has experienced no eye injuries. It is likely that her conjunctivitis is *(bacterial? viral? caused by a foreign body?)*. Explain. _____

_____

(b) A Gram stain and culture indicates infection with *Neisseria gonorrhoeae*. Her conjunctivitis is likely to be *(acute? chronic? hyperacute?)*. Leslea's condition *(is? is not?)* sight threatening. She *(is? is not?)* likely to have antibiotics prescribed.

B3. Complete this exercise about several other types of conjunctivitis.

(a) Viral conjunctivitis typically manifests with *(copious? minimal?)* production of tears and minimal exudate that is *(pus filled? watery?)*.

(b) List conditions or environments linked with viral conjunctivitis. _____

_____

(c) Herpes infections of the conjunctiva typically are *(bilateral? unilateral?)*. Circle medications helpful for herpetic conjunctivitis:

Antibiotics   Antivirals
Corticosteroids

(d) Conjunctivitis caused by *(C. trachomatis A to C? Herpes simplex? N. gonorrhoeae?)* is the leading cause of preventable blindness in the world. Other serotypes of this microbe cause conjunctiva in newborns born by *(cesarean section? vaginal delivery?)*. This form of eye infection occurs in approximately 1 in *(12? 1200?)* newborns in the United States.

(e) Conjunctival redness and swelling of eyelids that occurs 7 days after birth most likely is caused by ophthalmia neonatorum caused by:

(1) Silver nitrate treatment

(2) *N. gonorrhoeae?*

(3) *C. trachomatis*

B4. Abigail has hay fever. Describe the cause, symptoms, and treatment of hay fever.

_____

_____

_____

B5. Describe the cornea and its disorders in this exercise.

(a) The cornea *(is? is not?)* penetrated by blood vessels. State the significance. _____

_____

_____

(b) Sensations of the cornea are carried by the *(optic? trigeminal?)* nerve. The cornea is *(highly? minimally?)* sensitive to pain. List several examples of causes of corneal pain.

_____

_____

_____

(c) Explain how corneal trauma can affect the eye._____

_____

_____

(d) Define keratitis. _____

_____.

Define types of keratitis by matching them to the correct description:

Acanthamoeba   Herpes simplex
M. tuberculosis

(d1) The most common cause of corneal ulceration in the United States; may occur in neonates after vaginal delivery by infected mother: _____

(d2) Protozoan infection in soft contact lens users: _____

(d3) Nonulcerative keratitis: _____

_____

(e) List early symptoms of keratitis.

_____

_____

(f) Kayser-Fleischer rings that accompany Wilson's disease are related to deposits of *(copper? iron? lead?)* in the iris.

(g) Arcus senilis is most likely to occur in *(newborns? adolescents? elderly persons?)*. Typically this condition *(does? does not?)* lead to visual loss.

(h) Uveitis can lead to serious consequences. Explain. _____

_____

_____

C. GLAUCOMA (pages 1270-1274)

C1. Mr. Fuller, who is African American and 33 years old, has received a diagnosis of glaucoma. Complete this exercise about him.

(a) In glaucoma, the volume of *(aqueous humor? vitreous body?)* is excessive. In most cases glaucoma results from *(overproduction? obstructed outflow?)* of aqueous humor. Review the normal pathway of aqueous humor in Chapter 53, Question A3(g).

(b) Mr. Fuller's eyes are checked by a procedure that involves a puff of air blown against his cornea. This is known as *(applanation? noncontact? Schlotz?)* tonometry. Circle the normal intraocular pressure(s): *(10? 17? 28?)* mm Hg. Glaucoma involves a(n) *(increase? decrease?)* in intraocular pressure.

(c) Mr. Fuller's glaucoma is "open-angle," also known as *(wide? narrow?)*-angle glaucoma. Circle factors that increased his risk for this type of glaucoma.

   (1) His age

   (2) Being African American

   (3) Having a father with glaucoma

   (4) Having diabetes mellitus

(d) It is more likely that Mr. Fuller's diagnosis was made *(on an eye screening provided at his work site? as a result of severe pain?)*. Explain._____

   _____

   _____

(e) What causes open-angle glaucoma?

   _____

   _____

   _____

(f) Glaucoma is *(rare? a leading cause of blindness?)* in the United States. Explain how untreated glaucoma could result in blindness for Mr. Fuller. _____

   _____

   _____

(g) How is the condition of Mr. Fuller's optic nerve assessed? *(Funduscopy? Gonioscopy? Tonometry?)* How is the appearance of his optic disk likely to change in glaucoma?

   _____

   _____

(h) Most treatment of open-angle glaucoma is *(surgical? pharmacologic?)*, using *(systemic? topical?)* agents.

(h1) Choose the two classes of drugs that decrease Mr. Fuller's production of aqueous humor:

   Acetylcholine

   Beta blockers

   Carbonic anhydrase inhibitors

   Prostaglandins

(h2) Choose the two classes of drugs that increase outflow of aqueous humor.

   Acetylcholine

   Beta blockers

   Carbonic anhydrase inhibitors

   Prostaglandins

C2. Discuss another form of glaucoma in this exercise.

(a) *(Closed? Open?)*-angle glaucoma results from obstruction of the aqueous humor pathway by the iris. This form of glaucoma occurs in a *(large? small?)* percentage of patients with glaucoma.

(b) Also known as *(narrow? wide?)*-angle glaucoma, this condition is exacerbated by *(constriction? dilation?)* of the iris, which then "bulges" and narrows the angle between the iris and the cornea (text Figure 54-3). List several factors that can trigger episodes of closed-angle glaucoma.

   _____

   _____

(c) List two procedures that can identify a reduced corneal-iris angle. _____

   _____

(d) Circle typical manifestations of closed-angle glaucoma.

   (1) Eye pain

   (2) Blurred vision

   (3) Halos around lights

   (4) Nausea and vomiting

   (5) Excruciating headache

(e) Describe typical treatment for acute closed-angle glaucoma._____

   _____

   _____

D. CATARACTS (pages 1274–1275)

D1. Discuss cataracts in this exercise.

(a) A cataract is a disorder of the *(aqueous humor? cornea? lens? retina?)*. It is much more common in *(younger? older?)* persons. Cataract surgery is very *(common? rare?)*.

(b) List several factors that contribute to development of cataracts. _____

_____

(c) Identify two or more factors that can cause congenital cataracts. _____

_____

_____

D2. Cataracts typically develop *(rapidly? slowly?)*. Describe aging changes in the lens that lead to cataract.

_____

_____

_____

D3. List typical manifestations of senile cataracts.

_____

_____

_____

D4. Discuss treatments of cataracts.

(a) Medical

_____

_____

_____

(b) Surgical

_____

_____

_____

E. DISORDERS OF THE VITREOUS AND RETINA (pages 1275–1282)

E1. Describe the vitreous body (or humor) in this exercise.

(a) Vitreous is *(watery? gel-like?)* and fills about *(one? five?)*-sixth(s) of the eyeball. At what points are vitreous normally attached to the wall of the eyeball? _____

_____

_____

(b) Explain what causes "floaters" in the eyes?

_____

_____

(c) How might vision be disturbed by entrance of blood into the vitreous body?

_____

_____

E2. Identify retinal structures perfused by two different sources of blood supply.

Choriocapillaris of the choroid
Central retinal artery branches

(a) Most posterior portions of the retina, such as pigment cells, rods and cones of the photoreceptor layer, and the all-important fovea: _____

(b) Anterior two layers of the retina (bipolar and ganglion layers): _____

(c) Develops later in fetal life and may not be completed before birth in premature infants:

_____

E3. Explain the clinical significance of the following.

(a) Why funduscopic examination of retinal blood vessels can provide clues about more generalized blood vessel health.

_____

_____

(b) Why cardiac arrest may lead to permanent visual impairment. _____

_____

(c) What is indicated by a "choked disk" seen funduscopically. _____

_____

_____

(d) What is indicated by a cherry-red spot in the fovea surrounded by a pale retina.

_____

_____

_____

E4. Identify retinal disorders that fit each description.

Anopsia
Cotton-wool spots or exudates on the fundus
Detached retina
Macular degeneration
Retinitis pigmentosa
Retinopathy of prematurity
Retinal stroke
Scotoma

(a) Previously called "retrolental fibroplasia" because of growth of fibrous tissue in the vitreous (posterior to the lens), this condition has almost 100% incidence in infants with birth weight < 1.5 pounds:

_____

(b) Hereditary disease causing destruction of rods by a defect in phagocytes of the pigmented layer; manifestations begin with loss of night vision in early youth and ultimately can lead to gross visual loss:

_____

(c) Blindness in one eye; can be caused by occlusion of the central artery of the retina:

_____

(d) Caused by occlusion of branches of the central retinal artery; may result in scotoma:

_____

(e) Local blind spot resulting from ischemia:

_____

(f) Retinal opacities with irregular outlines; result of microhemorrhages, such as in diabetic or hypertensive retinopathies:

_____

(g) May be "wet" or "dry"; causes bilateral loss of central vision; large pale yellow spots ("drusen") suggest greater severity of the disorder; more common in elderly:

_____

(h) May result from shrinking of the vitreous or cataract surgery that exerts traction on the retina; robs photoreceptors of their only blood supply: _____

E5. Choose the two true statements.

(a) Detachment of the photoreceptor layer of the retina from the pigment epithelium of the retina **does not** cause sensory loss.

(b) The central retinal artery is a branch of the **ophthalmic** artery, which in turn is a branch of the **internal carotid** artery.

(c). When neovascularization occurs in response to impaired retinal circulation, the new blood vessels tend to be **stronger** walled than were the original vessels.

(d) In persons with chronic hypertension, retinal arteries **thicken** and appear more **pale** than do normal arteries.

E6. Mrs. Giovanni, age 34 years, has type 2 diabetes and sees her physician about "changes in my vision, especially glare."

(a) She receives a diagnosis of background retinopathy. This disorder involves:

(1) Formation of fragile blood vessels that may grow into the vitreous and obscure vision

(2) Thickening of retinal capillary walls with small hemorrhages confined to the retina and also macular edema

(b) Mrs. Giovanni should have eye examinations performed at least once every (_year? 5 years?_). If she becomes pregnant, the frequency of her eye examinations should (_increase? decrease?_).

(c) Control of her blood cholesterol levels and blood pressure (_is? is not?_) likely to reduce visual impairment in Mrs. Giovanni.

E7. (_Background? Proliferative?_) retinopathy that may accompany diabetes is more sight threatening. Describe two mechanisms of this disorder that can cause blindness.

_____

_____

_____

E8. Arrange from anterior to posterior the location of these hemorrhages.

Intraretinal   Preretinal   Subretinal

_____ → _____ → _____

Which of these conditions is most likely to result from proliferative diabetic retinopathy?

_____

E9. Identify treatments used for retinal disorders.

Cryotherapy   Photocoagulation
Pneumatic retinopexy   Scleral buckling

(a) Treatment for detached retina involving silicone "buckles" that adhere retina to sclera: _____

(b) Injection of gas (in lieu of silicone) to reattach areas of detached retina:

_____

(c) Argon laser applied to leaking microaneurysms or a grid (checkerboard) method used to treat diffuse areas of leakage, for example in patients with diabetic retinopathy: _____

(d) Method to destroy areas of retinal neovascularization that block light pathways, for example for newborns with retinopathy of prematurity or for older adults with the wet form of macular degeneration: _____

F. DISORDERS OF NEURAL PATHWAYS AND CORTICAL CENTERS (pages 1282–1285)

F1. Contrast functions of the primary visual cortex (area 17) and visual association areas (18 and 19).

_____

_____

_____

F2. Explain how persons with scotomas can adapt to them.

_____

_____

_____

F3. Refer to the left side of textbook Figure 54-9 and circle correct answers about visual pathways.

(a) An optic nerve transmits nerve impulses from (one? both?) eye(s), whereas an optic tract carries nerve impulses from (one? both?) eye(s).

(b) In the optic chiasma, axons from the ganglion layer of both retinas (do? do not?) synapse. The term *chiasma* indicates that axons cross here, specifically those from the (nasal? temporal?) portions of the retinas.

(c) A lesion that destroys the entire left optic tract will result in loss of the (right? left?) visual field of (the right? the left? both?) eye(s).

F4. Refer to Figure 54-9 and match terms related to visual defects with their descriptions.

Anopia   Hemianopia
Heteronymous   Homonymous
Quadrantanopia

(a) The same type of visual loss (such as loss of the right visual field) in both eyes:

_____

(b) The opposite type of visual loss in the two eyes: _____

(c) Total blindness in an eye, for example by destruction of an optic nerve: _____

(d) Loss of one quarter of a visual field, such as occurs with partial lesions of an optic radiation or the primary visual cortex:

_____

(e) "Tunnel vision" caused by a pituitary tumor; involves bilateral loss of temporal fields of view or: _____
(See also Chapter 53, Question A10[a].)

F5. Explain what causes the following visual cortex alterations.

(a) Contrecoup injury of the primary visual cortex _____

_____

(b) "Seeing stars" _____

_____

(c) Cortical blindness _____

_____

(d) Visual agnosia _____

_____

_____

F6. Describe simple testing methods that you could use to estimate a client's visual field.

_____

_____

_____

_____

F7. Ms. Billingsly checks pupil reflexes as she assesses her client, Mr. Bellman.

(a) Mr. Bellman has cortical blindness caused by a stroke involving his (anterior? middle? posterior?) cerebral artery. As Ms. Billingsly directs a penlight into Mr. Bellman's right eye, which of his pupils is/are likely to constrict?

(1) The left
(2) The right
(3) Both the left and right
(4) Neither

This result indicates that pupillary reflex requires intact pathways to the (midbrain? optic radiations and cerebral cortex?). This reflex is a simple check on the integrity of the midbrain.

(b) The bilateral pupillary reflex is described as _____. The motor portion of the reflex involves (sympathetic? parasympathetic?) fibers in cranial nerve (III? V? VII?). Destruction of any part of this pathway would cause pupils to remain dilated, a condition known as (miosis? mydriasis?). Mr. Bellman's pupil constriction is known as (miosis? mydriasis?).

G. DISORDERS OF EYE MOVEMENTS
(pages 1285–1288)

G1. Explain how coordinated eye movements of both eyes help you to read the words on this page.

_____

_____

G2. Refer to textbook Figure 54-11 and identify the name of the disorder of eye movements that fits each description.

Amblyopia   Esotropia   Exotropia
Cyclotropia   Diplopia   Hypertropia
Hypotropia   Strabismus

(a) Double vision: _____

(b) Uncoordinated eye movements that result in diplopia: _____

(c) Sometimes called "lazy eye," it involves diminished vision that is uncorrectable by lenses but has no detectable organic cause:

_____

(d) Upward deviation of the eye: _____

(e) Torsional deviation of the eye: _____

(f) Weakness of the right lateral rectus muscle (or damage to CN VI) is likely to lead to medial deviation of that eye, a condition known as: _____ (Figure 54-11A).

G3. Circle correct answers related to strabismus.

(a) In which type of strabismus is there no primary muscle impairment? (_Concomitant [nonparalytic]? Nonconcomitant [paralytic]_)

(b) In which type of strabismus is deviation equal in all directions of gaze? (_Concomitant/nonparalytic? Nonconcomitant/paralytic?_)

(c) The onset of strabismus, particularly the (_paralytic? nonparalytic?_) type, typically is in (_childhood? adulthood?_). By the age of 3 to 6 (_days? weeks? months?_), infants should have synchronized eye movements, with eyes in alignment during all of their waking hours.

(d) Almost all adult strabismus is of the (_paralytic? nonparalytic?_) type. List several causes. _____

_____

_____

G4. Describe three methods for assessing extraocular movements in children.

_____

_____

_____

G5. At what age should children begin treatment for amblyopia? _____ Describe treatment methods.

(a) Patching

_____

_____

(b) Pharmacologic

_____

_____

CHAPTER 55

Alterations in Hearing and Vestibular Function

■ Review Questions

A. ALTERATIONS IN AUDITORY FUNCTION (pages 1291–1302)

A1. Review the anatomy of the external, middle, and inner ear in Chapter 53, Question C2.

A2. List several causes of external ear infection (otitis externa). _____
_____

A3. Choose the two true statements about the external ear.

(a) Most otitis externa infections are caused by gram-**positive** bacteria or fungi.

(b) Pain upon movement of the pinna is **more** likely to be a sign of otitis media (OM) than of otitis externa.

(c) Scratching is likely to **exacerbate** pruritus in the external ear.

(d) Impacted cerumen usually produces no symptoms until the canal is **completely occluded**.

A4. Circle methods that are likely to help prevent or cure OM.

(a) Antibiotics

(b) Antifungals

(c) Corticosteroids

(d) Keeping the external canal warm and moist

A5. Identify structures associated with the middle ear.
Eustachian tube   Ossicles
Tympanic membrane

(a) Three-layered membrane: the outer membrane is continuous with the external ear, and the inner layer is continuous with the middle ear: _____

(b) Tube connecting the nasopharynx with the middle ear: _____

(c) Ear bones that transmit sounds from the eardrum to the oval window: _____

A6. Refer to textbook Figure 55-1 and identify structures seen through an otoscope.

(a) Arrange from superior to inferior:
Cone of light   Handle of the malleus
Pars flaccida

_____ → _____ → _____

(b) Most of the tympanic membrane consists of the pars *(flaccida? tensa?)*.

(c) The apex of the cone-shaped tympanic membrane is known as the *(chorda tympani? umbo?)* and consists of the tip of the handle of the *(malleus? stapes?)*.

A7. Describe the eustachian tubes in this exercise.

(a) List three functions of these tubes.
_____
_____
_____

(b) Explain how eustachian tubes help your ears to "pop" when you experience a change in altitude. _____
_____
_____
_____

(c) The opening of each of these tubes into the nasopharynx normally is *(open? closed?)*. How can this tube be opened? _____
_____

(d) Describe two reasons the eustachian tubes of young children may collapse.
_____
_____

(e) State two reasons infants are more likely to experience OM than are older persons.
_____
_____

A8. Circle the risk factors for OM in Evan, who is 8 months old and bottle fed. He and his 3-year-old brother Devon attend a large suburban day-care center. Devon has a history of three episodes of OM. Evan had AOM with antibiotic treatment earlier this month. Neither their parents nor other close relatives smoke.

A9. Circle the correct answers in these statements about acute otitis media (AOM).

(a) The most common causative agent of AOM is:

(1) *Escherichia coli*

(2) *Moraxella catarrhalis*

(3) Respiratory syncytial virus

(4) *Streptococcus pneumoniae*

(b) Most cases of AOM *(do? do not?)* follow respiratory infections. Describe the likely pathway of the microbes in this infection?

_____

(c) If Evan (Question A8) experiences AOM, which three manifestations are most likely?

(1) Body temperature of 99.0°F

(2) Being fussy at feeding time

(3) Tugging on his affected ear

(4) Rhinitis (runny nose)

(5) Bulging yellow or red eardrum seen by otoscopy

(6) Translucent eardrum with blue fluid or bubbles behind it

(d) Which of the following techniques can isolate a middle ear culture and relieve the pain of AOM? _____ Which measures the degree of mobility of the eardrum? _____

Acoustic reflectometry   Tympanocentesis
Tympanometry   Tympanostomy

A10. Write a rationale for the following treatments of OM.

(a) Why antibiotics—including those given prophylactically—are used judiciously:

_____
_____

(b) Why a switch of prescription to a different antibiotic is in order if no improvement is shown after a 3-day regimen of the first antibiotic: _____
_____
_____

(c) Myringotomy: _____
_____
_____

(d) Tympanostomy with the directive that the child keeps his or her head out of water:

_____
_____

A11. Circle the two true statements about OM.

(a) Recurrent OM is defined as three new AOM episodes within **1 year,** and these accompany almost every upper respiratory infection.

(b) In otitis media with effusion (OME), signs of infection are **severe.**

(c) In both AOM and OME, **hearing loss** may occur.

(d) **Most** cases of OME resolve without treatment within 3 months of onset.

A12. Complete this exercise about the complications experienced by Phillip, who has a history of recurrent OM.

(a) Explain how OM may be related to Phillip's delayed language development.

_____
_____

(b) List three complications of OM that may contribute to Phillip's hearing loss.

_____
_____

(c) Briefly describe two complications that can lead to destruction of some of Phillip's cranial bone tissue. _____
_____
_____
_____
_____
_____

A13. Stephanie is a junior in college and is experiencing gradual hearing loss diagnosed as otosclerosis.

(a) Both her mother and grandfather have this condition, which is an *(autosomal dominant? autosomal recessive? sex-linked?)* disorder.

(b) Arrange in correct sequence the typical events in the progression of this condition.

Bone becomes spongy and soft
Overgrowth of hard bone develops
Reabsorption of bone

_____ → _____ →

_____

(c) Eventually, Stephanie is likely to experience immobilization of her *(malleus? stapes? tympanic membrane?)*. What type of surgery could correct this condition?

_____

(d) A hearing aid *(is? is not?)* likely to help Stephanie.

A14. Choose the two true statements about the inner ear

(a) The inner ear is also known as the **labyrinth**.

(b) **Subjective** tinnitus refers to ringing in the ears in which the sound can be heard by an observer.

(c) Nicotine and caffeine **can** cause tinnitus.

(d) **Profound hearing loss** is defined as a loss greater than 20 to 25 decibels (dB) in adults.

A15. Identify the inner ear disorder that fits each description.

Boilermaker's deafness
Conduction deafness
Presbycusis
Mixed conductive and sensineural hearing loss
Sensineural deafness

(a) Hearing loss that accompanies aging:

_____

(b) External or middle ear conditions:

_____

(c) Disorders affecting the inner ear, auditory pathways, or the primary cortical hearing area: _____

(d) Hearing loss caused by ototoxic drugs:

_____

(e) Ménière's disease: _____

(f) Caused by chronic exposure to intense, reverberating sound: _____

A16. Circle known ototoxic drugs.

Aminoglycoside antibiotics such as kanamycin
Aspirin
Cancer drugs such as cisplatin
Erythromycin
Loop diuretics such as furosemide (Lasix)

A17. Mr. Franklyn, age 79 years, has presbycusis.

(a) His condition is *(common? rare?)* among older adults. Explain why it is underdiagnosed. _____

_____

(b) He is more likely to have difficulty distinguishing:

(1) Vowels (low-pitched sounds), as in "bard," "bird," "bored"

(2) Consonants (high-pitched sounds), as in "sin," "thin," "fin"

(c) In conducting a patient history, the nurse needs to question Mr. Franklyn and also _____. List several questions to be included in a patient history.

_____

_____

_____

(d) Both a Weber test and a Rinne test involve use of _____. In the Weber test, the instrument is placed on Mr. Franklyn's *(forehead? mastoid process?)*, and Mr. Franklyn hears sounds better in the right ear. This result indicates sensineural loss is in the *(right? left?)* ear.

A18. Describe the following diagnostic tests for hearing loss.

(a) ABR: _____

_____

_____

(b) EOAE: _____

_____

_____

A19. List several communication techniques that you can use to be better understood by hearing-impaired persons. _____

_____

_____

_____

A20. Discuss the use of cochlear implants in profoundly deaf persons. _____

_____

_____

A21. Describe Wernicke's area of the brain in this exercise.

(a) This area is located in the dominant hemisphere, usually the *(right? left?)* side, in the *(primary auditory? auditory association?)* cortex.

(b) Circle the manifestations of damage to Wernicke's area:

(1) Inability to speak intelligibly

(2) Inability to read normally

(3) Inability to understand what is spoken or read

(c) In other words, clients with damage to Wernicke's area have *(expressive? receptive?)* aphasia and agnosia of speech.

B. DISORDERS OF VESTIBULAR FUNCTION (pages 1302-1307)

B1. Describe vestibular function in this exercise.

(a) State two functions of the vestibular receptive organs. _____

_____

(b) Describe functions of the following neural connections with the vestibular organs:

(b1) Cerebellum: _____

_____

_____

(b2) CN III, IV, VI: _____

_____

_____

(b3) Chemoreceptor trigger zone: _____

_____

_____

B2. Match vestibular alterations with cases.

Benign positional vertigo   Labyrinthitis
Ménière's disease   Motion sickness
Nystagmus   Subjective vertigo

(a) Elaine exhibits slow-fast-slow eye movements (vestibulo-ocular reflexes) even when her head is held still; this condition is worsened when she is tired:

_____

(b) Jenny is on a boat in a violent storm; her pulse and blood pressure increase, and she is sweating; she becomes nauseous and vomits:

_____

(c) Marie's disorder is caused by excesses of endolymph fluid and manifests with hearing loss, vertigo, and ringing of the ears:

_____

(d) Duanne spins in place a dozen times and then feels dizzy, as if she is falling:

_____

(e) Laurie, a "regular" at the amusement park, feels nauseous as the careening roller coaster curves and dives; she recovers and is ready for more action within a few minutes:

_____

(f) Over the course of an hour, Kathy develops vertigo, is nauseous, and vomits; her condition appears to be an acute vestibular neuritis that completely resolves during the next 10 days: _____

B3. Circle all true statements about inner ear disorders.

(a) Nystagmus is **always** pathologic if it occurs when the head is held still

(b) Most cases of vertigo involve **brainstem (central)** disorders.

(c) The incidence of benign positional vertigo (BPV) **decreases** with age.

(d) In BPV, portions of **otoliths** of the utricle break off and form debris that **increases** sensitivity of a semicircular duct

(e) In the progression of Ménière's disease after initial episodes, **hearing** is likely to worsen and **vertigo** tends to improve.

B4. Explain how the following treatments can improve inner ear disorders.

(a) Low-sodium diet and diuretics for Marie (Question B2[c]) or endolymphatic shunt surgery: _____

_____

_____

(b) Canalith repositioning for Laurie (Question B2[e]): _____

_____

_____

(c) Avoidance of alcohol and aminoglycosides such as streptomycin or gentamicin:

_____

_____

_____

B5. List three possible causes of disorders of central vestibular function. _____

_____

_____

B6. Match tests of vestibular function with descriptions.

Caloric stimulation   Electronystagmography
Romberg test   Rotational tests

(a) A check for balance and postural stability, the person stands with feet together, arms raised forward, and eyes closed:

_____

(b) Electrodes placed lateral to eyes evaluate nystagmus eye movements: _____

_____

(c) Ice water instilled into each ear checks for vestibular response: _____

(d) Rotation in a Barany chair (like a barber's chair) is followed by abrupt stoppage; postrotational reflex nystagmus and related limb movements are measured:

_____

B7. Identify mechanisms of action of drugs used to treat vestibular disorders.

Anticholinergics   Antidopaminergics
Antihistamines

(a) Depress nausea and vomiting; an example is phenothiazines: _____

(b) Depress the vestibular system; examples include scopolamine and atropine:

_____

(c) Depress the illusion of motion; examples include Antivert, Dramamine, Phenergan:

_____

B8. Describe how physical therapists can work with clients to improve vestibular disorders:

_____
_____
_____

CHAPTER 56

Structure and Function of the Skeletal System

■ Review Questions

A. CHARACTERISTICS OF SKELETAL TISSUE (pages 1311-1317)

A1. Describe the skeletal system in this exercise.

(a) List five or more functions of this system.

_____

_____

_____

_____

(b) Contrast the axial with the appendicular skeleton. _____

_____

_____

(c) List types of tissues that form the skeletal system. _____

_____

_____

A2. Contrast collagen (C) and elastic (E) fibers in this exercise.

(a) Formed primarily of elastin, which gives these fibers great stretchability: ____

(b) Fibrous protein that provides great tensile strength to tendons: ____

A3. Identify the type of cartilage that fits each description.

Elastic   Fibrous   Hyaline

(a) The most abundant type of cartilage in the body, it forms most of the fetal skeleton:

_____

(b) Found on the ends of bones (articular cartilage) and connecting ribs to sternum:

_____

(c) Found in areas where flexibility is needed, for example in the external ear: _____

_____

(d) Provides strength and support in intervertebral disks and the pubic symphysis: _____

A4. Complete this exercise about cartilage tissue.

(a) Cartilage _(is? is not?)_ necessary for skeletal growth. Cartilage cells are known as _____cytes. Most cartilage is covered by a membrane known as the _____.

(b) Blood vessels _(do? do not?)_ perfuse cartilage. Explain how cartilage receives its oxygen and nutrients. _____

_____

A5. Refer to textbook Figure 56-2 and describe bone tissue in this exercise.

(a) _(One? Two?)_ third(s) of bone tissue is composed of inorganic salts made primarily of _(calcium? potassium?)_. The remainder of bone includes bone cells, blood vessels, nerves, and _____ fibers.

(b) _(Compact? Cancellous?)_ or trabecular bone is relatively lightweight and forms the bulk of rounded ends of long bones. _(Compact? Cancellous?)_ bone forms the strong outer portion of the shafts of long bones.

(c) Arrange in correct sequence from first to last in bone formation:

Osteoblasts   Osteocytes
Osteogenic cells

_____ → _____ →

_____

(d) Which cells (in Question A5[c]) synthesize collagen and other proteins that make up osteoid (prebone) tissue? _____
These cells then secrete the enzyme _____, which results in calcification of osteoid.

(e) Which cells (in Question A5[c]) are mature bone cells? _____ These cells lie in microscopic lakes known as _(canaliculi? lacunae?)_ and produce bony matrix in concentric layers called _____.

(f) Each unit of 4 to 20 lamellae forms a unit known as a(n) _____ that surrounds a central canal containing _____.

Explain how bone cells in lacunae receive nutrients. _____

_____

_____

(g) Explain how blood vessels reach bone tissue. _____

_____

_____

(h) Osteo_____ are cells that function in the resorption of bone. These cells are formed from *(osteoblasts? monocytes?)* under the influence of the hormone *(calcitonin? PTH?)*.

A6. Explain why tetracycline is contraindicated during pregnancy and in children younger than 6 years of age.

_____

_____

_____

A7. Describe functions of the following membranes attached to bone.

(a) Fibrous periosteum:_____

_____

_____

(b) Osteogenic periosteum:_____

_____

_____

(c) Endosteum:_____

_____

_____

A8. Refer to Table 56-2 and fill in the blanks below with names of the correct chemicals.

Calcitonin   Parathyroid hormone
Vitamin D

(a) _____ and _____ tend to increase the blood level of calcium, whereas _____ decreases the blood level of calcium.

(b) ____ stimulates osteoclasts and bone resorption, whereas _____ inhibits osteoclasts.

(c) Which of these chemicals increase(s) renal excretion of phosphates? _____

(d) _____ is synthesized by the thyroid gland.

(e) Hypocalcemia serves as a trigger for release of the hormone _____, whereas hypercalcemia stimulates release of the hormone _____.

A9. PTH raises the blood level of calcium by drawing calcium from which three sources?

_____

_____

_____

A10. Discuss vitamin D in this exercise.

(a) Vitamin D is a(n) *(amine? steroid?)* hormone. Name three food sources of vitamin D. _____

_____

_____

(b) Name a human organ that synthesizes a relatively inactive form of vitamin D. _____ Identify organs that activate vitamin D. _____ _____.

(c) Explain why elderly persons may be at higher risk for activated vitamin D deficiency. _____

_____

_____

(d) Circle the form of vitamin D that is most potent in intestinal absorption of calcium and promoting action of PTH in activating osteoclasts:

(1) 7-dehydrocholesterol

(2) 25-hydroxyvitamin D_3

(3) 1,25-hydroxyvitamin D_3

(4) 24,25-hydroxyvitamin D_3

(e) PTH and prolactin *(stimulate? inhibit?)* formation of 1,25-hydroxyvitamin D_3, whereas calcitonin *(stimulates? inhibits?)* formation of this active form of vitamin D.

A11. Circle the correct answers in these statements.

(a) There *(are? are no?)* known syndromes of calcitonin excesses or deficiencies.

(b) Salmon calcitonin (CT) is *(more? less?)* potent and clinically effective than human CT. Name one condition for which CT might be prescribed. _____ Explain why._____

_____

_____

(c) In parts of the world or seasons with limited sunlight, human vitamin D production is likely to be *(decreased? increased?)*.

B. SKELETAL STRUCTURES
(pages 1317-1320)

B1. Identify the type of bone that fits each description.

Flat   Irregular
Long   Short

(a) Vertebrae, mandible, and maxillae are examples: _____

(b) Wrist bones are examples; falls on the wrist often lead to fractures because carpals are composed mostly of spongy bone:

_____

B2. Refer to textbook Figure 56-1 and match the part of a long bone with the related description.

Diaphysis   Epiphysis   Metaphysis

(a) Broad, rounded end of a long bone that serves as a site for articulation:

_____

(b) Shaft of a long bone composed primarily of compact bone surrounding the medullary cavity: _____

(c) Located between the diaphysis and the growth plate in bones of young persons:

_____

B3. Circle the correct answers in these statements.

(a) Bones of *(children? adults?)* have relatively more red marrow and less yellow marrow.

(b) *(Ligaments? Tendons?)* connect bone to bone, whereas *(ligaments? tendons?)* connect muscles into periosteum of bones. Ligaments and tendons have a(n) *(abundant? limited?)* blood supply.

(c) *(Diarthroses? Synarthroses?)* are joints with limited or no motion. Which is a joint in which bones are joined by cartilage (as in costosternal joints)?

Synchondrosis   Syndesmosis   Synostosis

(d) Most joints of the body are *(diarthroses? synarthroses?)*; also known as *(cartilaginous? synovial?)* or *(freely movable? immovable?)* joints.

B4. Describe the structure of a synovial joint.

_____
_____
_____

B5. Circle the two true statements.

(a) The synovial membrane **does** normally cover the articular cartilage.

(b) Normal synovial fluid is **clear or pale yellow** and has the consistency of **egg white**.

(c) The synovial membrane has a **rich** blood supply that helps it to heal **rapidly** when injured.

(d) Synovial membranes are **well** innervated by nerve fibers that transmit pain.

B6. Mr. Dennis has an injured right hip, yet he feels pain in his right knee. Explain.

_____
_____
_____

B7. Contrast a bursa with a bunion.

_____
_____
_____

B8. The medial and lateral menisci are located in the *(shoulder? hip? knee?)* joints and are composed of *(fibrous? hyaline?)* cartilage. Explain why menisci are slow to heal if they are torn.

_____
_____
_____

CHAPTER 57

Alterations in Skeletal Function: Trauma and Infection

■ Review Questions

A. INJURY AND TRAUMA OF MUSCULOSKELETAL STRUCTURES (pages 1321–1334)

A1. The musculoskeletal system makes up about ____% of the body. List structures that compose the musculoskeletal system.

_____

_____

_____

A2. Complete this exercise about musculoskeletal injuries.

(a) Trauma is a *(common? rare?)* cause of musculoskeletal injury. Trauma from _____ is the leading cause of death in adults under the age of 45 years.

(b) Most sports injuries in children younger than 15 years that require emergency room care result from *(organized? unorganized?)* sports. Most athletic injuries occur from *(overuse? sudden trauma?)*.

(c) _____ are the most common cause of injury in individuals older than 65 years. Fractures are *(more? less?)* likely in elderly who have osteoporosis. List three bones most likely to be fractured in such falls.

_____

_____

_____

A3. Select the soft tissue injury that fits each description.

Contusion   Hematoma
Laceration   Puncture wounds

(a) Does involve tearing of skin: _____

(b) An injury that does not result in tearing of the skin, although the area may be bruised: _____

(c) Of these injuries, most likely to lead to gas gangrene (tetanus): _____

(d) Large accumulation of blood that causes the area to become "black and blue":

_____

A4. Contrast joint injuries in this exercise.

(a) Ligaments connect *(bones? muscles?)* to bones, and tendons connect *(bones? muscles?)* to bones.

(b) *(Sprains? Strains?)* involve no externally evident injury and heal relatively quickly. Circle regions that are likely sites for strains:

Cervical vertebrae   Elbows
Feet   Lumbar vertebrae
Shoulders

(c) For the first 24 hours after a joint is strained, *(cold? heat?)* should be applied to reduce pain and swelling.

(d) The joint most often sprained is the _____ and this more commonly involves turning of the foot *(in? out?)*ward. In Grade(s) *(1? 2? 3? 4?)* knee sprains, the medial collateral ligament is totally ruptured.

(e) Explain why affected joints are immobilized for several weeks. _____

_____

_____

(f) A subluxation is a *(partial? complete?)* dislocation. Once a joint is dislocated, it is *(more? less?)* likely to be dislocated again. Which two joints are most likely to experience congenital dislocations? _____ and _____

(g) Write two types of loose bodies that are most commonly found in joints.

_____

_____

A5. Describe injuries to specific joints in this exercise.

(a) Rotator cuff injuries affect the *(elbow? knee? shoulder?)* joints. Such injuries are likely to occur by trauma in _____ or

_____ players or by slow onset overuse in elderly persons.

(b) Menisci are located in *(elbow? knee? shoulder?)* joints. They are composed of C-shaped *(bone? cartilage? fat?)* tissue. List several functions of menisci.

_____

_____

(c) Explain why torn menisci heal slowly.

_____

Why is reconstructive surgery advisable before degeneration of menisci is complete?

_____

_____

(d) Which types of sports tend to cause patellar dislocation? _____ and _____
List examples of treatments for this disorder.

_____

_____

_____

(e) Chondromalacia refers to _____ of articular cartilage.

A6. Identify the type of fracture likely in each client.

Fatigue   Pathologic   Sudden injury

(a) Mrs. Blumstein, age 84, fractures an osteoporotic hip as she rises from her chair:

_____

(b) Bonnie, a 34-year-old long-distance runner, experiences a tibial fracture caused by overuse: _____

(c) Mr. Steves fractures his radius by a fall on the ice:_____

A7. Choose the two true statements about fractures.

(a) An **open** fracture involves movement of part of the bone through the skin.

(b) A **distal** fracture of the tibia is closer to the knee joint than to the ankle joint.

(c) Comminuted fractures involve a break of a bone into **more than two** pieces.

(d) Greenstick fractures occur more often in **elderly** and involve a **complete** break across the bone.

A8. Complete this exercise about fractures.

(a) Define the term *reduction* with regard to fractures. _____

_____

_____

A *(comminuted? oblique? spiral? transverse?)* fracture is not likely to lose its position after it is reduced.

(b) In addition to pain, what other signs and symptoms may accompany fractures?

_____

_____

(c) List three types of deformities that may occur with fractures: _____, _____, _____. Explain what causes these deformities. _____

_____

_____

(d) Define the term *crepitus* with regard to fractures. _____

_____

_____

(e) Explain how fracture reduction may be accomplished without pain within minutes after the break occurs. _____

_____

A9. Arrange phases of fracture healing in correct sequence; then match the phases to the descriptions.

Callus   Fibrocartilaginous callus
Hematoma   Ossification
Remodeling

_____ → _____ →

_____ → _____ →

_____

(*Hint*: refer to textbook Figure 57-6.)

(a) Torn blood vessels and soft tissue combined with bone fragments form this mass, which provides a fibrin scaffolding for granulation tissue:_____

(b) A relatively soft collar forms at the fracture site a few days postfracture: ____

_____

(c) Osteoblasts form a bridge between bone fragments; calcification begins to harden this tissue by a month after fracture:

_____ and

_____

(d) Osteoclastic removal of excess callus shapes the new bone: _____

A10. Circle factors that lengthen the time required for fracture healing.

(a) Age:

(1) 76 years

(2) 16 years (such as Terence in questions A12[c]–[g])

(b) Bones with ___ surface areas at fracture sites:

(1) Large

(2) Small

(c) Shape of bones:

(1) Short bones

(2) Long bones

(d) General health:

(1) Diabetic

(2) Nondiabetic

(e) Circulation:

(1) Normal

(2) Compromised

(f) Type of bone fractures:

(1) Cortical bone

(2) Spongy (cancellous) bone

A11. What information must be gathered as part of a patient history for fracture diagnosis?

_____

_____

_____

A12. List the three main objectives for treatment of fractures: _____, _____, _____. Circle the one of these that is most critical to achieving union of fracture fragments. Now describe these more fully in this exercise.

(a) Surgical reduction with internal fixation of bone fragments is known as *(closed? open?)* reduction.

(b) If a fracture is suspected, a splint *(should? should not?)* be applied before the client is moved. The splint should cover *(only? joints proximal and distal to?)* the fractured bone.

(c) Three hours ago, Terence (age 16 years) received his leg cast for a right tibial fracture. Circle the answers that indicate that his cast may be too tight:

(1) Paresthesia of his foot and toes

(2) Diminished pulse in his right dorsalis pedis artery

(3) Capillary refill of 2 seconds

(d) Terence's right leg should be kept *(with foot on the floor? elevated above heart level?)* during the next day. Explain.

_____

_____

(e) While his right leg is in the cast, Terence should perform isometric exercises with his *(right? left?)* leg and range of motion exercises with his *(right? left?)* leg. Explain.

_____

_____

(f) Within days, edema in Terence's right tibialis anterior muscles and arteries surrounded by nondistensible fascia causes compression of these tissues with pain, tingling, and some paralysis. This condition is known as _____ syndrome.

(g) Describe limb-lengthening devices such as the Ilizarov external fixator and explain why they are used. _____

_____

_____

(h) Which form of traction involves pins, wires, or tongs, and is used for long periods of traction?

(1) Manual

(2) Skeletal

(3) Skin

A13. Identify types of impaired healing likely from a fracture that occurred on January 1.

Delayed union   Malunion   Nonunion

(a) Not healed by June 15: _____

(b) Still not healed by November 15:

_____

(c) Abnormal angulation of the fracture is visible on an x-ray: _____

A14. Explain how electrical stimulation devices may facilitate fracture healing.

_____

_____

_____

A15. Identify types of complications that may follow fractures or other musculoskeletal injuries. One answer will be used twice.

Compartment syndrome   Fracture blisters
Fat embolism syndrome   Reflex sympathetic
                          dystrophy

(a) May occur from small globules of fat released from bone marrow (especially from a femur) that pass through major veins and lead to potentially fatal pulmonary emboli (PE): _____

(b) Epidermis and dermis are separated by twisting injuries; localized edema with possible infection resulting: _____

(c) Severe aching or burning pain occurs that is intense relative to the degree of the injury; excessive sweating and pallor also may manifest: _____

(d) A fasciotomy may be required for resolution of this condition: _____

(e) Assessment of arterial blood gases (ABGs) and changes in behavior are most associated with diagnosis of this condition: _____

A16. Describe signs or symptoms within a few days of the injury that may point to fat embolism syndrome. Build on these key terms or phrases:

(a) Signs of diminished cerebral blood flow

_____
_____
_____

(b) Chest pain, dyspnea and sympathetic responses, such as _____

_____
_____

(c) Rash _____

_____
_____

A17. Explain how fat embolism syndrome can be fatal.

_____
_____
_____

B. BONE INFECTIONS (pages 1334–1337)

B1. Circle clients at risk for iatrogenic bone infections.

(a) Ruth, age 55 years, who had hip replacement surgery last week

(b) Margaret, age 61 years, who has skeletal traction for a fractured femur

(c) Mr. Vonnahme, a person with diabetes who has a deep foot ulcer

(d) Paula, who is recovering from an abdominal hysterectomy

B2. List several measures that nurses can take to reduce the risk for iatrogenic bone infections.

_____
_____

B3. Circle or fill in the correct answers about osteomyelitis.

(a) Osteomyelitis involves infection of bone (*cortex? marrow?*).

(b) List four possible origins of such infections.

_____
_____
_____
_____

(c) The most common microbe causing such infections is the bacterium _____, which normally is present on skin surface. Describe two mechanisms that account for this infection. _____

_____

(d) Osteomyelitis is more likely to result from (*blood-borne infections? bone contamination from an open wound?*).

(e) Osteomyelitis from blood-borne infections occurs more commonly among (*children? middle-aged persons?*). In children, such conditions are likely to occur (*in vertebrae? at growing points of long bones?*), whereas _____ are the most common sites in adults.

(f) Explain why subperiosteal abscesses may accompany osteomyelitis.

_____
_____
_____

B4. Describe the pathogenesis of osteomyelitis. Include these terms: *phagocytes, enzymes, purulent, ischemia, necrosis, sequestra.*

_____
_____
_____

B5. Ruth (Question B1[a]) has osteomyelitis 10 weeks after her initial hip surgery.

(a) At this point she has (*acute? chronic?*) osteomyelitis. What is the hallmark sign of this condition? _____
Treatment is likely to be (*oral? IV?*) antibiotics.

(b) Ruth's hip infection requires additional hip surgery. Explain the possible reasons. _____

_____

B6. What is likely to be the underlying cause of Mr. Vonnahme's osteomyelitis (recall from Question B1[c] that Mr. Vonnahme is a person with diabetes who has a deep foot ulcer)?

_____

_____

_____

B7. Describe miliary tuberculosis in this exercise.

(a) What is the meaning of the term "miliary"?

_____

The incidence of this condition is currently greater _(in the United States? globally?)_ and is on the _(increase? decrease?)_ in the United States.

(b) Which bones are most commonly the target of miliary TB? _____

(c) How is diagnosis confirmed? _____

C. OSTEONECROSIS (pages 1337-1338)

C1. Max, age 58 years, has been taking corticosteroids for several years for his rheumatoid arthritis. He now has a diagnosis of osteonecrosis. Describe his experience.

_____

_____

_____

(a) Osteonecrosis refers to _(damage? injury? death?)_ of bone tissue caused by lack of adequate _(blood? nerve?)_ supply.

(b) Which parts of a bone does this condition commonly affect?_____

_____

Why not the cortical bone? _____

_____

_____

(c) Max's necrosis is of the femoral head within the hip joint. Is this a typical site for osteonecrosis? _(Yes? No?)_ Explain.

_____

_____

(d) Osteonecrosis is _(often? seldom?)_ idiopathic, which means _____. List several factors that can lead to the ischemia that underlies osteonecrosis. _____

_____

(e) Which of the factors you just listed would increase Max's risk for osteonecrosis?

_____

(f) Identify the prominent symptom Max is most likely to experience: _____

(g) What treatment will Max most likely need for his osteonecrosis? _____

Osteonecrosis accounts for about ___ % of hip replacements in the United States.

C2. Explain what causes the "soap" that may create lesions in necrotic bone and be visible on x-rays for a lifetime.

_____

_____

_____

Alterations in Skeletal Functions: Congenital Disorders, Metabolic Bone Disease, and Neoplasms

■ Review Questions

A. ALTERATIONS IN SKELETAL GROWTH AND DEVELOPMENT (pages 1341–1353)

A1. Choose the two true statements.

    (a) With aging, bone resorption is likely to **outpace** bone formation.

    (b) The skeleton develops from **ectoderm**.

    (c) The vertebrae begin to develop by the end of the **first** month of embryonic development.

    (d) Ossification of bone begins during the **ninth month** of fetal development.

A2. Answer these questions about normal bones and bone growth.

    (a) Arrange these parts of a long bone from the rounded end of the bone to the narrow middle shaft:

        Diaphysis   Epiphysis   Metaphysis

        _____, _____,
        _____

    (b) At the epiphyseal growth plate, _____ cells are replaced by bone cells. At what age do these cells typically stop dividing?

        _____

    (c) Vitamin *(C? D?)* is required for calcification of bone, whereas vitamin ___ helps form the protein fibers in bone.

    (d) Osteo*(blasts? clasts?)* form new bone cells in concentric rings or _____. As bones increase in diameter, the marrow (or _____) cavity is enlarged by osteo*(blasts? clasts?)* that erode bone of the inner cortex.

A3. Complete this exercise about abnormal musculoskeletal development.

    (a) Explain why early musculoskeletal assessment of newborns is important.

        _____

        _____

    (b) The typical fetal position in utero involves *(flexion? extension?)* of shoulders, elbows, hips, and knees. (Refer to textbook Figure 58-2.) Most *(flexion? extension?)* contractures present at birth normally disappear in newborns by the age of 4 to 6 *(days? weeks? months?)*.

    (c) List factors that can contribute to torsional deformities, such as toeing-in or toeing-out.

        _____

    (d) Toeing-*(in? out?)* or *(abduction? adduction?)* of the metatarsals is the most common congenital foot deformity. *(Fixed? Supple?)* foot deformities are more easily corrected.

    (e) Feet are turned inwards by *(internal? external?)* tibial torsion, which is more common in *(single? multiple?)* births. How is a Denis Browne splint corrective?

        _____

    (f) Toeing-*(in? out?)* is more associated with external *(femoral? tibial?)* torsion. This condition *(is? is not?)* normally corrected when the child becomes adept at walking.

    (g) When a child lies in the prone position with legs flexed and ankles apart, the degree of *(internal or medial? external or lateral?)* rotation of femurs can be measured (textbook Figure 58-4, bottom left). Excessive rotation of this type is also known as femoral _____. Children with this condition are more comfortable sitting in the _____ position, which *(improves? exacerbates?)* the condition.

(h) External femoral torsion *(is? is not?)* common. Write one cause of it.

_____

_____

A4. Contrast knock-knees and bowlegs in this exercise.

(a) When Tyler, age 31 months, stands with his inner ankles touching, his knees are at least 2″ apart. His condition is *(bowlegs? knock-knees?)*, also known as genu _____. (Note: *genu* = knees.) This disorder is *(very common? uncommon?)* in toddlers. It is *(sometimes? always?)* pathological.

(b) When Toby, age 6 years, stands with his knees touching, his inner ankles are several inches apart. This condition is known as _____ or genu _____ and is more associated with laxity of the *(medial? lateral?)* collateral ligament(s). It *(rarely? usually?)* requires treatment.

(c) Explain why severe genu varum or valgum should be diagnosed early.

_____

_____

_____

(d) Tiffany has a diagnosis of Blount's disease in her right leg; this is a condition in which the _____ of the tibia fails to form on the medial side. Blount's disease is more likely to lead to *(bowlegs? knock-knees?)*. Incidence is greater in *(small? large?)* children and in *(early? late?)* walkers. It is usually *(bi? uni?)*lateral.

A5. Choose the two true statements about flatfoot.

(a) This condition involves absence of the **transverse** arch of the foot.

(b) Until age 2 or 3 years, **all** children have flat feet.

(c) In **supple** flatfoot, the foot has no arch whether the child is sitting or standing.

(d) Well-fitting shoes with arch supports **may help** adults with flatfoot.

A6. Circle the answers that match a term with a correct description.

(a) Flexible flatfoot: associated with cerebral palsy or juvenile rheumatoid arthritis

(b) Syndactyly: webbing of fingers

(c) Polydactyly: presence of an extra bone in a finger

(d) Thalidomide: a teratogenic drug known to cause absence of limbs or limb parts, especially if mothers took the drug during the second month of gestation

A7. Complete this exercise about hereditary and congenital deformities.

(a) Osteogenesis imperfecta (OI) is more commonly an autosomal *(dominant? recessive?)* disorder. An autosomal *(dominant? recessive?)* form (also known as Type __) is more lethal because bones are so fragile they can fracture in utero. There *(is? is no?)* known treatment for OI.

(b) In almost all cases of congenital clubfoot, the forefoot is turned *(inward? outward?)* so that the foot resembles a horse's hoof (textbook Figure 58-11). This condition is known as equino*(valgum? varus?)*. (Note: *equus* = horse). List one health practice an expectant mother can take to lower risk for congenital clubfoot.

A8. Katelyn is a white 24-month-old who was born breech. She has developmental dysplasia of her left hip (DDH) with generalized joint laxity. Katelyn is her parents' first child, and there is no known family history of this condition.

(a) Circle factors in Katelyn's history above that increase her risk for DDH.

(b) DDH is *(quite common? extremely rare?)*. Katelyn's DDH in her left hip is *(more? less?)* common than right-sided DDH.

(c) Select the diagnostic test for DDH that fits each description:

Barlow's sign   Galeazzi test
Ortolani's sign   Trendelenburg's test

(c1) Indicates dislocation of a hip when hips are abducted with flexed knees:

_____

(c2) A positive sign is an audible click as the head of the femur is moved back into the acetabulum following Barlow's sign: _____

(c3) Measures the length of the femurs by comparing the height of the flexed knees: _____

(d) Luxation refers to a hip that is *(dislocated? dislocatable?)*, whereas subluxation refers to a _____ hip.

(e) Katelyn exhibits a typical gait associated with DDH. Describe it.

_____

_____

(f) Treatment for DDH involves maintenance of Katelyn's left hip joint in a(n) _____ position.

A9. Select the condition that fits each description.

Congenital clubfoot (CCF)
Developmental dysplasia of the hip (DDH)
Legg-Calvé-Perthes disease (L-C-P)
Osteogenesis imperfecta (OI)
Osgood-Schlatter disease (OS)
Slipped capital femoral epiphysis (SCFE)
Scoliosis

(a) Three hereditary or congenital disorders:

_____, _____,

_____

(b) Also known as congenital hip location; present to some degree in 1% of all newborns; limited abduction of thigh with a "hip click" and asymmetrical gluteal folds suggest this condition

_____

(c) A deformity known as "talipes" _____

_____

(d) A disorder in which bones lack collagen and are so brittle that they can fracture; skull bones are thin and misshapen, causing children to have triangular faces; may affect other sites of collagen, such as skin, joints, muscles and teeth _____

_____

(e) Mr. and Mrs. London's 15-month-old baby has multiple fractures that cause health care personnel to investigate child abuse.

_____

(f) Three forms of juvenile osteochondrosis in which new bone growth centers degenerate:

_____, _____,

_____

(g) Three conditions in which the head of the femur is not properly seated in the hip socket (acetabulum): _____,

_____, _____

(h) Trevor, age 5 years and white, has a disorder in which the bone-forming center in the head of his left femur becomes ischemic; as the femoral head degenerates and necroses, the head develops an abnormally flattened shape. _____

(i) Kathleen has pain and swelling in the front of her knee region (tibial tuberosity) as cartilage there is abnormally ossified; associated with growth periods and typically resolves afterward

_____

(j) Onset of signs and symptoms usually is during the teen years, more often in boys with rapid growth periods; although a hip problem, pain may refer to knees; early treatment is critical to prevent lifelong crippling _____

A10. Complete this exercise about Trevor (Question A9[h]) and his Legg-Calvé-Perthes (L-C-P) disease.

(a) Circle the factors that increase risk for L-C-P.

(1) White (Caucasian)

(2) Male

(3) Short stature

(4) Well-nourished

(b) Arrange in correct sequence the stages in pathogenesis of L-C-P.

(1) Avascular stage, during which the ossification center becomes necrotic; lasts several months to a year

(2) The synovial membrane becomes inflamed and leads to buildup of synovial fluid; this stage lasts 1 to 3 weeks

(3) Necrotic bone is resorbed, and immature new bone replaces it; this stage lasts 1 to 3 years

(4) The healed or residual stage involves formation of normal bone

___ → ___ → ___ → ___

(c) Trevor's L-C-P is *(bi? uni?)*lateral. Is this typical? *(Yes? No?)*

(d) What is likely to be the goal of treatment for Trevor? _____

He is fitted with an Atlanta Scottish Rite brace, which keeps his left hip joint in *(abduction? adduction?)*. He will need to *(increase? relieve?)* the force of weight bearing on this hip joint.

(e) The success of Trevor's treatment is likely to be *(greater? less?)* because he received a diagnosis at the age of 5 years, rather than at 10 years. Explain._____

_____

_____

A11. Suzannah, age 12 years, has right thoracic scoliosis, which is a(n) *(anterior-posterior? lateral?)* deviation of the spinal column; her *(concavity? convexity?)* is on the right side.

(a) Scoliosis is much more common in *(boys? girls?)* and is severe in about one of *(2? 20? 1000?)* cases. Severe cases have a curvature of greater than ___ degrees.

(b) *(Postural? Structural?)* scoliosis can be corrected by exercise; *(postural? structural?)* scoliosis cannot.

(c) Suzannah's scoliosis is structural; the cause of most cases of structural scoliosis is _____; it has been associated with joint *(laxity? tightness?)*. The most common age group for onset of idiopathic scoliosis is: _____

    (1) Adolescent

    (2) Infantile

    (3) Juvenile

(d) Suzannah's mother first questioned if her daughter might have scoliosis. What indicators may she have noticed?

_____

_____

(e) Suzannah's curvature is 32 degrees as measured by a _____meter. The fact that she is pre-menarche at the age of presentation *(increases? decreases?)* her risk of progression. Given her 32-degree curvature, which clinical approach is likely?

    (1) Surgery

    (2) Bracing

    (3) "Wait and see" approach

(f) Describe the Milwaukee brace used to treat scoliosis. _____

_____

_____

(g) *(Bracing? Surgery?)* halts the progression of scoliosis, whereas *(bracing? surgery?)* decreases the curvature.

B. METABOLIC BONE DISEASE
(pages 1353–1360)

B1. Choose the two true statements about bone remodeling.

(a) This is a process that occurs through adolescence **but not** later in life.

(b) **Structural** remodeling refers to deposit of new bone on the outer aspect of the shaft.

(c) **Internal** remodeling involves replacement of spongy (trabecular) bone.

(d) About eight times more **compact** bone compared to **trabecular** bone is replaced each year.

B2. Complete this exercise about processes involved in bone remodeling.

(a) Osteo*(blasts? clasts?)* tear down or resorb old bone, and osteo*(blasts? clasts?)* lay down new bone. Both of these types of cells are derived from _____ cells in marrow.

(b) One cycle of bone resorption and formation requires about 4 *(days? weeks? months? years?)*. With aging, which process occurs more? Bone *(formation? resorption?)*.

(c) Mechanical stress stimulates osteo-*(blasts? clasts?)*. Write one or more factors that would decrease mechanical stress so that new bone would not be laid down.

_____

_____

(d) Which vitamin is required for laying down organic matter (collagen) in bone? Vitamin *(C? D?)*. Give an example of foods that are good sources of this vitamin. _____ Absence of such food leads to the condition named _____, in which bones are *(softer? more brittle?)* than normal. Which vitamin is needed for calcium absorption from foods? Vitamin ___

(e) Which hormone stimulates osteoclasts to tear down bone and release Ca²⁺ into blood? _____ This hormone triggers production of interleukin-___, which plays a key role in this process. Too much of this chemical can cause excessive bone breakdown, as in _____ disease.

(f) Name a hormone that helps to build bones.

_____

(g) Osteo_____ is a term that means bone mass is less than normal for a person of a particular age, race, or gender. List several causes of this condition.

_____

_____

B3. The term "osteoporosis" literally means _____ bone such that bone resembles a _____. This is a *(common? rare?)* condition affecting about *(25,000? 25 million?)* Americans. Describe osteoporosis (OP) in this exercise.

(a) Bone mass reaches its maximum at about age 30 years. By age 50 years, a typical age for menopause, a woman is likely to have lost ____% of her bone mass; by age 70 years, her loss probably will be about ____%. Postmenopausal women have a 1 in __ risk of an osteoporotic fracture.

(b) Circle the factors that increase risk for OP. Being:

   (1) African American

   (2) Asian

   (3) A child

   (4) Female

   (5) A woman whose mother, sister, and aunts have OP

   (6) A woman receiving hormone replacement therapy (HRT)

   (7) A coffee drinker (more than 2 cups caffeinated coffee a day)

(c) Identify factors that increase risk for OP in the following clients:

   (c1) Gwen, age 24 years, 5'6" and 98 pounds, is a nonpurging bulimic. She works out "40 to 50 hours a week to try to stop from getting any more fat on me." Much of her diet consists of diet cola.

   (c2) Mrs. McAllister, age 46 years, takes aluminum-containing antacids for her peptic ulcer and corticosteroids for flare-ups of her Crohn's disease; she had a hysterectomy last year, in which her ovaries also were removed, but she wears an "estrogen patch."

   (c3) Mr. Latimer, age 64 years, eats a 12- to 14-ounce steak and drinks two 6-packs of beer with cheese and crackers every night; he is a self-proclaimed "couch potato" and "two-pack-a-day man."

(d) The rate of bone loss is greater *(early? late?)* in menopause because osteoclastic activity is *(increased? decreased?)*. During this time *(cortical? trabecular?)* bone is lost, increasing the risk of fractures in bones with large amounts of this type of bone. Name two such sites: _____ and _____

(e) Hip fractures are more likely to occur *(in early menopause? later in life?)* from Type *(I? II?)* OP.

(f) Are osteoporotic bones likely to be painful? *(Yes? No?)* Describe the first clinical signs or symptoms likely for osteoporosis.

_____

_____

(g) How is a "dowager's hump" related to OP?

_____

_____

(h) Describe the following assessment tools for OP.

   (h1) DEXA_____

_____

   (h1) ABONE _____

_____

(i) With aging, height typically *(increases? decreases?)*. This change occurs primarily in length of the:

   (1) Leg bones

   (2) Vertebral column

(j) Given risk factors for OP, make a list of seven or more healthy behaviors designed to prevent this condition. _____

_____

_____

(k) Match types of chemicals used in the treatment of OP to the correct descriptions below:

Biphosphonates   Calcitonin
Estrogen   Fluorides

   (k1) Decreases osteoclast activity; now available in a nasal spray: _____

   (k2) Chemicals (such as Fosamax or Actonel) that bind to bone tissue to prevent osteoclastic bone destruction:

_____

_____

   (k3) Present in water supplies, it may help to prevent OP: _____

   (k4) The single most powerful treatment to reduce incidence and progression of OP:

_____

B4. Contrast the appearance of bones that have lost virtually all of their content of:

(a) Minerals _____

_____

_____

(b) Organic matrix_____

_____

_____

B5. Complete this exercise about vitamin D.

(a) It is a *(fat? water?)*-soluble vitamin that is absorbed from foods with the help of bile or synthesized in _____.

(b) Vitamin D deficiency in the United States results mainly from *(deficient dietary intake? impaired absorption?)*. List three countries in which vitamin D often is lacking in the diet. _____

_____

B6. Describe osteomalacia (OM) in this exercise.

(a) Osteomalacia is a condition in which bones are deficient in *(minerals? organic matrix?)*, specifically in _____ or _____. As a result bones are *(softer? more brittle?)* than normal. This condition is also known as adult _____.

(b) List several types of medications that can lead to OM. _____

_____

(c) Circle the typical signs or symptoms of OM:

Bowlegs   Hip fractures
Muscle weakness   Pain
Severe hypocalcemia

(d) What are Milkman's fractures?

_____

_____

(e) Write two effective and inexpensive treatments for OM. _____

_____

_____

B7. Explain how kidney disorders can lead to osteomalacia by circling or filling in the correct answer.

(a) Kidneys, along with the liver, normally are sites of _____ of vitamin D.

(b) In chronic renal failure (CRF), kidneys excrete *(more? less?)* than normal phosphate and *(more? less?)* than normal calcium ions. Resulting *(hyper? hypo?)*calcemia acts as a stimulus for *(increased? decreased?)* secretion of parathyroid hormone, which then stimulates bone *(formation? resorption?)*. This is known as _____ rickets.

(c) Vitamin D-resistant rickets involves excessive loss of _____ from kidneys. State one additional cause of phosphate deficiency. _____

_____

B8. Describe rickets in children in this exercise.

(a) Rickets involves *(brittle? softened?)* and deformed bones caused by *(de? over?)*mineralization. Symptoms of this condition are most commonly identified in children *(6 months to 3 years? 3 to 6 years? 6 to 10 years?)* old.

(b) What causes nutritional rickets?

_____

_____

(c) Use these key phrases to describe characteristics of rickets in children

(c1) Buddha-like appearance _____

_____

(c2) Rachitic rosary _____

_____

(c3) Skull _____

_____

(c4) Hypocalcemia _____

_____

(d) Write two effective and inexpensive treatments for rickets. _____

_____

_____

B9. Alice, age 42 years, has been diagnosed with Paget's disease. Write a one-sentence description of this condition.

_____

_____

(a) Paget's disease typically begins in *(children? adults?)*. _____

(b) Explain Alice's manifestations of headache, vertigo, and hearing loss.

_____

_____

(c) Explain how Alice's waddling gait is related to Paget's disease. _____

_____

_____

(d) Alice is at increased risk for pathological fractures. Define this term.

_____

_____

(e) What condition poses the greatest risk of death for Alice? _____

_____

_____

(f) Alice is experiencing severe pain. Is this typical of Paget's disease? _____

_____

B10. Which is the most common metabolic bone disease in the United States?

Osteomalacia   Osteoporosis
Paget's disease   Rickets

C. NEOPLASMS (pages 1360–1364)

C1. Choose the three true statements about bone tumors.

(a) Most bone cancers are **metastatic** rather than primary cancers.

(b) Benign tumors typically grow **slowly** and do not metastasize.

(c) Bone cancers are **more** common among children younger than 10 years than among adolescents.

(d) A chondroma is a **malignant** tumor of **cartilage.**

(e) Osteochondromas are **rare** forms of benign bone tumors.

(f) Osteoclastomas are **benign,** but **metastasizing,** bone tumors.

C2. Most bone tumors—whether benign or malignant—are accompanied by pain that *(is? is not?)* relieved by rest. Write another major manifestation of bone tumors.

_____
_____
_____

C3. Complete this exercise about bone cancer.

(a) Malignant tumors are likely to have *(well? poorly?)* defined borders. They are associated with a *(low? high?)* mortality rate.

(b) Which technique is most accurate for determining the extent of tumor in bone marrow?

Biopsy   CT scan
Magnetic resonance imaging   X-rays

Which technique is most useful for grading a tumor?

Biopsy   CT scan
Magnetic resonance imaging   X-rays

(c) Explain the significance of identifying and treating bone cancer before the affected bone has a pathologic fracture.

_____
_____

(d) Which intervention is typically most effective for controlling metastases?

Chemotherapy   Radiation   Surgery

C4. Saidee, age 18 years, has been diagnosed with osteosarcoma of the right proximal tibia. Complete this exercise about her.

(a) Arrange the incidence of osteosarcoma in these age groups from greatest to least:

Adolescents   35-year-olds   Elderly

_____, _____,

_____

(b) This is *(the most common? a rare?)* form of bone cancer. The location of Saidee's tumor *(is? is not?)* a site of rapid bone growth and a common location of osteosarcomas in adolescents.

(c) Saidee experienced pain in her leg as the first sign of her tumor. Tumor pain is more likely to have a(n) *(sudden? insidious?)* onset.

(d) Metastases to *(lungs? lymph nodes?)* tends to occur early in the disease.

(e) Osteosarcoma *(does? does not?)* respond well to radiation. Saidee will have limb-salvage surgery. Describe this procedure.

_____
_____
_____

C5. Complete this exercise about primary bone cancers.

(a) Circle the correct answers about Ewing's sarcoma

(a1) The greatest incidence of Ewing's sarcoma is among:

(1) Females younger than 25 years

(2) Males younger than 25 years

(3) Females older than 25 years

(4) Males older than 25 years

(a2) Ewing's sarcoma *(is? is not?)* highly malignant. It develops from cells in the:

(1) Marrow cells

(2) Periosteum

(3) Cortex of bone

(a3) Ewing's sarcoma usually is found in

(1) Shafts of long bones

(2) Epiphyses of long bones

(3) Vertebrae

(a3) Explain why diagnosis of Ewing's sarcoma may be difficult.

_____

_____

(b) Circle answers about chondrosarcoma.

    (b1) This type of tumor occurs more in

        (1) Children or adolescents

        (2) Middle-aged or elderly adults

    (b2) Chondrosarcoma tends to be

        (1) Rapid growing and metastasizing early

        (2) Slow growing and metastasizing late

    (b3) Circle the bones that are most likely to be sites of chondrosarcoma:

        (1) Pelvis

        (2) Femoral head

        (3) Carpals

        (4) Distal radius

C6. Complete this exercise about metastasizing bone cancers.

(a) About *(1%? 10%? 50%?)* of all people with cancer will have bone metastases during the course of their disease. Explain why bone metastases are so common.

_____

_____

_____

(b) Metastases are likely to occur

    (1) In extremities

    (2) Within or close to the trunk

(c) Circle the three most common types of cancers that metastasize.

Breast	Colorectal
Lung	Prostate
Stomach	Tongue

(d) What causes the pain of metastasis?

_____

_____

(e) Explain why the following diagnostic or treatment approaches are used.

    (e1) Blood tests for alkaline phosphatase and calcium _____

_____

_____

    (e2) Radiation therapy _____

_____

_____

    (e3) Biphosphonates _____

_____

_____

    (e4) Intramedullary rods _____

_____

_____

(f) Death is more likely to result from effects of metastases to

    (1) Bone

    (2) Vital organs

CHAPTER 59

Alterations in Skeletal Function: Rheumatic Disorders

■ Review Questions

A. SYSTEMIC AUTOIMMUNE RHEUMATIC DISEASES (pages 1367–1376)

A1. Circle the two true statements about arthritis.

  (a) There are **more than 100** different types of arthritis.

  (b) Arthritis is a **rare** cause of disability in the United States.

  (c) Arthritis **cannot** be cured, but **much** can be done to control its progress.

  (d) In **all** types of arthritis, inflammation is the initial event in the disorder.

A2. Complete this exercise about rheumatoid arthritis (RA).

  (a) The incidence of RA is greater in *(women? men?)*, especially those in *(adolescence? middle age?)*.

  (b) The exact cause of RA *(is? is not?)* known. The rheumatoid factor (RF) is present in body fluids of *(few? most? all?)* people who have RA. Where is RF produced?

  _____.

  (c) The RF *(is? reacts with?)* a fragment of the IgG autoantibody. The result is known as an immune _____. Explain why some people begin to develop antibodies (RF) that react with their own IgG. _____

  _____

  _____

A3. Refer to text Figures 59-1 and 59-2 and select the key word or phrase that describes each major event (a–g) in the progression of RA.

  Ankylosis
  Immune complex
    formation
  Pannus formation
  Reactive hyperplasia

  Extra-articular changes
  Granulation tissue
  Lysosomal action
  Phagocytosis

  (a) RF from synovial membranes combines with altered IgG in the synovial joint:

  _____

  (b) Inflammation begins as polymorphonuclear cells, lymphocytes, and macrophages are attracted and "eat up" immune complexes:

  _____

  (c) Macrophages and white blood cells release enzymes that destroy joint cartilage and underlying bone: _____

  (d) As more inflammatory cells are drawn to the scene of destruction, the synovial membrane proliferates: _____

  (e) Excessive numbers of blood vessels (granulation tissue) grow within the synovial membrane, leading to a red, warm, swollen, and spongy joint: _____

  (f) Pannus exacerbates the inflammation and interferes with joint movement:

  _____

  (g) Ligaments stretch and alter joint stability with possible dislocation; muscles associated with the joint atrophy from disuse; weakness and fatigue result: _____

A4. Circle correct answers about RA.

  (a) Pannus formation is found in *(RA only? many forms of arthritis?)*. This growth of blood vessels is *(helpful by nourishing? destructive to?)* joint tissues.

  (b) Limitation of joint motion early in the course of RA is caused by *(fibrosis of? pain in?)* joints.

  (c) Joints most affected by RA are *(large, such as hip and shoulder? small, such as hands and feet?)*, and the effects typically are *(unilateral? bilateral?)*.

  (d) Which joints are least likely to be affected by RA?

  Distal interphalangeal
  Metacarpophalangeal
  Proximal interphalangeal

(e) Swan-neck deformity affects *(great toes? thumbs?)*. Subluxation also may occur; this is *(dislocation? spraining?)* of a joint.

(f) If vertebrae are affected by RA, they are most likely to be *(cervical? lumbar? thoracic?)*, leading to *(lower back? neck?)* pain. The *(hip? knee? shoulder?)* is a commonly affected large joint, accompanied by severe atrophy of *(hamstrings? quadriceps?)* muscles.

(g) Which of the following are included in criteria for RA by the American Rheumatism Association (ARA)?

Anemia   Evening stiffness
Cloudy synovial fluid   Nodules
Swelling of at least three joints for at least
    6 weeks
X-ray changes of hand joints

A5. Describe treatments for RA in each category.

(a) Patient education _____
_____
_____

(b) Rest and exercise _____
_____
_____

(c) Assistive devices _____
_____
_____

(d) Apheresis_____
_____
_____
_____

A6. Explain why early, aggressive treatment for RA is important.
_____
_____
_____

A7. Identify medications used to treat RA.

Corticosteroids   COX-2 inhibitors
Methotrexate
Nonsteroidal anti-inflammatory drugs (NSAIDs)

(a) Should not be repeated more than several times a year because of long-term side effects: _____

(b) Inhibit an enzyme that contributes to inflammation but reduce gastrointestinal side effects because they do not inhibit prostaglandin synthesis: _____

(c) Anti-inflammatories, including aspirin and ibuprofen: _____

(d) Reduce discomfort but do not prevent joint destruction: _____

(e) Potent, fast-acting drug that modifies the course of RA: _____

A8. Select the name of the surgery that fits each description.

Arthrodesis   Arthroplasty
Synovectomy   Tenosynovectomy

(a) Total joint replacement: _____

(b) Common surgery for RA that involves repair of damaged tendons: _____

A9. Identify the disorder that fits each description.

Polymyositis   Scleroderma
Systemic lupus erythematosus

(a) Ms. Kelsey has proximal muscle weakness with some muscle pain: _____

(b) Mr. Isaac's rare disorder involves thickening of skin with fixation to tendons and muscles: _____

(c) The name of Ms. Wu's disorder indicates that many systems are affected, including skin with a red rash that was thought to resemble a wolf bite: _____

A10. Complete this exercise about Ms. Wu's systemic lupus erythematosus (SLE) (Question A9[c]).

(a) Because she is a woman, Ms. Wu's risk of SLE is considerably *(higher? lower?)* than that for men; *(androgens? estrogens?)* seem to protect against lupus. This condition also is more common in *(African Americans and Asians? whites?)*.

(b) Ms. Wu is likely to have hyperactive *(B-lymphocytes? T8 lymphocytes?)* that lead to production of _____ against her own tissues. As a result, lupus is categorized as an _____ disease.

(c) Ms. Wu's autoantibodies combine with _____ to form immune complexes. How are consequences of this process similar to those in RA? _____
_____

(d) Explain why SLE is called "the great imitator." _____
_____

List five or more of Ms. Wu's organs likely to be targeted by SLE. _____

_____

(e) Explain what is likely to cause these manifestations of SLE in Ms. Wu:

   (e1) Fatigue _____

   (e2) Increased tendency to bleed

   _____

   (e3) Protein in her urine_____

   (e4) Small strokes _____

   _____

(f) Ms. Wu exhibits the classic "butterfly rash" of SLE. Where is this located? _____

(g) Diagnosis of SLE requires *(one single? many?)* test(s). The most common test for SLE is for high levels of *(antinuclear antibodies [ANA]? lactic dehydrogenase [LDH]? rheumatoid factor [RF]?).*

A11. Select the three true statements about SLE.

   (a) Symptoms of medication-induced SLE are likely to **subside** when use of the implicated drugs is discontinued.

   (b) **Both** SLE and RA are characterized by exacerbations and remissions.

   (c) Joint pain occurs in some patients with SLE, but it is an **uncommon** manifestation of SLE.

   (d) X-rays of joints of patients with SLE typically **do** show joint destruction.

   (e) SLE **frequently** affects kidneys, pericardium, or lymph nodes.

   (f) Discoid SLE primarily affects **intervertebral disks.**

A12. Circle the drugs that may be used to treat SLE and RA.

   Corticosteroids   NSAIDs
   Hydroxychloroquine (antimalarial)

B. ARTHRITIS ASSOCIATED WITH SPONDYLITIS (pages 1376-1379)

B1. "Spondylo-" refers to _____, and "ankyl" means _____. Describe these conditions in this exercise.

   (a) Spondyloarthropathies exert their main effects on the *(axial? appendicular?)*

skeleton, primarily joints involving *(ligaments that insert into bone? a synovial membrane?).* These conditions *(are? are not?)* inflammatory.

   (b) Rheumatoid factor (RF) *(is? is not?)* involved in spondyloarthropathies. Approximately 90% of people with ankylosing spondylitis (AS) have the HLA-_____ antigen genetic marker, which is *(sometimes? never?)* present in persons without AS.

B2. Identify the spondyloarthropathy that best fits each description.

   Ankylosing spondylitis   Enteropathic arthritis
   Psoriatic arthritis   Reiter's syndrome

   (a) Most likely to involve inflammation of the uvea (middle layer of the wall of the eyeball) and the urethra: _____

   (b) Almost all cases involve inflammation of the sacroiliac joint: _____

   (c) A skin condition involving rapid turnover of epidermal cells; joints are involved in 5% to 7% of persons with this skin disorder:

   _____

   (d) Classic sign is bamboo-like spine seen on x-ray: _____

   (e) Inflammatory bowel disease, such as Crohn's disease: _____

   (f) Forms of reactive arthritis, for example, occurring considerably after an infection:

   _____, _____

B3. Mr. Murray, age 68 years, has severe, debilitating AS. His thoracic spine has such a pronounced anterior curvature that he can barely maintain balance in walking. Seldom can he hold his head high enough to look ahead. His weight is 105 lbs, 35 lbs less than his ideal weight.

   (a) Describe the primary problem with AS.

   _____

   _____

   (b) Explain how this pathogenesis leads to the rigid "bamboo spine." _____

   _____

   _____

   (c) List reasons Mr. Murray may be at increased risk for:

      (c1) Fractures_____

   _____

   _____

(c2) Shortness of breath and recurrent infections _____
_____
_____

(c3) Lower back pain and hip pain
_____
_____

(c4) Insomnia_____
_____
_____

(d) About *(one? four?)* in five persons with AS will experience manifestations as severe as Mr. Murray's.

(e) Circle interventions that may help Mr. Murray.

(1) Sleeping on his side

(2) Getting flu shots

(3) Taking a cold shower before exercising

(4) Swimming

(5) Weight loss

(6) NSAIDs

B4. Which conditions are likely to dramatically improve in persons with HIV infection? Explain.

Psoriatic arthritis   Rheumatoid arthritis
Reiter's syndrome   Systemic lupus
                                    erythematosus

_____
_____
_____

B5. Complete this exercise about reactive arthritis.

(a) The trigger for reactive arthritis is least likely to be *(rheumatoid factor? bacterial infection? a silicone implant in a joint?)*. Such arthritis is sero*(negative? positive?)*.

(b) In reactive arthritis, such as rheumatic fever, bacteria *(can? cannot?)* be isolated from cultures of synovial fluid. The onset of symptoms is likely to occur *(days? months?)* after an infection.

(c) Identify the microorganism most likely to cause reactive arthritis in these patients:

Chlamydia   Salmonella or Shigella
Streptococcus

(c1) Claudia, age 46 years, who contracted bacterial dysentery earlier this summer:
_____

(c2) Bill, age 19 years, who presented at the university clinic 6 months ago with SARA (sexually active reactive arthritis)

manifested by severe urethritis:
_____

(c3) Amy, age 18 years, who has a defective mitral valve resulting from rheumatic fever at age 15 years: _____

(d) List four extra-articular organs that may be affected by seronegative inflammatory arthropathies._____
_____
_____

C. OSTEOARTHRITIS SYNDROME
(pages 1379–1384)

C1. Refer to Chart 59-3 and identify categories of disorders that can lead to osteoarthritis.

Anatomic   Idiopathic
Metabolic   Neuropathic
Post-traumatic

(a) Mr. Jeffrey, age 48 years, has frequent gout attacks related to his high serum urate levels: _____

(b) There is no known cause for Ms. Wright's OA: _____

(c) Junior, age 8 years, has a flattened head of the femur as a result of slipped capital femoral epiphysis: _____

(d) Mr. Plummer's type 2 diabetes has led to decreased proprioception in his feet and resultant injury known as Charcot foot:
_____

(e) Torn menisci and other knee injuries have resulted from Joost's years of downhill skiing: _____

C2. Contrast osteoarthritis (OA) with RA in this exercise.

(a) More common form of arthritis: ___

(b) Typically more destructive to joints: ____

(c) Likely to have an earlier onset: ____

(d) Sometimes known as degenerative joint disease or wear and tear arthritis: ____

(e) Affects joints but is not systemic: ____

(f) Joints are warm and spongy, rather than hard: ____

(g) Involves pannus formation: ____

(h) Not always inflammatory: ____

(i) Primarily involves inflammation of the synovial membrane with subsequent damage to other joint structures: ____

C3. Describe the pathogenesis of OA in this exercise.

   (a) The primary tissue injured in OA is:

      Articular cartilage   Bone
      Ligaments   Synovial membrane

   (b) Cartilage contains cells known as
      _____. Describe four chemical
      components of cartilage matrix surrounding
      these cells. _____
      _____
      _____
      _____

   (c) One function of articular cartilage is to
      (increase? decrease?) friction at joints.
      Deformation is a(n) *(abnormal? normal?)*
      function of articular cartilage that
      (maximizes? minimizes?) the joint surface
      area over which the load is distributed.
      Explain what happens if cartilage cannot
      deform properly. _____
      _____
      _____

   (d) Describe how articular cartilage is injured in
      each case.

      (d1) In Joost's knee joints (Question C1[e])
          _____
          _____

      (d2) Mrs. Shea, whose hip is immobilized
          after a fracture. _____
          _____

   (e) When articular cartilage is injured,
      chondrocytes are thought to respond by
      releasing _____, which causes release
      of _____-digesting enzymes; these
      destroy cartilage components such as
      _____ and _____. As cartilage
      erodes, the space between bones *(narrows?*
      widens?). (See Figure 59-9.)

   (f) Describe two changes in bone underlying the
      cartilage destroyed in osteoarthritis:

      (f1) Bone scleroses or hardens into an ivory-
          like mass, a process called _____

      (f2) Bones spurs known as _____ form
          (Figure 59-9) and can lead to joint
          enlargement with grinding sounds
          (known as _____) as joints are
          moved.

C4. Osteoarthritis affects *(only large? only small?*
both large and small?) joints. Circle the two
most common sites for osteoarthritis (OA) out

of the three sites listed in each case. (Identify
these sites on yourself.)

   (a) Hip joint   Knee joint   Sacroiliac joint

   (b) Cervical vertebrae   Lumbar vertebrae
      Thoracic vertebrae

   (c) First carpometacarpal joint
      First metacarpophalangeal joint
      First metatarsophalangeal joint

C5. Refer to text Table 59-2 and identify sites of OA
likely to cause the following manifestations.

   Distal interphalangeal joints
   Hip   Knee
   Proximal interphalangeal joints
   Spine

   (a) Genu varus or genu valgus along with
      quadriceps atrophy: _____

   (b) Radicular pain as spinal nerves are
      compressed: _____

   (c) Heberden's nodes: _____

C6. Discuss nonpharmacologic treatments for
osteoarthritis.
_____
_____
_____

C7. Circle the medications used for osteoarthritis
and contrast with those used for RA (Question
A7).

   Corticosteroids   COX-2 inhibitors
   Hyaluronate (joint lubricant)   Methotrexate
   NSAIDs

D. METABOLIC DISEASES ASSOCIATED WITH RHEUMATIC STATES (pages 1384–1386)

D1. List several common metabolic disorders other
than gout that can affect joints.
_____
_____
_____

D2. Circle the two true statements about gout.

   (a) Gout **is** a systemic disorder.

   (b) Incidence of gout is highest in **middle-aged
women.**

   (c) Tophi are **deposits of crystals** in tissues.

   (d) Gout is caused by deposits of **calcium
carbonate** crystals in soft tissues.

D3. Complete this exercise about the pathogenesis of gout.

(a) Excessive amounts of uric acid in blood is known as _____. Write a value for serum level of urate that indicates hyperuricemia. _____ mg/dL.

(b) Explain how joints are inflamed in gout. _____
_____

(c) Tophi are nodules that consist of _____ deposited in joint tissues. Tophi typically appear *(immediately? about 10 weeks? about 10 years?)* after the initial gout attack.

(d) Typically, the first gout attack involves *(one? many?)* joint(s). Subsequent attacks *(almost always follow within days? may not occur for years?)*. Gout is most likely to affect *(shoulder and hip joints? toes and external ears?)*. Explain._____
_____
_____

D4. Discuss management of an acute gout attack in Mr. Jeffrey (Question C1[a]).

(a) Treatment of an acute attack is focused on reducing *(serum urate levels? joint inflammation?)*. Which anti-inflammatory is used as a "last ditch" effort to control Mr. Jeffrey's gout attack?

Colchicine   Corticosteroids   NSAIDs

Explain. _____
_____
_____

(b) Uricosuric medications *(are? are not?)* helpful in treating acute gout. Explain.
_____
_____

How do these medications treat chronic gout? _____
_____

(c) Explain why Mr. Jeffrey should not take aspirin for pain relief. _____
_____
_____

(d) How can allopurinol help Mr. Jeffrey?
_____
_____
_____

(e) Uric acid is a chemical produced by the breakdown of chemicals known as _____ such as adenine and guanine.

List several foods that are high in purine content and thus should be avoided by Mr. Jeffrey._____
_____
_____

E. RHEUMATIC DISEASES IN CHILDREN AND THE ELDERLY (pages 1386–1389)

E1. Explain why a team approach is important in managing rheumatic diseases in children.
_____
_____
_____

E2. Identify the rheumatic disorder that fits each description.

Juvenile dermatomyositis
Pauciarticular arthritis
Polyarticular arthritis
Still's disease

(a) A common form of juvenile rheumatoid arthritis (JRA) in which no more than four joints are affected; onset younger in girls:
_____

(b) Form of JRA that closely resembles the adult form; more than four joints affected:
_____

(c) A form of JRA characterized by episodic high fever, rash, high white blood cell count, and enlargement of liver, spleen, and lymph nodes; in most cases, joints are involved:
_____

(d) Idiopathic inflammatory disorder causing calcifications, vasculitis with skin rash, and proximal muscle weakness:
_____

E3. Circle the three true statements about rheumatic diseases in children.

(a) NSAIDs are first-line drugs for treating JRA.

(b) The prognosis for most children with JRA is **poor.**

(c) The incidence of SLE in children is **higher** than in adults.

(d) Renal involvement in childhood SLE is **more** common and **more** severe than in adults.

(e) Children with SLE **should** receive immunizations containing live vaccines.

(f) Juvenile spondyloarthropathies are more likely to affect extremities than the sacroiliac or vertebral joints.

E4. Arthritis is a *(common? rare?)* complaint among elderly persons. Explain how arthritis can affect quality of life in older adults.

_____
_____
_____
_____

E5. The prevalence of RA, gout, and polymyalgia rheumatica **all** *(increase? decrease?)* with aging.

E6. Mrs. Thielens, age 60 years, has received a diagnosis of polymyalgia rheumatica. Circle the correct answers about her condition.

(a) To meet criteria for this disorder, she must have experienced pain and stiffness for at least 1 *(week? month? year?)*, and her sedimentation rate must be *(higher? lower?)* than normal.

(b) When a test dose of corticosteroid (prednisone) is administered to patients with polymyalgia rheumatica, pain relief is achieved in 1 to 2 *(days? weeks?)*. Patients with RA have a *(more rapid? slower?)* response to steroids.

(c) It is likely that Mrs. Thielens *(will? will not?)* need ongoing steroid therapy to control her condition. List two reasons patients often discontinue this treatment.

_____
_____

(d) Discontinuation of Mrs. Thielens' steroid therapy must be carried out *(abruptly? gradually?)*. Explain. _____

_____
_____

E7. How is giant cell arteritis related to polymyalgia rheumatica?

_____
_____
_____

Giant cell arteritis affects *(blood vessels? cartilage? synovial membranes?)*. Circle a serious consequence of giant cell arthritis.

Blindness   Deafness   Stroke

E8. Explain why elderly persons should be involved in the management of their rheumatoid disorders.

_____
_____
_____

CHAPTER 60

Control of Integumentary Function

■ Review Questions

A. STRUCTURE OF THE SKIN
(pages 1393–1400)

A1. Skin may be one of the most underestimated organs in the body. What functions does your skin perform while it is "just lying there" covering your body?

_____

_____

_____

A2. Choose the three true statements.

(a) Skin is the **first line of defense** of the body in a potentially harmful environment.

(b) Skin is **thicker** on the palms and soles than elsewhere on the body.

(c) The outermost layer of the skin is the **dermis.**

(d) Hair, nails, and glands are all formed from **dermis.**

(e) Epidermis is composed of **stratified squamous** epithelium.

A3. Epidermis contains four distinct cell types. Name the type of cell that fits each description. Choose from these answers:

Keratinocyte   Langerhans' cell
Melanocyte   Merkel's cell

(a) These cells contribute to the sensation of touch: _____

(b) Part of immune responses, these cells recognize, process, and (as dendritic cells) present foreign antigens to T cells:

_____

(c) These cells produce the pigment that gives skin brown or black color and protects skin from UV light: _____

(d) The most numerous cell type in skin, they produce the protective protein, keratin:

_____

A4. Arrange epidermal layers from deepest to most superficial. Stratum:

Corneum   Germinativum   Granulosum
Lucidum   Spinosum

_____, _____, _____,
_____, _____

(a) Which is the thickest layer and composed of all flattened, dead cells? _____

(b) Which layer is present only in skin of palms of hands and soles of feet? _____

(c) Which of these layers is the site of formation of all new epidermal cells? _____

A5. Identify the chemical that fits each description below.

Melanin   Sebum   Tyrosinase

(a) An enzyme missing in albinos: _____

(b) Oily substance produced by glands surrounding hair follicles; lubricates hair and skin: _____

A6. Choose the two true statements.

(a) As epidermal cells develop, they are pushed to more **superficial** layers.

(b) Melanocytes **do migrate** to more **superficial** layers.

(c) African Americans' skin contains **more melanocytes** than the skin of white people.

(d) The basal lamina connects the **epidermis** to the **dermis.**

A7. Circle the correct answers in each statement.

(a) The dermis is *(thicker? thinner?)* than the epidermis. The dermis is composed of *(connective? epithelial?)* tissue and is *(vascular? avascular?).*

(b) Most sensory receptors are located in the *(papillary? reticular?)* region of the dermis.

(c) *(Pacinian? Meissner's?)* corpuscles are located in the *(epidermis? dermis? subcutaneous tissue?).*

322

(d) Subcutaneous tissue *(does? does not?)* typically contain fat tissue.

(e) *(Apocrine? Eccrine?)* sweat glands are more numerous and empty directly *(onto the surface of skin? into hair follicles?).*

(f) Acne is an inflammation of *(sebaceous? sweat?)* glands.

(g) *(Arrector pili muscles? The eponychium?)* is/are responsible for "goose bumps."

(h) Hairs consist of *(collagen? dead keratinized cells?).*

CHAPTER 61

Alterations in Skin Function and Integrity

■ Review Questions

A. MANIFESTATIONS OF SKIN DISORDERS (pages 1401–1404)

A1. Match each type of primary lesion below with the correct category.

Flat with color change   Elevated and solid
Elevated and fluid-filled

(a) Acne pustule: _____

(b) Vesicle caused by herpes simplex or bulla as in second-degree burn: _____

(c) Papule such as a mole (nevus) or nodule: _____

(d) Macule such as a freckle: _____

A2. Circle the correct answer in each statement.

(a) *(Patches? Petechiae?)* are smaller lesions.

(b) A callus involves *(a? hyper?)*plasia of dead cells in the stratum corneum.

(c) *(Blanched? Erythematous?)* lesions are reddened.

(d) A(n) *(excoriation? lichenification?)* is a raw line of broken epidermis.

A3. Choose the two true statements about the sensation of itch.

(a) It is known as **pruritis.**

(b) Itch and pain are thought to be **closely** related and both types of impulses travel through **spinothalamic** tracts to the brain.

(c) Histamine, bradykinin, and substance P **reduce** itching sensations.

(d) Scratching itchy areas of skin usually **helps** to heal the area.

(e) **Heat** applications are usually helpful in controlling itching.

A4. Choose the two answers that match a term with a correct description.

(a) Morphine: a painkiller that also relieves itching

(b) Xerosis: dry skin

(c) Emollients: protein-containing chemicals that protect skin from drying

(d) Room humidifiers: help to prevent water loss from skin

A5. Mrs. Taylor, age 24, is African American. She is at *(higher? lower?)* risk for skin cancer because the increased _____ in her skin protects from UV rays. Areas of her face appear "ashy" (gray and dry). Explain what may be the cause.

_____

Mrs. Taylor's skin is *(more? less?)* likely to wrinkle as she ages compared to white skin.

B. SKIN DAMAGE DUE TO ULTRAVIOLET RADIATION (pages 1404–1406)

B1. Incidence of skin cancer has *(increased? decreased?)* over the past 2 decades. Complete this exercise about UV-induced skin damage.

(a) Which type of ultraviolet rays are the "sunburn rays?"

(1) UVA (long rays)

(2) UVB (medium length rays)

(3) UVC (short rays)

(b) Tanning salons deliver:

(1) UVA (long rays)

(2) UVB (medium length rays)

(3) UVC (short rays)

(c) Explain the relationship between the ozone layer and skin cancer. _____

_____

_____

(d) Exposure to UV rays causes skin vessels to vaso*(constrict? dilate?)* leading to sunburn. UV exposure leads to a decrease in Langerhans' cells. State the impact of this effect._____

_____

_____

(e) Drugs that cause an exaggerated response to UV light are known as:

(1) Photosensitive drugs

(2) Sunscreens

B2. Mary Beth is going running and swimming at the beach. Circle the behaviors that will help to reduce her risk of skin damage and possible skin cancer?

(a) Use of a sunscreen with an SPF of:
15   8

(b) Applying the sunscreen:
Once in the morning   Every 2 hours

(c) Spending 4 hours at the beach from:
7 AM to 11 AM   11 AM to 3 PM

C. PRIMARY SKIN DISORDERS
(pages 1406–1429)

C1. Primary skin disorders are those that begin *(in? outside of?)* the skin.

C2. Match the pigmentary skin disorder to the description by filling in the blanks.

Albinism   Melasma   Vitiligo

(a) Congenital disorder in which deficient levels of melanin cause light skin and hair as well as lack of iris pigmentation that may seriously affect vision: _____

(b) Darkening of the face; related to increase of estrogen and progesterone during pregnancy or with oral contraceptives:

_____

(c) Sudden appearance of white (depigmented) patches on black skin: _____

C3. Complete this exercise about fungal skin infections by circling the correct answers or filling in the blanks.

(a) Ringworm is a *(superficial? deep?)* skin infection. Name three sources of the fungi that cause these infections:

_____,
_____,
_____.

(b) Most of these microbes secrete enzymes that digest _____, causing skin scaling and nail disintegration.

(c) Treatments include:

(1) Topical agents that are typically *(more? less?)* effective than oral agents

(2) Oral agents that are likely to be *(more? less?)* toxic than topical agents. Explain.

_____
_____

(d) Fingernail infections are *(more? less?)* easily treated than toenail infections. Explain.

_____
_____

C4. Tinea, also known as _____, is a(n) *(arthropod? bacterial? fungal?)* infection. Identify the location of the following fungal infections.

(a) Tinea unguium; an onychomycosis:

_____

(b) Tinea capitis; most often caused by *Trichophyton tonsurans*: _____

(c) Tinea corporis, often transmitted from pets to children; circular patches look like donuts or targets: _____

(d) Tinea pedis, also known as "athlete's foot"; itchy and smelly: _____

(e) Tinea incognito can affect many body parts and is caused by widespread use of

_____

C5. Match the chemicals used for diagnosis or treatment of skin disorders with related descriptions.

Acyclovir   Corticosteroids
Griseofulvin   Potassium hydroxide
Malathion   Tetracycline
Tretinoin or isotretinoin

(a) An oral agent that protects new skin cells from fungal infections: _____

(b) Agent used to prepare skin scrapings for microscopic examination for fungal infections: _____

(c) Agents that reduce itching and erythema:

_____

(d) Antiviral agent: _____

(e) Vitamin A product that can be used to treat acne; has teratogenic effects:

_____

(f) Antibiotic used for skin infections (e.g., acne); exerts teratogenic effects on skeletal and tooth development: _____

(g) A treatment for arthropod infestations:

_____

C6. Explain why the following clients are likely to have developed candidiasis:

(a) Alecia had a severe *Streptococcus* respiratory infection for 2 months. For 6 weeks of that time, Alecia took a broad-spectrum antibiotic. Now she has a case of vaginal candidiasis.

_____

_____

_____

(b) Frank has AIDS. His CD4 T-cell count is currently 52 cells/µL. _____

_____

_____

C7. Complete this exercise about skin infections by circling the correct answers or filling in the blanks.

(a) Impetigo is most common among *(adults? children?)*. It is a *(superficial? ulcerative?)* infection, typically caused by *Staphylococci* or GABHS, which stands for _____ *streptococci*.

(b) Acne is a condition that affects the hair follicles and *(oil? sweat?)* glands of skin. These may involve *(blackheads? whiteheads?)*, which are melanin-containing plugs that block pores of glands. About *(10% 100%?)* of teenagers develop acne vulgaris. *(Androgens? Estrogens?)* have been implicated in acne. Circle the behaviors that are likely to lessen effects of acne vulgaris:

(1) Avoidance of chocolate

(2) Scrubbing of the face

(3) Use of cosmetics that are water based

(4) Use of sweatbands or hats.

(c) Warts are *(benign? malignant?)* conditions in which the epidermis is stimulated to become *(thicker? thinner?)*. Warts are caused by the HPV (or human _____ virus). This type of virus can also cause genital warts which *(can? cannot?)* be sexually transmitted.

(d) Herpesviruses typically affect *(sensory? motor?)* neurons where they may lie dormant for months or years. Herpes infections present with prodromal symptoms that include _____. The acute phase involves *(fluid-filled vesicles? solid macules?)* that *(do? do not?)* dry up and crust.

(e) Herpes simplex-1 (or HSV-1) virus is most likely to cause ___, whereas HSV-2 typically causes ___:

(1) Fever blisters

(2) Genital herpes

(3) Chickenpox or shingles

(f) Currently there *(is? is not?)* a cure for HSV. _____ may be used to prevent recurrences. Sunscreens *(can? cannot?)* prevent HSV-1 on lips.

C8. Mrs. Yaskolski, age 86, has shingles. Describe her condition in this exercise by filling in the blanks or circling the correct answers.

(a) Shingles is caused by herpes _____ virus that can be reactivated decades after it caused _____. List two categories of persons at high risk for shingles:

_____, _____

(b) Mrs. Yaskolski has lesions along the dermatome of her C8 spinal nerve. Vesicles are likely to appear *(bi? uni?)*laterally along this single dermatome. The lesions are likely to crust over and fall off within 2 to 3 *(days? weeks? months?)*.

(c) These lesions *(are not? can be?)* contagious. If the ophthalmic division of the trigeminal nerve is affected by shingles, Mrs. Yaskolski could experience _____. Postherpetic neuralgia can last for as long as a *(week? month? year?)*.

(d) Describe treatments that may help to manage shingles. _____

_____

_____

C9. Match the type of skin disorder with the correct description.

Allergic contact dermatitis	Atopic eczema
	Lichen planus
Irritant contact dermatitis	Nummular eczema
	Pityriasis rosea
Psoriasis	Toxic epidermal necrolysis
Urticaria	

(a) A type I hypersensitivity reaction that is usually hereditary; begins on the cheeks of children with oozing and crusting vesicles; treatments include bathing and moisturizers:

_____

(b) Round patches on the extremities, typically chronic with weeks to years between exacerbations: _____

(c) Also known as hives; involves reddened wheals with intense itching caused by release of the vasodilator histamine; can result from reactions to food, heat or cold, or pressure: _____

(d) Can be triggered by contact with metal in jewelry, some antibiotics, poison ivy, and latex gloves and condoms: _____

(e) Soaps and detergents are causes: _____

(f) Drug reaction (possibly to sulfa drugs) that may be life-threatening; Nikolsky's sign involves separation of epidermis from dermis by lateral pressure: _____

(g) Drug reaction that leads to mossy skin lesions; usually self-limiting: _____

(h) A hyperkeratosis with thick red plaques covered by silvery-white scales; has no cure but a variety of helpful treatments exist: _____

(i) Rash with oval lesions; may form a "Christmas tree" pattern on the back: _____

C10. Classify each of the following skin infections according to the type of causative microbe.

Arthropod   Bacteria
Fungi   Virus

(a) Acne and rosacea: _____

(b) Candidiasis: _____

(c) Shingles: _____

(d) Verrucae: _____

(e) Head lice or pubic lice ("crabs"): _____

(f) Cold sore: _____

C11. Arthropods are tiny animals with jointed appendages. Describe arthropod infections in this exercise by circling the correct answers or filling in the blanks.

(a) Rocky Mountain spotted fever is caused by *(lice? mites? ticks?)*. Name another condition caused by these arthropods: _____ Manifestations are caused by *(the tick bite itself? microbes carried by the tick?)*. They require that the tick feed on human blood for several *(minutes? hours? days?)*. These *(can? never?)* lead to systemic effects and possibly death.

(b) Scabies is caused by *(lice? mites? ticks?)*. Skin creases are sites where the arthropods *(commonly? rarely?)* burrow. Eggs hatch *(within? on the surface of?)* the skin. Mites *(can? cannot?)* live on sheets or clothing.

(c) Pediculosis refers to infections with *(lice? mites? ticks?)*.

(1) They *(can? cannot?)* be transmitted to humans by other animals. What precautions can reduce transmission from human to human? _____

(2) List several sites that lice can infest. _____

(3) The fertilized eggs are laid *(on the surface of the skin? along hair shafts?)*. The unhatched eggs are known as *(nits? stylets?)*; their presence can provide a positive diagnosis.

(4) Each adult louse can feed from human blood for 1 to 2 *(hours? days? months?)*.

D. NEVI AND SKIN CANCERS (pages 1429–1433)

D1. Choose the two true statements.

(a) Almost all adults **do** have nevi (moles).

(b) Nevi are **benign.**

(c) Nevi develop primarily from **keratinocytes.**

(d) Nevi typically have **poorly** defined borders.

(e) **Junctional** nevi have the ability to transform to malignant melanomas.

D2. Incidence of skin cancer has *(increased? decreased?)* significantly over the past several decades, especially among *(fair? dark?)*-skinned persons with _____ hair. List several reasons for the increased incidence. _____

D3. Arrange these types of skin cancers from most to least serious and likely to metastasize:

Squamous cell carcinoma   Basal cell carcinoma
Malignant melanoma

_____, _____, _____

(a) Which is the most common form of skin cancer, and generally appears pink and pearly in white-skinned persons? _____

(b) Which is the most common type of skin cancer in blacks? _____

D4. Dixie, age 52, is seeing a dermatologist for a mole on her upper chest that has changed over the past several months. Complete this exercise about her.

(a) Dixie has red hair with freckles on her face and upper back. She has visited tanning salons "to get a good base before summer" for about 10 years. In her late teens, she worked as a lifeguard for 4 years. Her mother died of metastatic malignant melanoma. Circle the factors in this history that are risk factors for malignant melanoma. Because of these risk factors, Dixie has a *(3.5? 20?)*-fold increased risk of malignant melanoma.

(b) Dixie's lesion has a diameter of 9 mm × 13 mm, is slightly raised, brown, with uneven borders. Which criteria of the ABCD rule used to diagnose malignant melanoma does her lesion meet? _____

_____

(c) She is diagnosed with superficial spreading melanoma. This type of lesion is a *(common? rare?)* form of malignant melanoma that typically occurs on areas of skin that *(are? are not?)* sun-exposed. With continued growth, it *(is? is not?)* likely to ulcerate and bleed.

(d) The fact that the lesion has a depth of 2.2 mm sets Dixie's likelihood of 8-year survival at about ___%. Treatment *(is? is not?)* likely to include surgical excision.

D5. Write two preventive measures regarding skin cancers.

_____

_____

E. BURNS (pages 1433–1437)

E1. List five or more categories of causes of burns.

_____
_____
_____
_____
_____
_____

E2. Complete this exercise about burns. Use these answers:

(1) First-degree
(2) Second-degree, full-thickness
(3) Second-degree, partial-thickness
(4) Third-degree

(a) Arrange in correct sequence the depth of burn from most to least extensive:

_____, _____, _____,

_____

(b) A mild sunburn is an example; involves only the epidermis; healing usually occurs within 1 to 2 weeks: _____

(c) Involves formation of blisters that actually protect underlying skin; white skin appears bright pink or red: _____

(d) Blister formation occurs and possibly some loss of sensation because all the dermis is involved; white skin appears mottled pink, red, or waxy white; some scar formation is typical: _____

(e) May extend into muscles and bone; skin is hard, dry and may vary in color from white to black; likely to require skin grafting and to leave permanent scars: _____

E3. Joel, age 19 years, has extensive third-degree burns covering all of his lower extremities and his buttocks from an incident in which his jeans caught on fire. Complete this exercise.

(a) Is Joel likely to experience pain from the burns? _____

(b) About what percentage of Joel's TBSA is burned? ___% The American Burn Association grading of Joel's burn severity would be *(minor? moderate? major?)*.

(c) Circle the more likely manifestations of Joel's burns and then write a brief rationale.
(1) Cardiac output of *(3? 5?)* L/min.

_____
_____

(2) Hematocrit of *(42? 56?)*.

_____
_____
_____

(3) *(Increased? Decreased?)* risk of thromboses.

_____
_____

(4) *(Increased? Decreased?)* risk of stomach ulcer. _____

_____

(5) *(Increased? Decreased?)* urinary output.

_____

(6) Increase of fluid within *(plasma? interstitial [between cells] areas?)* _____

_____

(7) *(Increased? Decreased?)* levels of oxygen in blood. _____

_____

(8) *(Increased? Decreased?)* risk for infection, including sepsis. _____

(d) Joel is likely to be receiving *(no? enormous amounts?)* of IV fluids and nutrients. Explain. _____

_____

_____

_____

E4. Describe treatments for Joel's burns by using the following key words in sentences or paragraphs.

(a) Water over burns

_____

_____

_____

(b) Cold (not ice)

_____

_____

_____

(c) IV fluids and antibiotics

_____

_____

_____

(d) Eschar

_____

_____

_____

(e) Autograft

_____

_____

_____

(f) Contractures

_____

_____

_____

F. AGE-RELATED SKIN MANIFESTATIONS (pages 1437–1442)

F1. Choose the two true statements.

(a) Congenital melanocytic nevi are considered **harmless** lesions.

(b) Strawberry hemangiomas and port-wine stains are both disorders of **blood vessels.**

(c) **Port-wine stains** typically resolve by age 5 to 7 years.

(d) Port-wine stains **can** lead to neurologic problems.

F2. Describe skin disorders of infants in this exercise.

(a) Contrast the appearance of simple diaper rash with that of severe diaper rash.

_____

_____

_____

(b) Use of cloth diapers with plastic pants is *(more? less?)* likely to lead to diaper rash than use of disposable diapers.

(c) Prickly heat (heat rash) is more likely to occur when skin is *(moist? dry?)*.

(d) Cradle cap typically occurs when hair is washed *(too often? infrequently?)*.

F3. Complete Table 61-1 (page 330 of the Study Guide) contrasting skin disorders related to infectious diseases of childhood.

F4. Arrange, in correct sequence, events in the typical course of chickenpox.

Scab formation   Vesicle formation
Macules on trunk, spreading to extremities and head

_____ → _____ →

_____

F5. Determine the probable diagnosis in each case below and determine which condition has a greater potential for serious complications. Select from disorders listed in Table 61-1 of the Study Guide.

(a) Jimmy, age 13 months, is brought to the clinic on Monday. His mother reports that Jimmy "slept and cried a lot and pulled at his ears" last week, and she thought he had had a fever. His rash started on Saturday on his back and abdomen; it has now progressed to his arms and legs. Lymph nodes in Jimmy's neck and behind his ears are normal. Probable diagnosis: _____

_____

Table 61-1. Skin Disorders Associated With Infectious Diseases of Childhood

Disorder	Cause	Appearance	Location	Fever	Complications
Roseola	Herpesvirus-6			105°F	Usually none
Rubella (3-day or German)		Punctate	Starts on trunk; spreads to arms, legs		
Rubeola (7-day or hard)		Confluent; Koplik's spots		100°F+	
Chickenpox (or shingles)	Varicella virus				Rarely
Scarlet fever					Possibly otitis media, heart or kidney defects

(b) Anabelle is 4 years old. Her father reports that she had "strep throat" 2 weeks ago and she's been "throwing up over the past 2 days." Now Anabelle has a pink rash extending from her trunk to her thighs. Her tongue is pink with a white coating. Probable diagnosis: _____

F6. Complete Table 61-2 relating observable changes in aging of the integument to their causes.

Table 61-2. Skin Changes Related to Normal Aging

Changes	Causes
Decreased sensation of touch	
	Decrease in Langerhans' cells
Dry, itchy, easily broken skin	
Less padding and insulation of skin	

F7. Choose the name of the common skin lesion in elderly that fits each description.

Actinic keratoses   Lentigines
Senile angiomas   Skin tags

(a) Cherry-red or purple, dome-shaped papules: _____

(b) Brown to black macules in sun-exposed areas; known as liver spots: _____

(c) Precancerous dry, brown-to-red scaly areas in sun-exposed areas: _____

Answers

Chapter 1

CONCEPTS OF HEALTH AND DISEASE

A1. See page 3.
A2. Coronary artery disease, cancer, and stroke
A3. Angry gods or evil spirits in the past to current awareness of effects of microbes, genetic mutations, and lifestyle factors (e.g., diet, exercise, stress)
A4. Smallpox introduced by Spanish conquistadors to Aztecs; other Europeans who also introduced smallpox as well as other infections to Native Americans.
A5. No, although emotions may contribute to illness.
A6. The stigma associated with disease (e.g., AIDS or other sexually transmitted diseases) may lead to delay in seeking treatment. Misunderstanding of causes of disease has perpetuated social conditions that contribute to disease.
B1. (a) Hippocrates; (b) Galen; (c) Harvey; (d) van Leeuwenhoek; (e) Jenner; (f) Nightingale; (g) Pasteur; (h) Röentgen; (i) Wald; (j) Fleming; (k) Salk
B2. See page 11.
B3. Access to worldwide travel (for example, in spread of AIDS and "mad cow disease" or variant BSE); development of resistant strains of microbes; tobacco with enhanced levels of nicotine content
B4. For discussion
B5. For discussion
C1. (a) WHA (1977)
   (b) WHO (1948)
   (c) USDHHS Healthy People 2010
C2. (a) Some of Tasha's systems have not yet fully matured, for example, her immune system. She still lacks the intestinal flora that provide a major source of vitamin K (needed for normal blood clotting).
   (b) Joyce's compromised mobility may interfere with her access to food, water, proper hygiene, and good health care. If she takes aspirin or other nonsteroidal anti-inflammatory drugs (NSAIDs), these can interfere with normal clotting mechanisms and may cause gastric bleeding that may lead to anemia.
C3. (a) Disease, function
   (b) Deviation (or alteration), symptoms; adapt (or compensate)
   (c) Causes (or study of causes); more than one
   (d) Risk; acquired
   (e) Pathogenesis
   (f) Tissues
C4. Erythema (reddened skin), fever, skin lesions, emesis (vomiting), and syncope (fainting), all of which can be observed or measured by another person
C5. See page 14.
C6. By careful analysis of information gathered from a history and physical as well as diagnostic tests
C7. 95%
C8. (a) Validity
   (b) Reliability
   (c) Sensitivity
C9. (a) Carrier
   (b) Subclinical
   (c) Exacerbations
   (d) Chronic, Acute (or Exacerbations).
D1. (a) (2)
   (b) (2)
   (c) (1)
   (d) (1)
D2. (a) Longitudinal or cohort
   (b) The Massachusetts city; 1950, heart (or coronary artery); 5,000
   (c) 121,000; 25; breast cancer
D3. (a) Its progression and outcome **without** medical intervention
   (b) Probable outcome with or without specific interventions
D4. (a) Tertiary
   (b) Primary
   (c) Secondary
   (d) Secondary
   (e) Primary
   (f) Tertiary

Chapter 2

DEVELOPMENTAL ASPECTS: CONCEPTS OF HEALTH AND DISEASE IN CHILDREN

A1. (a), (b); but (c) sudden infant death syndrome; (d) supine (face up)
A2. (a) 7.2
   (b) (2)
B1. (a) Birth
   (b) 2.54; 191 (Note: 36 inches × 2.54 cm/inch = 91.44 cm); 6 feet or 72 inches or 182.88 cm
   (c) 14, 21
   (d) Two
   (e) Head and proceeds towards the lower extremities
B2. Zygote, Morula, Blastocyst, Gastrula
B3. (a), (d); but (b) trophoblast forms placenta; (c) cells form different types of tissues; (e) ectoderm forms these structures.
B4. (a), (d); but (b) in third week; (c) sixth week.
B5. (c), (d); but (a) liver, then spleen; (b) fourth.
B6. (b), (c); but (a) immature hairs that form during fifth month; (d) thin fluid—not mucus—that helps keep alveoli from collapsing.
B7. (c), (d); but (a) second half; (b) after LMP.
B8. Is (since <10th percentile). See p. 24.
B9. (a) Is not
   (b) Weight
   (c) Asymmetric
   (d) Mucus-containing stool
   (e) Neurologic, muscular, skin; Ballard

B10. High; higher; hypo (because insulin tends to cause glucose to move from blood into cells), higher, LGA.

B11. May 25.

C1. (a) 5%-10%
   (b) 50; 20
   (c) 34.5-34.8; greater; 46.5
   (d) Neuroglia; triples
   (e) Faster

C2. (a) Their airways are small and soft (collapse easily because of little supporting cartilage).
   (b) The auditory tube is straight and short (but microbes are just as long as they are in older people).

C3. (a), (c); but (b) pulse decreases; (d) does not; rather, it is smooth.

C4. (a) Small bladder size and inability of the immature kidneys to concentrate urine.
   (b) Small capacity of stomach, rapid emptying of the stomach; in first several days, poor sucking reflex, so a small intake of food increases hunger.

C5. (b), (e); but (a) 1 and 5 minutes; (c) scores range between 0 and 10; (d) score of 0 to 3 indicates severe distress.

C6. 4; yes, until a score of 7 or higher has been measured.

C7. (b), (c); but (a) does not; (d) abnormal labor or delivery.

C8. (a), (c); but (b) clavicle; (d) vertex refers to a "head first" birth.

C9. (b), (d); but (a) C5-C8 and T1; (c) C7-C8, T1, and affects forearm, wrist, and hand.

C10. (c), (d); but (a) common: 1 in 5; (b) 67%.

C11. (a) Increase, respiratory distress syndrome; higher
   (b) Lower; increase
   (c) Apnea

C12. (a) RDS and IVH
   (b) Breakage of fragile, immature vessels in ventricles of the brain; do not
   (c) Necrotizing enterocolitis; increased; small (ileum); ischemia
   (d) Air within the (intestinal) wall

C13. (a), (d); but (b) lactase is the enzyme that digests milk sugar [lactose]; (c) only if child has proven milk intolerance.

C14. (a) Fluoride and iron
   (b) Comes and goes
   (c) Colic
   (d) Inorganic

C15. (a) SIDS
   (b) Injuries

C16. (a), (b), (d), (e), and (f)

C17. Motor vehicle accidents

C18. (a) Measles, mumps, and rubella
   (b) Diphtheria, pertussis (whooping cough), and tetanus

D1. (a), (d); but (b) 28 pounds, not 36 (birth weight quadruples); (c) in extremities rather than in trunk.

D2. (a) (3)
   (b) (3)
   (c) (2)
   (d) (4)

D3. Myelin formation over neurons is required for maximal function of the nerves that control sphincters. Muscle development contributes to sphincter function. Cognitive development accompanying brain development allows a child to understand reasons and mechanisms for control of body functions.

D4. Increased mobility (related to stronger bones and muscles and improved neurologic control) allows the child to move and explore more, possibly leading to dangerous situations.

E1. (b), (d); but (a) slower; (b) true because Stephanie is likely to weigh 40 kg = 88 pounds at age 12; (c) although weight tends to double during these 6 years, height will increase by only about 30%: 116 cm = 46 inches to 150 cm = 60 inches.

E2. (a), (b); but (c) girls enter puberty about 2 years earlier than boys; but (d) typically form peer relationships.

E3. Skin disorders, asthma, epilepsy, certain cancers, developmental or learning disabilities.

F1. (b), (c); but (a) 2 to 3 years; (d) extremities before trunk.

F2. (a) Decreases, increases, increases
   (b) Increases
   (c) 13
   (d) Increases
   (e) Secondary
   (f) Accidents
   (g) Automobile accidents
   (h) Leukemia
   (i) White; males

F3. (a), (d); but (b) decreased; (c) 50%.

Chapter 3

DEVELOPMENTAL ASPECTS: CONCEPTS OF HEALTH AND DISEASE IN OLDER ADULTS

A1. (b), (c)

A2. (a)

A3. (c), (d); but (a) 10%; (b), 4.2%

A4. An enzyme that helps to maintain the ends of chromosomes (telomeres), which are required for continued cell replication and therefore oppose changes associated with aging.

B1. (b), (d)

B2. (a), (b); but (c) dryness; (d) breakdown

B3. (a), (b); but (c) less; (d) trabecular (spongy)

B4. (b), (c); but (a) 80%; (d) is not

B5. (b), (c); but (a) opposite; (d) increase in thickness of left ventricle

B6. Sit on the side of the bed before standing, and support herself while standing up.

B7. (a), (b)

B8. (a) Decreases
   (b) Decrease
   (c) Increase
   (d) Decrease
   (e) Neither (stay intact)

B9. (a) Presbyopia (trouble focusing on close-up objects)
   (b) Glare and abrupt changes in light
   (c) Difficulty distinguishing blue tones from green
   (d) Difficulty distinguishing high frequency tones as in speech (so that reading lips can be helpful); shouting distorts sounds
   (e) Tendency for cerumen to impact external auditory canals
   (f) Decreased sense of taste
   (g) Decrease in gastric production of intrinsic factor increases risk for vitamin B$_{12}$ deficiency and pernicious anemia

B10. (b), (c), (e); but (a) hearing loss of old age; (d) stomach

B11. (b), (c)

C1. (a) IADL
   (b) IADL
   (c) IADL
   (d) ADL
   (e) ADL
   (f) ADL
   (g) ADL

C2. (a) Overflow
   (b) Stress
   (c) Neurogenic
   (d) Urge
   (e) Functional

C3. (c), (d); but (a) is not; (b) transient

C4. (a) Vision and balance
   (b) Posture, gait, and muscle strength
   (c) Orthostatic hypotension and effects of hypertension and related drugs (such as diuretics) that dehydrate and may lead to dizziness. (See details on page 52 of the text.)

C5. (a), (d), (e); but (b) visual; (c) loss of interest or pleasure in life

C6. Depressed mood may not occur nor may other typical signs of depression (see the APA list, page 54). Instead, somatic signs and symptoms, cognitive changes, or anxiety may present in these patients.

C7. (a), (d); but (b) fewer; (c) weeks

C8. (a), (c); but (b) the most common; (d) acetylcholinesterase (the enzyme that destroys acetylcholine); (e) they are not synonyms

C9. See page 56.

C10. (a) Folstein
   (b) Erikson
   (c) Katz
   (d) Hall

D1. (a) Two to three
   (b) Stays about the same
   (c) More
   (d) Higher
   (e) Decreased, decreased

D2. Use of many prescription and OTC medications, which may interact with each other and cause other disease problems. Example: NSAIDs cause water retention and can exacerbate hypertension.

D3. Associating dosage with a specific activity, such as "take with breakfast," providing pillboxes or blister packs; educating (verbally and in writing) the person about the medication; having prescriptions that are cost effective.

Chapter 4

CELL AND TISSUE CHARACTERISTICS

A1. Most diseases begin at the cellular level.

A2. Water, Proteins, Lipids, Carbohydrates

A3. (a) Lipids
   (b) Carbohydrates
   (c) Potassium
   (d) Water

A4. Form structures of cells such as muscles, fibers in bones, hemoglobin, and antibodies, as well as enzymes that are required for synthesis of carbohydrates and lipids.

A5. (a) Transfer
   (b) Proteins
   (c) Introns
   (d) The nucleolus

A6. Active (euchromatic) sections of cells stain more intensely (i.e., are heterochromatic). The nucleolus is large and prominent in active cells.

A7. (a) Rough ER
   (b) Smooth ER
   (c) Golgi
   (d) Golgi
   (e) Golgi
   (f) Golgi
   (g) Lysosomes
   (h) Peroxisomes
   (i) Mitochondria
   (j) Mitochondria
   (k) Smooth ER
   (l) Smooth ER

A8. (a), (b), (e); but (c) autophagocytosis; (d) mitochondria fit this description

A9. (a)

A10. (a) Flagella
   (b) Cilia
   (c) Actin and myosin
   (d) Centrioles
   (e) Basal bodies

A11. (a) Diabetic changes in microtubules alter ability of white blood cells to migrate to sites of infection.
   (b) The drug restricts the action of microtubules in this disease involving excessive inflammation.
   (c) Airways without functional cilia cannot clear bacteria and other debris.
   (d) These structures indicate disruption of the cytoskeleton of brain neurons.

A12. (a), (c); but (b) hydrophobic; (d) integral

A13. Cystic fibrosis

A14. Cell coat; is

B1. (a) Endocrine; distant from
   (b) Down, decreasing
   (c) Ion
   (d) G, cAMP
   (e) Immunity

(f) Can; the nucleus
B2. (a) S
   (b) G_2
   (c) G_0
B3. (a) Prophase
   (b) Metaphase
   (c) Telophase
B4. They regulate cell division. (See text page 75 for details.)
B5. (a) Anabolism
   (b) Three, two; ATP
   (c) Does not; begins, pyruvate; small
   (d) Lactic; pyruvic; glucose, gluconeogenesis
   (e) Does; citric or tricarboxylic, mitochondria
   (f) Transport; cyanide
   (g) 90; CO_2, H_2O
C1. The cell membrane normally forms a barrier that controls whatever enters and leaves the cell and determines chemical composition of fluids and electrical potential inside and outside cells. Errors in these functions provide the basis for many disorders.
C2. Active; "downhill" with; diffusion, osmosis, and facilitated diffusion
C3. (a) Diffusion
   (b) Facilitated diffusion
   (c) Facilitated diffusion
C4. (a) Phospholipid bilayer. See question A12A above.
   (b) Increases
   (c) Water
C5. (a), (d); but (b) 14 times greater outside; (c) primary
C6. (a) Drinking
   (b) Lysosome
   (c) Leukocyte (white blood cell) or a macrophage
   (d) Exo
C7. (a) Positive
   (b) Electrical changes
   (c) Acetylcholine; high
C8. (a), (c); but (b) millivolts; (d) greater concentration on one side than on the other; (e) permeable
D1. (a) More
   (b) Do not undergo
   (c) Slightly, not mature and can undergo mitosis
D2. Cancer cells, Blood-producing cells in bone marrow, Cells lining the stomach, Skeletal muscle cells
D3. Epithelium, connective, muscle, and nervous; nervous
D4. (a), (d); but (b) avascular; (c) endoderm
D5. (b), (c); but (a) simple columnar; (d) lines urinary bladder
D6. (a) Exo
   (b) Loose
   (c) Parenchymal
   (d) Fat; brown
   (e) Dense regular; muscle to bone
   (f) Dense irregular; bone
D7. (a), (d); but (b) cannot; (c) smaller
D8. (b), (d), (e), (g), (h); but (a) forms muscle cell membrane; (c) from one Z line to another; (f) troponin; (i) single-unit
D9. (a) Axons (*Remember as*: **A** for **A**way from.)
   (b) Afferent

(c) Oligodendrocytes, microglia
D10. (a) Desmosomes
   (b) Gap (nexus) junctions
D11. (a) Polysaccharides; proteoglycans; gels, compression
   (b) Hyaluronic acid; embryonic development, wound repair
   (c) Collagen; ability to stretch
   (d) Adhesion; high; few

Chapter 5

CELLULAR ADAPTATION, INJURY, AND DEATH AND WOUND HEALING

A1. Cells respond to changes in the internal environment; (a)
A2. (a) Decrease in hormones
   (b) Ischemia
   (c) Disuse
A3. (a) Hyperplasia
   (b) Hypertrophy
   (c) Metaplasia
   (d) Hypertrophy (because cells cannot undergo mitosis)
   (e) Hypertrophy (because cells cannot undergo mitosis)
   (f) Hyperplasia (because cells can undergo mitosis)
   (g) Dysplasia
A4. May. The liver's epithelial cells can increase in number (hyperplasia).
A5. The bladder's (detrusor) muscle works extra hard to empty urine through the narrowed urethra. This work causes smooth muscle cells of the bladder to grow in number and size.
A6. (a) Tay-Sachs disease
   (b) Fatty liver
   (c) von Gierke's disease
   (d) Lead poisoning
A7. Excessive breakdown of RBCs (as by incompatible blood transfusion); toxins that destroy RBCs excessively; a "sick liver" (hepatitis or cirrhosis) that is unable to remove bile pigments from RBCs; blocked bile routes (from liver to intestine) through gallstones or a tumor pressing on the bile duct system, so that bile backs up into the liver
A8. A brown chemical that builds up in aging cells. No
A9. Coal miners; coal dust (carbon particles) that interfere with gas exchange in lungs.
B1. (a) Nutritional imbalances
   (b) Chemical injury (and often accompanying nutritional imbalances)
   (c) Ionizing radiation
   (d) Electrical injury
   (e) Temperature extremes
   (f) Mechanical forces
B2. (a) Vasoconstricting
   (b) Increase
   (c) Skin at entrance and exit sites
   (d) Nonionizing

B3. (c), (d); but (a) less; (b) localized irradiation for cancer treatment

B4. An enzyme needed to repair sunlight-induced DNA damage; increased, increased

B5. Liver

B6. (a) Eating or inhaling lead paint or by playing in lead-contaminated soil
(b) 1–2
(c) Anemia; lead colic
(d) Is
(e) Finger stick

B7. Free radical injury, hypoxia, and alteration of calcium homeostasis within cells; free radical injury

B8. Electron(s); smoking, excessive radiation, unwashed foods that were treated with pesticides

B9. (a) Protein
(b) DNA
(c) Lipid

B10. (b), (c), (e); but (a) low oxygen level; (d) irreversible

B11. (a) Lactic; decrease
(b) Little, Na^+/K^+; Na^+, swell; increases, digestive

B12. An organ (could be heart, liver, brain, or muscle) is damaged (possibly by hypoxia) causing cells to open up and release contents (including these enzymes) into blood. The higher the serum levels of these enzymes, the more damage that tissue has sustained.

B13. (a) Low, active (ATPase)
(b) Increase, activate

B14. Reversible; liver and heart

B15. Apoptosis accounts for death of some cells as other cells form to replace them. It functions to eliminate cells during embryologic development to make room for the next stage of development. Apoptosis decreases cell number as a normal part of aging. It accounts for death of endometrial cells (lining the uterus) that are sloughed off during menses when hormone levels fail to support the lining and diminishes breast size after cessation of breast-feeding.

B16. Does. Inadequate apoptosis may be involved in cancer. Apoptosis may destroy neurons in Alzheimer's disease, Parkinson's disease, and amyotrophic lateral sclerosis (ALS or Lou Gehrig's disease). Also some forms of hepatitis as well as thermal and radiation injury.

B17. Unlike
(a) Caseous
(b) Liquefactive
(c) Coagulative

B18. Large; (a), (d)

B19. (a) (5)
(b) Clostridium
(c) Fractured bones, skin, GI tract, vagina
(d) Anaerobic, high

C1. Labile, Stable, Permanent
(a) Permanent
(b) Labile
(c) Stable

C2. (b), (d); but (a) stroma; (c) slower, worse

C3. (a) Inflammatory, Proliferative, Remodeling
(b) (3), (4), (1), (2)

C4. (a) Macrophages are critical to wound healing: their roles include cleaning up debris, releasing growth factors such as TAF, and attracting fibroblasts.
(b) Stimulate growth of new blood vessels (= *angio*).
(c) These WBCs (mainly neutrophils) ingest bacteria and cell debris.
(d) The key cells during the proliferative phase, they secrete the collagen used to form collagen fibers.
(e) With fibroblasts, they form soft, pink granulation tissue that serves as the foundation for a scar.

C5. (a) G and B, because granulation tissue is a sign of the beginning of healing but excessive amounts are "proud flesh" and may need to be removed.
(b) B, because a keloid is excessive scar tissue.

C6. (a), (b); but (c) 10%; (d) 70%-80%

C7. (a) Vitamin B
(b) Vitamin A
(c) Vitamin C (also vitamin A)

C8. (a), (b); but (c) decreases; (d) decrease, delay

C9. Overall, this is true because sutures approximate (bring together) the two sides of the wound, prohibiting entrance of most microbes. However, sutures themselves are foreign bodies that can serve as routes for infection. So sutures are removed (unless they are the type that dissolve) a number of days after suturing.

C10. See page 112 of the text.

Chapter 6

GENETIC CONTROL OF CELL FUNCTION AND INHERITANCE

A1. (a) DNA, protein
(b) Transcription
(c) Messenger
(d) The same; only part

A2. Mitochondria; Leber's hereditary optic neuropathy

A3. (a) Phosphate, sugar (deoxyribose), nitrogenous base
(b) Deoxyriboses and phosphates, deoxyriboses
(c) Thymine, guanine
(d) Helic; only one strand is
(e) Proteins

A4. (a) Three, mRNA; amino acid
(b) Lysine; synonyms
(c) RNA; ribose; uracil; U A G
(d) RNA polymerase; introns; may differ
(e) Smallest; 20; an mRNA codon
(f) Most, nucleus; endoplasmic reticulum (ER), translation
(g) 100–300

A5. (d), (e); but (a) only a small number; (b) induction; (c) structural

A6. (a) DNA, base
(b) Do not
(c) Morphism, cannot

B1. (a), (d); but (b) similar; (c) males

B2. (a) meiosis and mitosis
(b) meiosis

    (c) meiosis
    (d) mitosis
    (e) meiosis

B3. Bivalent formation with crossing over between homologous chromosomes. (Also independent assortment [the way in which homologous chromosomes align] during Metaphase I.)

B4. 4; 1, 3

B5. (a) Cytogenetics.
    (b) Venous blood (lymphocytes).
    (c) The picture that shows all pairs of chromosomes from one cell.
    (d) One with the centromere near the end of an arm
    (e) By a "p" (for petite)
    (f) They allow the DNA in the end of the chromosome to be completely replicated (see Study Guide Chapter 3, Question A4.)

C1. (a) Phenotype, genotype
    (b) Penetrance
    (c) Locus, allele
    (d) Multiple-gene, single-gene; multifactorial

C2. Parent

C3. (a) a
    (b) Mother's (AA); father's (Aa)
    (c) Heterozygous, does not
    (d) Round
    (e) Pedigree

D1. See page 127 of the text.

D2. mRNA; polypeptide (or protein)

D3. (a) The same; close together, are
    (b) X; only one, more (because they have no other X chromosome to override the harmful gene)

D4. Iron (Fe), liver

D5. Both parents or only one

D6. (a) Another species, such as a mouse; gene
    (b) Radioactive DNA or RNA; gene (or DNA sequence)

D7. (a) Insulin, growth hormone
    (b) Bacteria, DNA, human gene
    (c) Bacteria

D8. A gene that is defective (in the patient with cystic fibrosis) can be replaced by normal DNA that is introduced into the patient within the genome of an adenovirus. The virus does not become part of the human genome but does deliver the normal gene product so that patients with cystic fibrosis produce normal mucus.

D9. DNA from the suspect is cleaved with restrictive enzymes, separated, and characterized by probes to reveal banding patterns.

Chapter 7

GENETIC AND CONGENITAL DISORDERS

A1. See Study Guide Chapter 6, Questions C1 and C3.

A2. (b), (c); but (a) some do not appear for decades after birth; (d) may affect many different parts

A3. (a)

A4. (a) 4; 2, 2

(b) 2, 4
    (c) Circles, squares
    (d) Grandmother, mother
    (e) Yes; the partnered daughter on the left and one single son
    (f) Yes: grandmother to her son is shown here; this is not a sex-linked disorder

A5. (See the table.)

A6. (a) Only one parent
    (b) 50%
    (c) Can (in cases of reduced penetrance)

A7. (a) Connective; skeletal, cardiovascular, special senses [eyes]; cardiovascular; tall, thin
    (b) Two, different; NF-1, café-au-lait; eyes; hearing

A8. (a), (c); but (b) usually do not; (d) lysosomal

A9. (a) Recessive (See Table 7-1, page 133 of the text)
    (b) X; males
    (c) Cannot

A10. (a) 50% of children have the autosomal dominant disorder (short limbs); 50% are normal.
    (b) Besides the 25% normal (CC: shown), 50% are likely to be carriers (heterozygous = Cc), and 25% (cc) to have the autosomal recessive disorder, CF.
    (c) Because hemophilia is sex-linked, probabilities are described for children of each gender: 50% of females are normal, and 50% are carriers ($X^H X^h$); 50% of males are normal, and 50% have hemophilia ($X^h Y$). **Note:** no carriers among males.

A11. Pyloric stenosis, clubfoot, diabetes mellitus, congenital heart disease, congenital hip dislocation, and coronary artery disease. (See Table 7-1, text page 133 regarding Fragile X syndrome and Tay-Sachs disease.)

A12. (b), (c); but (a) 47,XX,+21; (d) 47.

A13. (a) Frequently
    (b) Increases
    (c) Smaller, larger
    (d) Leukemia; Alzheimer's

A14. Amniocentesis, chorionic villi sampling, percutaneous umbilical blood sampling.

A15. (a) Turner's
    (b) Klinefelter's
    (c) Fragile X syndrome

A16. (a) Robertsonian translocation
    (b) Deletion

B1. (b), (d); but (a) **first** trimester, specifically during weeks 3 to 8 of gestation; (c) embryonic or fetal abnormality

B2. (a) Is not
    (b) Few
    (c) Lipid, small
    (d) X

B3. (c), (d); but (a) **cause** some abnormalities; (b) throughout the gestation period

B4. No

B5. (a), (d); but (b) urine tests positive for only a short time; (c) increase, which may cause premature birth

B6. (a) Neural tube (such as spina bifida, myelomeningocele, and anencephaly)

(b) Cereals, grains, orange juice, dark leafy vegetables

(c) Tooth

B7. (a) Microorganisms

(b) Protozoan, cats

(c) Viral, German measles

(d) Herpes

C1. See page 144 of the text.

C2. (a) In, alpha fetoprotein

(b) Decrease, increase, human chorionic gonadotropin

C3. (a) Chorionic villi sampling; note: the others can all be performed at about 16 to 18 weeks

(b) Ultrasound

(c) Dermatoglyphic analysis

(d) Amniocentesis

C4. (a) Chromosomes; amniocentesis or CVS

(b) Can; can

Chapter 8

ALTERATIONS IN CELL DIFFERENTIATION: NEOPLASIA

A1. (a) Female incidence: breast, lung, colorectal, uterus

(b) Male deaths: lung, prostate, colorectal, lymphoma. Female deaths: lung, breast, colorectal, pancreas

A2. (c), (d); but (a) cardiovascular disease; (b) differentiation

A3. G_1, S, G_2

A4. (c)

A5. (c), (b), (a)

A6. (a) Lose

(b) Do not

B1. (c), (d); but (a) some; (b) connective or muscle

B2. (a) B

(b) B

(c) M

(d) M

(e) M

B3. (a) More

(b) Each other

(c) Lesser; decreased; infiltrate other regions; enzymes

(d) Markers, less

B4. Kidney carcinomas often metastasize to lungs where they are discovered. Examination of the lung tissue revels that the cancer cells have characteristics of kidney cells, which points to kidneys as the site of the primary tumor.

B5. (a) By infiltration of endometrial (uterine lining) cancer through all layers of the uterine wall, through the peritoneum, and then by seeding into the abdominopelvic cavity to peritoneum of GI organs, and then infiltration into walls of those organs.

(b) Veins

B6. (a) Testicular veins carry cancer cells from testes, empty directly into inferior vena cava to the right side of the heart, to pulmonary artery, and then to **lungs**.

(b) Veins from intestine (including colon) empty into the portal vein and directly into **liver**.

B7. (Not even) 1; see mechanisms on text page 158.

B8. (a) Platelets

(b) Type IV collagenase

(c) Tumor-angiogenesis factors

(d) NM 23

B9. (a) (2)

(b) Hormones, good blood supply, and undifferentiated state of tumor cells

(c) One billion

B10. (a) Blockage of the bowel by the tumor, breakage of vessels by straining, and pressure of the tumor against blood vessels

(b) Growth of the tumor may exert pressure on ureters, bladder, or urethra

(c) Pressure of the tumor against nerves, ischemia, or metastasis of the tumor into pelvic bones

(d) Cachexia related to production of cachectin (TNF) or interleukin-1 by macrophages or immune cells, anorexia due to cancer treatment. Fluid in abdomen (ascites) may be due to blockage of venous flow or inflammation with increased permeability of the cancerous organs.

(e) Bone metastasis or effects of ectopic production of PTHrP, causing osteolysis and movement of Ca^{++} into blood

C1. (c)

C2. (b), (d); but (a) multifactorial; (c) viruses are implicated in some cancers; (e) many

C3. (b), (c); but (a) irreversible; (d) is; (e) different from

C4. (a) Do not

(b) Antioxidants, inhibit

(c) Dominant

C5. Breast.

C6. Smoked meats (especially those with nitrates), foods fried in reused fat, high-fat diet, lack of dietary fiber, alcohol, smoking and exposure to second-hand smoke, hormones. (See Chart 8-1, page 164 of the text.)

C7. Chemicals released during smoking are procarcinogens that are activated by metabolism in the liver; a lifetime of such assault to the liver can lead to serious liver damage. The activated carcinogens may trigger cells in the liver, pancreas, stomach, or intestine to gradually transform to cancer cells. There is usually a delay of about 5 to 30 years between exposure to chemical carcinogens and development of recognizable cancer.

C8. (a) Vaginal

(b) Skin

(c) Leukemia

(d) Lung

C9. Some cancers are directly caused by viruses. However, viruses play more important functions in cancer research; human cells have been found to have some DNA sequences (proto-oncogenes) similar to DNA in viruses that cause cancer in laboratory animals.

C10. (a) Hepatitis B virus

(b) Human T-cell leukemia virus-1

(c) Human papilloma virus

(d) Epstein-Barr virus

D1. (a) As cells become more abnormal, their cell surfaces change so they lose cohesiveness and are more likely to shed (exfoliate).

(b) Breast and testicular self-examinations, and colorectal screening

D2. PSA is a tumor marker, an antigen found on certain cancer cells, such as those of the prostate. An increase in PSA in circulating blood points to increase in the number of cancer cells from Mr. Rodenberger's prostate cancer.

D3. (a) Carcinoembryonic antigen

(b) Alpha-fetoprotein

D4. High, high

D5. (a) S (**Hint:** remember "S" for staging and "S" for spread of the tumor); lymph nodes

(b) G (grading studies the pathology of cancer cells to indicate degree of malignancy); Grade IV.

D6. 90. See page 169.

D7. In people with a family history of cancer; for example, breast or colon cancer.

D8. (c)

D9. (a) Adjuvant

(b) Ionizing, rapidly; radiosensitive

(c) Multiple fractionated; cancer cells die, but normal tissue is more likely to recover between treatments.

(d) Hypoxic cells have fewer free radicals of oxygen to be susceptible to radiation.

(e) Rapidly dividing skin and bone marrow cells are vulnerable to radiation.

D10. (a) Unsealed internal radiation

(b) Brachytherapy

(c) External beam radiation

D11. (a) Only a specific proportion (percentage) of the cancer cells are killed with each course of treatment.

(b) Combination

(c) Specific; S; CMF

(d) Venous blood

D12. (a) Bone marrow suppression causes platelet count to drop to its lowest point—in this case, after 21 days of chemotherapy.

(b) Severity of the drug for causing vomiting and diarrhea

(c) Mouth sores (*stoma* = mouth) due to effects of chemotherapeutic drugs on rapidly dividing epithelial cells.

(d) Cessation of menses due to effects on the endometrial lining of the uterus

(e) Caustic effects of the chemotherapy may alter normal cells so that they too become malignant over time.

D13. Chemotherapy destroys rapidly dividing body cells, including

(a) hair cells

(b) cells lining the GI tract (causing nausea, vomiting, diarrhea, and anorexia)

(c) WBC-forming cells in marrow (increasing her risk for infection)

(d) RBC-forming stem cells in bone marrow (causing anemia and related fatigue)

D14. It blocks estrogen receptors on some cells, such as in the breast or endometrium.

D15. Methods that alter the person's response to cancer

(a) A

(b) A

(c) P

(d) P

D16. (a) Hematopoietic growth factors

(b) Monoclonal antibodies

(c) Interferons

(d) Interleukins

D17. (a) An HLA-matched donor's cells

(b) To destroy her malignant blood cells and stem cells

(c) Neutrophils, erythrocytes, platelets

(d) Stem cells are taken from circulating blood (veins) rather than from marrow, so PBSTC is less invasive, less costly, and involves less risk of leukocytopenia.

D18. Germ-line; has not. See page 175.

E1. (c), (d); but (a) secondary to injuries/accidents; (b) blood, neuroglia, or connective tissue

E2. (a) Less, difficulty in

(b) Higher; high

(c) Of preschool age

(d) Are known to

Chapter 9

STRESS AND ADAPTATION

A1. (a) Claude Bernard

(b) Walter Cannon

(c) Hans Selye

A2. (a) Increase, dilate; negative, opposite

(b) Negative; stability; elevated; lower

B1. See pages 183–184.

B2. Adrenal enlargement, atrophy of the thymus, and gastric ulcer.

B3. General adaptation syndrome.

(a) Alarm, Resistance, Exhaustion

(b) Alarm

(c) Resistance; exhaustion

B4. Mild headaches, insomnia, upset stomach, GI ulcer, joint and muscle problems, cardiovascular and renal diseases

B5. (a) Eustress (perhaps mixed with some distress about this life transition), dis; exo

(b) External, decrease (although they may have strengthened her coping skills)

B6. Nervous (releasing neurotransmitters), endocrine (releasing hormones), and immune (releasing chemical mediators)

B7. This is true of mild, short-lived stress, but not true of severe, prolonged, uncontrolled distress, which can become pathologic.
B8. (a) Thalamus
  (b) Reticular activating system, cerebral cortex
  (c) Limbic system
  (d) Hypothalamus, locus ceruleus–norepinephrine pathway
  (e) Locus ceruleus–norepinephrine pathway
  (f) Hypothalamus
B9. (a) Sympathetic, catecholamine; increasing, decreasing, increasing, dilating
  (b) Glucocorticoid, increases, decreases, decreases
  (c) Low; negative
  (d) Stimulates, increases; positive
  (e) Inhibits, thrive
  (f) ADH, retain, increase
  (g) Decrease, menstruate (amenorrhea); decrease, decrease.
B10. (a) Catecholamines, such as NE and epinephrine, and glucocorticoids, such as cortisol; receptors
  (b) Lymphocytes, pituitary, adrenal
B11. For discussion
B12. (a) (2); timing of onset
  (b) (2); age
  (c) (2); health status
  (d) (1); psychological factors
B13. Insomnia: inability to fall asleep or stay asleep. Increased somnolence: tendency to sleep excessively
C1. (a) Chronic intermittent
  (b) Chronic sustained
C2. The compensatory sympathetic response of vasoconstriction of vessels in kidneys (as well as GI organs and skin) can further injure Mr. Clement's already compromised kidneys. Because patients with diabetes are at increased risk for heart disease, the high blood pressure may cause cardiac overload.
C3. Stress (such as that related to examinations or a significant social event) can increase risk for infections (such as cold sores or flu) that might not occur if presickness stress levels had been lower.
C4. (a) Avoidance, depression, alcohol or drug abuse, survival guilt
  (b) Sleep disturbances, intrusions
C5. (a) War, bombings, or other violence (including rape and child abuse); airplane or automobile crashes; tornados; floods; hurricanes
  (b) Fear, sympathetic, decreased; decreased cortisol levels
  (c) Decrease
  (d) Relaxation; guided imagery; music, art, or massage therapy; biofeedback; and psychotherapy
C6. Decreases, constriction; electrothermal
C7. Human stress responses vary; suitable (nonstressful) measurement methods for humans are limited and many are invasive, such as checking blood for antibody levels and lymphocyte count.
  (a) Heart rate and blood pressure
  (b) Electrodermal skin resistance

  (c) Catecholamines (epinephrine and norepinephrine)
  (d) Cortisol
C8. No causal link has been established. However the link between stress and disease is compelling. See question B1 and page 183 of the text.

Chapter 10

ALTERATIONS IN TEMPERATURE REGULATION

A1. (d), (e)
A2. (a) Does; fluid in his middle ear and the small size of his ear canal
  (b) 104.0°F; 1.8
  (c) Dilation
A3. (a) G
  (b) G
  (c) G
  (d) L
  (e) L
  (f) G (because less blood volume is available to reach skin surface)
A4. (a) Convection
  (b) Conduction
  (c) Evaporation
  (d) Radiation
B1. (a) Resetting the temperature set point in the hypothalamus
  (b) 40 (104); convulsions or higher ambient temperature
  (c) Pyrexia; decrease; resetting the temperature set point
  (d) Exo; endo, interleukin, tumor necrosis factor
B2. (a) Injured heart cells or macrophages may release pyrogens.
  (b) Cytokines may be released by the lymphocytes present in excessive numbers in Hodgkin's disease.
  (c) Neurogenic fever
B3. Slight fever does activate the immune system (leukocytes and interferon) and retards growth of some microbes.
B4. (a) Relapsing
  (b) Remittent
B5. Increase; increases.
B6. Prodrome → Chill → Flush → Defervescence
  (a) Chill
  (b) Flush, defervescence
B7. Increased body temperature activates the dormant virus.
B8. Fever of unknown origin with a temperature of 101°F or higher for at least 3 weeks. See page 201.
B9. More poorly; 38°C = 100.4°F
B10. Elderly persons typically maintain a lower baseline temperature, which may mean that a temperature of 100.2°F is considerably elevated. Oral temperature may not be accurate due to tongue tremors and mouth breathing associated with PD. Mr. Baker's anticholinergic medication taken for PD may

decrease his ability to sweat; his diuretic medication reduces the volume of blood that can cool his body.

B11. Heat cramps→ heat syncope→heat exhaustion→heat stroke
(a) Heat syncope; heat cramps
(b) Heat stroke

B12. Rapidly; 43°C (109.4°F); brain, heart, lungs.

B13. (a) Increases
(b) Decrease, constriction, pyrogens
(c) Are not

B14. Bad or serious (not cancerous); is; rapid; skeletal muscle; anesthetics or muscle relaxants may trigger episodes.

C1. (a) Water
(b) Severe; is not
(c) Low blood pressure, decreased metabolic rate and oxygen consumption, loss of consciousness. Note: shivering and rapid heart rate accompany mild hypothermia; hyperglycemia is likely to occur.
(d) Active, unable

Chapter 11

ALTERATIONS IN NUTRITIONAL STATUS

A1. See pages 209–210.

A2. By eating (p.o. or per os = by mouth); by enteral feeding through a tube into the GI tract; by parenteral feeding (a line directly into vein); and by use of stored foods (from liver, muscle, adipose deposits).

A3. Fats, alcohol, carbohydrates or proteins

A4. (a) Carbohydrates
(b) Fats
(c) Fats
(d) Carbohydrates (specifically, glucose)
(e) Fats
(f) Proteins
(g) Fats
(h) Carbohydrates
(i) Fats
(j) Fats
(k) Proteins
(l) Proteins

A5. (a) Synthesis; uses; ATP; enzymes
(b) Catabolic; 100 to 115 (400 to 460 at 4 kcal/g); can be supplied by amino acids and the glycerol portion of triglycerides that are converted to glucose. See A5(d).
(c) Triglycerides (fats) in adipose stores and glycogen (complex carbohydrate) in liver and skeletal muscle
(d) Glycogenolysis, gluconeogenesis; glucagon
(e) All except insulin (which lowers blood glucose level)

A6. "Water weight" is lost as hydrated glycogen stores are catabolized before water-free fat stores are lost.

A7. See page 213.

A8. Heat.

A9. (a) 7
(b) 3.5 hours
(c) About 1.25 (75 minutes)

A10. No. Health consequences would occur. See page 216.

A11. (a) (1)
(b) (1)
(c) (2)
(d) (1)
(e) (2)
(f) (2)
(g) (2)
(h) (2)
(i) (1)
(j) (1)
(k) (1)

A12. (a) Dietary intake
(b) Health history
(c) Physical examination
(d) Anthropometric measurement
(e) Laboratory studies

A13. (a) to (c) Compare your answers with those of a colleague. (Watch decimal points when squaring meters.)
(d) Obese; see Table 11-7 in text.

B1. (a) 25
(b) 55; 3 (18%)
(c) Both genetic and environmental
(d) Women

B2. See text pages 220–221.

B3. Fat distribution
(a) 0.933 (42″/45″); upper; upper body or abdominal
(b) Visceral. Hypertension, heart disease, stroke, type 2 diabetes, some forms of cancer, arthritis, sleep apnea, social and psychological effects, and others listed on text page 222.

B4. See text pages 221–223.

B5. (a) (1), because older than 45 years; (2), because his waist is over 40″; (3) because HDL is less than 35 mg/dL and LDL is more than 160 mg/dL; not (4) because BP is less than 140/90 mm Hg; not (5), (6), or (7) because his BMI is just over 30. Calculation of his BMI: 220 pounds = 100 kg; 6′ = 72 inches × 2.54 cm/inch = 182 cm = 1.82 m. $1.82 m^2 = 3.31 m^2$. BMI = 100 kg/3.31 = 30.2 kg/m^2.
(b) 300–500 (based on a BMI between 27 and 35); 30
(c) One half, most days each week
(d) See text page 223.
(e) Is not.

B6. Common; 14; triceps, 120; that obese children grow up to be obese adults, and psychosocial concerns for children, such as low self esteem and discrimination

B7. Highly educated parents, obese parents

C1. (a) Physical health problem
(b) Willful eating behaviors
(c) Lack of food availability

C2. (a) Marasmus
(b) Marasmus

(c) Kwashiorkor
(d) Kwashiorkor
C3. (a) Fat
(b) Fat
(c) Protein
(d) Protein
(e) Carbohydrate, fat, protein
C4. Respiratory, cardiac, and other muscle weakness, problems with digestion and absorption, diminished immunity and healing. (See details on page 225.)
C5. Slowly; is, should not
C6. (a) Females; 56
(b) Reproductive (amenorrhea) and skeletal (osteoporosis).
C7. (b), (c), (d); but (a) not quite low enough to meet DSM-IV-TR criterion of 85%. (e) and (f) are a part of the anorectic profile but are not listed as part of the DSM-IV-TR criteria.
C8. Decreased estrogen production stops the monthly thickening (then sloughing) of the uterine lining. Because estrogen protects against bone loss, estrogen deficiency in the anorectic can mimic osteoporosis of elderly, complete with kyphosis and fractures.
C9. (a) Binge eating two or more times a week; self-induced vomiting
(b) Purging
(c) Action of gastric acid on teeth and on the esophageal lining
(d) Repeated bouts of emesis are likely to result in aspiration of vomitus into lungs with resulting infection.
(e) Bulimia, since not as dramatically low as that of an anorectic
C10. See page 227.

Chapter 12

ALTERATIONS IN ACTIVITY TOLERANCE

A1. See page 231.
A2. (a) Lower, raise
(b) Improve
(c) Better, increase
(d) Decreased depression and improved self-esteem and quality of life, especially if she exercises with friends
A3. (a) Aerobic; endurance; red, many; oxygen
(b) Isometric, does not; resistance; strength, white, fast-twitch; few
(c) Isometric
A4. (a) Motivation and mental endurance
(b) Cardiopulmonary fitness (which can lead to lack of muscle strength, flexibility, and endurance; energy sources; and motivation and mental endurance)
(c) Muscle strength, flexibility, and endurance and possibly energy sources and cardiopulmonary fitness

(d) Energy sources, which can also result in lack of cardiopulmonary fitness; muscle strength, flexibility, and endurance; and motivation and mental endurance
A5. (a) Heart (cardiac output), lung function, transport of O_2 and CO_2 within blood, and arterial blood flow into muscles along with their ability to extract oxygen
(b) Each minute; 5 (range of 4–8); 2–6 (range of 15–22 L/min)
(c) (2)
(d) Sympathetic; norepinephrine
(e) Increases; more; increases
(f) Systolic; skeletal muscles; pulse; increases; 48 to 70
(g) Perfusion; increase
(h) Increase
(i) Dilate; constricted; increased
(j) Red
A6. (a) Flexibility
(b) Strength
(c) Endurance
A7. (a) (2)
(b) (3)
(c) (1)
(d) (2)
A8. (a) ↑
(b) ↑
(c) ↑
(d) ↓
(e) ↑
A9. (a) Rating of perceived exertion
(b) Metabolic equivalents
(c) Maximal heart rate
(d) Fatigue severity scale
(e) Human activity profile
(f) Ergometric tests
B1. (a) Tiredness is relieved by a good night's sleep, whereas fatigue persists.
(b) See text page 236.
(c) Central: related to a CNS problem; peripheral: related to muscle or nerve problem
(d) Deconditioned persons are more likely to develop fatigue.
B2. (b), but (a) insidious; (c) is not; (d) does not
B3. It may interfere with job, socializing, ADLs, and quality of life in general. See Table 12-1.
B4. (a) Months'; 1, 3
(b) (1), (3), (5) (pharyngitis and cervical lymph nodes), (6) (malaise and fatigue); but (2) typically without swelling, (4) often occurs but not a diagnostic criterion
(c) Unknown (idiopathic); infections (viral, bacterial, or fungal) possibly activating immune changes in NK cells, interleukin-2, or interferon; hormonal, neural, or psychological disorders
(d) (2)
(e1) Guaiac test
(e2) Serum Na^+ and K^+
(e3) CBC
(e4) Lyme disease

(e5) Blood glucose

(e6) BUN

(f) See text page 240.

C1. Skeletal muscles of legs contract and return blood to the heart (reducing venous stasis and potential clot formation). Bones are strengthened by stimulation of body weight and the pull of gravity on bones.

C2. (a) Thorax, arms, and head; increased; 7-8; decreased

(b) Decreased; increased, de; increase

(c) Increased, decreasing; increase

(d) Orthostatic (postural); autonomic (sympathetic), a

(e) Nausea, sweating and tachycardia (both related to sympathetic activity), and possibly fainting upon standing

C3. (a) Workload to meet oxygen demands associated with decreased circulating blood volume due to dehydration and decreased cardiac filling (caused by shortened diastole in tachycardia)

(b) Stasis; DVT and PE

(b1-3) Venous stasis, irritated vessel lining (due to pressure against the mattress), and hypercoagulability due to stasis and also hypercalcemia which enhances clot formation.

C4. See text pages 242–244.

C5. (b), (d), (e); but (a) 12% or one-eighth, (c) faster; (f) soft and spongy and more prone to fracture

C6. Decreased capillary flow in skin and subcutaneous tissue overlying bony prominences (related to increased pressure), increased moisture of skin (due to compensatory sweating), and effects of shearing forces on skin; for example, by being moved in bed

C7. (a) ↓

(b) ↑

(c) ↑

(d) ↓

(e) ↓

C8. Implement an interdisciplinary approach that addresses both physical and psychosocial needs; reduce sensory deprivation; and create a safe environment that reduces risk of complications acquired in the health care setting (nosocomial).

Chapter 13

BLOOD CELLS AND THE HEMATOPOIETIC SYSTEM

A1. (a) Plasma, Buffy coat, Red blood cells

(b) Buffy coat

(c) Red blood cells

A2. Plasma proteins are produced in a healthy liver. These include albumins that normally act as "blotters" that hold water in plasma. Low plasma albumin levels cause fluid to leave plasma and leads to edema and ascites. Plasma protein gamma globulin (antibodies) normally provide some immunity from infections. The plasma protein fibrinogen is needed for blood clotting.

A3. (a) Red blood cells; carrying O_2

(b) Leukocytes; infection control

(c) Neutrophil; bone marrow; myeloblasts; indicates a blood disorder

(d) Mature, immature; marginating; early; lysosomes

A4. (a) Lymphocytes

(b) Monocytes

(c) Basophils

(d) Eosinophils

(e) Lymphocytes, monocytes

A5. Bleeding; 150,000 to 400,000

A6. Blood formation.

(a) Liver and spleen, bone marrow

(b) RBC; fat; pelvis, ribs, and sternum

(c) Pluripotent stem, do; differentiate

(d) Aplastic anemia and leukemias; transplant

(e) Cytokines; red; G-CSF; lymphocyte

B1. (a) White blood cell (a little high)

(b) Red blood cell

(c) Differential WBC

(d) Blood smear

B2. High; inflammation indicated by the release of fibrinogen that elevates ESR.

B3. Hip bone. See page 257.

Chapter 14

ALTERATIONS IN HEMOSTASIS

A1. Stoppage (or standing) of blood flow

A2. Vasospasm → Platelet plug formation → Coagulation → Clot retraction → Fibrinolysis

A3. (a) Constrict; less than a minute

(b) Thromboxane A_2 (TXA_2); platelets; prostacyclin

(c) Megakaryocytes; can, growth factors

(d) Week (8–9 days); thrombo

(e) Spiny; collagen; vWF

(f) Increases; fibrin

A4. (a) Blood; blood vessel

(b) Blood vessels

(c) K

(d) Calcium (Ca^{++})

A5. (a) IV (Ca^{++})

(b) X

(c) VIII

A6. (a) Fibrinogen (made in the liver) is the inactive form of fibrin, which is insoluble and constitutes the meshwork of clots (thrombi).

(b) Thrombin is the active enzyme that converts fibrinogen to fibrin to *form* clots (**coagulation**); plasmin is the active enzyme that *breaks down* fibrin clots (**fibrinolysis**).

(c) An anticoagulant (heparin or Coumadin) prevents (or limits) clot formation, whereas fibrinolytic agents (e.g., tPA or urokinase) break down clots that have *already* formed.

A7. Possibly, because the decision was made to give him tPA. Other factors, such as ECG readings, would contribute to the diagnosis. The chemical tPA can also be given to break down clots involved with

CVA (stroke), for DVT or PE, or for keeping coronary bypass grafts open or patent.

A8. (a) Warfarin (or Coumadin)

(b) Heparin

(c) Plasminogen

(d) Tissue plasinogen activator

(e) Plasminogen activator inhibitor

A9. (a) Calcium ions, coagulation factors VII-XII, fibrinogen, thrombin

(b) Antithrombin III, heparin, protein C, warfarin (Coumadin)

(c) Tissue plasminogen activator, protein C, thrombin (regulates coagulation by triggering clot formation but also activating plasminogen activators to break down clots)

B1. Blood clots can stop unwanted bleeding. However, inappropriate clot formation (thrombi) can be harmful, even lethal (eg, in cerebral or coronary arteries).

B2. Veins. (a–b) See Chart 14-1.

B3. (a) Damaged blood vessel lining, platelet adhesiveness and aggregation

(b) Damaged blood vessel lining, platelet adhesiveness and aggregation

(c) Damaged blood vessel lining, platelet adhesiveness and aggregation

(d) Platelet adhesiveness and aggregation (related to high platelet count)

(e) Stasis of blood flow (leading to increased clotting factors)

(f) Stasis of blood flow (leading to increased clotting factors)

(g) Increased clotting factors

(h) Increased clotting factors (and possibly stasis of blood flow related to immobility resulting from illness).

B4. Long-term sitting (eg, in a car, plane, or bus) increases risk of PE because venous return is impeded from legs into iliac veins (at flexed hips)—especially in obese persons. Taking frequent walks and drinking adequate fluids keeps circulation moving and helps prevent PE formation. His age also puts him at risk for slower circulation so clotting factors "get more friendly with each other."

C1. (a) (3). Note from Table 13-2, page 253, that a normal thrombocyte count is 150,000-400,000.

(b) (2)

(c) (3)

C2. (a) Blood backs up from the liver into abdominal organs, enlarging the spleen so that it sequesters more platelets than normal.

(b) Sulfa is a type of drug that destroys platelets.

(c) Chemotherapy leads to bone marrow suppression with decreased production of megakaryocytes.

(d) Thrombotic thrombocytopenic purpura (TTP).

C3. Newborns lack the normal flora in the colon required to synthesize vitamin K. After ingesting food in the digestive tract, Kareenya will begin to establish an intestinal flora that will produce vitamin K.

C4. (a) The liver is the source of many clotting factors, including prothrombin, fibrinogen, and factors V, VII, and IX to XII.

(b) Aspirin and NSAIDs often taken as analgesics are platelet inhibitors.

(c) Antibiotics can destroy the normal intestinal flora that produce vitamin K.

(d) Hemophilia A, an X-linked recessive disorder that occurs almost entirely in males.

(e) Van Willebrand disease, the most common hereditary bleeding disorder, which may not manifest until dental extraction leads to prolonged bleeding.

C5. Factors that can lead to hypocoagulability are splenomegaly, lack of vitamin K, lack of Factor VIII as in the most common form of hemophilia, taking 0.5 aspirin each day, heparin or Coumadin. Factors that lead to hypercoagulability are aneurysm (stasis), smoking, smoking and taking oral contraceptives, dehydration (stasis of thickened blood), diabetes mellitus

C6. Disseminated intravascular coagulation

(a) See Chart 14-3.

(b) Massive clotting occurs in "unneeded" areas (leading to organ ischemia and failure), using up clotting factors so they are not available for needed clots (leading to extreme bleeding and bruising).

(c) Bleeding; see page 268.

(d) Kidneys, heart, lungs, and brain

C7. (a) Thin-walled, dilated capillaries and arterioles

(b) Bruising in the elderly

Chapter 15

THE RED BLOOD CELL AND ALTERATIONS IN OXYGEN TRANSPORT

A1. Transport oxygen; transport carbon dioxide; the biconcave disk shape provides much cell membrane surface area for diffusion and deformability allows RBCs to squeeze through narrow capillaries.

A2. HbF; it allows fetal blood to transport more oxygen through the relatively inefficient fetal circulatory system

A3. (a) Meats (or green, leafy vegetables); transferrin; ferritin; ferritin

(b) (3)

A4. (a) Pluripotent stem cells → Erythroblasts → Normoblasts → Reticulocytes → Erythrocytes

(b) Reticulocytes

(c) 120, 1; nucleus

(d) Kidneys

(e) Hypoxia

A5. Failing kidneys do not produce erythropoietin, so RBC production is limited. LaVerne's Hb level is well below a normal range of 12 to 15g/dL. Fatigue is a classic sign of anemia and it becomes more intense as anemia worsens. Erythropoietin (EPO) therapy can help.

A6. Bilirubin; observe his sclera ("whites of the eyes") and note if they appear yellow. Significant RBC destruction (as by transfusion reactions or HDN [see question E2]) or obstructions of bile pathways.

A7. Maturing RBCs lose their mitochondria, which are the site of aerobic metabolism in other body cells. When 2,3-DPG binds to Hb, it causes oxygen to be released into tissues.

A8. (a) 4
(b) 14 (not 42, which would be hematocrit)
(c) 4
(d) 120

A9. (a) 37% to 47% (for women)
(b) (3), because it focuses on the newly formed ("adolescent") RBCs, which will rise more dramatically than the entire RBC count or hematocrit
(c) 15; 1 is a normal count, but the goal of therapy is an increased reticulocyte count. Values for reticulocytes are in "% of total RBCs," so can never exceed 100%. A number greater than 100 would indicate an error in documentation.

A10. (a), (d); but (b) jaundice may *accompany* anemia if the cause of anemia is breakdown of RBCs, but jaundice is a sign of hyperbilirubinemia; (c) false because males have the effect of testosterone stimulating blood cell formation, and the female population as a whole has a lower RBC count related to regular menstrual flow among much of the female population.

B1. (a) Hemorrhage (bleeding), RBC destruction
(b) Nutritional (iron, folic acid, or vitamin B_{12}); bone marrow

B2. (a) Fatigue, weakness, angina, or dyspnea; increased; pallor; increased
(b) Size
(c) Fracture or brain injury

B3. (a) Acute; dilute; normal
(b) Chronic; is; reduced; hypochromic

B4. (a), (d); but (b) one of 12 = 8%; (c) less

B5. (a) Hypoxia-triggered events in which RBCs sickle because of defective hemoglobin; sickled cells occlude vessel and cause painful ischemia and organ damage.
(b) Cold exposure, physical exertion, dehydration, infection
(c) (3)
(d) (4), because HbF is typically replaced by HbS by then
(e) The spleen, which normally destroys encapsulated microorganisms when a child's ability to produce antibodies is still undeveloped; microbes may enter blood stream (septicemia).
(f) Is not; are

B6. (a) B_{12} deficiency
(b) Folic acid deficiency
(c) Hemorrhagic
(d) Chronic disease
(e) Iron-deficiency
(f) Hemolytic
(g) Aplastic
(h) Sickle cell (also a form of hemolytic)
(i) Thalassemia (also a form of hemolytic because RBC membrane is fragile)
(j) Spherocytosis

B7. Women.
(a) Because of blood lost in menstruation.
(b) Others with increased blood loss: people with gastric irritation and bleeding, hemorrhoids or polyps, and those having blood drawn frequently. Persons requiring more iron for increased growth, such as pregnant women or growing children. Additionally, those with decreased dietary intake of iron, such as individuals who cannot chew meat and lack other dietary sources of iron.

B8. (a) Red blood; myelin; stomach (or gastric); small (ileum)
(b) Cancer cells compete with normal cells for folic acid, and methotrexate, often used in chemotherapy, blocks activation of folic acid; neural tube.

B9. (a), (b); but (c) it is not likely that a newborn baby will have been exposed to factors such as radiation, chemotherapy, or toxins that typically cause bone marrow destruction; (d) splenomegaly is more likely to "snag" RBCs and cause hemolytic anemia.

C1. (c), (d); but (a) when hemoglobin reaches 8 to 10 g/dL = hematocrit of 24-30%; (b) rapid massive hemorrhage or acute anemia

C2. (a), (c); but (b) AA or AO; (d) Oliver would have experienced a number of months of exposure to A and B blood (as people cough or sneeze around him) before he would have developed A and B antibodies in his serum.

C3. (a), (d); but (b) do not; (c) destruction of donor's RBCs because they are transfused into the recipient in a mass that will cause a local antigen-antibody reaction as recipient's antibodies attack them; donor's antibodies are diluted out in the recipient's plasma, so do not usually cause a reaction.

C4. Symptoms of a transfusion reaction include chills, difficulty breathing, fever, hives, nausea and vomiting. Other symptoms are a sensation of heat (not cold); tachycardia (not bradycardia); flushed face (not pale); hypotension (not hypertension).

D1. (d)

D2. (a) All except (6).
(b) All
(c) (2)

D3. (a) Primary
(b) Relative
(c) Secondary
(d) Secondary. Note in considering parts (d) and (e): hypoxia stimulates erythropoietin in both cases.

E1. (a) Declined; HbA
(b) Less; are; common

E2. (a) Second or third; negative
(b) Higher; kernicterus; brain; photo, fluorescent lights; urinary and digestive.
(c) Negative.

(d) Antibodies (that will destroy fetal Rh-positive cells that have entered mother's circulation)

E3. Decrease; iron-deficiency anemia

Chapter 16

DISORDERS OF WHITE BLOOD CELLS AND LYMPHOID TISSUES

A1. (a) Myeloid
   (b) Lymphocytes; lymph nodes, thymus, and spleen, as well as lymph and lymph vessels
   (c) Bone marrow; thymus
   (d) Natural killer
A2. See Chapter 13, Question A6(c).
A3. They are all growth factors that stimulate development of different types of blood cells. (See Chapter 13, Question A6[e], and page 292 of the text.)
A4. Afferent lymphatic channels → Lymph node → Efferent lymphatic channels → Collecting trunk → Neck veins
A5. Good news: lymphatics carry fluid and protein back towards blood and clean the fluid along the way. Bad news: lymph pathways can serve as routes for metastasis of cancer cells.
B1. (a) 6,000; leukopenia
   (b) Neutrophils
   (c) One; penia
B2. (a) Felty's syndrome
   (b) Congenital neutropenia
   (c) Drugs that interfere with normal marrow function
   (d) Drugs that interfere with normal marrow function
   (e) Aplastic anemia
   (f) Bacterial or viral infection
   (g) Metastatic solid tumor cancer
   (h) Hemopoietic cancer
B3. Chemotherapy not only destroys rapidly dividing cancer cells, but it also kills normal body cells that rapidly divide, such as those lining the mouth, stomach, intestine; hair-forming cells; and bone marrow. Destruction of blood-forming cells in marrow decreases RBCs → fatigue; destruction of WBCs leads to infections that may exacerbate ("make worse") her mouth sores (ulcerations); the drop in platelet count causes bleeding that exacerbates anemia.
C1. Epstein-Barr virus
C2. Incubation period (4 to 8 weeks) → prodromal (several days) → manifestations (2 to 3 weeks) → recovery phase (2 to 3 months)
C3. EBV → BCD → ATC
C4. (b), (c), (d)
C5. 20 to 30; lymphocytes and monocytes **both** have single, relatively round nuclei that designates them as "mononuclear" (without the segmented lobes seen in neutrophils, eosinophils, or basophils). EBV

affects the lymphocytes in IM. The disease is called lymphocytic mononucleosis.
C6. The excessive number of immature WBCs are very mobile and tend to infiltrate those organs (ie, enlarge them) that are ordinarily sites that remove old blood cells.
C7. (b), (c); but (a) middle to upper socioeconomic levels; (d) do not; (e) mostly by asymptomatic persons who shed the virus for 18 months after the infection.
D1. Huge numbers of immature ("-blasts") WBCs form and circulate in blood and in the lymphatic system; proliferation of these cells prevents normal blood cells from forming. See B2(h) above. In persons of all ages; common
D2. (a) Acute
      (1) R
      (2) W
      (3) P
   (b) Gradual
   (c) Lymphocyte; spleen, lymph nodes, and central nervous system; myelocytic, bone marrow
   (d) Are not; exposure to high levels of radiation and chemotherapy drugs, chromosomal changes
D3. (a) Rapid formation of immature (blast) WBCs
   (b) Owing to the presence of huge numbers of immature WBCs, blood becomes so sluggish that it comes to a standstill.
   (c) Immature WBCs have crossed the blood-brain barrier into the brain, affecting the N/V center, and producing extra intracranial fluid that exerts pressure on the cranial nerves; one effect is papilledema of the optic nerve.
   (d) Chemotherapy destroys WBCs and leads to excessive breakdown of purines to uric acid.
   (e) Necrosis of huge numbers of WBCs leads to life-threatening imbalances in blood electrolytes (see page 298).
   (f) The BMT donor's immune system regards the recipient's cells as foreign and mounts an immune response.
D4. Induction → intensification or consolidation → maintenance
D5. (a) Chemotherapeutic agents do not cross the blood-brain barrier to destroy WBCs that have entered the CNS.
   (b) Antibiotics treat infections caused by leukopenia.
   (c) It is used to treat renal complications from excessive uric acid in urine.
D6. (a) ALL
   (b) AML
   (c) CLL
   (d) CLL
   (e) CML
E1. Bone marrow; lymph tissue; decreased; increased
E2. (a) H
   (b) N-H (*Hint*: remember that Non-Hodgkin's is a longer term than Hodgkin's and involves more lymph nodes initially than Hodgkin's does.)
   (c) H, N-H
   (d) N-H
E3. Epstein-Barr virus (EBV); mononucleosis

E4. Reed-Sternberg; mirror-image, double nucleus that stains with eosin

E5. (a) The stage determines the treatment and points to the prognosis.
(b) Low-grade fever, night sweats, and unexplained weight loss

E6. A combination of chemotherapy. See page 303.

E7. Radiation of her mediastinum (central thoracic region) to control lymphoma there damaged her coronary arteries, reducing blood flow through them over the years.

F1. (a) B; immunoglobulins (Igs)
(b) Osteoclasts; destruction
(c) Heart and nerves; kidneys

F2. Multiple myeloma and treatments both injure bone tissue leading to signs and symptoms of pancytopenia: fatigue, infections, and bleeding problems. As osteoclasts destroy bone tissue, calcium is released into blood (causing hypercalcemia) and deposited in kidneys, destroying them and leading to CRF. Bone tissue is rigid and rich with sensory nerves. Any invasion of cancer into bone (+ effects of treatment) damages bone tissue, stimulating pain nerves there.

Chapter 17

MECHANISMS OF INFECTIOUS DISEASE

A1. (a) Normal microflora; mutualism
(b) Host, virulent, colonized
(c) Pathogenic; opportunistic infection

B1. (a) Viruses
(b) Prions
(c) Viruses
(d) Bacteria
(e) Bacteria
(f) Mycoplasma
(g) Fungi
(h) *Rickettsiae*
(i) *Chlamydiae*
(j) Parasites

B2. (a) Cocci; spirochetes
(b) Clusters, pairs; species
(c) Increase; acid-fast
(d) (2)
(e) (2)

B3. (a) Superficial, cool
(b) Antibiotic therapy kills the normal microflora but does not touch fungi (see B1[g]). As a result, yeast overgrowth causes a "yeast infection."

B4. (a) Protozoa; by direct contact between humans, through infected fecal contamination of food or water, or through arthropod vectors
(b) Roundworms, tapeworms, and flukes; developing nations
(c) Ecto; lice

C1. Study all the factors that contribute to the spread of disease with the goal of interrupting the spread of the infectious agent, as well as predicting and preventing future outbreaks.

C2. (a) Incidence
(b) Epidemic
(c) Endemic

C3. (a) Inhalation
(b) Ingestion
(c) Ingestion
(d) Penetration
(e) Direct contact
(f) Penetration

C4. Direct contact: passage of HIV, rubella, or other viruses across the placenta during pregnancy; infection leading to blindness caused by *Neisseria gonorrhoeae* or trachoma as the baby passes through the mother's infected vagina during birth. Ingestion: HIV infection through breast milk.

C5. (a) Mucus and cilia, coughing, antibodies, and phagocytic cells of alveoli
(b) Low pH (acidity) of the stomach
(c) Intact skin provides a mechanical barrier with its tightly packed epithelial cells.

C6. (a) Fomites
(b) Zoonoses
(c) Nosocomial

C7. Incubation → Prodromal → Acute → Convalescence and recovery (See also Chapter 16, C2 about stages of infectious mononucleosis)
(a) Incubation
(b) Prodromal
(c) Convalescence and recovery
(d) Prodromal

C8. (a) Blood
(b) Diverticulitis
(c) Fulminant
(d) Digestive
(e) Gastric ulcers

C9. (a) Evasive factors
(b) Evasive factors
(c) Invasive factors
(d) Adhesive factors
(e) Toxins

D1. (a) Pathogenic microbe (or pathogen)
(b) Signs and symptoms (or manifestations)

D2. (a) Serology
(b) Culture
(c) Genome sequences
(d) Antigen detection (antigens on the pathogen bind to specific antibodies)

D3. Antimicrobial agents, immunologic approaches, and surgery

D4. Destroy or interfere with some key component of the anatomy or metabolism of the harmful microbe without destroying or interfering with host (human) cells, which would cause side effects

D5. (a) Cephalosporins
(b) Aminoglycosides
(c) Sulfonamides

D6. See text page 327

D7. (a) Antibiotic
(b) Antiviral

(c) Antiparasitic

(d) Antifungal

D8. (a) Immunizations (against measles, mumps, rubella and diphtheria, pertussis and tetanus)

(b) White; phagocytosis, antibody production, leukocytosis, and fever

(c) Cytokines

(d) Intravenous immunoglobulin; bodies

D9. (a) Debridement

(b) Gas gangrene

(c) Infected heart valve

(d) Appendectomy

Chapter 18

IMMUNITY AND INFLAMMATION

A1. (a) S

(b) S

(c) NS

(d) NS

A2. See text page 332.

A3. (a) Antigens; stimulate

(b) Bacteria, fungi, pollen, protozoans, transplanted organs, viruses. (Note that penicillin is a hapten that must complex with body proteins to form an antigen.)

(c) Epitope

(d) Hundreds of

A4. (a), (c), (d), (e); but (b) humoral or antibody-mediated immunity

A5. (a) Gen; antigen presenting; macrophage

(b) Kines, divide (or clone)

(c) Bodies; plasma; humoral

(d) Cell, cytotoxic

A6. Exposed to a myriad of antigens, lymphocytes become programmed to respond to each type of antigen. "Memory" T and B lymphocytes are formed from each clone and remain in the body for a long time, ready to respond when the specific antigen presents itself again.

A7. (a) Major histocompatibility; 6; nonself; gens

(b) Autoimmune; destroy

A8. (a) Nearly every cell of the body; cytotoxic

(b) APCs such as macrophages and B cells; CD4 helper

A9. Human leukocyte, white; HLA-B and HLA-C; is (except for identical twins); very similar

A10. Monocytes; liver; brain and spinal cord (CNS); APCs, CD4; cytokines; phagocytosis

A11. They are both APCs, so both present antigens to lymphocytes; lymphoid, Langerhans'

A12. B

(a) Bacteria and their toxins; causing production of antibodies, humoral

(b) Antibodies (or immunoglobulins); plasma, memory

A13. (a) Proteins, 4, 2

(b) D, E, and G

(c) Antigen, forked, antigen; variable; domain; constant

A14. (a) IgM

(b) IgG

(c) IgA

(d) IgE

(e) IgD

A15. (a) Viral; direct killing action, cell-mediated or CMI

(b) T, B; rejection, delayed

(c) Bone marrow; thymus, CD8

(d) 4, II, cytokines, macrophage or white blood

(e) 8, I; release of cytokines, as well as perforins that punch holes in infected cells and toxic enzymes that destroy cells

(f) Natural killer, are; directly; do not; they recognize MHC molecules on normal cells

A16. (a) Bone marrow and thymus; the remainder are peripheral organs

(b) Thorax, anterior to his heart; smaller

(c) Cortex to medulla; do not; MHC or self

(d) Trunk and proximal ends of his extremities; B and T

(e) Stomach; left; red, B, T

(f) Tonsils (including adenoids) and MALT tissues in mucosa of airways.

A17. (a) Are made by **and** act on; T; nearby, receptors; more than one.

(b) IL-1, IL-6, and TNF

(c) IL-1 to IL-7, IL-11, and CSFs

(d) IL-2

(e) They stimulate cells near cells infected with viruses (or other microbes) to produce anti-viral proteins; IFNs are not pathogen specific.

(f) TNF

A18. (a) S

(b) S

(c) NS

(d) NS

A19. (a) A

(b) A

(c) P

(d) P

A20. B. (See A5[c]). See text page 346.

A21. The second: the secondary or memory response. See text Figure 18-13.

A22. T; Helper, cytotoxic

A23. (a) Proteins, C9, humoral

(b) Dilate, increased; anaphylaxis

(c) Opsonization; chemotaxis

(d) Cytolysis

A24. Antigens, as well as antibodies and cytokines are short-lived; tolerance to self-antigens, which normally prevents autoimmune diseases.

B1. (a) IgGs

(b) Deficient, because most IgGs cross the placenta from mother to fetus during final weeks of pregnancy.

(c) Will, because any antibodies in mother's blood can cross the placenta into fetal blood; although Celia's blood tests positive for HIV (because she does have the antibodies), Celia may not have received sufficient HIV viruses from mother to be infected. Further testing can determine her HIV status.

(d) Cannot; Jill has been exposed to antigens and is producing antibodies against them.

(e) Through breast milk; reduce diarrheal infections in Miji

B2. Cell-mediated immunity, antibody-mediated immunity, T cell count, IL-2 cytokine production

C1. Inflammation is designed to mobilize defenses against infection, but does cause some discomfort and sometimes serious side effects.

C2. (a) Dilation of blood vessels that bring more (warm) blood into the area

(b) Increased permeability of vessels to allow more white blood cells and defensive chemicals to reach tissues

(c) Edema and chemical stimulation of nerves by release of prostaglandins and bradykinin

C3. A number of hours (4 to 24)

C4. (a) Neutrophils; adhesion, margination; 1.5

(b) Diapedesis or emigration; enzymes

(c) Increases; cytosis; bands; left

(d) Baso, eosino; basophils, dilates

(e) Mono; longer; macrophages; lymph nodes

C5. Chemotaxis → adherence/opsonization → engulfment → intracellular killing

C6. Cytokines, bacterial and cellular debris, complement fragments

C7. (a) Increase

(b) Increases

(c) Increases

(d) Increases

(e) Decreases (lethargy sets in)

C8. (a) Prostaglandin

(b) Bradykinin

(c) Platelet-activating factor

(d) Leukotrienes and platelet-activating factor

C9. Watery; leukocytes, proteins, and tissue debris

C10. Chronic; granulomatous; granulomatous, cheesy (like cottage cheese)

Chapter 19

ALTERATIONS IN THE IMMUNE RESPONSE

A1. Protect against microorganisms and cancer, and facilitate healing

A2. Immunodeficiency disorders; allergies or hypersensitivity reactions; transplantation reactions; autoimmune disorders

A3. (a) S

(b) S

(c) P

(d) S

(e) S

(f) P

A4. (a) Combined B-cell and T-cell deficiencies

(b) T-cell (cellular) deficiency

(c) T-cell (cellular) deficiency

(d) Phagocytic dysfunction

(e) Combined B-cell and T-cell deficiencies

(f) B-cell (humoral) deficiency

A5. (c), (d), (f); but (a) many such genes are on X-chromosomes; (b) IgGs; (e) less

A6. (a) IgA; 50%; does not

(b) IgG; polysaccharide, polysaccharide

(c) IgMs are too large to pass across kidney membranes. (Look again at textbook Figure 18-3.)

A7. Secondary; few persons survive primary T-cell deficiencies very long. Autosomal (chromosome 22). Failure of thymus and parathyroids to develop (with hypocalcemia); heart defects; increased risk of infections

A8. (a) Viruses (measles, CMV, HIV, herpes type 6), cancers (Hodgkin's and other lymphomas); opportunistic; negative, or diminished skin test reactions to antigens such as the Tb test or to the yeast *Candida*

(b) Severe combined immunodeficiency syndrome; both B and T; 2; bone marrow and gene-treated stem cell

(c) Poor muscle coordination, dilated vessels in eyes or in sun-exposed skin; is; helper, respiratory.

(d) Bleeding, Hodgkin's and leukemia; *Varicella*.

A9. Autosomal recessive; homozygous (recessive genes from both parents); cannot. Increased susceptibility to infections caused by pathogens that are not opsonized and phagocytosed normally, vascular diseases, and autoimmune diseases similar to lupus.

A10. Synthesis of complement proteins in the liver is reduced.

A11. (a) Chronic granulomatous; do not kill ingested; blue

(b) E, chemotaxis; *Staphylococcus aureus*

A12. Diabetes mellitus and AIDS. Also at risk are patients who received transplants or who are taking immunosuppressants such as cyclosporine.

A13. Chemotherapy to ablate diseased bone marrow, followed by transplant with a compatible donor. See text page 365.

B1. Induce an immune response.

(a) Inhalation, ingestion, injection, or skin contact

(b) Large, complex compounds such as proteins; antibodies (Igs)

(c) The same

B2. (a) I, II, and III; B; I; II and III

(b) IV; cytokines or lymphokines; delayed, days

(c) II and III

(d) III; arthus. Joints by rheumatoid arthritis; joints and kidneys in SLE (lupus); kidneys by damage to glomerular vessels

B3. (a) Mast, IgE, ragweed pollen

(b) Inflammatory; histamine, complement, ACh, leukotrienes, PGs, kinins

(c) I; immediate

(d) Rhinoconjunctivitis; seasonal

(e) Atopic (hereditary); high

(f) Antigens (pollen and other allergens), G

B4. (a) Proteins; E; I

(b) Children; rash or hives, dilation of blood vessels with drop in blood pressure (anaphylaxis);

difficulty breathing (dyspnea) as airways constrict.
(c) Nonatopic
(d) Being tested for allergies and avoiding those foods that cause allergic reactions; being prepared with treatments such as antihistamines

B5. Hemolytic (disease of the) newborn; II, Rh antibodies; G (because IgMs are too large to cross the placenta); anemia and hyperbilirubinemia (if severe, can lead to kernicterus)

B6. Purified protein derivative, subcutaneously; has enough sensitized T cells to cause a hypersensitivity reaction; IV

B7. IV
(a) Cosmetics or medications applied to skin; metals (e.g., in jewelry such as rings or necklaces); poison ivy
(b) Check the location(s) of the affected area and get a good history.
(c) Swollen, red, and warm. Avoid contact with the allergen; use topical creams to treat symptoms.

B8. Widespread use of latex for clinical procedures (see page 371); Type IV, delayed-hypersensitivity reaction or Type I (IgE); I (IgE). Avoidance of latex

C1. (a) (1)
(b) 95%; match closely
(c) (2)
(d) T, B; blood vessels; arthus, humoral
(e) Increase. **Note:** in healthy kidneys, creatinine is filtered from blood into urine; in failing kidneys, this chemical builds up in blood.

C2. Hyperacute → acute → chronic; hyperacute

C3. (b), (c); but (a) less; (d) commonly

C4. (a) Nausea, bloody diarrhea, and abdominal pain
(b) Bleeding and coma
(c) Rash and itching beginning on palms and soles, but often spreading and leading to skin peeling (desquamation)

C5. Removal or destruction of T cells from the transplanted tissue; T-cell-blocking drugs (e.g., cyclosporine)

D1. (a) Ability of the immune disease to distinguish its own antigens from non-self antigens and to *not* mount an immune response against one's own tissues.
(b) CD4 helper T-cell receptors recognize MHC (major histocompatibility) molecules that identify "self" and are presented along with "non-self" antigens.
(c) T cells that would react with self are eliminated (negative selection) centrally in the thymus; self-reactive B cells are eliminated centrally (in bone marrow); self-reactive T or B cells that escape thymus or bone marrow may be removed or inactivated peripherally from blood or lymph.

D2. See Chart 19-2 in the textbook.

D3. (a) Specific antigens are highly associated with autoimmune conditions including joint disorders such as ankylosing spondylitis, Reiter's syndrome, rheumatoid arthritis, and lupus.
(b) Because not all persons with a genetic predisposition do develop an autoimmune disorder; also a virus or chemical attached to the antigen-MHC complex may alter it and cause CD4 cells to fail to recognize MHC as self.
(c) The autoimmune disease lupus occurs more commonly in women, thus suggesting a role of estrogen in development of lupus.
(d) Results in failure to delete T cells that react to self.
(e) These can trigger an immune response by a short-circuit that omits need for antigen processing and presentation by an APC.

D4. (a) Strepto; heart
(b) Streptococcal, mimicry, HLA; increased, failure

D5. Antibodies; enzyme-linked immunosorbent assay

Chapter 20

ACQUIRED IMMUNODEFICIENCY SYNDROME

A1. (d), (e); but (a) in Sub-Saharan Africa; (b) higher; (c) 1981, although first evidence of HIV cases worldwide was in central Africa in 1959

A2. Blood, semen, and vaginal fluids; breast milk. (See also p. 381 under Universal Precautions: HIV has not been shown to be transmitted by any of the other fluids in question A2.)

A3. Their use alters perceptions of risk and reduces inhibitions to risk-taking behaviors.

A4. (b), (c); but (a) acquired—meaning not hereditary; (d) 25%, but 90% of children with HIV have acquired the virus from their mothers.

A5. (b)

A6. 1 in 333 (or 3 chances out of 1000)

A7. (a), (c), (d); but (b) can; (e) very unlikely, but it does happen rarely

B1. (b)

B2. CD4+ T lymphocytes and macrophages

B3. (a), (d), (e); but (b) RNA; (c) RNA

B4. (b) → (h) → (e) → (d) → (g) → (f) → (c) → (a)

B5. Latent cells serve as reservoirs for viruses that may not be released for years. Other CD4+ T cells are killed by the HIV virus, open up, and release millions of new HIV viruses (virions) into the bloodstream. These viruses may then infect (and kill) other CD4+ T cells.

B6. (b)

B7. (b), (c); but (a) not the first test because it is more expensive and slower than the ELISA test; (d) opposite

B8. The antibody against HIV. See page 384 of the text.

B9. Carl: category 2C; Terry: category 1A; Kelsey: category 3C
(a) Carl and Kelsey because both are in clinical category C.
(b) Kelsey's invasive cervical cancer, recurrent pneumonia, and pulmonary tuberculosis

B10. (a) Acute
(b) Acute

(c) Latent
(d) Overt AIDS (or symptomatic)

B11.

Name of Microbe	Class of Microbe	System (s) Commonly Infected
Candida albicans	Fungus	D-E, NS, R
Cryptosporidium	Protozoan	D-I
Cytomegalovirus (CMV)	Virus	D-E, D-I, NS, R
Herpes simplex (HSV)	Virus	D-E, D-I, NS
Mycobacterium avian complex (MAC)	Bacterium	D-I, R
Mycobacterium tuberculosis	Bacterium	NS, R
Pneumocystis carinii (PCP)	Fungus	R
Toxoplasma gondii	Parasite	NS, R

B12. (a) *Cryptosporidium*; also CMV, MAC
(b) *Candida*
(c) PCP
(d) *Mycobacterium tuberculosis*
(e) Candida, CMV, HSV
(f) *T. gondii*
B13. AIDS dementia complex, PNL caused by the JC virus, and *T. gondii* infection
B14. Kaposi's sarcoma (KS). Non-Hodgkin's lymphoma (NHL) and invasive cervical cancer (in women)
B15. (a) HIV-wasting syndrome
(b) Lipodystrophy
(c) Mitochondrial disorders
B16. (a) Cleavage, which requires protease (B4[c])
(b) Reverse transcription (B4[e])
B17. For prevention of infections; should not; MMR, pneumococcus, and flu.
B18. See text page 391 and information from organizations supportive of persons living with AIDS.
C1. (c), (d); but (a) less, because they have pores large enough to allow passage of the HIV virus; (b) is not
C2. See text page 392 and discuss with your colleagues
D1. (b), (c); but (a) perinatally; (d) for all pregnant women
D2. (a), (c)
D3. Different from; early; less, do

Chapter 21

CONTROL OF THE CIRCULATION

A1. The heart, blood vessels, and blood.
A2. (a), (b); but (c) direct blood flow through the heart; (d) pulmonary artery; (e) one eighth
A3. (a) Venules and veins→arteries and arterioles→heart (See Figure 21-2 in text)
(b) Arteries→capillaries→veins
(c) Superior vena cava→right side of the heart→pulmonary artery
A4. The same amount of
B1. (a) Right

(b) Ventricles; pumps; reservoirs
(c) Myo
B2. Fibrous pericardium→Parietal pericardium→Pericardial cavity→Visceral pericardium→Myocardium→Endocardium
B3. (a) S
(b) C
(c) C
(d) C
B4. Connective tissue that separates atria from ventricles. Serves as an attachment point for valves and helps produce orderly contractions by "forcing" electrical impulses to pass through the AV node. (See Chapter 25.)
B5. (a) Aortic
(b) Bicuspid
(c) Bicuspid, tricuspid
(d) Aortic, pulmonary
(e) Bicuspid, tricuspid
B6. (a) Electrical; atria, QRS complex
(b) (3)→(1)→(2)→(5)→(7)→(6)→(4)→(8)
(c) (1) A
(2) F
(3) Rapid ventricular filling occurring between D and H
(4) H
(d) AV; semilunar
(e) Early; stroke
(f) Great arteries; 120
(g) Elastic recoil; 80
(h) (1) B. 120 mL − 50 mL = 70 mL.
(2) A. 70/120 = close to 60%.
(i) Decrease, increase.
B7. (a) Normal
(b) Weak, bulging (as right atrial blood backs up in jugular veins)
B8. (a) 70 mL/beat × 72 beats/minute = about 5000 mL/minute = 5 L/minute
(b) 300%
(c) More, increasing; more
(d) Greater, actin (and) myosin; Frank
(e) Dehydration, hypovolemic shock, lack of exercise
(f) Increase, decrease; inversely.
B9. (a) Her cardiac muscle is "overstretched" (beyond the optimum for the Frank-Starling law), so her stroke volume decreases whereas EDV and preload increase.
(b) Contractility
(c) 0.5 (= 120 cycles/60 seconds); 0.33 (= 180 cycles/60 seconds); diastole, fill; low
C1. Externa→media→intima; media.
C2. (a) Capillaries
(b) Arterioles
(c) Arteries
(d) Venules
(e) Veins
C3. Requires relatively little energy; arrangement of muscle filaments; channels that respond to calcium and neurotransmitters. Calmodulin binds and

releases the calcium ions needed for muscle contraction.

C4. (a) 16; vasoconstriction as a result of sympathetic nerve impulses or epinephrine, atherosclerosis, or stenosis

(b) Blood pressure (P), resistance (R); P/R

(c) Higher (see Chapter 13); high, increases

(d) Aorta, capillaries; blood flows swiftly through the aorta to reach organs, but maximum time is permitted within capillaries for exchange of gases and nutrients.

(e) Within the center; laminar; in curving or branching

(f) More; increases; Laplace's

(g) Veins

C5. (a) 120, 80; pulse (pressure), 40 mm Hg (= 120 – 80)

(b) It is the basis for Korotkoff sounds heard when BP is taken, and pulse pressure can be palpated when "pulse is taken," for example, over the radial artery.

(c) 120 mm Hg (= 120 – 0); because ventricles lack the elastic recoil found in the great arteries, diastolic pressure is 0 mm Hg.

(d) Dissipates; cannot.

C6. Cardiac output and vascular resistance; factors "m" through "r" on Figure 21-1.

(a) ↑ CO

(b) ↑ Stroke volume

(c) ↑ Venous return

(d) ↑ Exercise

(e) ↑ Blood volume

(f) ↑ Heart rate

(g) ↑ Sympathetic impulses

(h) ↑ Norepinephrine and epinephrine

(i) ↓ Vagal impulses

(j) ↑ ADH

(k) ↑ Aldosterone

(l) ↑ NaCl in diet

(m) ↑ Peripheral vascular resistance (PVR)

(n) ↑ Vasoconstriction

(o) ↑ Angiotensin II

(p) ↑ Viscosity of blood

(q) ↑ Erythrocyte count

(r) ↑ Plasma protein

C7. (a) L

(b) S

(c) L

(d) S

(e) S

(f) L

C8. Increases; (d)→(b)→(a)→(c).

C9. (a) Constrictor

(b) Constrictor

(c) Dilator

(d) Constrictor

(e) Constrictor

(f) Dilator (See textbook Figure 21-25)

D1. Both are located in carotids and the aorta (See textbook Figure 21-26) and both signal a need for altering BP. However, chemoreceptors respond to

changes in chemical (O_2, CO_2, H^+) levels in blood, and baroreceptors respond to changes in BP.

D2. (a) Medulla, vasomotor, sympathetic; elevate; stimulating vasoconstriction that increases SVR and increasing heart rate.

(b) Orthostatic ("standing up straight").

D3. (a) P: DE; S: IN

(b) P: NA; S: IN

(c) P: NA; S: IN

D4. (a) NE

(b) NE

(c) NE

(d) NE

(e) NE

(f) NE

(g) ACH

(h) ACH

D5. (a) β_2

(b) α_1

(c) β_1

D6. Brain ischemia signals the vasomotor center to increase heart rate and to vasoconstrict vessels in skin, GI organs, and kidneys. BP skyrockets during the body's attempt to reestablish adequate cerebral perfusion. When the cause is head injury with brain swelling, high ICP (intracranial pressure), and compression of cerebral arteries, then this is a Cushing reflex.

D7. (b)→(a)→(c)→(d).

E1. (a) Precapillary sphincters

(b) Nutrient flow

(c) Interstitium

E2. (a) Pulling, interstitium into plasma

(b) Pushing, directly, plasma into interstitium

(c) Arterial, venous; lymphatic

(d) Decrease, lower

(e) Increase

E3. Decreased, edema (due to decrease in plasma COP); albumin

E4. Removal of lymph nodes lowers her defenses against infection; interference with lymph pathways by node surgery leads to stasis of fluid in her arm.

E5. Just superior to medial aspects of clavicles at the junctions of subclavian veins with internal jugular veins

E6. Increased capillary pressure (by hypertension or heart failure); increased capillary permeability (due to inflammation); decreased plasma protein (as by liver damage, malnutrition, or burns); and blockage of lymph flow (due to tumors or surgery to remove nodes).

Chapter 22

ALTERATIONS IN BLOOD FLOW IN THE SYSTEMIC CIRCULATION

A1. (a) Infarction

(b) Ischemia

(c) Perfusion

(d) Patent

A2. Good news: fats are needed for energy, for building cell structures (such as phospholipids in cell membranes and myelin covering over neurons), and for synthesis of steroid hormones such as estrogen or cortisone. Bad news: excessive fat can lead to atherosclerosis.

A3. (a) LDL; bad; high; low density lipoprotein
(b) In this disorder, LDL receptors are decreased, yet most (70%) removal of LDLs from blood requires LDL receptors on cells. As a result, the body must call on the limited number of non–receptor-dependent mechanisms, and blood levels of LDLs are likely to rise.
(c) HDL; good; high; decrease
(d) VLDLs
(e) Apo; some play roles in metabolism (getting rid) of cholesterol

A4. (b), (c); but (a): secondary; (d): LDLs

A5. (a) Dominant; can; 50; 2
(b) High because > 240 and 160, respectively; low
(c) Cholesterol deposits (xanthomas) along tendons are a sign of this disorder.
(d1) Increased, increase.
(d2) Fruits, vegetables, and fish
(d3) Cholesterol and fats; saturated, 140 (= 7% of 2,000 calories)
(d4) 25

A6. (a) Statins (Lipitor, Zocor, Mevacor)
(b) Cholestyramine and colestipol
(c) Niacin and cholestyramine and colestipol

A7. (a) High cholesterol, smoking, diet high in saturated fats and calories, and inactivity; his blood pressure is still in the normal range, but is relatively high for his age.
(b) Male gender, probable family history of heart disease
(c) Chemicals in cigarette smoke damage the lining of blood vessels and contribute to platelet aggregation and clot formation.
(d) Studies have indicated that fatty streaks may be present even in adolescence.

A8. (a) Increased, blood vessels; meats; folic acid, and vitamins B_6 and B_{12}
(b) LDLs, increasing; C-reactive
(c) *Chlamydia pneumoniae*, herpesvirus hominis, cytomegalovirus

A9. All four factors

A10. (a) Obstruction
(b) Ischemia
(c) Emboli
(d) Aneurysm

A11. Vasculitis
(a) Secondary to other disease
(b) Immune process
(c) Physical agent

A12. (a) Raynaud's phenomenon
(b) Acute arterial occlusion
(c) Polyarteritis nodosa
(d) Thromboangiitis obliterans
(e) Giant cell temporal arteritis
(f) Atherosclerotic occlusive disease

A13. Acute arterial occlusion, atherosclerotic occlusive disease, Raynaud's phenomenon, and thromboangiitis obliterans

A14. Mr. Vonnahme (f) has pain on exercise that subsides with rest.

A15. Chemicals in cigarette smoke act as vasoconstrictors and enhance clot formation.

A16. (b), (d), (e) where clots form due to stasis of blood in abnormally dilated vessels; but (a) dilatation; (c) brain; (f) the ascending aorta

A17. A dissecting abdominal aortic aneurysm. Clues: the ripping pain, and syncope (from hypovolemic shock as blood accumulates within the wall of the aorta); B

A18. Rupture of the weakened wall; replacement of the aneurysm section of the vessel with a synthetic graft.

B1. Contraction of the gastrocnemius and other skeletal muscles of the legs; inspiration that increases size of lungs and decreases intrathoracic pressure, "inviting" blood to move through the inferior vena cava back to the heart; and valves in veins that prevent backflow of blood.

B2. (a) Superficial, perforating or communicating, and deep
(b) Valves in perforating veins prevent such flow
(c) Deep; secondary; deep venous thrombosis

B3. All except male gender

B4. Superficial; they lack the support of muscle and connective tissues possessed by deep veins.

B5. Avoid prolonged standing; elevate feet when sitting; applying support hose before standing.

B6. (a) Superficial, lower
(b) Venous, arterial
(c) Lung (because blood from legs cannot enter the portal vein to directly reach the liver)

B7. (a) Varicose veins
(b) Peripheral arterial disease
(c) Deep venous thrombosis
(d) Chronic venous insufficiency

B8. (a) Venous stasis
(b) Hypercoagulability and some venous stasis related to pressure of the fetus
(c) Vessel injury with some venous stasis during recovery period
(d) Vessel injury
(e) Hypercoagulability
(f) Venous stasis (and some hypercoagulability related to dehydration)

B9. Pulmonary embolism, which can be lethal

B10. Prevention is best. Early ambulation after childbirth or surgery; avoiding severe flexion at hips or knees or prolonged standing; antiembolism stockings; anticoagulants, thrombolytic agents; insertion of devices into the inferior vena cava to filter emboli before they become pulmonary emboli.

C1. (d)

C2. (a) Scar tissue from burns; tight dressing; limb compression in accident or unconscious state
(b) Trauma to extremity, including fractures and bone surgeries; postischemic swelling; excessive IV fluids. (See more on page 452)

C3. (a), (c) because major arteries are located outside of compartments, (e); but (b) is; (d) is not because BP in that extremity would fall owing to gravity.

C4. (a) Decubitus ulcers, decubiti, or bedsores; ischemia of skin and underlying tissues by forces that impair blood or lymph flow.

    (b) Over bony prominences in the lower part of the body, such as sacrum and coccyx, ischial tuberosities, and greater trochanters

    (c) Immobilizing conditions such as spinal cord injury or stroke; diminished mental capacity such as Alzheimer's disease or coma; malnourishment, dehydration, edema, compromised circulation, and incontinence of bowel or bladder

    (d) Sliding of one tissue over another with stretching and damage of skin, underlying tissues, and blood vessels

C5. (a) Reposition in bed every 2 hours; avoid applying shearing forces; assist with fluid and nutritional intake; observe skin while cleansing it and applying moisture barriers, keep bed linens and pads clean, dry, and wrinkle free.

    (b) Reposition in the wheelchair or move to bed every hour with padding that cushions bony prominences; especially observe skin over ischial tuberosities. Other interventions as in C5(a).

C6. (a) Stage III

    (b) Stage I

Chapter 23

ALTERATIONS IN BLOOD PRESSURE REGULATION: HYPERTENSION AND ORTHOSTATIC HYPOTENSION

A1. (c), (d), but (a) the most common; (b) open; (e) after

A2. (a) (2), (3), but (1) rigid aorta

    (b) (1)

    (c) (1), (2)

    (d) (1), (2), (3) as (3) systolic BP increases and diastolic BP decreases as blood sloshes back into the left ventricle

    (e) (3)

    (f) (1)

A3. (a) (2) (= 40% of circumference); over

    (b) 170; 10

    (c) Systolic; diastolic, K5; Korotkoff

    (d) (3).

    (e) A lower BP in a few minutes can suggest that Mrs. Shaw initially had "white coat hypertension." A repeated high BP may indicate worsening of Mrs. Shaw's hypertension. Her home equipment or her technique may not be accurate.

    (f) (4)

A4. Less

B1. (a) Man

    (b) Lower

    (c) African

B2. (a), (b); but (c) typically no signs or symptoms, but increased urinary output may occur as damaged kidneys lose their ability to concentrate urine; (d)

less than 120/80 mm Hg, or less than 130/80 mm Hg for patients with diabetes

B3. See text page 464.

B4. No. Less than normal urinary output of sodium (and, osmotically, water) when BP increases. See also Question B6(b).

B5. Increase in sympathetic nerve impulses, stroke volume, and PVR; kidney malfunction with increased sodium and water retention; and hormones such as the RAA mechanism or ADH. Also contributing: family history of hypertension; high dietary sodium, calorie, and alcohol intake; low dietary potassium; obesity; pregnancy or oral contraceptives; and smoking

B6. (a) 50/40; close to 80; 10

    (b) It decreases natriuresis; the increased salt and water retention may have aided survival of workers in severely hot environments, but it also contributes to hypertension. Barriers to finances and health care and other factors on text page 468.

    (c) Dietary Approaches to Stop Hypertension through a diet low in processed foods, red meats, and sweets

    (d) (1)

    (e) 2; higher; increase, increase

    (f) 4 AM; night; less

B7. All except (f), increase in dietary potassium, not supplements

B8. (a) Decreases, larger; increase; systolic; 140, 90

    (b) Increases until age 50 and then stays the same or decreases

    (c) Increase

    (d) Left ventricular hypertrophy develops, increasing oxygen demands; but diastolic BP (needed for coronary perfusion) does not increase.

B9. (a) Kidneys, heart, brain (stroke), eyes, extremities—any part of the body because hypertension increases risk for arteriosclerosis.

    (b) Systolic

    (c) LVH does regress with therapy that reduces systolic BP.

    (d) Nephropathy can decrease urinary output; fluid retention increases blood volume, venous return, and workload of the heart (see Question C2[a]).

B10. Few, other than BP checks and tests to rule out causes of secondary hypertension. So BP screening is critical for early diagnosis.

B11. (a) 20% = 1,200/6,000 g of sodium

    (b) No, but it can decrease weight, which reduces BP, and excessive weight is a risk factor for heart disease.

    (c) Does

    (d) Swimming

B12. (a) Central adrenergic inhibitors

    (b) Calcium channel blockers

    (c) β_1-blockers (not β_2-blockers, which bronchoconstrict)

    (d) Diuretics

    (e) Angiotensin-converting enzyme inhibitor

    (f) α_1-receptor antagonists

B13. (a) Low, step-wise; one
     (b) Diuretics or β_1-blockers
C1. (b), (d); but (a) only 5% to 10% with the rest being primary = essential; (c) some forms such as renal artery stenosis and coarctation of the aorta are more common in younger persons
C2. (a) Hypertension caused by any condition that reduces renal perfusion and activates the RAA mechanism; stenosis
    (b) Renin. Constrictor; aldosterone, retain; hypo. (See Figure 31-2C.)
    (c) (2), (3), (4)
    (d) Is
    (e) Medulla; catecholamines; pheochromocyt(oma); sympathetic; headache; (2), (3)
    (f) Narrowing; arms
C3. (c), (d), (f); but (a) No, a fast and fatal form of secondary hypertension; (b) 120; (e) immediately in intensive care
C4. (a) Preeclampsia/eclampsia
    (b) Gestational hypertension
    (c) Chronic hypertension
C5. (a), (d), (f); but (b) less; (c) less; (e) increased, indicating liver damage
C6. Sometimes. Women with PIH lose protein in urine; this lowers plasma protein which leads to edema; decreased glomerular filtration rate (GFR) leads to smaller urinary output; some women with PIH have impaired renal sodium excretion.
C7. (b), (c), (d), (e); but (a) multiple fetuses
C8. Eclampsia superimposes seizures with no other explanation onto signs and symptoms of preeclampsia.
C9. (a) Increase, increase
    (b) Does not; decrease; does, decrease
    (c) High; angiotensin, epinephrine, ADH, or thromboxane (vasopressin)
C10. (a), (b), (c); but (d) can injury the baby; (e) not unless on a salt-restricted diet before the pregnancy
D1. (a) Higher; higher
    (b) Secondary, kidney disorders
    (c) 95th; significant, should
D2. (a), (d); but (b) systolic; (c) 140, not "100 + age"
D3. See text page 479.
E1. (a) Lower; decreases
    (b) Thorax (aorta) and neck (carotids); increase, constriction; increase
E2. A drop in BP when the person stands (or sits) up
    (a) Excessive sweating, vomiting or diarrhea or production of large volumes of urine (diuresis)
    (b) Antihypertensives, antipsychotics, or diuretics
    (c) Altered autonomic (sympathetic) nerves slow down reflexes
E3. (a) 2
    (b) Low blood pressure decreases cerebral perfusion. Her pressure is low because of fluid loss from bed rest, increased respiratory work, possible fever with infection, and leg muscle weakness that decreases venous return. Elderly people are at greater risk for orthostatic hypotension.
    (c) See text page 483.

Chapter 24

ALTERATIONS IN CARDIAC FUNCTION

A1. (a) Parietal pericardium, visceral pericardium
    (b) 30 to 35, 2 to 3
    (c) That accumulation of excessive fluid will compress the heart and prevent filling of the heart, and that this will lower stroke volume and cardiac output.
A2. (a) Constrictive pericarditis
    (b) Cardiac tamponade
    (c) Acute pericarditis
    (d) Pericardial effusions
    (e) Acute pericarditis
A3. (b), (c); but (a) sharp pain; (d) expands the pericardial cavity, compressing the heart; (e) withdrawal of fluid from this cavity
A4. (a) Increases, decreases; decreases; decreases 2 to 4
    (b) Less; is; extra compression of the heart decreases stroke volume and systolic blood pressure to even lower values than normal during inspiration
B1. (a) Left
    (b) Right
B2. Lower. Coronary arteries normally perfuse during diastole; perfusion decreases when diastolic pressure drops lower than 60 mm Hg and in association with tachycardia, which especially reduces the time spent in diastole.
B3. (b), (c), (e); but (a) fatty acids by aerobic; (d) endothelins do, but EDRF is a vasodilator
B4. (a) 75
    (b) Proximal (related to turbulent flow where coronary arteries branch)
    (c) After arising in the morning, high, sympathetic
    (d) Increases
    (e) Inhibits; do not
B5. (a) Cardiac catheterization
    (b) Electrocardiography
    (c) Nuclear imaging
    (d) Exercise stress testing
B6. (a) and (c); veins would lead to the inferior vena cava and right side of the heart, not to the aorta and coronary arteries.
B7. (a) Atherosclerotic plaque and vasospasm
    (b) Stress, exercise, exposure to cold, excessive production of thyroid hormone that increases metabolic demands
B8. (a) Stable; choking (angina) of the chest (pectoral region); ischemia; squeezing or suffocating
    (b) II; III, stable.
    (c) His "silent myocardial ischemia" (unknown until a month ago) may be related to his lack of sufficient exercise to cause angina at that point; he may have developed adequate collateral circulation to prevent ischemic pain; and his perception of pain may be diminished as a normal aging change or a neuropathy.
    (d) Sit; lying down would increase venous return, preload (and therefore workload of the heart).

(e) See text page 499.

(f) Nitroglycerin would be absorbed from the GI tract into blood but then metabolized (destroyed) in the liver before it could be effective as a dilator.

B9. (a) Long-acting nitrates
(b) Nitroglycerin
(c) Calcium antagonists
(d) Lipid-lowering drugs
(e) β-adrenergic-blocking drugs
(f) Antiplatelet drugs

B10. (a) Unstable; vasospasm; increase
(b) Some; (2)
(c) (4), (3), (2), (1)
(d) (3), (4)
(e) (4)

B11. Intact myocardial cells; directly; days
(a) Myoglobin
(b) Troponin I
(c) Total creatine kinase; CK-MB levels specifically indicate injury to cardiac muscle cells.

B12. (b), (d); but (a) left more than right; (c) is not

B13. (a) Severe pain and irritation of the vagus nerves may occur.
(b) These are due to sympathetic responses that occur under stress and when cardiac output decreases.

B14. (a) A half hour (i.e., 20 to 40 minutes)
(b) 20; stunned; may
(c) Ischemic; soft, week; rupture
(d) Months; is not; ECG; aneurysm
(e) Peri

B15. (a) Aspirin, heparin; beta blockers and vasodilators
(b) S-T, Q
(b1) Oxygen
(b2) Intravenously; dilator, decreases
(b3) Streptokinase; tPA
(b4) Reduces workload of the heart during defecation
(b5) Reduces fluid retention and preload
(c) Some, (namely nitroglycerin, β-adrenergic-blocking drugs, antiplatelet drugs)
(d1) Balloon
(d2) Radiation
(d3) Surgical
(d4) Coronary artery bypass graft; saphenous, internal mammary. See text pages 505–506.

B16. See text page 506 for more details.

C1. MI is caused by coronary artery disease (CAD) leading to ischemia; the other disorders are not.

C2. (a), (b); but (c) not fatal; (d) bed rest

C3. Idiopathic: cause unknown
(a) Hypertrophic
(b) Dilated
(c) Restrictive
(d) Hypertrophic
(e) Peripartum
(f) All

D1. (a) Bacteria; do; acute
(b) Endocardium, portal of entry
(c) Microbes, cellular debris, and fibrin

(d) (2) → (3) → (1)
(e) Is; see text page 511.

D2. (a) Group A (beta-hemolytic) streptococcal; can; poor
(b) Is systemic; central nervous system, joints, skin
(c1) Skin
(c2) Central nervous system
(c3) Joints
(d) Temporary (for about a month).
(e) Permanent; after decades; mitral (see textbook Figure 24-20).
(f) Penicillin, years, dental

D3. (a) Rheumatic fever
(b) Kawasaki's disease
(c) Bacterial endocarditis
(d) Bacterial endocarditis
(e) Kawasaki's disease

D4. (a), (d), (e); but (b) not itchy; (c) no discharge; (f) in subacute or convalescent phase

E1. (a) Rheumatic fever
(b) Mitral and aortic because they are exposed to high pressure on the left side of the heart.
(c) Workload of the heart is increased and may lead to heart failure; if mitral or aortic valves are involved, blood accumulates in lungs causing pulmonary edema and dyspnea.
(d) Opening, closing; regurgitation

E2. (a) Mitral valve stenosis
(b) Mitral valve stenosis
(c) Mitral valve regurgitation
(d) Mitral valve prolapse
(e) Aortic valve stenosis
(f) Aortic valve regurgitation
(g) Aortic valve regurgitation
(h) Aortic valve regurgitation

E3. Auscultation for heart murmurs with a permanent record by phonocardiography; ECG changes; echocardiography (ultrasound) to detect changes in heart function; and client history of fatigue, dyspnea, palpitations

F1. (a) Weeks
(b) Pulmonary artery and aorta
(c) AV, septa
(d) Atrial; ovale

F2. (a) Umbilical arteries
(b) Ductus venosus
(c) Ductus arteriosus and foramen ovale

F3. Umbilical arteries → placenta → umbilical vein → ductus venosus → foramen ovale

F4. (a) Lower
(b) Fluid, hypoxic; constrict, high; ductus arteriosus
(c) Increase, decrease; lowers, increases; foramen ovale; remain open
(d) Thinning, lowering; constriction
(e) Banding

F5. (a) Many; 50; 16
(b) (1), the left side of the heart develops greater pressure because postnatal systemic circulation has higher resistance.
(c) (1)

(d) (2), because blood enters systemic circulation without having passed through lungs

F6. Poor perfusion deprives tissue of oxygen and nutrients necessary for growth; fatigue may reduce ability to feed and also limit muscle development as children are inactive.

F7. (a) Tetralogy of Fallot and transposition of the great vessels
(b) Atrial septal defect
(c) Tetralogy of Fallot
(d) Coarctation of the aorta
(e) Transposition of the great vessels
(f) Patent ductus arteriosus
(g) Ventricular septal defect
(h) Endocardial cushion defects
(i) Pulmonary stenosis, transposition of the great vessels

F8. See text page 527.

Chapter 25

DISORDERS OF CARDIAC CONDUCTION AND RHYTHM

A1. (a) Can; faster
(b) SA node → AV node → Bundle and bundle branches → Purkinje fibers
(c) SA node; right
(d) SA node, AV node; Wenckebach's
(e) Slow; ventricles can completely fill before their contraction is initiated
(f) AV node; because atria and ventricles are otherwise completely separated, ventricles are protected from excessively high rates that arise in the atria (see Question B7[a])
(g) Within the interventricular septum
(h) Rapid; this increases the likelihood that all parts of the ventricles will contract virtually simultaneously to swiftly eject blood

A2. (a) Sudden change in voltage involving depolarization and repolarization
(b) –90, K^+, Na^+
(c) Na^+, –55; +20, rapidly; 0, de; QRS complex
(d) Downward, negative
(e) Plateau; slow movement of K^+ out of the cell along with influx of Ca^{++} into the cell so cardiac muscle can sustain a contraction 3 to 15 times longer than skeletal muscle; ST segment
(f) Dramatically, out of, ceases
(g) Does; diastole

A3. (a) (1); cannot
(b) Relative refractory period; ectopic

A4. (a) 12; see textbook Figure 25-6
(b1) T wave
(b2) QRS complex
(b3) PR interval
(b4) RR interval
(c) (3)
(d) 0.2

B1. (a) Excitability
(b) Conduction, refractoriness

(c) Automaticity, excitability

B2. 60–100, SA; AV node, 40–60; 20–40

B3. Sites other than the normal structure (SA node) that set the rate of the heart; stimulants such as caffeine, or heart disease

B4. Slow conduction and unidirectional conduction block

B5. SA. Not necessarily, because variations in sinus rhythm normally parallel breathing patterns: inspiration causes the heart rate to increase (textbook Figure 25-9D)

B6. (a) Brady; increase in vagal impulses, sleep, having the heart of a trained athlete
(b) Tachy, probably related to her fever and possibly sympathetic nerves related to stress of a fever
(c) The AV node or the Purkinje system takes over pacing the heart.

B7. Atria
(a) Atrial flutter
(b) Sick sinus syndrome
(c) Atrial fibrillation
(d) Paroxysmal atrial tachycardia

B8. (a), (c); but (b) less; (d) AV node

B9. (a) Common
(b) (1)
(c) Stasis of blood in the ineffective atria increases risk of clot formation.

B10. All answers

B11. (a) Premature ventricular; (1), (3)
(b) Fibrillation
(c) Tachycardia; decreases, decrease

B12. (c), (d); but (a) more; (b) longer than normal

B13. First-degree → Second-degree: Wenckebach's phenomenon → Second-degree: Mobitz type II → Third-degree
(a) Third-degree
(b) Second-degree: Wenckebach's phenomenon
(c) First-degree and second-degree: Wenckebach's phenomenon

B14. See text pages 543–544.

B15. (a) Class II
(b) Class III
(c) Class IV
(d) Class I
(e) Cardiac glycosides

B16. (a), (d); but (b) unsynchronized; (c) stop disorganized impulses to allow the SA node to initiate a heart beat

B17. Implantable, defibrillators, ventricular.

Chapter 26

HEART FAILURE AND CIRCULATORY SHOCK

A2. (a1) Increase
(a2) Increase
(a3) Increase
(b) Constrict, hyper, stenosis
(c) Digitalis, epinephrine, sympathetic nerve impulses

A3. (a) Overstretched, increases; decreases, inadequately

(b) Cardiac output, ejection fraction, stroke volume

(c) (3), (4), (5), (6)

(d1) Constrictor; decrease, decreases, increases; exacerbates

(d2) Aldosterone, cortex; Na^+ and H_2O

(d3) Increase

(d4) Hyper, ischemia with decreased contractility

A4. CHF is heart failure that leads to congestion (or retrograde blood flow).

A5. (a) EWD

(b) EWD

(c) EWD

(d) ICF

(e) ICF

(f) ICF

A6. Low. Anemia in which even a normal cardiac output does not provide enough oxygen to tissues. Hyperthyroidism (or thyrotoxicosis = sudden increase in thyroid hormone) increases metabolism; tissues then require unusually large amounts of oxygen.

A7. (a) Forward, ejection; ischemia

(b) Backward, filling; edema

(c1) D

(c2) S

(c3) S (as blood backs up in left ventricle, overstretching it)

(c4) D (because filling time is reduced)

A8. (a) Left: APE, DN, F, ICP-P, PSOB

(b) Right: AA, Asc, F, HS, ICP-S, JVD

A9. (a) Shortness of breath while lying flat because blood backs up into the heart, overloading it (increasing preload)

(b) Sweating: a sympathetic response

(c) Skin is cool related to vasoconstriction, and clammy because it is both cool and sweaty (sympathetic responses).

(d) Increased need to urinate at night as fluid from edematous legs returns to the heart and increases perfusion of kidneys

(e) Deep breathing when PCO_2 is high, and slight breathing when PCO_2 is low

(f) Limited exercise tolerance related to dyspnea

A10. (a) IV

(b) Her cachexia may be caused by fatigue, depression, and congestion of blood in GI organs that have led to anorexia and malnutrition.

(c) Edema may be manifested by a weight gain of 2.2 pounds for 1 liter of fluid; she also may be gaining some weight from her tube feeding.

A11. (a) Pulmonary capillary wedge pressure

(b) Echocardiography

(c) Thermodilution method

(d) History and physical examination

A12. (a) Dietary modifications

(b) Angiotensin-converting enzyme inhibitors

(c) Digitalis

(d) Diuretics; also dietary modifications, digitalis (by increasing effectiveness of heart contractions), and angiotensin-converting enzyme inhibitors

I (by increasing renal flow and urinary output)

A13. (d), (f), (g), (h); but (a) productive cough; (b) tachycardia as a compensatory mechanism; (c) agitation; (e) moist (diaphoretic) skin

A14. (a) Left.

(b) Prevent total assessment of bluish tinge (cyanosis) of lips and nail beds

(c) Assist her in sitting up so that blood will move out of her lungs and to lower (i.e., dependent) body parts by gravity

(d) Remove excess fluid from lungs; but the decrease in circulating blood volume can lower diastolic blood pressure so that inadequate coronary perfusion occurs

(e) Reduces anxiety and pulmonary vasoconstriction

A15. Heart. (a), (b); but (c) chemical released by the body that causes shock; (d) increase

A16. (a) Dilators, decrease, decrease, decrease; out of, into

(b) Increase, constrictors, increase

(c) An intra-aortic balloon pump, increase

(d) Heart failure that does not respond to medication or surgery

(d1) Cardiomyoplasty

(d2) Heart transplantation

B1. Inadequate oxygenation of tissues; functional heart, effective vessels, adequate blood, and tissues that can make use of the oxygen

B2. (a) Increases; tachy, increased

(b) Constriction, much; increases, Frank, increase

(c) (3)

(d) Increased; cool, clammy

(e1) Interstitium into blood

(e2) Sympathetic, angiotensin and ADH (vasopressin); aldosterone and ADH

(e3) Thirst, ADH

(f) Increase; increase

B3. (a) Lactic; anaerobic

(b) Decrease; sodium; Na^+; swelling; enzymes

B4. (a) Tachy

(b) Constriction, pale, moist

(c) Hypo

(d) Agitation

(e) Decreased

(f) Thirst

B5. (a), (b), (e), (f)

B6. (a) Hemorrhage; 25 to 30 (3 pints of 10 to 12 pints total); moderate.

(b) Cardiac output because vasoconstriction maintains his MAP temporarily

(c) (4) because his circulating blood volume is already decreased. If his shock is severe and prolonged, then dopamine may be given to restore blood to kidneys and GI organs.

(d) Mimic, α

B7. Normal, decreases, dilate; decreased, dilators; anaphylactic, neurogenic, septic

B8. (a) Histamine, increases; decreases; urticaria or hives

(b) Histamine constricts smooth muscle of airways.

(c) It constricts blood vessels but dilates airways.

B9. (a) Hypovolemic

(b) Neurogenic

(c) Hypovolemic

(d) Septic

(e) Anaphylactic

(f) Cardiogenic

(g) Obstructive

(h) Obstructive

(i) Neurogenic

B10. TNF, interleukin-1, and interleukin-8; (d through g); but (a) fever; (b and c) warm, flushed skin; (h) leukocytosis

C1. (a) (2); vasoconstriction of renal blood vessels is a compensatory mechanism for shock; measuring her urinary output, and checking her blood levels of BUN and creatinine

(b) Vasoconstriction of vessels to the stomach and duodenum increases risk for ulcers

(c) Acute respiratory distress syndrome; days; stiffer; is

(d) 50

C2. Multiple organ dysfunction syndrome; decompensated; is. Hypoxia, lactic acid buildup, compensatory vasoconstriction (which causes more hypoxia), and complications such as ARDS, DIC, renal failure, and malnutrition (partly related to peptic ulcer)

D1. (a) (4 to 8), (12), (13); but (2) tachycardia; (10) grunt on expiration; (11) cool hands and feet

(b) Weight assesses fluid retention associated with heart failure: 1 pound means 1 pint.

(c) All except supine positioning; upright position will decrease preload and heart workload.

D2. (a), (c); but (b) common; (d) carefully prescribed exercise; (e) are not typically

Chapter 27

CONTROL OF RESPIRATORY FUNCTION

A1. (1) Ventilation (inspiration and expiration), (2) Perfusion of blood through pulmonary capillaries, and (3) Diffusion of O_2 and CO_2 across alveolar-capillary membrane

A2. Nose or mouth → Pharynx → Larynx → Trachea → Bronchi → Bronchioles → Alveolar ducts → Alveolar sacs

A3. Warming, humidifying, and filtering air

A4. Slows down or paralyzes cilia, which allows particles to accumulate in lungs; stimulates growth (hyperplasia) of goblet cells, which increase secretions and risk of infections

A5. Pharynx. Food there (specifically in the oropharynx) must be kept out of the larynx to prevent airway obstruction and risk of aspiration pneumonia.

A6. Larynx; glottis; epiglottis

A7. (c), (d); but (a) larynx; (b) follows. Note: See Chapter 21, Question D7.

A8. The right bronchus is more vertical and slightly wider than the left.

A9. Do not; bronchospasms can collapse airways.

A10. (a), (b); but (c) transit and respiratory zone; (d) II, open or not collapse

A11. Bronchial

A12. Pleural cavity (which normally contains only a few drops of serous fluid); Parietal pleura → Pleural cavity → Visceral pleura

B1. (a) 760; 29.9 = 760 mm/25.4 mm/inch. (Recall this when weather reports state that the barometric pressure is 29.9.)

(b) Oxygen; 152; partial pressure

(c) 3, 456 (152 × 3); 2280

(d) Water vapor; alveoli in Jillian's lungs—which should have 100% humidity unless she is dehydrated

B2. (a) Intrapulmonary (or intra-alveolar)

(b) Intrapleural; negative; elastic recoil tends to cause lungs to collapse, yet the chest wall (because of flexibility of ribs and "give" of other tissues) tends to pull away from lungs

(c) Intrapulmonary (or intra-alveolar)

(d) Both pressures

B3. (a) Closed; sternum, thoracic vertebrae, ribs, intercostal muscles, and diaphragm; trachea

(b) Diaphragm; phrenic; cervical; inferiorly, 1 cm

(c) Increases; decreases; sucked into; in

(d) Passive; relaxes, up; increase; pushed out of; recoil

(e) External, in, lift; in, ex

B4. Internal intercostals and abdominal muscles. (Note that scalenes and sternocleidomastoids would aid with forced inspiration.)

B5. (a) Ease of; (1).

(b1) Surfactant-producing cells do not usually mature until weeks 26 to 28 of gestation; infant respiratory distress syndrome (IRDS)

(b2) Interstitial lung disease causes lungs to stiffen (lose compliance).

B6. (a), (e); but (b) lipoproteins; (c) outside; (d) dry

B7. (a) Small; Poiseuille's

(b) Ex; ex

(c) Trachea and bronchi, larger; trachea and bronchi

(d) Compressing

B8. (a) Tidal volume

(b) Vital capacity

(c) Functional residual capacity

(d) Minute volume

B9. (a) 500

(b) 4600

(c) 2300

(d) 6000

B10. (c), (d); but (a) lung volumes; (b) volume exhaled in 1 second

C1. (a) Base. Because of gravity, alveoli in the base are more collapsed (much like balloons that are almost empty), so they can accommodate more air (i.e., are farther from being fully inflated).

(b) Posterior or dependent, for the same reason as in C1(a)

(c) Blood; base

(d) Less; pulmonary vessels are thinner, more compliant, and the pulmonary capillary bed is much less extensive than the systemic bed.

(e) Less; 22/8, 120/70

(f) Artery; vein; left, because blood flows retrograde into pulmonary veins and capillaries

C2. Constrict

    (a) Blood is shunted away from hypoxic areas of the lungs to regions that are well ventilated.

    (b) If all lung areas are hypoxic (as in chronic bronchitis), pulmonary vasoconstriction will force blood back into the right ventricle and overload it, possibly leading to right-sided failure (cor pulmonale: see Chapter 29, Question D8.

C3. (a) Surface area for gas exchange (because emphysema involves destruction of alveolar walls)

    (b) Diffusion distance (related to extra fluid between alveoli and pulmonary capillaries)

    (c) Partial pressure of gases (because PO_2 is lower at high altitudes)

    (d) Diffusion distance, which is increased in pulmonary edema. Also solubility and molecular weight of gases: CO_2 is considerably more soluble than O_2 so readily diffuses out of blood and into alveoli

C4. Tidal; 350; 150, anatomic

C5. (a) Dead air space

    (b) Shunt

C6. Ventilation without perfusion

C7. (a) About the same as

    (b) A, about 40; B, about 45; C and E, about 80 to 100; D and F, 35 to 45 (or ideally, 38 to 42)

    (c) Radial. No, ABGs should be the same as aortic or alveolar values (as shown in E to C of Fig. 27-1); Jeremy's values indicate inadequate gas exchange.

    (d) 98; 4; 75; venous; about 98

    (e) Blood plasma; hyperbaric, carbon monoxide

    (f) Increase in temperature and CO_2, decreased pH (as in lactic acidosis), and also increased blood level of 2, 3-DPG, which is an intermediate chemical in breakdown of carbohydrates; right, more

    (g) PO_2; SO_2; only PO_2 because SO_2 is a percentage (% of Hb that is saturated with SO_2) that cannot exceed 100

C8. (a) (2)

    (b1) H_2CO_3

    (b2) HCO_3^-

    (c) See Study Guide Figure 27-2A.

    (d) It is the enzyme that catalyzes the first reaction shown in Study Guide Figure 27-2A.

    (e) Increase

    (f) 30

D1. (b) (pons and medulla)

D2. (c), (d); but (a) apneustic; (b) hypercapnia, or elevated blood level of PCO_2

D3. Hypoxia (with PO_2 less than 60 mm Hg) serves as his major stimulus for ventilation.

D4. (a) Stretch; in, ex; Hering-Breuer

    (b) Trachea and bronchi; vagus, medulla

D5. See page 602.

D6. Difficulty breathing (or perception of that). See text page 602.

D7. Tachypnea: rapid, somewhat shallow breathing; hyperventilation: rapid, deep breathing

Chapter 28

ALTERATIONS IN RESPIRATORY FUNCTION: RESPIRATORY TRACT INFECTIONS, NEOPLASMS, AND CHILDHOOD DISORDERS

A1. (a) Viruses

    (b) The common cold; 2 to 4

    (c) More than 200 types of viruses; rhino

    (d) Can; infected fingers

    (e) Have not; related to the large number of types of viruses that cause the common cold

A2. Your fingers can pick up viruses by contact with infected surfaces and then spread the viruses to mucous membranes of your nose or eyes.

A3. (e)

A4. (a) Frontal, ethmoid and sphenoid, maxillary

    (b) Paranasal, nose; polyps can block the openings (ostia) into nose.

    (c) Mucous, do; do not

    (d) Acute; is not

    (e) (1), (2), (4)

    (f) (1), (3)

A5. (a) 3, rapidly; 2, 7

    (b) Fever, chills, malaise, muscle ache, headache, "runny nose" (rhinitis), sore throat, and nonproductive cough

    (c) 4–6; 8–11

    (d) (2)

    (e) (2), (4); but (1) antivirals; (3) warmth discourages viral growth, which is optimal at cooler temperatures of about 35°C (95°F).

    (f) Is (she is in a high-risk group related to her age); each fall

A6. (c), (d); but (a) elderly; (b) type A

A7. (a) Alveoli, bronchioles

    (b) Is (sixth most common)

    (c) Aspiration of esophageal or gastric contents; inhalation of fumes

    (d) Virulent organisms, a large amount of microbes, or inadequate host defenses

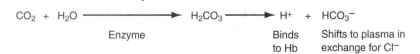

Figure 27-2A

(e) Cough reflex, cilia, lymph tissue, phagocytic cells, T cells, and antibodies (Igs)

A8. (a) Community; 3

(b) *Streptococcus*; pneumo; positive; capsule

(c) Decreased, increased (as a compensatory mechanism); is

(d) To identify the causative microbe and to determine appropriate antibiotic therapy

(e) Antigens from 23 types of pneumococcal capsular polysaccharides; yes, she is over 65

A9. Sickle cell is likely to cause destruction of the spleen (See Chapter 15, Question B5[e]). The spleen's macrophages and antibody production normally combat pneumococci.

A10. Common; negative; in warm, standing water; an epidemic of this pneumonia started with an infected hotel air-conditioning system at a 1976 convention of the American Legion in Philadelphia.

A11. Hospital; nosocomial; bacterial

A12. (a) SACG

(b) B

(c) VFMP

A13. (b), (d), (f) ; but (a) a parasite that may be a protozoan or a fungus; (c) abrupt with a high fever, dyspnea, and a nonproductive cough; (e) frequently, especially during the first year of life

A14. (a) Common; crowded; is

(b) Capsules; acid-fast

(c) Lungs; miliary; avium; GI

(d) (2)

A15. (c) →(b) → (a) →(d) →(e) →(f)

A16. (a) Immunosuppressed clients lack the normal T-cell mediated responses that prevent further spread of TB bacilli (in Ghon's lesions) as they are encapsulated with scar tissue and calcified.

(b) Calcified scar tissue is evident on x-rays.

(c) Primary TB typically has no symptoms; see symptoms of progressive primary or reactivated TB on pages 616–617.

(d) Purified protein derivative (ppd) of TB bacilli antigens are injected into skin, and the site checked for response in 2 to 3 days. (See page 617.)

(e) Previous exposure to TB bacilli, but not necessarily that the person has active TB

(f) Negative because they cannot mount a cell-mediated response to TB antigens

(g) Check for reactions to common microbes to which most people have been exposed; negative responses to these indicate that the negative TB test came from immunosuppression and that the person may actually have been exposed to TB.

(h) The most widely used drug for TB treatment; long (months or years); TB bacilli become resistant to one drug

A17. (a) Blastomycosis

(b) Histoplasmosis

(c) Histoplasmosis

(d) Coccidioidomycosis

B1. (a) Leading

(b) 80%; 50 (to) 90

(c) Many bronchogenic carcinomas are so poorly differentiated that they become sites of ectopic production of such hormones.

(d) Is not; chronic cough, dyspnea, and wheezing

(e1) Blood in sputum

(e2) Related to pressure of the tumor on the recurrent laryngeal nerve (a branch of cranial nerve X that supplies vocal cords)

(f) Lung cancer may have spread to distant sites, and cytological studies will indicate that the primary tumor was in a lung.

(g) Metastasized

(h) 13% to 15%

B2. (a) Squamous cell carcinoma

(b) Large cell carcinoma

(c) Adenocarcinoma

(d) Small cell carcinoma

(e) Adenocarcinoma, squamous cell carcinoma

C1. (b), (c), (e) ; but (a) more slowly; (d) Type II; (f) age 8 years

C2. (a) Fluid

(b) Before

(c) Compliant because tissues are soft; easier

(d) Abnormal, inspiration

(e) 80-100; 25-30; 50-70

C3. (a) Restrictive; helps to increase her lung volume

(b) Intra, wheezing or whistling, ex

(c) Obstructive, extra; slower; in, inspiratory stridor

C4. (a) Born prematurely by cesarean of an insulin-dependent mother; see text page 627.

(b) Increases, decreasing; higher

(c) Such a membrane forms inside alveoli, decreasing gas exchange

(d) Do; tachy, restrictive

(e) Surfactant administration and symptomatic relief

C5. Bronchopulmonary; premature infants who were on mechanical ventilators; lung damage increases pulmonary vascular resistance, and blood flows retrograde into the right ventricle

C6. Common; young children have not yet built immunity to common pathogens, and airways are of small diameter

C7. (a) Younger; viral

(b) (1)

(c) (3), (4)

C8. (a) Epiglottitis

(b) Epiglottitis

(c) Epiglottitis

(d) Croup

(e) Bronchiolitis

(f) Bronchiolitis

(g) Croup

C9. (a–c) All answers

Chapter 29

ALTERATIONS IN RESPIRATION: ALTERATIONS IN VENTILATION AND GAS EXCHANGE

A1. See Study Guide Chap. 27, A12 and B2.

A2. (d)

A3. 2 to 4 (Note: 4 to 5 mL = 1 tsp), serous; effusions. (1 to 2) Increased capillary pressure or permeability (as occurs in inflammation); (3) decreased blood colloidal osmotic pressure (due to deficient plasma protein); and (4) blocked lymphatic pathways

A4. (a) Hemothorax
(b) Empyema
(c) Chylothorax
(d) Hydrothorax
(e) Hemothorax
(f) Pneumothorax

A5. (a) Dyspnea; dullness or flatness; diminished
(b) Removal of fluid from the pleural cavity as a diagnostic procedure or to allow lung re-expansion

A6. (a) Traumatic
(b) Tension
(c) Spontaneous

A7. (c), (d), (e); but (a), (b) both increase as compensatory mechanisms

A8. (a) O
(b) O
(c) C

A9. Similar to: (c), (d), (e), as in Question A7

A10. Reinflating the collapsed lung (or portion of it)

B1. (a), (c); but (b) dilate; (d) increasing

B2. (a) Inflammatory; during the night
(b) 10 to 20; mast, E
(b1) Constriction
(b2) Permeability
(b3) Increased; decrease
(c) Macrophages, several types of white blood cells; may not be

B3. (a) Younger, do; house dust mite allergens, cockroach allergens, and animal dander
(b) Common, cold
(c) Viruses
(d) Tobacco smoke, smog, occupational fumes, gases, dusts
(e) Do sometimes
(f) Aspirin, NSAIDs, beta blockers such as propranolol (Inderal)

B4. (c–d, f–h); but (a), (b), (e) opposite because the patient with asthma has difficulty with expiration

B5. Lung hypoxia causes vasoconstriction and increased resistance of pulmonary vessels, retrograde flow into the right ventricle, and overload and hypertrophy of the right ventricle (see Chapter 27, Question C2[b]).

B6. (a) (2)
(b) Yellow

B7. (a) Education regarding avoidance of exposure, relaxation and breathing techniques
(b) Metered-dose inhaler

(b1) Dilators, sympathetic or adrenergic, parasympathetic or cholinergic or vagal; relax; blood
(b2) Inflammatories
(b3) Leukotriene

B8. Four visits to ER in 1 year, one in the past month; has been intubated for asthma

B9. (b), (d); but (a) severe, chronic; (c) common

B10. A cold with runny nose, nonproductive cough, irritability, rapid heart rate and rapid, difficult breathing with prolonged expiration

B11. See text page 645.

B12. (a) 26; 14
(b) Smoking
(c) Are not
(d) (1), (3), (5); but (2) true of asthma but not COPD; (4) true of the COPD emphysema but not asthma

B13. (a) Breakdown, decreased
(b) Smoking; inflammatory cells (such as neutrophils or macrophages), elastase, protein; hyper

B14. (a) CB
(b) CB
(c) CB
(d) CB
(e) Emph
(f) Emph. Chronic bronchitis causes excessive fluid in ankles (edema) and abdomen (ascites) so less weight loss.
(g) Emph

B15. (a) History and physical examination, pulmonary function tests (PFT), chest x-rays (CXR), and lab tests
(b1) Ex
(b2) 7 to 8
(b3) Less
(b4) Greater. Exhalation is compromised.

B16. (a), (b), (d), (f)

B17. (a), (b), (d); but (e) to maintain PO_2 at 55 to 65 mm Hg, or SO_2 at more than 90%

B18. (a) Dilatation; infection; decreasing
(b) Tumors, foreign bodies, or mucus plugs in airways
(c) Cystic fibrosis, immunodeficiency states, lung infection, or exposure to toxic gases
(d) Permanent; destruction; bi
(e) Infection and inflammation lead to dilatation of airway walls, pooling of secretions, and new infection
(f) Fever; large, blood (hemoptysis), microbes and leukocytes (purulent), is; loss; clubbing

B19. (a) Common; autosomal recessive; no
(b) 7, CFTR, Cl⁻; exocrine; high; thick
(c) Lungs and pancreas; infections, *Pseudomonas*; bronchiectasis
(d) Pancreas; steat; lower
(e) Vas deferens

B20. So that early treatment can delay onset and limit severity of CF
(a) Sweat

(b) Trypsinogen, pancreas; elevate (as the trypsinogen accumulates in the pancreas); 95%

(c) CFTR; is not; can

B21. 33; pancreatic, airways. See text page 652.

C1. (a), (c), (f); but (b) collagen and elastic connective tissues in the interstitium-located between airways or alveoli and blood vessels; (d) may be; (e) commonly

C2. (a), (e), (f); but (c), (d), (g) note that interstitial lung disease differs significantly from COPD, although both involve dyspnea, tachypnea, cyanosis, and hypoxemia

C3. (a) Inorganic: silica, asbestos, talc, particles from coal, ore, slate, sand, pottery

(b) Organic: hay, feathers, sugar cane, cotton, mold in air conditioners (see text Table 29-3)

C4. See text page 655.

C5. Lungs, skin, and eyes; unknown; by history and physical examination, chest radiograph, lung biopsy, and by ruling out other diseases

D1. (a) Air, fat, or amniotic fluid (in maternal blood)

(b) Deep venous thromboses, lower

(c1) Immobilization after surgery, fracture, heart attack, CHF, or SCI

(c2) Surgical injury or inflammation of veins (phlebitis)

(c3) Pregnancy, use of oral contraceptives, HRT, smoking

(d) Direct obstruction to flow through pulmonary vessels and reflex vasoconstriction related to pulmonary hypoxemia

(e) Chest pain, dyspnea, and tachypnea; hypoxemia; large

D2. (a) D-dimer testing

(b) Pulmonary angiogram

(c) Lower-limb compression ultrasonography

(d) Ventilation-perfusion scan

D3. (a) III

(b) II

(c) I

D4. 28/8, 15 (= 8 + [1/3 of 20]); low, thin and compliant

D5. Secondary

(a) PHPV

(b) EPPV

(c) PHPV

(d) IPBV

D6. Signs or symptoms of the underlying cause; also dyspnea, fatigue (because blood is not getting oxygenated), and signs of cor pulmonale (right-sided heart failure)

D7. (a) 26 (Note: 15 would be normal; 94 is a normal value for mean systemic arterial BP.)

(b) Rare, million; 20

(c) Same as in Question D6 except no signs of an underlying cause

(d) Oxygen, anticoagulants, dilators (such as Epoprostenol), and calcium channel blockers that both dilate and decrease heart workload

D8. Lung; (c) → (b) → (f) → (a) → (d) → (e) → (g)

D9. Hypoxia stimulates kidneys to produce erythropoietin, which stimulates erythrocyte production causing skin redness.

D10. (a) Acute respiratory distress; burns and related infections, fat emboli (from fractures), chest trauma and lung injury, heat trauma, reactions to smoke and other inhaled gases, hypovolemic or septic shock leading to DIC, and multiple transfusions

(b) Increase, decrease, decrease; increase

(c) Oxygen

E1. Hypoxemia, hypercapnia

E2. Partial (pressure), arterial; see Study Guide Chapter 27, question C7 for C-F.

E3. (b) (c); but (a) fresh air (20% oxygen); (d) disorders outside the lung

E4. (a) Shunt (also cyanosis, hypercapnia, and hypoxemia)

(b) Impaired diffusion

(c) Cyanosis

(d) Hypercapnia

(e) Hypoxemia

E5. See text page 664.

E6. (a) Central, H^+, high blood levels of CO_2

(b) Decreases; peripheral, common carotid

(c) Increase; because a low level (<60 mm) of PaO_2 serves as the major "drive" for ventilation in persons with COPD, she is likely to hypoventilate and build up her $PaCO_2$ levels.

E7. (a1) Are hyperinflated or airway resistance is increased, as in COPD

(a2) In malnutrition, anemia, hypoxia, heart failure, electrolyte imbalances, or degenerative neuromuscular diseases

(b1) Increases; fever; hyperactivity

(b2) Carbohydrates, parenteral; 1.0; CO_2 production

E8. (a) Acidosis, 7.25. (See Study Guide Chapter 27, question C8.)

(b) Markedly, 38 to 42 (or 35 to 45); decrease; dilatation

Table 29-1A. Blood and Alveolar Gas Values

	Venous Blood: Normal	Alveolar Air: Normal	Arterial Blood: Normal	Arterial Blood: Respiratory Failure
PO_2	(A) PvO_2: **40**	(C) PaO_2: **about 100**	(E) PaO_2: **80-100**	(G) PaO_2: **<50**
PCO_2	(B) $PvCO_2$: **46**	(D) $PaCO_2$: **35–45** (ideally, 38–42)	(F) $PaCO_2$: **35–45** (ideally, 38–42)	(H) $PaCO_2$: **>50**

(c) Decreasing the work of breathing, strengthening respiratory muscles, oxygen therapy to keep PaO_2 about 60 mm Hg, and possibly mechanical ventilation

F1. (a) All (1 to 5)

(b) Inspiring air with high levels of CO_2 can increase his $PaCO_2$ and decrease his alkalotic arterial pH.

(c) They reduce sympathetic symptoms such as palpitations.

Chapter 30

CONTROL OF RENAL FUNCTION

A1. (a) At waist level; retroperitoneally; renal surgery does not require operative entry into the peritoneal cavity

(b) Capsule → Cortex → Medulla

(c) Pelvis, ureters

(d) Renal artery → Intralobular artery → Afferent arteriole → Glomerular capillary → Efferent arteriole → Peritubular capillary → Intralobular vein → Renal vein

A2. (a1) Glomerulus; Bowman; corpuscle

(a2) Tubule; peritubular

(b) Basement membrane; prevents

(c) Mesangial; phagocytosis and contraction to control blood flow through glomeruli

(d) PCT → DLLH → ALLH → DCT → CD

A3. (a) Glomerular filtration

(b) Tubular reabsorption

(c) Tubular secretion

A4. (a) 125; glomerular filtration; blood cells and plasma proteins

(b) 124; 1, 60, 1440 (= 60 mL/hour × 24 hours/day)

(c) 60; higher; af; decreased, decrease, increased

A5. (a) Interstitial fluid and blood, Na^+; reabsorption; co; secondary

(b) Opposite, counter, secretion; bicarbonate, phosphate, and ammonia

(c) Passive; PCT

(d) Higher, more; transport, does

A6. More

(a) Smaller, concentrated

(b) Countercurrent; opposite, vasa recta; hyper

A7. (a) Increase; on Figure 30-2: H_2O in circle, ↑ blood volume and BP and ↓ UO

(b) DCT, Na^+; K^+, H^+; on Figure 30-3: Na^+ and H_2O in circles on left, K^+ and H^+ in circles on right; ↑ blood volume and BP and ↓ UO

(c) Decrease; raise; right atrium, opposes

(d) DCT, Ca^{+2}; mimics; increase; on Figure 30-4: Ca^{+2} in circle on left, PO_4^{-3} in circle on right; ↑ Ca^{+2} and ↓ PO_4^{-3}

A8. 25%

(a1) Antidiuretic hormone (vasopressin), angiotensin II, sympathetic nerve activity

(a2) Dopamine, nitric oxide

(b) Autoregulation, decreasing

(c1) Macula densa.

(c2) Afferent and efferent arterioles; angiotensin; aldosterone

(d) Increase

A9. Well; poorly; inulin; not at all

A10. Uric; aspirin, sulfinpyrazone, probenecid, and certain diuretics

A11. (a) Urea; 8 to 20; high

(b) Proteins, decreased, de

(c) Intestine, liver, kidneys

(d) Degradation of proteins in blood released by GI bleeding (related to long-term use of analgesics for arthritis); tissue wasting (caused by muscle inactivity or anorexia related to the pain of arthritis; dehydration (which increases blood concentration of urea) associated with high blood glucose; and increased risk for renal damage (indicated by a GFR that is 20% of normal: see Question A4) related to diabetes

(e) Increase; she may need lower dosages of her medications because her kidneys do not eliminate these drugs

(f) A low red blood cell (RBC) count may result from reduced erythropoietin production by failing kidneys and from iron deficiency anemia (related to anorexia); epoetin-a will stimulate RBC production.

(g) Failing kidneys do not activate vitamin D (calcitriol) needed to maintain calcium levels, and they excrete excessive calcium because they excrete little phosphate (see Chapters 31 and 34).

B1. Casts, cloudy (high turbidity), glucose, pink color, 400-mL total volume in a 24-hour urine sample

B2. (a) 1.025 (concentrated urine); colorless

(b) Such kidneys lose the ability to concentrate urine

(c) High, acid

B3. Normal

(a) Is not; 120; good

(b) Less, increase; poor

(c) 1.0; one third; higher as GFR and creatinine clearance decrease with age

(d) 10:1, 1.2

B4. Creatinine. The other chemicals may increase because of many other factors besides renal function: BUN by high protein intake, GI bleeding, and dehydration; levels of K^+ and H^+ by fluctuations of aldosterone; serum K^+ increases with tissue damage; and H^+ increases with respiratory disorders and ketoacidosis.

B5. (a), (d); but (b), noninvasive; (c), into blood which carries the dye to kidneys for imaging

C1. Increase; pulmonary edema, cerebral edema, hypertension

C2. Most diuretics cause K^+ loss, so additional K^+ through diet or a supplement are recommended to avoid hypokalemia.

C3. (a) Loop diuretics

(b) Aldosterone-antagonists

(c) Osmotic diuretics

(d) Loop diuretics and thiazide diuretics

Chapter 31

ALTERATIONS IN FLUID AND ELECTROLYTE BALANCE

A1. (a) Intracellular fluid
   (b) Intracellular fluid
   (c) Plasma or serum
   (d) Interstitial fluid and plasma or serum
A2. (a) Bicarbonate, chloride, proteins
   (b) Glucose
   (c) Osmosis
   (d) (1)
   (e) Iso
   (f) Swell
   (g) Pleural, pericardial, or peritoneal cavities, synovial cavities, or the lumen of the GI tract; third
A3. 60; 40, 20; interstitial fluid
A4. (a) Capillary (or BP); pushes out of; hypertension, CHF, high steroid level
   (b) Capillary, pulls into; decrease of production of plasma proteins (starvation or liver failure) or loss of protein (burns or renal failure)
   (c) Increase; inflammation or burns
   (d) Lymphatic; removal of lymph nodes in cancer surgery
A5. (a) (2)
   (b) (1), which is a relatively small protein and also the most common plasma protein
   (c) (1)
   (d) (1)
   (e) (2)
   (f) (2)
   (g) (3)
B1. (a) Increases, constrict
   (b) Retention
   (c) Vasoconstriction and retention of sodium and water
B2. Creates osmotic pressure; takes part in buffer systems; involved in nerve impulses
B3. 20 times; medication including sodium bicarbonate, IV solutions; kidneys
B4. (a) Save Na^+
   (b) Save Na^+
   (c) Lose Na^+
   (d) Lose Na^+
   (e) Lose Na^+
   (f) Save Na^+
B5. (a) Kidneys
   (b) Lungs
   (c) Adrenal cortex
   (d) Hypothalamus
B6. 60 to 40; 20-year-old woman, lean person, person with body temperature of 99.0°F, 2-month-old infant (See page 703.)
B7. (a) Food and drink; metabolism (burning up)
   (b) 1500, 1 (1500 mL per day/1440 minutes/day)
   (c) GI tract; skin and exhalations
B8. Early
   (a) Hypothalamus, sup; de; aorta, carotids, major veins, left atrium, and mouth

(b) ADH, pos; in
B9. (a) Hypo
   (b) Psychogenic
   (c) (3)
B10. (a) More; increases, decreased; opposite of
   (b) Pressin, constrict
B11. Decreases
B12. (a1) Little; 15 (normal is 1.5 L); increase, concentrated; nasal spray
   (a2) Nonsugary; large; sugary; insulin
   (a3) Central; adequate, do not
   (b1) Over; retention, edema, hypo, anemia
   (b2) Stress and pain, head injuries, drugs (text Table 31-3), certain cancer cells, and HIV
B13. Na^+
   (a) ADH, increases (hypernatremia), 135-145
   (b) Aldosterone
B14. (a) Hypernatremia
   (b) FVE
   (c) FVD
   (d) FVE
   (e) Hypernatremia
   (f) FVD or hypernatremia
   (g) Hyponatremia or hyponatremia
B15. (a) FVE
   (b) FVD
   (c) Hypernatremia or FVD
   (d) Hypernatremia
   (e) Hyponatremia
   (f) FVD
   (g) FVD or hyponatremia
   (h) Hyponatremia
B16. (a) (1)
   (b) (2)
C1. (a) ICF; 3.5 to 5.0 mEq/L
   (b) Cantaloupe, dried fruits such as prunes or figs, avocado, orange juice, and bananas
   (c) Into; into
   (d) Kidneys; increases; H^+ also enters urine, and Na^+ and H_2O are reabsorbed from urine into blood
   (e) H^+; 0.7 such as 4.5 to 5.2 (mEq/L)
   (f) Non–potassium-sparing diuretics; Mg^{++}.
C2. (a) Deficient; hyper
   (b) Hypo
   (c) Hyper; hypo
C3. (a) Hypokalemia; cardiovascular, 3.0
   (b) Exacerbate = make worse; brady
   (c) Decreases (such as from −70 to −90 mV), decrease; muscle weakness, fatigue, tingling of nerves (paresthesia)
   (d) Dietary sources of K^+ (see items in answer C1b) or K^+ supplements; ensure that urine output is adequate to avoid hyperkalemia and possible cardiac arrest
C4. (a) Hyper; common; rare
   (b) Is, because her level is greater than 6 mEq/L
   (c) K^+ level > 5.0 mEq/L and risk of cardiac arrest with extremely high K^+ levels (such as 8.0 mEq/L)

(d) Exacerbate because acidosis tends to cause hyperkalemia (Study Guide Figure 31-1E)

(e) Not if they have their major ingredient as K^+ (which most do)

D1. Bones; Mg^{+2} and PO_4^{-3}

   (a) D, PTH (parathyroid hormone)

   (b) Skin, liver, kidneys; PTH; calcitriol, also known as $1, 25-(OH)_2D$

   (c) Posterior of thyroid gland (in the neck); hypo; Mg^{+2}

D2. (a) Increase; bones, food in intestine, and urine in kidneys

   (b) Increases, decreases, renal; decrease

   (c) Mg^{+2}

D3. Congenital agenesis of parathyroids, thyroid or other neck surgery, autoimmune disorders, copper (Cu) excesses (e.g., Wilson's disease), or hypomagnesemia; Ca^{+2}, PTH, PO_4^{-3}; Ca^{+2}, PTH, Mg^{+2}

D4. (a) Failing kidneys do not secrete PO_4^{-3}, but they secrete excessive amounts of Ca^{+2}, which leads to hypocalcemia, which is the major stimulus for PTH growth and secretion.

   (b) PTH then pulls minerals Ca^{+2}, PO_4^{-3}, and Mg^{+2} from bones, weakening them.

D5. See page 723 of the text.

D6. (a) High; normal is 8.5 to 10.5 mg/dL = 4.5 to 5.3 mEq/L

   (b) Cheese, milk, turnip or collard greens, almonds, peanuts

   (c) Bone; rare

   (d) Urine

   (e) Ionized

D7. (a) Hypo

   (b) Hyper: lack of stimulation of osteoblasts by movements causes bones to give up Ca^{+2}

   (c) Hyper: these chemicals break down and demineralize bone

   (d) Hypo

   (e) Hyper: kidneys fail to eliminate Ca^{+2} or to activate vitamin D

D8. Rapid. Transfused blood has calcium chelated (tied up) to citrate to prevent clotting in the blood bank. The recipient's liver requires some time to remove the citrate and free ionized Ca^{+2}.

D9. (a) Less, more; 7.0, hypo

   (b) Low serum Ca^{+2} triggers PTH production, which demineralizes bones.

   (c) Tapping on the face (over facial nerve), which causes muscle spasms of nearby muscles (a positive sign of hypocalcemia)

   (d) These are signs of hypocalcemia and also related to buildup of other toxic substances in the brain caused by ESRD.

   (e) Paresthesia, carpopedal; larynx (blocking her airway)

   (f) If acute, administration of IV calcium compounds; for chronic hypocalcemia; attempts at improvement of the underlying cause (renal function); and provision of calcium and activated vitamin D

D10. (a) Hyper

   (b) Hyper

   (c) Both hyper and hypo

D11. (a) Bones; ICF, increase

   (b) 2.5 to 4.5; no immediate

   (c) (1), (2), (3), (4)

   (d) Milk and other foods that are calcium-rich, listed in answers to D6(b)

   (e) Lower

   (f) ATP, red

D12. (a) Hypo

   (b) Hypo

   (c) Hyper

   (d) Hyper

D13. Magnesium is a cofactor to many aspects of metabolism that are dependent on ATP, including protein synthesis, and nerve conduction.

D14. (a) PO_4^{-3}, Mg^{+2}

   (b) PO_4^{-3}, Mg^{+2}

   (c) PO_4^{-3}, Mg^{+2}

   (d) Ca^{+2}, Mg^{+2}

   (e) Ca^{+2}, Mg^{+2}

Chapter 32

ALTERATIONS IN ACID-BASE BALANCE

A1. (b), (d); but (a) release; (c) less; (e) as bicarbonate

A2. $CO_2 + H_2O \rightarrow H_2CO_3 \rightarrow H^+ + HCO_3^-$. Write CA above the first arrow.

A3. (a) Lactic, ketoacids

   (b) Sulfuric, hydrochloric, and phosphoric

A4. (a) 7.4; 7.35 to 7.45

   (b) 20:1; Henderson-Hasselbach

   (c) 24-31, 27

   (d1) 45, 40

   (d2) 1.35; $40 \times 0.03 = 1.2$; less

   (e1) About 27 to 1.35 = 20 to 1.

   (e2) About 24 to 1.2 = 20 to 1 (see textbook Figures 32-3 and 32-4)

   (f) 2.4; in (actually double) to 48 mEq/L; increase also; 48/2.4 = 20/1

   (g) Metabolic; $NaHCO_3$; H_2CO_3 = dissolved CO_2; respiratory

A5. Buffers attempting to maintain the 20:1 ratio just described; lungs altering amounts of CO_2 exhaled; and kidneys altering amounts of H^+ or HCO_3^- excreted; buffers, lungs, kidneys

A6. (a) HCO_3^-; 20, 1

   (b) Carbonic acid (H_2CO_3); Cl^-; $H_2CO_3 + NaCl$

A7. (a) Protein

   (b) Bicarbonate-carbonic acid

   (c) Plasma potassium-hydrogen exchange

   (d) Ammonia buffer system

   (e) Plasma potassium-hydrogen exchange

A8. (a) Raise; carbonic

   (b) H^+; HCO_3^-

   (b1) Na^+ and HCO_3^-

   (b2) Phosphate; Na^+ and HCO_3^-

   (b3) Ammonia; NH_3, NH_4, Na^+ and HCO_3^-

(b4) These prevent urine from being so acid as to injure renal tubules

A9. (a) K^+, H^+; alkal

    (b) Na^+, H_2O, K^+, H^+; alkal, acid

    (c) HCl; HCO_3^-; alkal

A10. (a) Yes (80 to 100 mm Hg is normal)

    (b) No, moderately high related to her COPD (38 to 42 mm Hg is normal)

    (c) No, somewhat acidotic which fits with her elevated PCO_2 (7.35 to 7.45 is normal)

    (d) High to compensate for her acidosis (24 to 31 mEq/L is normal) (See text Table 3-1, page 694.)

    (e) High, related to her high HCO_3^- ($\pm$ 3.0 is normal)

A11. His anion gap is calculated as $136 - 120 = 16$. This is slightly high, probably related to high lactic acid levels in his blood. His HCO_3^- level is raised as it buffers the increased PCO_2 from the run. His Na^+ and Cl^- levels have dropped somewhat from sweat production.

B1. (a) Compensation of metabolic acidosis

    (b) Correction of metabolic acidosis

    (c) Renal compensation for her respiratory alkalosis

B2. (a) Increases, decreases, decreases; weakness, fatigue, confusion, lethargy and stupor that can lead to coma; malaise, headache, anorexia, nausea, vomiting, abdominal pain

    (b) Decreases, increases, increases; muscle spasms or tetany

B3. (a) Mr. Hershey's high serum levels of BUN, creatinine, K^+, and H^+ relate to his renal failure, and his ECG changes, abdominal cramping and diarrhea related to high K^+.

    (b) Tyler's lethargy; Mrs. Litzinger's carpopedal spasms from alkalosis

    (c) Tyler's hyperventilation; Mrs. Litzinger's renal secretion of HCO_3^-

B4. (a) Metabolic acidosis

    (b) Metabolic acidosis

    (c) Respiratory acidosis

    (d) Metabolic acidosis related to lactic acid production

    (e) Metabolic acidosis

    (f) Metabolic acidosis

    (g) Metabolic acidosis

    (h) Metabolic acidosis

    (i) Metabolic alkalosis

    (j) Metabolic alkalosis

    (k) Metabolic alkalosis

B5. (a) Kussmaul's, metabolic; 5.0 as kidneys excrete H^+; can

    (b) Repeated vomiting causes metabolic alkalosis with loss of both K^+ and Cl^-.

    (c) Increased; slowly so the acid pH (with its effects) continues for hours or days

    (d) 7.5 (respiratory alkalosis), hyper; breathing into a paper bag so she rebreathes air high in CO_2

B6. The key is to determine which is the "problem" value because it "matches" the pH. Mr. Feinberg's high PCO_2 "fits" his low (acidic) pH. So this is respiratory acidosis. His high HCO_3^- must be due to

a compensatory mechanism (*when pCO_2 goes up, so will HCO_3^-*: see Questions A4[b] and [f]) because a high (alkalotic) HCO_3^- value does not "match" a pH of 7.33. Emily's high pH (7.54) is related to her loss of Cl^- (through emesis) that causes plasma HCO_3^- to increase (metabolic alkalosis). To compensate for her high HCO_3^-, she automatically increases pCO_2 by hypoventilating.

Chapter 33

ALTERATIONS IN RENAL FUNCTION

A1. (a), (d), but (b) less = oligohydramnios; (c) less

A2. Ureters are likely to kink, thus obstructing urine flow and causing urinary tract infections and possibly backflow that leads to kidney damage.

A3. (a) Renal tubules or collecting ducts; fluid-filled

    (b) 2 inches; they cause damage by compressing blood vessels or kidney tissue

    (c) Common; benign; do not; elderly

A4. (a) Nephrophthisis-medullary cystic disease complex

    (b) Autosomal dominant polycystic kidney disease

    (c) Acquired renal cystic disease

A5. (a) Compression of renal vessels activates the renin-angiotensin mechanism.

    (b) Cysts press on blood vessels, which bleed into cysts.

    (c) It is due to pressure within kidneys or against external structures.

    (d) Pressure of cysts causes urinary stasis, which predisposes to infection.

B2. (a) Infections; obstruction (and more infections: vicious cycle)

    (b) Stones, alkaline

    (c) Hydro; hydronephrosis; days

    (d) Acute; gradual

B3. Lithiasis.

    (a) Uric acid

    (b) Struvite

    (c) Calcium oxalate or calcium phosphate

B4. (d), (e), (f); but (a), (b), (c) all decrease risk for kidney stones

B5. (a) Colicky; left; uni

    (b) Drinking fluids can help to prevent formation of kidney stones; but after they have formed, large amounts of fluid can cause them to move into a ureter.

    (c) Are; is not; (1) (extracorporeal shock-wave lithotripsy)

    (d) The stent keeps the ureter open; the sandlike stone particles are strained and collected during urination to determine that they are passing.

    (e) Urinary outflow from the bladder is impeded so urine concentrates.

    (f) Immobilization causes calcium depletion from bones and leads to hypercalcemia.

    (g) Some dark, leafy vegetables, chocolate, and some nuts

C1. (c), (e); but (a) second most; (b) less; (d) lower to upper urinary tract
C2. (a) (2) has less estrogen and less protective mucin
(b) (1) has a shorter urethra which limits the washout phenomenon; also potential trauma to the urethra by sexual activity
(c) (1) obstruction leads to urinary stasis
(d) (2) has urinary stasis from neurogenic bladder (result of her MS), urethral irritation by catheter insertion, and possible growth of a biofilm on the catheter
C3. (a) These filaments allow bacteria to adhere to receptors on cells of the urinary tract.
(b) Ureters attach to the bladder at such an angle that urine is forced back into ureters during micturition. See text page 763.
C4. (a) (1) (indicated by lack of flank pain and only mild fever)
(b) 20; 15 and 24
(c) 3 to 7; drinking large volumes of fluid increases the washout phenomenon
C5. See text pages 755–766.
C6. See text pages 755–766.
D1. Endothelial layer of the capillary, basement membrane, epithelial layer forming the outer layer of the capillary, and the lining of Bowman's capsule; lack
D2. (a) Nephritic, common; is
(a1) Azotemia
(a2) Oliguria, hypertension, edema
(a3) Hematuria; pyuria
(b) Nephrotic
(b1) Proteinuria, hypoalbuminemia
(b2) Edema
(b3) Infections, coagulation disorders
D3. Her GFR is likely to decrease, which does decrease urinary output (see question D2(a)(2)). However, this may be offset by the damaged kidneys' loss of ability to concentrate urine. Large amounts of dilute urine may then result.
D4. (a) Are; bodies, gens; DNA in a person with lupus or chemicals in infective *Streptococci*
(b) Diffuse; segmental
(c1) Sclerotic
(c2) Proliferative
(c3) Membranous
D5. (a) Nephrotic syndrome (Note: normal protein in urine is less than 150 mg/day.)
(b) Focal segmental glomerulosclerosis
(c) Acute proliferative glomerulonephritis
(d) IgA nephropathy
(e) Chronic glomerulonephrosis
D6. (a) 3; glomerulus
(b) Thicker; glucose
(c) High; slightly; are
(d) Is
D7. Both. See Chapter 23.
E1. Tubules and inter
(a) More
(b) Less; Ca^{++}; fewer
(c) Increases; reabsorb; loss, hypo

E2. Tubules and surrounding interstitium
(a) Chronic
(b) Acute
E3. Renal perfusion is high (25% of cardiac output) and kidneys metabolize (destroy) many toxic chemicals in the body.
E4. Older adults are likely to have somewhat reduced renal function. She may take multiple medications, such as analgesics and diuretics.
F1. Young children; higher; uni; hyper; 90
F2. 60; hematuria; late; nephr; I

Chapter 34

RENAL FAILURE

A1. (a), (c), but (b) 42% to 88%; (d) prerenal
A2. (a) Prerenal
(b) Postrenal
(c) Intrarenal (or intrinsic)
(d) Intrarenal (or intrinsic)
A3. (a) Decrease; 20:1, not
(b) 20; tubules; tubules; concentrate
A4. (a) Nephrotoxic
(b) Nephrotoxic
(c) Intratubular obstruction
(d) Ischemia
A5. (b) (maintenance phase): his urinary output is low, and he has azotemia and hyperkalemia—all signs of low GFR.
A6. Uncorrected ARF has a high mortality rate, and reversal of injury requires early intervention. Older people are likely to have reduced renal reserves.
B1. (a) A high level of
(b) (1), (2), and (3)
(c) Improved
B2. (a) Renal insufficiency
(b) Diminished renal reserve
(c) Renal failure
B3. Both involve high BUN and high creatinine levels in blood, but uremia involves other multisystem signs or symptoms of renal failure (Table 34-1). Uremia occurs when more than two thirds of the nephrons have been destroyed.
B4. GFR falls, leading to fluid retention, edema, and hypertension. However, kidneys may also experience tubulointerstitial damage that causes inability to concentrate urine, polyuria, and dehydration.
B5. (a) ↑
(b) ↑
(c) ↑, ↓, ↓
(d) ↑, decreasing
(e) ↓, ↓
(f) ↓, ↑, ↓
(g) ↓
B6. (a) Inversely; PO_4^{-3}; Ca^{+2}
(b) Hyper (see B5[e], [f])
(c) Decreased; over
(d) Softer, low, decreases; vitamin D; H^+; dialysis, aluminum (Al)

B7. (a) Neurologic
(b) Neurologic
(c) Integumentary
(d) Reproductive
(e) Immune
(f) Gastrointestinal
(g) Cardiovascular
(h) Hematologic, cardiovascular (left ventricular hypertrophy as a compensatory mechanism for hypoxia associated with anemia and decreased oxygen supply to the myocardium)

B8. (a) To increase red blood cell count
(b) To treat hypertension; also if on hemodialysis. See Question B11(d).
(c) Kidneys do not eliminate drugs effectively, so blood levels of drugs tend to increase.
(d) Milk is high in phosphates and CRF patients typically have hyperphosphatemia.
(e) Aluminum-containing antacids can contribute to osteodystrophy.

B9. Technology and funding for treatments such as dialysis and transplantation have dramatically improved.

B10. (a) H
(b) P
(c) H
(d) H

B11. (a) 72 g/d =1.2 g/kg × 60 kg
(b) They contain potassium; these patients already have hyperkalemia.
(c) Yes
(d) The renin angiotensin mechanism contributes to thirst, and her daily intake of fluid is probably restricted to 2 to 3 cups a day.
(e) 12 pounds = 2.2 pounds/liter × 6 liters

B12. (b), (c), but (a) 90; (d) they are good sources of proteins with high biologic value

C1. (a) More; bone growth should be rapid because epiphyses are still open.
(b) Nutrition
(c) Peritoneal, at night
(d) He will be receiving immunosuppressants, and these reduce his defenses to infection.

C2. (a) Does; greater
(b) Is not; because of decreased muscle mass, serum creatinine levels (which derive from creatine in muscle) tend to be lower to start with
(c) Younger
(d) Altered immune function (decreased T-cell count) that decreases transplant rejection.

Chapter 35

ALTERATIONS IN URINE ELIMINATION

A1. Micturition
(a) Trigone; ureters; 12; do not; normally, the rise in pressure during micturition prevents backflow (reflux) at the vesicoureteral junction
(b) Urethra; males
(c) Transitional; it can stretch
(d) Has folds known as rugae
(e) Serous membrane (continuous with peritoneum), muscle, submucosa, mucosa
(f) Detrusor, great; stimulated, "go;" internal, flow out
(g) External, stay in; continence, restrict micturition to appropriate locations (such as a bathroom)

A2. (a) Sympathetic; in, detrusor; is not; adrenergic or anticholinergic (Hint: remember "S" for sympathetic, "S" for "stop urination")
(b) S2 to S4, pelvic; "go" (Hint: remember "P" for parasympathetic, "P" for "pee"); cholinergic; anticholinergic
(c) Voluntary, pudendal; decreased
(d) Motor, all three types; pons; detrusor, external sphincter; cerebral cortex

A3. Sympathetic; trigone and internal sphincter, does not (See Question A2[a])

A4. 400–500; 100–200; 50

A5. (a) Sphincter electromyography
(b) Postvoided residual volume (PVR)
(c) Cystometry
(d) Cystoscopy

B1. (a) Damage to sacral nerves interferes with normal sphincter function.
(b) This STD can irritate the lining of the urethra, narrowing the lumen.
(c) The enlarged rectoanal area presses anteriorly against the urethra.

B2. (a) Hyper; fatigue; frequent; infection; hydroureter and hydronephrosis
(b) Hyper; bladder spasms and urgency, as well as incontinence

B3. (a) Stroke (CVA), Parkinson's disease, or tumors
(b) Empty, flaccid, at; a
(c) Higher, T6-T7; spinal cord (because pathways between brain stem and S2-S4 control levels are cut off), hyper
(d) Diabetes and multiple sclerosis
(e) Constricts, increase
(f) Catheterization (intermittent or indwelling); adequate fluid intake to reduce risk of UTIs but not overfill the bladder; bladder retraining including manual methods; medications; or surgery such as urinary diversion or implantation of electrodes that stimulate bladder contractions

B4. (a) P; flaccid bladder
(b) S; inhibits
(c) S; incontinence

B5. (a) Overflow
(b) Stress
(c) Overflow
(d) Other cause (unfamiliarity with surroundings and confusion)
(e) Urge (overactive bladder)
(f) Other cause

B6. See text pages 808–809.

B7. Elderly: with aging, detrusor function declines, leading to larger postvoided residual (PVR) volumes; elderly women are more likely to have given birth to more children, leading to weakened pelvic support; older men have higher incidence of BPH; more likely to be taking diuretic therapy; may avoid drinking fluid (because of incontinence), which increases risk of constipation and related urinary obstruction; conditions such as failing vision or arthritis interfere with getting to the bathroom fast enough. Do not: usually related to embarrassment

C1. (b), (d); but (a) the most common; (c) 94%

C2. (a) Painless hematuria; frequency, urgency, and dysuria (difficult or painful urination)
    (b) Better
    (c) Backflow of urine into ureters (hydroureter) and kidneys leading to renal damage
    (d) Electrocautery; ileum

Chapter 36

CONTROL OF GASTROINTESTINAL FUNCTION

A1. (a) Intake, digest, and absorb foods; produce enzymes, hormones, and vitamins; eliminate wastes
    (b) Food or wastes pass through the GI tract but not through accessory organs (salivary glands, pancreas, liver, and gallbladder), which contribute secretions.
    (c) The hollow opening in the GI tract through which foods and wastes pass

A2. (a) Mouth, pharynx, esophagus, and stomach; pharynx
    (b) 10; lower; cardiac
    (c) Great; pyloric
    (d) Duodenum → jejunum → ileum
    (e) Cecum → ascending colon → transverse colon → descending colon → sigmoid colon → rectum → anus
    (f) Cecum

A3. (a) Mucosa → submucosa → muscularis → peritoneum
    (b1) Peritoneum
    (b2) Mucosa
    (b3) Submucosa
    (b4) Muscularis

A4. (a) Visceral, parietal; ascites
    (b) Mesentery; lesser

B1. (a) Smooth; rhythmic
    (b) Submucosal
    (c) Parasympathetic; vagus; pelvic; overexcite
    (d) Decrease, inhibit, stimulate; decrease
    (e) Are located within; sensory

B2. (a), (b); but (c): brainstem (or pons and medulla); (d): esophageal

B3. The pressure exerted by the lower esophageal sphincter normally is greater than pressure within the stomach.

B4. (a) 3 to 5; 20

    (b) Pyloric sphincter, sympathetic nerves, and hormones CCK and GIP
    (c) Atony and retention
    (d) Segmentation waves; they mix chyme with digestive enzymes.
    (e) Ileocecal
    (f) Auscultation of (listening to) the bowel with a stethoscope pressed against different regions of the abdomen
    (g) Within the (haustra of the) colon
    (h) Large; several times a day

B5. (a) Rectum; sacral; parasympathetic, internal
    (b) External

C1. Seven; local, neural, and hormonal; parasympathetic

C2. (a) Secretin
    (b) Cholecystokinin
    (c) Gastrin
    (d) Gastric inhibitory peptide and cholecystokinin
    (e) Gastrin

C3. (a) Enkephalins (natural opioids)
    (b) Histamine (Note: H_2 refers to "histamine$_2$.")

C4. (a) Small intestinal wall
    (b) Salivary glands
    (c) Stomach
    (d) Large intestine

C5. (a), (d); but (b): parotid (see Figure 36-1); (c): intestinal, mucus

C6. (a) Gastrin
    (b) Pepsinogen
    (c) Intrinsic factor
    (d) Mucus
    (e) Hydrochloric acid and intrinsic factor

D1. (a) They must be broken down into smaller pieces before they can be absorbed into blood or lymph.
    (b) Small intestine; large (250 m²) surface area provided by circular folds, villi, and brush border
    (c1) Produce mucus
    (c2) Enterocytes secrete brush border enzymes, which have direct access to disaccharides or dipeptides that can be digested and then absorbed "on the spot."
    (d) These lymph capillaries absorb fatty acids resulting from fat digestion.

D2. (a) Mouth; salivary glands and pancreas
    (b) Glucose and galactose; in lactose intolerance, lactose cannot be absorbed; it remains within the gut, attracting water and microbes, and contributing to diarrhea and flatulence.
    (c) Glucose and fructose; fructose; glucose
    (d) Pancreas; bile; A, D, E, K
    (e) Fat; inadequate digestion or absorption of fats (as in cystic fibrosis)
    (f) Inactive; before activation, they are moved away from organs that produce them so that they do not digest the organs themselves
    (g) Pepsinogen and pepsin; trypsinogen and trypsin
    (h) (1), (2)

Chapter 37

ALTERATIONS IN GASTROINTESTINAL FUNCTION

A1. Anorexia and/or nausea may precede vomiting, they may occur simultaneously, and they have many common triggers.
   (a) Good news: vomiting serves as a protective signal of disease and helps to eliminate ingested noxious agents; bad news: potentially fatal alterations in fluids and electrolytes and, if chronic, may cause damage to esophagus and teeth by exposure to acidic gastric contents
   (b) Hypothalamus, medulla
   (c) Sympathetic responses: pallor caused by vasoconstriction, sweating, and tachycardia
   (d) Vomiting; both will decrease (vasovagal responses)
   (e1) Motion sickness may involve emesis; anticholinergics such as Dramamine, Antivert, and Bonine decrease such nausea
   (e2) Hypoxia with shock, decreased cardiac output, or increased intracranial pressure can trigger vomiting
   (e3) Visceral afferent neurons transmit such changes in the GI tract
   (e4) A neurotransmitter that stimulates the vomiting center; Compazine (a dopamine antagonist) inhibits vomiting

A2. (a) Melena
   (b) Hematemesis
   (c) Blood urea nitrogen
   (d) Bright red blood
   (e) Occult blood

A3. To avoid a false-positive guaiac test result. Other foods and medications to avoid include high-fiber diet, horseradish, iron pills, aspirin, and anti-inflammatory drugs (that can cause GI bleeding).

B1. (a) Diverticulum
   (b) Achalasia
   (c) Aspiration
   (d) Odynophagia
   (e) Dysphagia

B2. (a), (c); but (b): are not; (d): do

B3. (a) Narrowing of the esophagus by scar tissue, spasm, and edema
   (b) Metaplastic response to acid irritation in which the superficial squamous epithelium is replaced by more protective columnar epithelium

B4. See text page 835.

B5. Common; an infant has a small esophagus, frequent regurgitation (with burping), and may eat in a reclining position

B6. (a), (b), (e)

B7. Dysphagia; late, poor

C1. Tight junctions between mucosal cells and a protective mucus layer with lipid that prevents passage of ionized, water-soluble chemicals.

C2. (a) Because aspirin and NSAIDs are both lipid soluble, they can enter mucosal cells, directly injuring them; they also inhibit synthesis of prostaglandins (PGs), which are needed for normal mucus and bicarbonate production and adequate gastric blood flow.
   (b) Alcohol (lipid soluble) also injures cells; smoking decreases PGs and also vasoconstricts.

C3. 9 PM; acute

C4. Parietal cells (Figure 36-10) normally secrete both intrinsic factor (needed for vitamin B_{12} absorption required for red blood cell production) and HCl. Injury to parietal cells leads to both of these disorders.

C5. It is the major microbe involved with noninvasive chronic gastritis and peptic ulcer and also is linked to stomach cancer.
   (a-b) Both help *H. pylori* move through the mucosa.
   (c) This enzyme helps *H. pylori* survive in the acid gastric environment.

C6. (a), (c); but (b): 1 in 10; (d): men than in women; (e): is no

C7. (a) *H. pylori* and use of aspirin and other NSAIDs; 70, 10 to 20.
   (b) Examples: endoscopy with biopsy test and/or stool specimen test for this bacterium, blood test for antibodies to *H. pylori*
   (c) (2), (4) (between meals and during the night)
   (d) Bleeding with hypovolemic shock
   (e) Signs of peritonitis (see text pages 840 and 856)
   (f1) Antacid
   (f2) Histamine (H_2) blocker
   (f3) Bismuth subsalicylate (Pepto-Bismol)
   (f4) Antibiotic

C8. (a) Curling ulcer
   (b) Zollinger-Ellison syndrome
   (c) Cushing ulcer

C9. (a) Decreasing; common (the major cause of cancer death)
   (b) Late
   (c) Subtotal gastrectomy

D1. (d), (e), (f); but (a): 1 in 5 to 10; (b): is not; (c): is

D2. (a) Both
   (b) Both
   (c) CD
   (d) CD
   (e) UC
   (f) Neither
   (g) CD
   (h) UC

D3. (a), (c); but (b): less; (d): dilation with stasis and absorption of toxic chemicals

D4. Anti-inflammatory drugs, including corticosteroids; immunosuppressants; nicotine patches

D5. (a) Condition acquired in a clinical setting such as hospital or skilled nursing facility
   (b) Antibiotic that attacks a wide variety of microbes, including the normal flora, and increases risk for virulent pathogens to thrive
   (c) Pain that occurs when pressure is applied to an area and then released

D6. (a) *E. coli* 0157:87 infection
   (b) *C. difficile* colitis
   (c) Diverticulosis

D7. (a) This spore-forming, toxin-producing bacterium is resistant to common antibiotics.
  (b) More, because smooth muscle tone of the colon may be lost, possibly causing dilation and perforation of the colon
  (c) Discontinue, and then start other drugs that eliminate *C. difficile*
D8. (a) More; related to less dietary fiber
  (b) Diverticulitis; (1) (lower left quadrant, site of sigmoid colon)
  (c) Vesicosigmoid fistula connecting the bowel to the bladder
  (d) Is not; rupture of the bowel would lead to barium spread throughout the peritoneal cavity
D9. (a) Common, young
  (b) Colicky, LRQ; increase
  (c) Appendectomy (surgical removal)
E1. (a) Wall of the intestine, parasympathetic
  (b) 200 to 300; diarrhea; large-volume
  (c) Sometimes; acute
  (d1) Large volume: secretory
  (d2) Small volume: infectious
  (d3) Small volume: inflammatory
  (d4) Large volume: osmotic
  (e) Is not; when prolonged in infants, elderly, or otherwise ill persons, who are especially vulnerable to dehydration and electrolyte imbalances
  (f) Should; bananas, rice, applesauce, and toast
  (g) They reduce intestinal motility and stimulate water and electrolyte absorption
E2. (a) Varies for different people (and their views of what should be normal): possibly daily to twice a week
  (b1-3) See text page 850.
  (c) Response to the urge to defecate, especially after a meal; intake of water and fiber; exercise; avoidance of regular laxatives or enemas
  (d) Fecal impaction
E3. (a) Volvulus
  (b) Paralytic ileus
  (c) Strangulation
  (d) Intussusception
  (e) Borborygmus
E4. Mechanical; removal of gas from the bowel (decompression) by nasogastric suction or surgery
E5. (a) Digestive disorder
  (b) Lymphatic obstruction
  (c) Mucosal malabsorption
E6. (a) Barley, oat, wheat
  (b1) Yellow-gray
  (b2) Because of their high fat content
  (b3) He is likely to have less absorption of fat-soluble vitamins, including vitamin K, which is required for clotting.
E7. (a) Common; benign; attached by a stalk
  (b) Mucosa; deficient; villous; does
E8. (a) Common (second leading cause of cancer death)
  (b) (1), (2), (3), (5), (7). Not risk factors: (4): her husband's cancer is not part of her family history, although it could be relevant if it is

related to the environment or diet that Mildred and he share; (6): these medications actually appear to reduce risk of colorectal cancer
  (c) Bleeding from the bowel; change in bowel habits (frequency, urgency, consistency); no pain until later stages
  (d) Later; C, 23
E9. (a) 3°
  (b) 2°
  (c) 2°
  (d) 1°
F1. This serous membrane lines the entire abdominopelvic cavity and forms the outside layer of the wall of most abdominopelvic organs (such as stomach, intestine, liver, uterus, bladder); normally a membrane free of microorganisms, a small area of infection can "spread like wildfire" over this large membrane.
F2. Any condition that introduces microbes into the normally sterile peritoneal cavity, such as rupture or perforation of the GI wall, PID, abdominal trauma, or surgery. See text page 856 for more.
F3. (a) (2)
  (b) (2)
  (c) (1)
  (d) (1)
F4. (a) To replace fluids and electrolytes lost by "weeping" from the inflamed peritoneum
  (b) To decompress the GI tract and reduce weeping into the peritoneal cavity and related abdominal distention

Chapter 38

ALTERATIONS IN HEPATOBILIARY FUNCTION

A1. (b), (d); but (a): cannot; if it can, may indicate hepatomegaly; (c): hepatic artery and portal vein
A2. Stomach, small intestine, large intestine, pancreas, and spleen; lacks, so blood backlogging from the heart (in heart failure → inferior vena cava → valveless hepatic veins → liver, can lead to hepato-megaly, a classic sign of right-sided heart failure
A3. (a) Kupffer's cells
  (b) Lobules
  (c) Hepatocytes
  (d) Sinusoids
A4. Bile canaliculi → right and left hepatic ducts → common hepatic duct → ampulla of Vater → sphincter of Oddi
A5. (a) Fibrinogen
  (b) Ketone
  (c) Amino acid
  (d) Urea
  (e) Bile
  (f) Glycogen
  (g) Albumin
A6. (a) The liver normally destroys (metabolizes) many drugs; with a failing liver, blood levels of such drugs will be elevated.

(b) Similarly, hormone levels rise, including female hormones normally present in small amounts, and this leads to breast enlargement in males.

(c) Many clotting factors are synthesized by a healthy liver; vitamin K is not absorbed if bile is not released from the liver.

A7. (a) Glycogenolysis

(b) Gluconeogenesis

(c) Beta oxidation

(d) Deamination, transamination

A8. Inhibits the enzyme 3-hydroxy-3-methylglutaryl-coenzyme A reductase (HMG-CoA), which is critical to cholesterol synthesis

A9. (a) Passes through the duodenum, jejunum, and ileum, where it is absorbed into blood into the portal vein and then back to the liver to start the cycle again (or is excreted in feces); enterohepatic

(b) Decrease in bile flow; obstruction within the liver (intrahepatic) or by obstruction of bile ducts (extrahepatic, as in last four structures of Question A4

(c) Pruritus, accumulations of cholesterol in skin (xanthomas), high blood levels of lipids including cholesterol, high serum levels of ALP, nutritional deficiencies of fat-soluble vitamins, and possibly signs of liver damage or failure

A10. Hemoglobin → biliverdin → free bilirubin → conjugated bilirubin* → urobilinogen**

A11. Bilirubin

(a) (3), (4)

(b) (4)

(c1) Posthepatic

(c2) Intrahepatic

(c3) Prehepatic

(c4) Prehepatic

(c5) Intrahepatic or posthepatic

A12. Damaged cells release their normal contents, including enzymes such as ALT or AST; ALT (alanine aminotransferase)

B1. Drugs including alcohol, toxins, infection or inflammation, immune responses, metabolic disorders, and tumors

B2. (a) Liver cells metabolize ("chew up") virtually all drugs and many of the body's hormones, especially if they are lipid-soluble. The more drugs to which the liver is exposed, the more potential damage to the drug-metabolizing "machinery" of liver cells. A damaged liver can leave high levels of unaltered drugs or their intermediates in blood. See Question A6 (a–b).

(b) Transformations

(b1) Inactivated; smooth ER membranes (known as microsomes); P450; increase, fewer

(b2) Lipid, water, kidneys; specific nutrients are required for Phase 2 liver functions

(c) Liver

(c1) 5

(c2) The Phase 2 pathways of the liver cannot meet demands to detoxify huge doses; toxic intermediates build up

(c3) Large overdoses can irreparably destroy the liver and be fatal.

(d) Insulin, thyroid hormones, and steroids such as estrogens, testosterone, cortisone, and aldosterone; increase; refer to Question A6(b) re Mr. Newman's increase in the normally minimal amount of estrogens in the male body

(e) Intake of numerous drugs can over challenge the liver and lead to increased levels of these drugs (and their toxic metabolites) in circulating blood; this is especially a problem in elderly clients, who are more likely to have impaired hepatic function and to take a variety of medications.

(f) Bile, pruritus; normally leads to recovery

(g) Are not; a person may have a genetic predisposition to mount an abnormal reaction to a drug

B3. Inflammation

(a) All (re bacteria: salmonellosis; protozoans: amoebiasis, malaria; viruses: infectious mononucleosis [Epstein-Barr virus], or hepatitis A, B, C, D, E.).

(b) Induction of immune responses against viral antigens

(b1) Does, does

(b2) Fewer, leads to a chronic or carrier state; sometimes; B, C, and possibly D

(c) Jaundice

(c1) Preicterus; malaise; myalgia; severe anorexia; nausea, vomiting, diarrhea; high serum levels of liver enzymes (AST and ALT)

(c2) Jaundice, high blood bilirubin, severe pruritus

(c3) Sense of well being, hearty appetite

(d) 2, 4

B4. (a) B

(b) E

(c) D, B

(d) C

(e) A, E

(f) B, C, D

(g) B, C, D; C

(h) 90%; 25%; HBV DNA.

(i) Is; all children younger than 18 years, all sexually active persons regardless of sexual orientation, all clients and staff at institutions for the developmentally disabled, inmates of long-term correctional agencies, patients on hemodialysis, persons traveling abroad; for others, see text page 872

B5. Interferons, such as alfa-2a or alfa-2b, and liver transplantation for end-stage liver disease

B6. (a) PSC

(b) PBC

(c) Both PBC and PSC

B7. (a) Is; 7, more

(b) 80% to 90%; acetaldehyde, more

(c) Ten million; women, increases, decreases

(d) 4 (Note: 4% beer = 4 g alcohol/100 g [or 100 mL] of beer = 10 g/250 mL = 8 oz glass; for wine with 12% alcohol content, the equivalent intake is approximately 13 oz/day for women)

(e) Excessive synthesis of lipids, ketones, and collagen fibers; impaired detoxification reactions and synthesis of proteins, leading to inflammation, cholestasis, and scarring

(f) If early in the disease, most changes are reversible, but some fibrosis and scarring may persist

B8. Fatty liver disease → alcoholic hepatitis → cirrhosis

(a) Yellow

(a1) Alcohol

(a2) Stimulates, decreases

(b) Spree drinking or an increase in alcohol intake; (1), (2), (4), (5); but (3): necrosis of central zone cells

(c) Small; as they enlarge (combined with fibrous bands), they block portal blood flow (leading to portal hypertension) and bile flow (cholestasis); yes, it signals end-stage liver disease.

B9. 85% to 90%

(a) Viral hepatitis, toxic reactions to drugs, biliary obstruction (including tumors), heart failure, and iron or copper deposits within liver

(b) Hepatomegaly indicates interference with blood flow through the fibrotic liver, backing up blood into the portal vein (portal hypertension); ascites occurs when portal vein blood backs up into veins of the abdomen, seeping fluid into the peritoneal cavity; the extra fluid leads to anorexia and masks weight loss; ankle edema is associated with decreased plasma protein (albumin) synthesis by the failing liver and decreased liver metabolism of aldosterone, which causes water retention.

B10. (a) Portal hypertension backlogs blood into esophageal veins, dilating them and increasing risk for rupture into the stomach (see Question B12[e]); a tendency to bleed exacerbates the condition.

(b) Like Mr. Nardella, he has ascites, but to such degree that fluid presses upon his diaphragm, causing dyspnea; diuretics reduce his fluid retention, and repeated paracentesis draws off abdominal fluid.

(c) The failing liver is not producing adequate clotting factors; splenomegaly (from backup of blood caused by portal hypertension) removes excessive numbers of platelets and red blood cells from blood; folic acid deficiency (from poor diet) may lead to megaloblastic anemia.

(d) Caused by backup of portal vein into rectal veins

B11. See text page pages 878 to 879 about portal hypertension and 881 for other aspects of liver failure.

B12. (a) Caput medusae

(b) Fetor hepaticus

(c) Asterixis

(d) Azotemia

(e) Esophageal varices (see Question B10[a])

B13. (a) 1 to 2; developing countries

(b) Hepatocytes; cirrhosis (and alcohol); HBV, HDV, and especially HCV (see Question B4[d])

(c) Late; 1

(d) Metastatic; colorectal, breast, lung, or urogenital

C1. (a) Concentrate

(b) Cholecystokinin (CCK)

(c) Cystic

(d) Dilates (and holds bile)

C2. (a) Cholesterol, bilirubin

(b) Abnormalities in composition of bile, cholestasis, and inflammation of the gallbladder

(c) (3), (4), (5)

(d) When bile flow is obstructed; right shoulder and back (via right phrenic nerve)

C3. (a) Cholelithiasis

(b) Choledocholithiasis

(c) Cholangitis

(d) Cholecystitis

C4. (a) Is

(b) Fatty meals

(c) Colicky; do not (pain subsides, then returns)

(d) (3)

(e) Cholangitis; if the duct ruptures, pancreatitis and possibly peritonitis (which may be fatal) may result

C5. Open surgery is a shorter procedure but is associated with greater inpatient and recovery time; laparoscopic surgery takes longer but has a much faster recovery time.

C6. Rare, insidious; 3

C7. (a) Duodenum, spleen; only when changes are great because the pancreas has functional reserve and can expand greatly without exerting undue pressure on other organs

(b) Many; starch, fats

(c) Pancreatic enzymes are secreted in an inactive form and activated once they are in the duodenum; in addition, the pancreas produces a trypsin inhibitor.

C8. (a) Gallstones in the common bile duct, alcohol abuse

(b) Alcohol stimulates pancreatic secretions, forming protein plugs that can block the passageway into the duodenum (sphincter of Oddi).

(c) Life threatening; pancreatic enzymes can autolyze the pancreas and digest surrounding tissues

(d) These are compensatory mechanisms that accompany hypovolemia related to shift of fluid through inflamed abdominal tissues with pooling in the abdominal cavity or retro-peritoneally.

(e) Amylase and lipase (because most of these are produced by pancreas cells); damage to pancreatic cells will release the normal contents of these cells into blood where the enzymes are then detected

(f1) To replace those he is "third-spacing"

(f2) To decompress the distended bowel and inhibit secretion of pancreatic enzymes

(f3) To prevent infection of necrotic tissue resulting from inflammation (f4) To "flush out" microbes from the peritoneal cavity, as well as necrotic debris that could sustain microbes

C9. (a) Thick mucus combined with protein plugs can block the passageway into the duodenum. Enzymes pass retrograde from duodenum into pancreas, digesting part or all of it.
   (b) See text page 886.
   (c) The pancreas makes more than 80% of the body's lipases, especially in response to fatty foods. Lowering fat intake lowers lipase levels, which will help to prevent digestion of fat in/on any abdominal organs and also reduce fat in the stool (steatorrhea).
   (d) These enzymes help to replace pancreatic enzymes that are "stuck" in the pancreas because of mucoprotein plugs.

C10. (a) 1%; elderly; after
   (b) Diet high in calories, fat, meat, salt, dried foods, refined sugar, and soybeans
   (c) Smoking and family history of some other cancers
   (d) Insidious; pain, jaundice, weight loss, dull epigastric pain or back pain
   (e) Protective factors include a diet rich in vitamin C and fresh fruits and vegetables, as well as avoidance of preservatives, smoking, and other factors listed in C10(b).

Chapter 39

MECHANISMS OF ENDOCRINE CONTROL

A1. See text page 891.
A2. (a) Estrogen exerts effects on the uterus, breasts, ovaries, hypothalamus, pituitary, and bones.
   (b) Increase of blood glucose is regulated by epinephrine, glucagon, cortisone, and growth hormone.
A3. Auto, juxta; blood plasma
A4. (a) Fatty acid derivatives
   (b) Amines or amino acids
   (c) Steroids
   (d) Peptides, polypeptides, and proteins
   (e) Amines or amino acids
A5. (a) Smooth; peptide, polypeptide, or protein; rough
   (b) Protein; Golgi
   (c) Inactive; aldosterone, cortisone, estrogen, thyroid hormone (thyroxine)
   (d) 99; aspirin competes for thyroxine's carrier and will lead to release of thyroxine into the unbound (active) state; this can exacerbate an already elevated thyroid hormone level (as in thyrotoxicosis)
A6. (a) Either degrades the hormone into an inactive form or activates some hormones
   (b) In the liver or at the site of the hormone's receptor

(c) MAO (monoamine oxidase) or COMP (catechol-O-methyltransferase)
   (d) They are conjugated in the liver, which inactivates them, and are then eliminated in bile.
A7. Hormones bind to cells that have specific receptors for the hormone.
   (a) As many as 100,000
   (b) Increase; induction; up
   (c) Water; cannot; surface; first; cAMP; second; second
   (d) Can (because they are lipid); intracellular
A8. (a) Hypothalamus
   (b) Anterior pituitary
   (c) Anterior pituitary
   (d) Adrenal cortex
   (e) Posterior pituitary; note that these are synthesized in hypothalamus
   (f) Kidney
   (g) Testes and adrenal cortex
A9. (a) Calcitonin
   (b) Insulin
   (c) Releasing hormones such as CRH, GnRH, and TRH
   (d) Catecholamines including epinephrine (adrenalin) and norepinephrine
   (e) GH
   (f) Gastrin
A10. (a) Blood vessels, hypothalamus, anterior pituitary; releasing
   (b) Anterior; thyroid gland, thyroid hormone (T_3T_4); negative or opposite, decrease
   (c) Cortex, cortisol; glucose; exo, decrease, suppression
   (d) Insulin and glucagon (by glucose), calcitonin and PTH (by Ca^{+2}), and aldosterone (by blood levels of Na^+ and K^+).
A11. (a) IRMA and RIA
   (b) See text page 900.
B1. Hypo; see text pages 900–901.
B2. (a) 3° if hypothalamus is destroyed or 2° if the pituitary is destroyed by radiation
   (b) 1°
   (c) 2°
B3. (c), (d); but (a): 70% to 90%; (b): sometimes
B4. GH → LH → FSH → TSH → ACTH (*Hint*: Remember the Mnemonic "Go Look For The Adenoma")

Chapter 40

ALTERATIONS IN ENDOCRINE CONTROL OF GROWTH AND METABOLISM

A1. (a) GH, insulin, T_3T_4, androgens
   (b) (1), (2); but (3): indirectly by stimulation of the liver to produce IGFs; (4): increases use of fats and decreases use of carbohydrates (Refer to Study Guide Figure 41-1, page 211.)
A2. (b), (c); but (a): throughout life; (d): increase
A3. (a) Male children: 6'1"; female children: 5'8"

(b) Actual height, velocity of growth, and parental height
(c) Short, normal; recombinant DNA
A4. (a) Laron-type dwarfism
(b) Psychosocial dwarfism
(c) Genetically short stature
(d) Panpituitarism
(e) Somatotrope
A5. (a) Somatopause
(b) Acromegaly
(c) Gigantism
A6. (a) Is not; growth plates in his long bones closed decades ago
(b) Rare, insidious; benign
(c) Organs (including the heart) grow abnormally large; cardiomegaly is likely to lead to cardiac ischemia. Excessive GH also causes release of free fatty acids from adipose tissue; possible acromegaly-related diabetes also would increase cardiac risk.
(d) His enlarged pituitary increases pressure on his optic nerves, blood vessels, and meninges.
(e) A transsphenoidal approach accesses the pituitary through the nose.
A7. (a) Thelarche
(b) Menarche
(c) Isosexual precocious puberty
B1. (a) Isthmus; lobules, thyroglobulin
(b) Tyrosine, iodide; triiodothyronine (T_3), three
(c) Protein, TBG; free
(d) De, in (see Chapter 39, Question A5[d])
B2. See Study Guide Chapter 39, page 203. Inhibit; triggers, hypothalamus
B3. All major; increases
(a) De
(b) In
(c) De; in
(d) In; in
(e) De, in; de
(f) In
(g) In; de
B4. (a–e) All hypo
B5. (a) Goiter
(b) Cretinism
(c) Myxedema
(d) Myxedema
(e) Hashimoto's disease
(f) Thyroid storm
(g) Graves' disease
B6. (a), (d); but (b): the most common; (c): an acute
C1. (a) On top of kidneys
(b1) M
(b2) C
(b3) C
(b4) C
C2. (a) Aldosterone
(b) Aldosterone
(c) Dehydroepiandrosterone sulfate
(d) Cortisol
C3. (a) Increases
(b) Breakdown

(c) Gluconeogenesis
(d) Decreases
(e) Decreases
(f) Decreases
(g) Anti-inflammatory
C4. Varies with time of day; ACTH (and consequently, cortisol) are higher in the morning and lower at night. This pattern is reversed for night workers and is altered with Cushing's syndrome.
C5. (a) Glucocorticoids affect parts of the brain that alter mood and behavior.
(b) Exogenous cortisone inhibits her production of CRH and ACTH, causing atrophy of her adrenal gland.
(c) This is dangerous because her atrophied adrenals cannot suddenly begin making cortisol; gradual weaning from steroids can prevent this problem; recovery may take a year or more.
C6. (a) 24-hour urinary free cortisol test
(b) Insulin hypoglycemic stress test.
C7. (a) Is; cortisol
(b) Increases; increases; increases; virilizing effects of her external genitalia
C8. (a) Secondary adrenal cortical insufficiency
(b) Secondary adrenal cortical insufficiency (she may have developed iatrogenic Cushing's syndrome)
(c) Incidental adrenal mass
(d) Addison's disease
(e) Cushing's disease (also a secondary adrenal cortical insufficiency)
(f) Cushing's syndrome
C9. (a) Primary (because the problem lies in the thyroid gland itself); 10%
(b) (1) and (3) (due to deficiency of aldosterone); but (2): a sign of Cushing's; (4): hypoglycemia and lethargy; (5): bronzed skin because his high ACTH levels mimic high melanocyte-stimulating hormone (MSH)
(c) Will
C10. Excessive; (b) (moon face and buffalo hump), (c) (purple striae); but (a): opposite, (d): osteoporosis, (e): hypertension related to the effects of steroids on fluid retention

Chapter 41

DIABETES MELLITUS

A1. Its high incidence (more than 15 million persons) and effects on so many systems (cardiovascular, renal, and special senses, especially eyes)
A2. Islets of Langerhans
(a) Glucagon; increases
(b) Insulin; decreases
(c) Somatostatin, insulin, glucagon; decreases
A3. (a) 76; 36
(b) (1), (3)
(c) (3); liver
(d) (1)
(e) Cortisol, epinephrine, glucagon
(f) (2)

(g) Increases; insulin; blood into cells, stimulates, glycogen (glycogenesis); lowers

A4. (a) Protein; C
   (b) Glucose; GLUT-2; pre-formed (followed by release of newly synthesized insulin)
   (c) Portal vein; 15
   (d) Adipose and skeletal muscle; insulin; 1; does not
   (e) Amino acids, protein; fatty acids, lysis
   (f) Inhibit, antagonizes; increase
   (g) Excessive GH (in acromegaly) and cortisol (in chronic stress or in Cushing's syndrome) both lead to chronic increase in blood glucose (Figure 41-1A and B) and overstimulation of beta cells, which can lead to diabetes.

B1. (a), (c); but (b): sweet, related to sugar in urine; (d): 10%

B2. (a) (2)
   (b) 1A, immune-mediated; insulin, do
   (c) Honeymoon; beta cells regenerate temporarily
   (d) Inhibits; 1, ketones or ketoacids (diabetic ketoacidosis or DKA)
   (e) Obese, high. A vicious cycle develops as beta cells become exhausted in attempts to maintain normal blood glucose; as glucose increases, beta cells are challenged to secrete even more insulin. See B2(f) also.
   (f) Stimulate (contributing to beta cell burnout), inhibit (exacerbating hyperglycemia); increase
   (g) Can
   (h) Are

B3. Cause
   (a) Gestational diabetes mellitus
   (b) Type 1 (type 1A)
   (c) Endocrine disorder
   (d) Drug disorder

B4. (a), (b), (d), (f), (i) ; but (c): older women; (e): more than five pregnancies; (g): obese; (h): glucosuria

B5. Even mild maternal hyperglycemia can be injurious to the developing fetus.

B6. (a) 2
   (b) Increased; high blood glucose (hyperglycemia) "spills over" into urine and "pulls" water (osmotically) into urine; decreased circulating blood can lead to hypoxia and fatigue
   (c) Polydipsia (clients "dip into water" as cells are dehydrated by polyuria)
   (d) 1; cells cannot access glucose, fats, or proteins
   (e) 1; fluid loss (polyuria), depletion of cellular fat and protein as these are "burned" for fuel, and possibly vomiting with episodes of ketoacidosis
   (f) More; glucose in skin and mucus "invites" microbes, including *Candida*; loss of sensation reduces awareness and early treatment of infection
   (g) Glucose moves into the lens.

B7. (a) Glucose tolerance test
   (b) Fasting blood glucose test
   (c) Random blood glucose test
   (d) Glycosylated hemoglobin (HBA$_{1C}$)test
   (e) Self-monitoring test

B8. (a) Blood

(b) Nutrition, exercise, and antidiabetic agents (oral hypoglycemic medications)
   (c) Does not; consistent
   (d) 100 (about 4 Cal/g)
   (e) 140 (7% of 2000); protein (to <200 Cal = 50 g)
   (f) See text page 938.

B9. 2
   (a) ISC, IHC (so may be toxic to liver), RFFA
   (b) IHC (no longer used because they "exhausted" liver cells and led to lactic acidosis), ISC
   (c) SBC, ISC

B10. (a) Insulin (required for individuals with type 1 diabetes); insulin is a protein and would be destroyed by gastric acid and enzymes
   (b) 100 units/1 mL
   (c) Maintains blood glucose at more normal levels with fewer peaks and valleys
   (d) Pork (porcine) pancreas preparations are more likely to cause buildup of antibodies against the insulin.
   (e) See text page 942.

C1. (a) Hypoglycemia
   (b) Diabetic ketoacidosis (See Study Guide Figure 41-1C).
   (c) Hyperglycemic hyperosmolar nonketonic syndrome and diabetic ketoacidosis
   (d) Hypoglycemia
   (e) Diabetic ketoacidosis and hypoglycemia
   (f) Hyperglycemic hyperosmolar nonketonic syndrome
   (g) Hyperglycemic hyperosmolar nonketonic syndrome
   (h) Hyperglycemic hyperosmolar nonketonic syndrome

C2. 260
   (a) (1), (2), (3), (4)
   (b) Ketones; acids, decrease; decrease
   (c) Fruity smell of her breath as blood with ketones passes through her lungs; ketones can be detected in her urine by a "dip stick" method; she may exhibit signs of DKA (text page 943)
   (d) Decrease; tachy. Hyperglycemic blood leads to polyuria with low circulating blood volume; heart rate increases (tachycardia) as a compensatory mechanism for low blood pressure.
   (e) Lower blood glucose and increase fluids (IV) gradually to prevent cerebral edema; raise blood pH; correct Na$^+$ and K$^+$ imbalances

C3. (a) (2), (3), (4)
   (b) (1), (2), (5); but (3) and (4): may occur as autonomic nervous system (ANS) compensatory mechanisms
   (c) (4)
   (d) (2) or (5) if available; (3) or (4) once he is conscious

C4. (a) Increase
   (b) Hypo
   (c) Increase; epinephrine, glucagon, cortisol, and growth hormone
   (d) Somogyi, hypo, hyper
   (e) Morning, exacerbate

C5. (a) Sorbitol; neurons (nerves)

(b) Basement, decreasing

(c) Higher, decreases

C6. (a), (e); but (b): kidneys; (c): common; (d): glomeruli

C7. (a) Feet and hands, proximally; "stocking-glove," bilateral

(b) Loss of sensation can lead to burns and exacerbations related to lack of awareness of infection; weakness can result in falls that injure joints.

(c) (3), (4), (5), (6); but (1) and (2): signs of peripheral neuropathies

(d) (1), (2), (3), (4), (6)

(e) Heart (heart attack), brain (stroke), feet and legs (peripheral vascular disease with ulcerations)

(f) His ability to sense on the plantar surface of his foot; loss of sensation of pain and foot injuries caused by neuropathy and increased risk of infection related to hyperglycemia

(g) Retinopathy; (1) (because onset of type 1 DM is likely to be early in life) and (2); (3) and (4) somewhat because they contribute to stress and related hyperglycemia

C8. Tight control of blood glucose levels, maintenance of normal lipid levels, and control of hypertension

Chapter 42

STRUCTURE AND FUNCTION OF THE MALE REPRODUCTIVE SYSTEM

A1. To produce, transport, and ejaculate sperm and to produce androgens (male sex hormones), mainly testosterone. (Urine is also eliminated through the urethra.)

A2. (c), (d); but (a) XY rather than XX; (b) is not evident until after this time

A3. (a) Testosterone

(b) Dihydrotestosterone

(c) Anti-müllerian hormone

A4. (a) Testes develop in the abdominal cavity (near kidneys) and normally descend into the scrotum during the last 2 months of fetal life. Dennis may have "undescended testes" (cryptorchidism), which can lead to infertility because sperm require the cooler (92°F–96°F) temperature of the scrotum for normal development.

(b) As testes descend, their blood and lymphatic vessels are pulled down with them. So testicular cancer cells enter lymphatic pathways that accompany testicular veins and ascend to nodes parallel to the aorta at about the level of the kidneys where testes originally developed. See A4 (a).

(c) When testes descend into the scrotum, they exert pressure on the inguinal canal, which may not close completely; females have no such descent so are much less likely to develop inguinal hernias.

(d) Sperm can be stored for 4 to 5 weeks within the widened end (ampulla) of the vas deferens (see textbook Figure 42-3).

A5. (a) Vaginalis; albuginea

(b) Dartos, cremaster

(c) Veins

A6. Seminiferous tubules → Rete testis → Efferent ductules → Epididymis → Vas (ductus) deferens → Ejaculatory duct → Urethra; only the urethra

A7. (a) Two, posterior; fructose, prostaglandins

(b) Seminal vesicles

(c) Inferior; an enlarged prostate (BPH or prostatic cancer) can impede flow of urine through the urethra

(d) Mucosal; main; alkaline; 6.0 to 6.5

(e) Muscle, ejaculation; serves as a sphincter preventing urine from passing from bladder into urethra (or semen from urethra to bladder) during ejaculation

A8. (a) Glans, prepuce; circumcision

(b) Corpora (or corpus = singular); spongiosum

B1. (a) Gonadotropin releasing hormone

(b) Follicle-stimulating hormone, luteinizing hormone

(c) Follicle-stimulating hormone

(d) Anti-müllerian hormone (or müllerian inhibitory factor), estradiol, and inhibin

(e) Luteinizing hormone

(f) Estradiol

(g) Inhibin

(h) Testosterone

(i) Testosterone

B2. (a), (b); but (c) four cells that each contain 23; (d) 60 to 70 days

B3. Spermatogonia → Primary spermatocytes → Secondary spermatocytes → Spermatids

(a) Primary spermatocytes, secondary spermatocytes

(b) Secondary spermatocytes, spermatids.

B4. (a) Contains enzymes that permit fertilization of the ovum

(b) Propels the sperm through female reproductive tract

(c) Provide energy for motion of the tail

B5. 100 to 400; days

B6. (a) Differentiates male genitalia and regulates descent of testes

(b) Develops secondary sex characteristics such as changes in hair, skin, and voice; facilitates full maturation of sperm

(c) Promotes and maintains musculoskeletal growth

B7. See text page 961.

C1. (a) (2)

(b) (1); corpora cavernosa and corpus spongiosum

(c) Parasympathetic; S2–S4

(d) Sympathetic; L1–L2

(e) Relaxation, erect

(f) At the base; squeezing of the penis during ejaculation

C2. (a) Detumescence

(b) Emission

(c) Ejaculation

C3. (a) Is not

(b) 2–5

C4. See text page 963.

C5. It can improve muscle strength and vigor and decrease bone turnover; side effects include effects similar to those of anabolic steroids (Question B7), such as acne, gynecomastia, and a decrease in the "good" cholesterol (HDL). Testosterone is contraindicated for men with prostate cancer.

Chapter 43

ALTERATIONS IN STRUCTURE AND FUNCTION OF THE MALE GENITOURINARY SYSTEM

A1. (a) Hypo; 300; more; 9 months
   (b) Be retracted over; the foreskin is so tight that it cannot cover the glans
   (c) Balanoposthitis
A2. (a) Cryptorchidism
   (b) Chordee
   (c) Peyronie's disease
   (d) Phimosis
   (e) Balanitis xerotica obliterans
A3. (a), (d); but (b) should not to avoid injury; (c) epithelial debris that is likely to accumulate under the foreskin if cleanliness is not maintained here, as in phimosis
A4. (a) Erection
   (b) Detumescence
A5. (a) Mixed
   (b) Diabetes mellitus, which diminishes neuronal function.
   (c) Cigarette smoking and hypertension cause vasoconstriction; hypercholesterolemia is related to arteriosclerosis.
   (d) Aging, use of antidepressants, depression regarding psychosocial issues such as divorce, and history of alcohol abuse
   (e) Testosterone and prolactin
   (f) Increases the second messenger GMP (see Question A4[a].)
A6. Prolonged, painful, involuntary erection
   (a) Fibrosis of penile tissue leading to erectile dysfunction; low-flow (stasis)
   (b1) Trauma, infection, or neoplasms
   (b2) Sickle cell disease and others in text, page 969.
   (c) Stasis of blood in cavernous sinuses during erection leads to deoxygenation, sickling, and additional stasis of blood here.
A7. (a) Middle-aged; highly; embarrassment
   (b) Poor hygiene, HPV, UV radiation, HIV or other causes of immunosuppression
   (c) Other countries; have not
   (d) Lymph node involvement; 20%–50%
B1. (a) Failure of one or more testes to descend into the scrotal sac
   (b) Common (one third of premature boys), rare (3% to 5%); uni
   (c) 0 to 3
   (d) A retractable testis is palpable at birth but retracts into the inguinal canal because of the exaggerated cremaster muscle action.

   (e) To enhance potential for fertility, reduce risk for testicular cancer, and for cosmetic appearance
   (f) Orchiopexy
B2. (a) Hematocele
   (b) Hydrocele
   (c) Varicocele
   (d) Spermatocele
B3. (a), (b), (f); but (c) do not; (d) from 15 to 35; (e) left, right
B4. Injury, inflammation, lymph obstruction, germ cell tumor, or side effect of irradiation
B5. (a) Scrotal palpation of a hydrocele is compared to the feel of a "bag of worms."
   (b) When the client forces expiration against a closed glottis, a venous rush is heard due to retrograde blood flow.
   (c) The varicocele disappears in the recumbent position as blood moves from testes into spermatic and renal veins and on into the inferior vena cava.
B6. (a) Spermatic artery, veins, lymphatics, nerves, and vas deferens
   (b) Neonates
   (c) Intra, can
B7. (a) Within the scrotum, posterior to testes; serve as sites for storage, maturation, and transport of sperm
   (b) Neisseria gonorrhoeae; young men
   (c) Pressure from the infected site causes back flow of infection into the ejaculatory duct and the vas.
   (d) Infection carried by lymphatics or blood vessels (septicemia)
   (e) Days; common; yes, because the causative microbe is Chlamydia
   (f) Bed rest; to encourage lymphatic drainage out of the epididymis by gravity; antibiotics, antipyretics, and analgesics; discouraged
   (g) One or both testes
B8. Mumps (infection of parotid gland(s)
   (a) Both involve pain and swelling in the scrotal area and commonly include fever; orchitis does not involve dysuria or urethral discharge.
   (b) About 30%
B9. (a) Testicular
   (b) It was the first type of cancer linked to a specific occupation (chimney sweeps); poor hygiene, exposure to UV light, or radiation therapy, for example to treat previous cancer of testes
   (c) 15 to 34; is
   (d) Cryptorchidism (See Question B1[e]); seminiferous; men in their 20s; highly
   (e) (1); but (2) and (3) both signs of metastasis
   (f) Monthly; in a warm shower
   (g) 95; III; Alpha-fetoprotein, human chorionic gonadotropin, lactic dehydrogenase
   (h) All, orchiectomy; is
C1. (a) Chronic prostatitis/chronic pelvic pain syndrome (the inflammatory type)
   (b) Acute bacterial prostatitis
   (c) Chronic bacterial prostatitis
C2. (c), (d)

C3. (c), (d); but (a) inferior; (b) inner periurethral; (e) make it worse; 5α-reductase inhibitors are likely to improve BPH

C4. African American descent, high levels of dihydroxytestosterone, family history of BPH, older men

C5. (a) Obstruction of urine outflow with retention of urine in the bladder

   (b) Infection of urine retained in the bladder leading to UTIs; overflow incontinence with related urgency; development of bladder hypertrophy with ischemia and infected diverticula; back pressure into ureters with possible hydronephrosis and renal failure

   (c1) Indicate UTI probably related to urinary stasis

   (c2) Indicates BPH rather than prostate cancer

   (c3) Negative screening for prostate cancer

   (c4) Volume over 100 mL indicates urinary stasis in bladder

   (c5) Flow rate <10 mL/sec indicates weak stream

   (c6) Compromised renal function because creatinine level is twice normal

C6. Moderate, because falls in the range of 8 to 20.

C7. (a) Is not; transurethral resection (of the) prostate; see text page 979

   (b) The transurethral incision of the prostate reduces pressure within the urethra.

   (c) Temporarily widens the urethra to allow urinary flow

C8. (b), (c); (a) common—the leading male cancer and second leading cause of cancer deaths; (d) late—is often asymptomatic until after metastasis

C9. (a) Pressure of the prostatic tumor that impedes urinary outflow

   (b) Metastases to lungs

   (c) Metastases to vertebrae and pelvis

C10. Digital rectal palpation of a hard mass; PSA (positive in 30% of prostate cancers but also in some cases of BPH); transrectal ultrasonography for identifying small masses

C11. Poorly; that his cancer has extended beyond the prostate and metastasized to at least one site. Prostatectomy or radiation

Chapter 44

STRUCTURE AND FUNCTION OF THE FEMALE REPRODUCTIVE SYSTEM

A1. Clitoris, urinary meatus, vaginal orifice, perineal body, anus

A2. (a) Introitus

   (b) Clitoris

   (c) Urinary meatus

   (d) Mons pubis

   (e) Vestibule

   (f) Labia majora, labia minora

A3. (a), (c); but (a) sexual sensations are related to changes in external genitalia; (b) recesses surrounding the cervix; (d) does not necessarily

A4. (a) 4; fermentation of glycogen in the vaginal epithelial lining by Döderlein's bacilli that are normally present in this lining

   (b) Discourages growth of microbes that cannot survive such acidity

   (c) Changes in estrogen (with oral contraceptives, pregnancy, or menopause); diabetes; antibiotics that destroy "normal flora"

A5. (a) Fundus, body, cervix

   (b) Rectum, uterus, bladder

   (c) (2)

   (d) (1)

   (e) Endometrium, myometrium, perimetrium

   (f) Myo; in dysmenorrhea, contractions of the myometrium are accompanied by pain

A6. (a) Fallopian tubes

   (b) Uterus

   (c) Fallopian tubes

   (d) Ovaries

B1. (a), (b); but (c) is not; (d) 28 days

B2. Is; fat is a source of estrogens; all

B3. (a) Gonadotropin-releasing hormone

   (b) Follicle-stimulating hormone, luteinizing hormone, prolactin

   (c) Estrogen, progesterone

B4. Follicle-stimulating hormone, luteinizing hormone

B5. (a), (b); but (c) decrease; (d) estradiol (B2)

B6. (a), (b), (d), (e), (f), (h); but (c) decrease; (g) ductile growth and development

B7. This hormone decreases myometrial contractions.

B8. Do; ovaries and adrenal cortex

B9. PF → SF → ODF → LH → CL → CA

B10. (a) Ovulation

   (b) Corpus luteum; pregnant

   (c) Functional

   (d) Estrogen; thin

   (e) Stretchability; dries; estrogen

B11. (a) Peri

   (b) Diminished; even if ovaries have stopped producing estrogen, adrenal cortex and fat tissues continue to produce some of the hormone

   (c) Hot flashes

   (d) Hot flashes, night sweats, and insomnia directly related to hormonal changes

   (e) Increased; estrogen protects bones by interfering with action of PTH

   (f) Both estrogen and progesterone; decreases risk of endometrial cancer

   (g) See text page 992.

   (h) Increased risk of blood clots and possibly breast cancer

C1. (a) Alveoli

   (b) Cooper's ligaments

   (c) Areolar tissue

C2. (a) Progesterone

   (b) Estrogen

   (c) Follicle-stimulating hormone (FSH), luteinizing hormone (LH), and prolactin

   (d) Oxytocin

C3. Alveolar (gland)

Chapter 45

ALTERATIONS IN STRUCTURE AND FUNCTION OF THE FEMALE REPRODUCTIVE SYSTEM

A1. External; does; *Candida albicans*; genital herpes, genital warts (HPV), chemical irritants, allergens, or atrophy of aging

A2. (a) Vulvodynia
(b) Cyclic vulvovaginitis
(c) Nevi
(d) Bartholin's cyst
(e) Vulvar dystrophy

A3. (c), (d); but (a): less; (b): is a precursor to

A4. (a) Normal flora; glycogen; 4.5
(b) Decreased, alkaline, increases; estrogen replacement helps to regenerate the vaginal lining and increase the population of Döderlein's bacteria; after using the toilet, it is advisable that a woman wipe from front to back to avoid fecal contamination of vagina or urethra

A5. (a) No, they indicate infection
(b) Candida
(c) Antibiotics can destroy the normal flora, allowing yeast to proliferate; stress can lower Sally's resistance to infection.

A6. See text pages 999 and 1000.

A7. (a) Common, 60; daughters of women who took DES, and young women exposed to human papilloma virus (HPV)
(b) To prevent miscarriage, 1940–1971; benign
(c) Vaginal bleeding
(d) Local excision, laser, loop electrode excision procedure (LEEP), radical surgery, and/or radiation
(e) Vaginal reconstruction.

B1. (a) (1); (2)
(b) A becomes B; transformation
(c) Meta, normal for the body but not for this region; can
(d) Trauma and infections (such as HPV)
(e) Nabothian; no, but they may have to be removed if they excessively enlarge the cervix

B2. (a) C
(b) A
(c) A

B3. (a) Years; cervical cells become increasingly abnormal (dysplastic) over an extended period
(b) Moderate; HSIL; has not
(c) I; 90% because it is localized (stage I) (*Hint*: Remember "s" stands for "stage," which indicates spread, whereas "grade" indicates the abnormality of cells microscopically.)
(d) There is a strong link between HPV and cervical cancer; HPV is associated with early age of first intercourse and multiple sexual partners and is rare among celibate women.
(e) Smoking, family history, DES exposure in utero
(f) Decreased; gynecological examinations with Pap smears can identify early stages of dysplasia
(g) Less

B4. (a) (2), (3)
(b) Endometrial tissue in her ovaries; old blood that resembles chocolate syrup; rupture may lead to peritonitis and adhesions
(c) Retrograde movement of endometrium through fallopian tubes, passage of cells via blood or lymph, or genetic or immune factors
(d) Cyclic rise in estrogen stimulates endometrial tissue to grow wherever it is located.
(e) Pain during sexual activity (dyspareunia) and infertility
(f) Observation by laparoscopy; surgery; high

B5. (a) Leiomyoma
(b) Adenomyosis
(c) Endometritis
(d) Endometriosis

B6. (a) More; older than
(b) (1), (3), (4), (5); but (2): unopposed estrogen
(c) (1), (2); but (3): painless; (4): not in early stages
(d) (4)
(e) 90%

C1. (a) Uterus (endometritis); Fallopian tubes (salpingitis); ovaries (oophoritis)
(b) *Neisseriae gonorrhoeae, Chlamydia trachomatis*; they ascend from the vagina, are harbored in the sloughing endometrium in the uterus, and may then ascend to tubes and ovaries
(c) (3), (4), (5); but (1): older; (2), single, nulliparous women; (5): if a combination of multiple sex partners with intrauterine device
(d) Exquisitely painful cervix, lower abdominal pain that starts after a menstrual period, adnexal tenderness, C-reactive protein in the blood; increase; is
(e) Antibiotics and anti-inflammatory agents such as ibuprofen

C2. (a) Fallopian tubes
(b) All answers
(c) Acute appendicitis, PID, ruptured ovarian cyst, and degenerating fibroid
(d) Lower
(e) Its wall is too thin to support a full-term pregnancy.
(f) Salpingectomy (removal); is not (because she had a salpingectomy rather than salpingostomy)

C3. (c), (d), (f); but (a): rare; (b): the most common form; (e): benign (well-differentiated)

C4. (a) (2), (3)
(b) Frequently; after; vague; gastrointestinal
(c) Are no; CA-125; chemotherapy; 50%

D1. (a) (3)
(b) (1)
(c) Gravity, pregnancy, childbirth, aging, coughing, lifting or straining with defecation
(d) (3) (*cyst* = bladder)
(e) (2)
(f) (3)

D2. (a) Kegel's exercises or use of pessary in the vagina to support the uterus
(b) See text page 1015.

E1. (a) Metrorrhagia
(b) Menorrhagia
(c) Amenorrhea
(d) Oligomenorrhea

E2. (a) Thinner
(b) Thicker; fails to
(c) Low, heavy, is not; teenagers and perimenopausal women
(d) History (including bleeding pattern) and physical examination
(e1) S
(e2) P

E3. Dys; S

E4. (d), (e), (f); but (a): is not; (b): mid-30s; (c): multifactorial, possibly including estrogen and prostaglandin E_1 deficiency, estrogen-progesterone imbalance, and aldosterone increase

E5. See text page 1018.

F1. (a) Mastitis
(b) Ductal ectasia
(c) Galactorrhea
(d) Fibroadenoma
(e) Fibrocystic disease

F2. (a) Second
(b) Biopsy
(c) Avoided; these foods contain xanthines, which are linked to fibrocystic disease.

F3. (a) Common (second leading cause of cancer deaths among women); 8; increased; more women take part in screening
(b) (2), (4), (5); but (1): older women; (3): women who have been nulliparous until at least age 30 years
(c) 55% to 85%
(d) (2)

F4. Monthly BSE, mammogram, physical examination by physician
(a) 1 mm, 1 cm; painless
(b) Because she is premenopausal, just after she completes menstruation each month
(c) Fine needle aspiration biopsy, excisional biopsy, ultrasound, MRI, PET

F5. (a), (d), (f); but (b): less; (c): first; (e): 96%

G1. (a) 1 year; 15; 1
(b) Secondary
(c) 30%–40% in each case

G2. (a) (1), (3)
(b) (1) (Note: *asthen* = weak), (3)
(c) See text page 1023.

G3. (a), (b), (d), (f), (i) ; but (c): LH, not FSH; (e): progesterone, not estradiol; (g): test for ovulation, not pregnancy; (h): 14, and if less, may account for infertility

G4. (b), (c); but (a): clomiphene citrate is an antiestrogen

G5. (a) PID can reduce fallopian tube motility, preventing ovum pickup at ovulation.
(b) Can prevent passage of sperm or ovum through the fallopian tube and possibly limit space for fetal growth within the uterine cavity.

G6. (a) Gamete intrafallopian transfer
(b) Zygote intrafallopian transfer
(c) Tubal embryo transplant
(d) Clomiphene citrate
(e) Human chorionic gonadotropin
(f) Partial zona dissection
(g) Assisted hatching

Chapter 46

SEXUALLY TRANSMITTED DISEASES

A1. (a), (b); but (c): increasing at an alarming rate; (d): less because not responsive to antibiotics

A2. Mouth, vagina and surrounding tissue of the vulva, urinary meatus (urethral opening), rectoanal area, and skin

A3. (a) (4)
(b) Cervical; smoking, immunosuppression such as by HIV, and hormonal changes as with oral contraceptives or pregnancy
(c) 100; 16, 18; different
(d) August 31 (6 weeks to 8 months); itching of the vulva, aceto-whitening of vulvar lesions, results of Pap smear, colposcopy, or biopsy
(e) There are no treatments that eradicate HPV, although some medications and surgeries can provide symptomatic relief (see text page 1031).
(f) By limiting sexual partners or use of a barrier such as a condom.

A4. Nine; chickenpox, shingles; simplex
(a) 2; fever blisters; also can
(b) 5; women; women have a larger surface area of genital mucosa
(c) Dorsal root (sensory) ganglia, sacral; are not
(d) Do not; do not; epidemic proportions
(e) Women: vulva, vagina, cervix; men: penis, scrotum; either gender: urethra or anus
(f) Malaise, myalgia, headache, fever, swollen lymph nodes

A5. (a1) A
(a2) Primary; some immunity is built up after the initial infection
(a3) 7 to 10
(a4) Is not known; they can reduce the incidence and severity of recurrent infections and decrease viral shedding and contagion during sexual activity
(a5) HSV can infect the corneas and lead to blindness
(b1) A
(b2) Cesarean; 60%

A6. (a) Virus
(b) Bacteria
(c) *Chlamydia*
(d) Virus

B1. Moniliasis, thrush, yeast infection

B2. (c), (e), (f); but (a): three; (b): usually not; (d): commonly

B3. In the mouth (thrush) and in warm moist folds of skin

B4. (a) Has an; over 6.0

    (b) Metallic, contraindicated; gastrointestinal, cardiovascular

    (c) Is; is

C1. *Chlamydia*; these three STDs are likely to exert widespread systemic effects

C2. (a) Primarily

    (b) Are many types; elementary, reticulate

    (c) Quite similar, chlamydia; 50%; cases go undiagnosed and untreated and may lead to more serious conditions such as pelvic inflammatory disease (PID), infertility, or cervical cancer

    (d) Conjunctiva, joints, and mucosa

    (e) Eye

    (f) Amplified DNA testing on urine or vaginal fluid samples

C3. (a) 650,000; days; oropharynx (throat), eyes, or skin

    (b1) Painful or burning upon urination

    (b2) Pain upon intercourse or other sexual activity involving the vulva

    (b3) Inflammation has spread to her fallopian tubes

    (c) Orogenital sexual abuse

C4. See completed Table 46-1 below.

Table 46-1. Comparison of Sexually Transmitted Diseases

Name of STD	Causative Microbe	Description
(a) **Condyloma acuminata**	**HPV virus**	Genital warts, pruritis; increased risk of cervical cancer; rapidly growing STD in the U.S.
(b) **Trichomoniasis**	Protozoan: turnip-shaped with flagellae	**Copious green or yellow discharge with odor; usual medication (Flagyl) leaves metallic taste; 5 million cases diagnosed in U.S. in 1999**
(c) **Chlamydia**	**Bacterial pathogen that resembles virus**	The most prevalent STD in the U.S.; often no symptoms, but women may have mucopurulent discharge and men, pruritis; may spread; causes blindness in 25%–50% of infected neonates
(d) Chanchroid	**Gram-negative bacteria: _Haemophilus_**	**Acute, painful ulcers; profuse discharge; buboes (lymphadenopathy); rare in U.S.; highly contagious**
(e) **Gonorrhea**	*Neisseria* bacteria (gram-negative diplococci)	**Creamy yellow discharge in men with urethral pain; may spread to other genitalia, or systematically; may cause blindness in infected neonates**
(f) **Bacterial vaginosis**	*Gardnerella vaginalis*	Thin, gray-white discharge with foul, fishy odor; "clue cells" seen on slides; very common; **not inflammatory, so an "-osis," not an "-itis"**
(g) **Syphilis**	Spirochete bacteria: *Treponema pallidum*	**Painless chancres in primary stage; rash and flu-like symptoms may occur in secondary stage; multisystem tertiary stage may occur 20 years later; new U.S. cases in 1999 under 7000**
(h) Genital herpes	**HSV-2 (or -1): neurotropic virus**	**Prodromal paresthesia; painful vesicles in acute stage, especially in primary infections; no cure**
(i) **Candidiasis**	*Candida (Monilia)*	Most women have this infection at least once; thick, cheesy, odorless discharge; antifungals can cure

Chapter 47

ORGANIZATION AND CONTROL OF NEURAL FUNCTION

A1. (a) Spinal cord, brain
(b) Neurons
(c) Efferent
A2. (a) (3)
(b) Ribosomes
(c) Axon; one, some
A3. Peripheral
(a) Myelin; white
(b) Insulator; increases, lacking; saltatory
(c) Is; neurons lacking myelin will die, possibly because the myelin sheath secretes neurotrophic compounds
(d) Regeneration; central; may account for the fact that CNS neurons do not regenerate well
A4. (a) Astroglia
(b) Astroglia
(c) Ependymal cells
(d) Microglia
(e) Oligodendroglia
(f) Satellite cells
(g) Satellite cells, Schwann cells
A5. (a) 2, 20; hyper
(b) Cannot; glial cells do store glycogen, and ketones can provide small amounts of energy.
(c) No; death is likely to begin after 4 to 6 minutes of anoxia.
(d) Hypoglycemia deprives the brain of a constant supply of glucose.
B1. Action potential
(a) Negative; −70 to −90
(b) Sodium; negative; −60; 0; overshoot (such as +20 mV)
(c) Potassium; −75 or −80 (an overshoot or hyperpolarization)
(d) A millisecond; early; no
B2. (a), (d); but (b): raise so less negative, such as from −90 to −70, and closer to threshold; (c): IPSP
B3. (a) ADH (vasopressin)
(b) Norepinephrine made by sympathetic nerves and the adrenal medulla
B4. (b) → (c) → (a) → (e) → (d)
B5. (a) Each neuron may be involved in thousands of synapses between different parts of neurons (see B2[a]); neurons can be both excited (EPSP) and inhibited (IPSP); the effects are additive.
(b) Billions of neurons may be involved in these complex networks.
(c) Chemical synapses are relatively slow, yet their transmission requires only 0.3 msec (thousandths of a second).
(d) These include a myriad of neurotransmitters, hormones, neuromodulators, and growth factors, as well as light and physical factors.
B6. (a) Dopamine, norepinephrine, serotonin
(b) Endorphins and enkephalins
(c) Gamma-aminobutyric acid, glycine
(d) Acetylcholine

(e) Dopamine
C1. (a), (c); but (b): before; (d): CNS
C2. (a) Meso (which forms bone and cartilage), vertebral column
(b) Ecto; all (1–6)
(c) Front or cephalic; fore; mid; hind; brain stem
(d) (1), (2), (3)
(e) (1), (2), (4)
C3. (b), (c); but (a): each spinal nerve but not cranial nerve; (d): efferent [motor] output association [OA] and lower motor neurons [LMNs]; (e): most
C4. (a) Special somatic afferent
(b) General somatic efferent, general somatic afferent
(c) Special visceral afferent, general visceral efferent, general visceral afferent
C5. White, outer
(a) Archi; shortest
(b) Paleo, middle
(c) Neo, brain stem and cerebrum; about 6 years of age; adequate myelination is required before a child can achieve bladder control or fine, coordinated movements
C6. Ascending portions increase awareness; descending regions speed reaction times and help to maintain posture.
D1. (a) Shorter; conus medullaris, L1 or L2; cauda equina (horse's tail)
(b) Between L3 and L4 (or L4 and L5); this site is inferior to the lower end of the spinal cord, so the cord is not injured during the procedure
(c) Gray; ventral, motor; lower, skeletal
(d) C5 and L1 to S2, which are origins of nerves that supply arms and legs
(e) Denticulate ligaments and filum terminale (both pia mater) and spinal nerve roots
D2. (a) 32; Cervical: 8; Thoracic: 12; Lumbar: 5; Sacral: 5; Coccygeal: 2+
(b) Sensory, motor; mixed
(c) Branches of spinal nerves, and all are mixed; ventral because they form plexuses that supply all except small regions posterior to the vertebrae
(d) Axons of sympathetic nerves en route to sympathetic ganglia
(e) Sensory neuron that enters the cord through a dorsal root and leads to a synapse with a motor neuron whose axon exits the cord through a ventral root
(f) Myotatic; reduces risk of over stretching muscles and helps to regulate muscle tone
(g) Hypo; spasticity (hypertonia)
(h) Nociceptive (harmful or offending) stimulus
E1. (a) Cerebrum, hypothalamus, thalamus
(b) Midbrain
(c) Cerebellum, medulla, pons
E2. (a) Pons
(b) Medulla
(c) Midbrain
(d) Cerebellum, medulla, and pons

(e) Medulla
(f) Cerebellum
E3. (a) IX–XII (9–12)
(b) V–VIII (5–8)
(c) III–IV (3–4)
E4. (a) Oculomotor, III, L
(b) Spinal accessory, XI, R
(c) Optic, II, R
(d) Vagus, X, L
(e) Hypoglossal, XII
(f) Facial (VII); note that glossopharyngeal (IX) would affect saliva (but not tear) production
(g) Facial (VII)
(h) Trigeminal (mandibular branch), V
E5. (a) Glossopharyngeal and vagus
(b) Facial (anterior of tongue), glossopharyngeal (posterior of tongue plus pharynx), and vagus (pharynx)
(c) Vestibulocochlear
(d) Vagus
(e) Abducens
(f) Olfactory
(g) Oculomotor
E6. (a) L2–S1 (and S2–S4)
(b) C5–C8 (and T1)
(c) C1–C4
E7. (a) H
(b) T
(c) T
(d) H
E8. (a1) Corpus callosum, W
(a2) Basal ganglia, G
(a3) Internal capsule, W
(b1) Temporal
(b2) Occipital
(b3) Parietal
(b4) Frontal
(c) Left; gradually throughout childhood
E9. (a) Basal ganglia
(b) Premotor area (6)
(c) Primary auditory cortex (area 41)
(d) Auditory association area (22)
(e) Somesthetic association areas (5 and 7)
(f) Limbic system
E10. (a) Dura mater, arachnoid, pia mater
(b) Pia mater
(c) Dura mater
(d) Cerebellum, medulla, pons
E11. Cranial bones; meninges (including the falx cerebri and tentorium cerebelli that limit shifting of cerebral hemispheres); and CSF
E12. (a) Capillaries of the choroid plexuses located in the four ventricles
(b) 0.5 to 0.75
(c) Lateral ventricles → third ventricle → cerebral aqueduct → fourth ventricle → subarachnoid space → arachnoid villi → cranial venous sinuses
E13. (a) Tight junctions of endothelial cells, basement membrane, and astrocytes
(b) All except epinephrine
(c) Ependymal

(d) CO_2, H_2O, O_2
F1. Subconscious regulation of viscera
F2. (a) S (for *Stress*)
(b) P (for *Peace*)
(c) S
(d) P
(e) P
(f) P
F3. (a), (d); but (b): opposing; (c): parasympathetic
F4. (a) III, VII, IX, and X
(b) Solid; P
(c) S
(d) S; many
(e) S; S
(f) S
(g) P
(h) Adrenal medulla, blood vessels of skin, hair muscles of skin, sweat glands
F5. (a) See text page 1085.
(b) See text page 1085.
F6. (a) Acetylcholine
(b) Acetylcholine
(c) Norepinephrine (or other catecholamines)
(d) Acetylcholine
(e) Norepinephrine (or other catecholamines)
F7. (a) Acetyl CoA + choline; nicotinic and muscarinic; muscarinic
(b) ACh-ase
(c) Tyrosine (an amino acid) → L-DOPA → Dopamine
(d) Methyl; does
(e) Active reuptake (recycling) by the presynaptic neuron, enzymatic destruction by MAO or COMT, or diffusion of the NT into surrounding tissues
(f1) MAO inhibitors inhibit MAO-catalyzed breakdown of NE.
(f2) Block reuptake of NE
(g) Adrenergic
(g1) (3)
(g2) Increases, decrease
(g3) Relax, dilate
(g4) Contract, constriction, increase
(h) Adrenergic

Chapter 48

SOMATOSENSORY FUNCTION AND PAIN

A1. (a) Three; peripheral, dorsal root; C6-C8
(b) Do, anterolateral, left
(c) Cerebral cortex, left, parietal; homunculus; (3)
(d) (1)
A2. (a) Anterolateral pathway
(b) Discriminative pathway
(c) Discriminative pathway
(d) Anterolateral pathway
(e) Discriminative pathway
(f) Discriminative pathway
(g) Anterolateral pathway

A3. (b), (d); but (a): faster; (c): L2 and L3

A4. (a) Touch, heat, pain, pressure, tickle, itch, muscle or joint awareness (proprioception), vision, hearing, taste, smell; selective sensitivity of receptors to specific forms of physical or chemical energy

(b) Ability to discriminate location of a sensory stimulus that depends on density of sensory receptors and factors such as emotions

(c) Level of sensory stimuli required for sensory perception

A5. (a) Meissner's corpuscles
(b) Pacinian corpuscles
(c) Free nerve endings
(d) Merkel's disks
(e) Ruffini's end organs

A6. (a) Lips; fingers
(b) Do not; sensation of temperature change is protective
(c) Awareness of body position and movement
(d) Dynamic

A7. A withdrawal reflex indicates that sensory and motor pathways involving level S1 of the spinal cord are intact.

B1. It is a warning signal of tissue injury but is also "a pain."

B2. (a) Reaction to
(b) 13.7
(c) Neuropathic; analgesic
(d) Virtually all; pattern

B3. (a) Fast, slow; Melzack, Wall; does not (which are now known to be more complex); it stimulated interest in pain and in approaches such as therapeutic touch in controlling pain
(b) Multiple factors, many including the brain, regulate pain. See text page 1101.

B4. Pain
(a) Skin, teeth, periosteum, meninges, and internal organs
(b1) Mechanical: intense pressure or puncture, muscle contraction or stretching of tissues
(b2) Heat or cold
(b3) Chemical: release of chemicals is associated with trauma, inflammation, or ischemia
(c) A δ
(d) Neo, fast; paleo

B5. (a), (b); but (c): initiate and prolong; (d): midbrain and leads to analgesia (pain relief); (e): producing analgesia

B6. Moves the body part away from an offending stimulus

B7. They are the body's own (endogenous) pain-killing chemicals; enkephalins, endorphins, and dynorphins

B8. Tolerance; threshold

B9. (a) Deep somatic; sharp, bright
(b) Visceral; splanchnic; autonomic nervous system (ANS) nerves are activated
(c) (1)
(d) Is not; see text page 1105
(e) Referred; pain from visceral receptors (in ischemic heart) enters dorsal roots at the same

level as somatic afferents (from skin in left arm and chest)
(f) Right, neck; these organs lie just inferior to the diaphragm, which developed embryologically in the neck with its nerve supply at C3 to C5
(g) Acute; 6; anxiety, muscle spasms, and sympathetic responses
(h) It serves as a warning signal and points to possible diagnoses, whereas chronic pain extends beyond a period of usefulness and can deplete resources.
(i) Chronic

B10. (a) (1)
(b) Questions or scales that describe quality, severity, duration, location, pattern, radiation of pain; questions about factors that trigger or relieve pain; Ms. Templeton's reaction to pain

B11. (d), (e); but (a): less; (b): less; (c): low because short-term

B12. See text page 1109.

B13. (a) Applications of cold packs should be limited to 15 minutes at a time (to prevent tissue ischemia).
(b) Possible overuse of heat (with burns) because of the potential age-related loss of sensation and limited mobility associated with arthritis

B14. Transcutaneous electrical nerve stimulation; noninvasive, can. See text page 1110.

B15. Acupuncture, ancient; acupressure, fingers

B16. Without
(a) Codeine, dynorphins, endorphins, morphine
(b) Aspirin, nonsteroidal anti-inflammatory drugs
(c) Acetaminophen
(d) Serotonin reuptake inhibitors

B17. (b), (d); but (a): are not; (c): should not

C1. (a) Paresthesia
(b) Hyperalgesia
(c) Hyperpathia
(d) Allodynia
(e) Athermia

C2. (a) Nerve compression or entrapment or specific neuralgias (trigeminal or postherpetic)
(b) Diabetes mellitus, chronic alcoholism, hypothyroidism, renal alterations, and neurotoxic drugs

C3. (a) Treat the underlying cause, such as diabetes or hypothyroidism.
(b) Palliative pain medications ease pain without curing the underlying cause (such as cancer)

C4. Acetaminophen is nephrotoxic; for a terminal condition, risk of opioid addiction is less of a concern.

C5. Severe, often repetitive pain along cranial or spinal nerves
(a) Trigeminal, cranial nerve V; unilateral; severe, lightning-like; light touch along the face; see text page 1114.
(b) Zoster, shingles; more because of decrease in numbers of large (type A) nerve fibers and decreased immunity
(c) Sympathetic nerves are involved, and these affect blood vessel diameter and sweat glands.

C6. 70%. See text page 1115.

D1. (a), (d); but (b): some but not most; (c): without

D2. Sudden onset of severe, intractable (not responsive to treatment) pain; also those that disturb sleep, occur with exertion, or are accompanied by drowsiness, changes in vision or mental status, paralysis, tingling, or numbness of extremities

D3. Factors that trigger, exacerbate, or relieve the headache, including meals, alcohol, stress, exercise, menstrual cycle, and medications

D4. (a) Tension-type
(b) Tension-type
(c) Migraine
(d) Migraine
(e) Chronic daily
(f) Cluster

D5. (a) 5 to 20 minutes
(b1) Double vision related to paralysis of eye muscles
(b2) Mixed type as with tension-type or chronic daily
(c) Can; (3), (4), (5)
(d) Nonpharmacologic: avoidance of triggers, regular patterns of eating and sleeping, stress reduction; pharmacologic: beta blockers such as propranolol, certain antidepressants, and other medications (listed on text page 1117)

E1. Research indicates that neonates respond to painful heel sticks, children as young as 3 years accurately report and remember pain, and the prevalence of pain increases among elderly.

E2. (a) Show pictures of faces with smiley or hurting expressions or show outlines to bodies on which Jewel can indicate location of pain
(b) Numeric or word graphic codes, and the child's self-report of pain

E3. Before; positive self-talk, imagery, modeling, and rehearsal

E4. They may not want to be a burden or to experience testing or treatment.

E5. See text page 1120.

Chapter 49

ALTERATIONS IN MOTOR FUNCTION

A1. For smooth movements to occur, such as flexion at the elbow, antagonistic movements, such as extension, must be simultaneously inhibited.

A2. See text page 1124.

A3. (a) Proteins that form the contractile elements of muscles
(b) Decreases the angle of a joint, takes part in withdrawal reflexes, antagonizes extensor, and permits fine manipulations
(c) A lower motoneuron (LMN) and the muscle fibers it innervates

A4. (a) Thousands
(b) Slow; oxygen in blood, slow
(c) Fast

A5. (a) Supplementary motor cortex

(b) Primary motor cortex
(c) Prefrontal association cortex
(d) Primary motor cortex.

A6. (b) → (a) → (d) → (c) → (f) → (e)

A7. (d), (e), (f); but (a): hands and face; (b): face; (c): left

A8. See text page 1127.

A9. (a) Less than normal
(b) Paresis; para
(c) LMNs

A10. (a) (1)
(b) UMNs, below
(c) Complete use; spasticity (because regions below T6 still have spinal cord reflexes because LMNs are intact there)
(d) Clonus or clonic movements
(e) Is; may (by first level reflexes involving tactile stimulation but not by psychic or visual stimuli because spinal pathways are severed)

A11. (a) LMNs, hyper, tetany
(b) LMNs, flaccid, atrophy

A12. L4, right

B1. (a) Duchenne's muscular dystrophy
(b) Denervation atrophy and disuse atrophy
(c) Myasthenia gravis
(d) Disuse atrophy
(e) Polyneuropathy
(f) Mononeuropathy

B2. (a) Males; DMD is an X-linked disorder
(b) Muscular, dystrophin
(c) (1), (4)
(d) High; shows muscle cell destruction with leakage of contents into blood
(e) Is not; fat and other connective tissue that replaces atrophied muscle leads to pseudohypertrophy
(f) Is not

B3. (a) Acetylcholinesterase
(b) Physostigmine and neostigmine
(c) Curare
(d) *Clostridium botulinum* toxin

B4. (a) Women
(b) (1), (2), (3); but (4): more distal movements are less affected; (5): myasthenia gravis is a neuromuscular junction disorder, not a sensory disorder
(c) Physostigmine and neostigmine
(d) Antibodies that may be attacking her NMJs
(e) Respiratory failure

B5. (a) Wallerian degeneration
(b) Schwann cells
(c) Chromatolysis
(d) Endoneurial tube

B6. (a) Herniated; (soft inner) nucleus pulposus; posterolaterally because ligamentous support is weakest there
(b) L4-L5 (the greatest weight-bearing region); common
(c) Pain; rare
(d) Positive
(e) (1), (3), (4)

B7. (a) (1), (2); but (3): hyperthyroid
- (b) (2), (3); but (1): numbness in thumb, index finger, and middle finger
- (c) Can be

B8. Poly

C1. (a) (2), (4)
- (b) Inhibitory; biceps; (2)
- (c) Extrapyramidal; extrapyramidal

C2. (a) Gray, cerebrum
- (b) Putamen; internal capsule; striatum (or neostriatum)
- (c) Nigra; dopamine
- (d) Parkinson's, deficient; hyper; stiffness, rigidity, and tremor; left
- (e) Do; these connections modulate voluntary movements, posture, and muscle tone, leading to efficient, balanced, graceful movements
- (f) GABA, ACh, norepinephrine, serotonin, enkephalin, glutamine
- (g) ACh

C3. (a) Chorea
- (b) Athetosis
- (c) Ballismus
- (d) Tardive dyskinesia
- (e) Tic
- (f) Dystonia

C4. (a) Is; 80%; see text page 1140
- (b1) Bradykinesia
- (b2) Cog-wheel movements
- (b3) Tremor
- (b4) Masklike face
- (b5) Dysphagia
- (b6) Autonomic manifestations
- (b7) Bradykinesia
- (c) Five
- (d1) A precursor of dopamine that can cross the blood-brain barrier; but 97% to 99% of L-dopa is decarboxylated to dopamine, which cannot cross the blood-brain barrier
- (d2) This decarboxylase inhibitor allows more L-dopa to enter the brain, so smaller dosages (with fewer side effects) are needed
- (d3) Decrease levels of (excitatory) ACh to balance low levels of (inhibitory) dopamine

C5. Does not; helps make movements smooth and coordinated

C6. Congenital defect; stroke or trauma that leads to ischemia; tumor

C7. (a) Truncal ataxia
- (b) Intention tremor
- (c) Dysdiadochokinesia
- (d) Dysmetria
- (e) Cerebellar dysarthria
- (f) Nystagmus

D1. (a) Lou Gehrig; are not; older; 2 to 5
- (b1) Shrinkage of muscles related to destruction of
- (b2) lateral corticospinal tracts (axons of UMNs) in the spinal cord, and
- (b3) hardening caused by scar tissue (gliosis) in these tracts
- (c) (2), (4), (6), (7)

- (d) An antiglutamate drug (riluzole)
- (e) By blinking eyelids or moving eyes

D2. (a) Before, women; is
- (b) CNS, myelin, decreases; oligodendrocyte; both
- (c) Multiple demyelinated areas of axons become hardened plaques with scar formation (gliosis) composed of proteins, enzymes, and various cells that indicate inflammation.
- (d) Is; T cells and antibodies may induce oligodendrocyte damage
- (e) (3), (4)
- (f) See text page 1144.
- (g) Four
- (h) See text page 1145.

D3. (a), (d)

D4. (a) Lumbar; they support the most weight
- (b1) A
- (b2) B
- (c) Intervertebral disks, ligaments, trunk muscles, and normal curvature of spine; and rib cage for the thoracic region

D5. Tetraplegia (or quadriplegia) refers to loss of function in all four extremities, trunk, and pelvic organs; in paraplegia, use of the arms and upper trunk is retained.

D6. (a) I
- (b) C
- (c) I
- (d) I

D7. (a) B
- (b) Left; contralateral; ipsilateral (See Figure 49-15)
- (c) Arms; elderly
- (d) Arms; cauda equina; is
- (e) Primary; is not; secondary

D8. (a) To preserve residual neurological function and prevent additional neurological damage
- (b) To maintain circulation to the injured cord (and to the rest of the body)
- (c) To reduce inflammation and edema that could impede blood flow and exert pressure on injured tissues
- (d) To promote axonal regeneration

D9. (b), (c), (e); but (a): more; (d): is not because tenodesis (natural finger flexion when wrists are hyperextended) requires use of arms and wrists as with C6 or lower SCIs

D10. (a) Is; spastic
- (b) A, absent; positive
- (c) Is (because SCI is T12 or higher, which affects trunk muscles)

D11. C3 to C5; intercostal muscles receive innervation from T1 to T7, and abdominal muscles from T7 to T12; both of these sets of muscles are required for coughing and deep breathing needed to clear mucus from lungs

D12. Low
- (a) Persist (because it arises from the medulla, which is not injured in the SCI); its slowing effect on the heart is not counterbalanced by sympathetic impulses

(b) Ann; because her injury is so high (C3) that more of her sympathetic nerves (all those originating below her injury) are deprived of their regulation from the brainstem. Sympathetic nerves (from about levels T1–T5) to the heart do not stimulate the heart (which also receives less venous return from paralyzed lower extremities); nerves from T1–L2 do not vasoconstrict blood vessels to maintain blood pressure; excessive blood in dilated skin vessels give up heat, which lowers the body temperature.

(c) Suctioning stimulates afferents of vagus nerves and leads to bradycardia (vagovagal response).

(d) Postural (orthostatic) hypotension; gradual elevation to the sitting upright position and wearing of compression hose

D13. (a) Ann and Mr. Tenley; their injuries are high (T6 or above) with large areas (below injury) of unregulated sympathetic nerves

(b) Full bladder or rectum or painful episodes (see others on text page 1153)

(c) Exaggerated; pallor, high

(d) Flushing, dilation; brady

(e) Lower, upper; is

D14. (a) The inability to regulate body temperature according to the environment occurs as connections involving the hypothalamus ("thermostat") and sympathetic nerves (to blood vessels in skin and sweat glands) are severed

(b) Immobility leads to edema, stasis of blood, and increased risk of clot formation.

(c) See text pages 1154–1155.

(d) See text pages 1154–1155.

(e) Once the period of spinal shock (areflexia) is over, persons with UMN disorders experience lack of awareness of bladder filling and have spastic bladder (micturition when bladder is full); persons with LMN lesions cannot void voluntarily or involuntarily because of the flaccid bladder.

(f) Spastic bowel if the lesion is above S2 to S4 of the cord, and flaccid bowel if below S2 to S4 of the cord

(g) See text page 1155.

Chapter 50

DISORDERS OF BRAIN FUNCTION

A1. (a) 2, 20

(b) Ischemia, hypoxia

(c) They depend on anaerobic metabolism; this can lead to lactic acid excess that results in acidosis.

(d) Focal; cardiac arrest, circulatory shock

(e) Seconds; 5

(f) Ionic pumps; Na^+ and water enter brain cells, causing them to swell; calcium ions also enter cells and cause release of destructive intracellular enzymes

(g) (3), (4)

(h) Distal

A2. (a) and (b), see text page 1161.

(c) Hypothermia decreases cerebral oxygen requirements and thus may help to reduce severity of cerebral hypoxia; for example, in near-drowning accidents.

A3. (a) CVA, trauma, hypoglycemic injury, Huntington's disease, ALS, and possibly Alzheimer's disease

(b) A glutamate receptor that operates channels controlling flow of Na^+ and Ca^{+2}

(c) Cells swell because of excessive inflow of Na^+ and H_2O; entrance of Ca^{+2} into cells releases intracellular enzymes that destroy neurons (see A1[f])

(d) ICF within; glutamate is allowed to exit from cells and injures surrounding cells

(e) Cerebral cortex, hippocampus; memory, cognition

(f) Decrease excitoxicity by decreasing release of glutamate

A4. (a1) Brain, 80; brain tumor or cerebral edema resulting from trauma or surgery

(a2) Cerebrospinal fluid (CSF), 10; excessive CSF production or obstructed outflow

(a3) Cerebral blood, 10; hemorrhage or obstructed venous outflow

(b) Brain (edema); blood (hemorrhage and possible obstruction to outflow by clot formation); and possibly CSF (by obstruction of outflow caused by brain edema, bleeding, and clots)

(c) Dramatically

(d) Decreased level of consciousness (LOC), evidenced by lethargy and confusion

(e) 85 (Her MAP is 110 + 30 = 140. *Hint:* see Chapter 23, Question A2. Her CPP = MAP – ICP = 140 – 55 = 85; normal (although both MAP and ICP are high as a result of the Cushing's reflex)

(f) Increased, systolic; widened; Cushing; vasoconstrictive; is not; ICP monitoring is available in many clinical settings

(g) Brady, high; dilation; increases cerebral blood flow

A5. (a) Dura, vertically, the two cerebral hemispheres; cingulate, anterior; medial, leg

(b1) A horizontal section of dura mater, it separates cerebral hemispheres from cerebellum; transtentorial

(b2) Opening or "notch" in the tentorium through which the midbrain passes; uncal

(c1) Blindness, respiratory arrest, dilated pupil (ipsilateral); possibly death by compression of vital structures in the medulla and posturing (decorticate or decerebrate)

(c2) "Clouding" of consciousness, death by compression of vital structures in the medulla, respiratory arrest, posturing (decorticate or decerebrate)

(d) Decorticate

(e1) Infratentorial

(e2) Brainstem

A6. (a) Interstitial
   (b) Vasogenic
   (c) Cytotoxic
A7. Steroids (controversial) and osmotic diuretics, such as mannitol
A8. (a) CSF; reduced reabsorption
   (b1) NC
   (b2) C
   (b3) NC
   (c) Infants; because sutures are still open
   (d) (2), (4), (5), (6)
   (e) Ophthalmoscopic observation of the optic nerve
A9. (a) Medulla, midbrain, hypothalamus, pons, thalamus
   (b) Ascending reticular activating system (ARAS); cerebral cortex
   (c) Hypothalamus, limbic system
A10. (b), (d); but (a): is not; (c): delirium; (e): lower
   (f): move (and rotate)
A11. Rostral, caudal
   (a) Midbrain
   (b) Medulla
   (c) Diencephalon
A12. High; eye opening (E), motor response (M), verbal response (V)
A13. See text page 1171. (a), (c), (d), (e); but (b): 30 minutes
A14. See text pages 1171–1172.
B1. (a) Vertebral arteries, basilar artery
   (b) Internal carotid arteries, middle cerebral arteries
   (c) Anterior cerebral arteries
   (d) Anterior cerebral arteries, basilar artery, middle cerebral arteries, posterior cerebral arteries, vertebral arteries
   (e) Posterior communicating arteries, posterior cerebral arteries
B2. (a) Superficial; because of their location on the surface of the cerebral cortex
   (b) Dura; internal jugular
   (c) Do not; an increase in central venous pressure (as by a Valsalva maneuver) can briefly increase ICP
B3. (a) Deep, local; auto, 60 to 140
   (b) (1), (3), (5)
   (c) Depresses; increased perfusion "flushes out" excessive H+
B4. (a) Vascular disorders that injure myocardial and brain tissue, respectively; in both cases impairment may be limited by rapid emergency treatment
   (b) Both are warning signs of decreased perfusion; treatments of angina and TIA may reduce the risk of infarctions in these organs
B5. (a) African American
   (b) 75
   (c) Hypertension
   (d) History
B6. (a) Blood sludging during a crisis increases risk of clot formation.
   (b) Stasis of blood in the left atrium increases the risk of cardiogenic emboli to the middle cerebral arteries.
   (c) Polycythemia leads to sluggish flow (with clot formation) and hypertension.
B7. Smoking cessation, avoidance of alcohol and cocaine, lowering blood cholesterol levels and weight (if obese), increasing exercise (if sedentary), control of hypertension and diabetes
B8. (a) Focal, minutes
   (b) The "halo" of brain tissue surrounding the core of the dead or dying cells resulting from a stroke; rapid emergency treatment that increases perfusion to the CVA area may allow penumbral cells to survive unimpaired. Note: a TIA is a penumbra without the central infarcted zone.
B9. (b), (d); but (a): thrombi; (c): are not; (e): focal, subcortical, "lacunar" syndromes, such as clumsy hand syndrome
B10. (b); see text page 1177.
B11. (a) L, middle cerebral artery
   (b) R, anterior cerebral artery
   (c) Posterior cerebral artery
B12. (a) Is not (because > 24 minutes)
   (b) Is; slurred speech, difficulty maintaining balance, posture, and muscle tone
   (c) Because ischemic (thrombotic) and hemorrhagic strokes require very different treatments, and early treatment may salvage penumbral areas.
   (d) Magnetic resonance imaging
   (e) Ischemic (not thrombolytic); recombinant tissue-type plasminogen activator (tPA), streptokinase, urokinase
   (f) See text page 1178.
B13. (c), (d); but (a): ages 30 to 60 years; (b): two thirds do not; (e): is
B14. (a), (c), (d), (e); but (b): severe headache
B15. (a) Occurs especially within the first 24 hours and leads to gradual brain deterioration
   (b) Rapidly deprives the brain of blood flow and is difficult to treat
   (c) Related to blockage of reabsorption of CSF into arachnoid villi
B16. (a) Capillary beds are lacking, so veins are subjected to higher pressure blood from arteries (rather than lower pressure from capillaries), so they are at higher risk for rupture.
   (b) Are, do
B17. (a), (c); but (b): speech; (d): left, right
B18. (a) Dysarthria
   (b) Expressive aphasia
   (c) Fluent aphasia
   (d) Wernicke's aphasia
   (e) Apraxia
   (f) Anomic aphasia
C1. See text page 1182.
C2. (a) Accidents involving vehicles and pedestrians
   (b) Comminuted
   (c) Nose
   (d) Concussion, contusion
   (e) Contusion

(f) Posterior
C3. (a1) Epidural; rapid
(a2) Right, left
(b1) Subacute
(b2) Arachnoid membrane; veins, slowly
C4. (a) Encephalitis, myelitis
(b) (2), (3)
(c) Rapidly, through CSF around brain and cord
(d1) B
(d2) V
(d3) B
(d4) B
(e1) Nuchal rigidity
(e2) Petechiae
(e3) Brudzinski's sign
(f) Glucocorticoids (steroids); see text page 1186.
(g) Viral; do
C5. (a) Neurons, neuroglia: astrocytes, neuroglia: ependymal cells
(b) Meningeal cells, pineal cells, pituitary cells
(c) Breast cancer cells, prostate cancer cells
C6. (b), (c); but (a): can, based on location and size; (d): benign, slow
C7. The brain does lack pain receptors, but headache associated with brain tumors is related to stretching of dura mater or blood vessels.
C8. (a), (c); but (b): less; (d): almost always
D1. Sensory, motor, and autonomic changes; hallucinations; confusion; loss of consciousness. They vary with location of cells affected and degree of spread to other parts of the brain.
D2. (b), (c); but (a): common; (d): interictal; (e): secondary
D3. (a) Is; are
(b) See text page 1190.
(c) Does not, one
(d) Do, both; common
(e1) A
(e2) S
(e3) M
(f) An aura is considered a simple partial seizure that may precede a more severe seizure; is
(g) Clonic
D4. (a) Tonic-clonic
(b) Atonic
(c) Absence
D5. (a) Are
(b) Protect the client from injury
(c) Avoids drug interactions and additive side effects
D6. Seizures that do not stop spontaneously, and if not treated, may be fatal
E1. Depression is one sign of dementia; antidepressants may be introduced for a differential diagnosis: they relieve depression but not the cognitive changes associated with dementia.
E2. (a) Cortical atrophy
(b) Sundown syndrome
(c) Neurofibrillary tangles
(d) Neuritic plaques
(e) Acetylcholine
(f) Amyloid precursor protein

E3. High; the APP gene is located on chromosome 21, and almost all persons with Down syndrome have three (trisomy) of chromosome 21 (and thus more APP gene)
E4. (a) 2
(b) 1
(c) 3
E5. See text page 1196.
E6. (a) Pick's disease
(b) Wernicke-Korsakoff syndrome
(c) Huntington's disease
(d) Creutzfeldt-Jakob disease
(e) Multi-infarct dementia

Chapter 51

SLEEP AND SLEEP DISORDERS

A1. Restoration of mental and physical function, processing information received during wakefulness, rest, repair, growth of tissues
A2. See text pages 1201–1202.
A3. (a) Height
(b) Higher
(c) Lower
A4. (a) Beta, alpha, theta, delta
(b) Beta
(c) Theta, delta
A5. (a) Non-REM
(b) REM
(c) REM
(d) Non-REM
(e) REM
A6. $4 \rightarrow 3 \rightarrow 2 \rightarrow REM$; $4 \rightarrow 3 \rightarrow 2 \rightarrow REM \rightarrow 2$
A7. (a) 3, 4
(b) 2
(c) 1
A8. Certain activities are increased (dreaming, eye movements, pulse, blood pressure, and respirations), whereas other activities are greatly diminished (muscle tone).
A9. (a) 24-hour diurnal rhythms, including patterns of sleep, wakefulness, body temperature, and hormone production
(b) See text page 1205.
(c) The circadian "clock" located superior to the optic chiasma in the hypothalamus with projections to the pituitary and brainstem; light and other stimuli can reset this clock; contains many melatonin receptors
A10. Pineal, night; it may help to regulate sleep-wake cycle and circadian rhythm
B1. (a) Weeks; see text page 1207.
(b) A sleep study; electrocardiogram (ECG), electroencephalogram (EEG), electromyograph (EMG), electro-oculogram (EOG); eye movements; percentage of hemoglobin that is saturated with oxygen
(c) Day after; the first evidence of sleep; 10; daytime sleepiness because he falls asleep so quickly

B2. (a), (b); but (c): less time; (d): the most common

B3. See text page 1208.

B4. (a) Advanced sleep phase syndrome
(b) Delayed sleep phase syndrome
(c) Chronic insomnia
(d) Narcolepsy
(e) Acute insomnia

B5. Use several alarm clocks, bright light, a brisk shower or walk outside

B6. (a) Faster, short
(b) Weakness REM
(c) Hypocretin is a neurotransmitter synthesized by neurons in hypothalamic control centers for wakefulness; low levels of hypocretin and its receptors may help to explain mechanisms of narcolepsy.

B7. (a) Relaxation techniques, restricting of the amount of time in bed, cognitive therapy, weight loss if obese, eliminating evening alcohol and caffeine
(b) Benzodiazepines, antihistamines, and sedating antidepressants

B8. (a) Efficiency
(b) Hygiene
(c) RLS; dopaminergic

B9. (a), (b), (c), (d), (f), (g); but (e): male; (h): hypertension

B10. (a) Sleep terrors
(b) Somnambulism
(c) Enuresis
(d) Somnambulism, sleep terrors
(e) Enuresis, somnambulism, sleep terrors

B11. (b), (c); but (a): REM; (d): should not, except to assure safety

C1. 16 to 17; one half; 13, decrease; 12 to 15

C2. Increase, are not
(a) 4 and 12, are; see text page 1215
(b) 4 to 30

C3. (a), (c); but (b): less; (d): higher

C4. See text page 1216.

Chapter 52

NEUROBIOLOGY OF THOUGHT, MOOD, AND ANXIETY DISORDERS

A1. Thought, mood, behavior

A2. Nature: neurobiology, including brain structure, neurotransmitters and functions, vs. nurture: psychosocial environment, including relationships

A3. (a) Genetic studies
(b) DSM-IV
(c) Psychotherapy
(d) Imaging studies

A4. See text pages 1220–1221.

A5. (a), (d); but (b): more; (c): lower

A6. (a) TCAs
(b) SSRIs
(c) MAOIs

B1. (a) Parietal
(b) Temporal
(c) Occipital
(d) Frontal
(e) Frontal
(f) Temporal (see Question B2[b])
(g) Frontal, temporal
(h) Frontal, parietal

B2. (a) Hippocampus
(b) Amygdala
(c) Hypothalamus

B3. (a) Implicit, explicit
(b) See answer to Chapter 47, Question B4.
(c) Thal → Amyg → Hip → Pre → Par → Fro

B4. (a) Gamma-aminobutyric acid
(b) Serotonin, norepinephrine and epinephrine (see Question A6)
(c) Serotonin
(d) Acetylcholine (see Chapter 50, Question E2[e])
(e) Dopamine (see Questions C5[c] and [d])

C1. (a) Disconnection between thought and language (not a "split brain")
(b) (1), (2)
(c) (2), (4)
(d) 30; deinstitutionalization has left many with schizophrenia without means of support or housing

C2. Positive symptoms are abnormal manifestations that are present, and negative symptoms indicate an absence of normal behaviors.
(a) N
(b) P

C3. (a) Word salad
(b) Derailment and tangentiality
(c) Alogia
(d) Anhedonia
(e) Delusions
(f) Hallucinations

C4. (a) Catatonic
(b) Paranoid
(c) Disorganized

C5. (b), (c); but (a): month (along with impaired functioning in at least one area for 6 months); (d): antagonists because dopamine is overactive

D1. (a) Depression (or a milder form: dysthymia), bipolar disorder (or its milder form: cyclothymia), and seasonal affective disorder
(b) Common, increasing; more, whites and Hispanics
(c) Mild; years
(d) Short
(e) Bipolar; 20s

D2. See text page 1228; 5, 2; see text page 1229

D3. (a) A
(b) M

D4. (a) ↓
(b) ↓
(c) ↓ (see Question B4)
(d) ↓
(e) ↑

D5. Elevated or expanded; see text page 1229

D6. More

D7. They permit neurotransmitters such as NE or 5-HT to "linger longer" in synapses so that postsynaptic neurons continue to be activated (see Question A6).

E1. (a) Common, 15; is not
(b) Fear that is unwarranted

E2. (a) Social anxiety disorder
(b) Obsessive-compulsive disorder
(c) Generalized anxiety disorder
(d) Panic disorder

E3. (a) Compulsions; is not; (4) and (5)
(b) 15 to 30 minutes; months

Chapter 53

CONTROL OF SPECIAL SENSES

A1. (a) Sclera → uveal tract (or vascular layer) → retina
(b) Frontal → sphenoid → maxillary
(c) Lacrimal glands and ducts → medial canthus → nasolacrimal duct
(d) Cornea → Anterior cavity → Lens → Posterior cavity

A2. (a) Conjunctiva
(b) Optic foramen
(c) Palpebrae
(d) Lysozyme
(e) Canthus
(f) Tarsal plate
(g) Pupil
(h) Vitreous body

A3. (a) Lens
(b) Iris
(c) Enhance visual acuity by absorbing light that would otherwise scatter
(d) Highly; vessels nourish the adjacent pigment layer of the retina (Figure 53-9)
(e) Lens shape, pupil diameter
(f) Parasympathetic, oculomotor; midbrain
(g) Ciliary processes → Posterior chamber (of anterior cavity) (then around iris) → Anterior chamber (of anterior cavity) → Trabeculae and canal of Schlemm
(h) Zonules (or suspensory ligaments)

A4. (a) Refraction; they pass from air (low density) into the conjunctiva and cornea (higher density), then through varying densities in aqueous humor, lens, and vitreous humor. As a result, the image of something much larger than your eye (bird or bird feeder) can be focused on a tiny spot (fovea) on your retina.
(b) Rounded or convex; ciliary, accommodation
(c) Anterior; myopia, near; biconcave
(d) Constriction or miosis, iris (constrictor), narrowing
(e) Thicker; presby; paralyzed; for better viewing of the fundus of the eye during eye examinations

A5. (a) Posterior; retina
(b) See Questions A3(c) and A3(d)
(c) E to B; B to E; optic

(d) Photoreceptor layer → bipolar layer → ganglion layer
(e) Photoreceptor layer; ganglion layer

A6. (a) C
(b) R
(c) R (because needed for formation of rhodopsin)
(d) R

A7. Posterior; macula lutea; does not, cones; point of sharpest vision

A8. Does not; sex linked; more in males; the person can detect the change in brightness of the lights (red on top, yellow in the middle, and green on the bottom)

A9. Left eye: nasal retina → Left optic nerve → Optic chiasma → Right optic tract → Right lateral geniculate nucleus of thalamus → Right optic radiations and occipital cortex

A10. (a) "Tunnel vision" (loss of temporal field of view of both eyes)
(b) Some visual loss from both eyes because left optic tracts transmit to the left cortex the impulses from the temporal side of the retina of his left eye and the nasal side of the retina of his right eye
(c) Lower half of the entire field of view of his left eye

A11. Constriction of both pupils shows that the pupillary reflex is intact in both eyes, indicating function of the pretectum regions of the midbrain (and bridging connections, which give the bilateral or "consensual" response), parasympathetic fibers in the oculomotor nerve, and sphincter of ciliary muscles in the eyes. If pupils stay "fixed and dilated," this indicates damage to brainstem, nerves, or ciliary muscles.

B1. Both eyes; see text page 1249

B2. (a) Superior rectus (inferior oblique is somewhat synergistic)
(b) Medial rectus
(c) Medial rectus (reciprocal contraction)
(d) Lateral rectus with some help from superior oblique and inferior oblique
(e) Levator palpebrae superioris
(f) All except lateral rectus (VI) and superior oblique (IV)

B3. Eye movements that are triggered by visual stimuli
(a) Conjugate, convergence
(b) Saccadic; nystagmus

B4. (a) Oculomotor nucleus
(b) Abducens nucleus (the nucleus on the right side of the pons)
(c) Trochlear nucleus

B5. Centers communicate by links from anterior to posterior (medial longitudinal fasciculus) and between right and left sides (posterior commissure).

B6. See text pages 1252–1253.

C1. (a) Pitch; 1000 to 3000
(b) Height, amplitude; 42 to 70

C2. (a) External ear, middle ear
(b) External ear
(c) Inner ear
(d) Inner ear
(e) Inner ear
(f) Inner ear

C3. (a) Air-filled spaces lined with mucous membrane
(b) Limits (or dampens) movements of the stapes, which protects the inner ear
(c) A lever system, composed of three bones, that amplifies sounds that strike the eardrum
(d) Concentrates sound waves that strike the relatively large eardrum onto the tiny surface area of the oval window, thus amplifying the effects of sounds

C4. (a) Temporal
(b) Oval
(c) Cochlea

C5. (a) External ear canal→ tympanic membrane → malleus → incus → stapes → oval window → perilymph of the scala vestibuli
(b) Scala vestibuli containing perilymph → vestibular membrane → cochlear duct containing the organ of Corti and endolymph → basilar membrane → scala tympani containing perilymph
(c) Tectorial membrane → hair cells → cochlear nerve fibers

C6. (b), (d); but (a): at apical end; (c): outer; (e): temporal

C7. (b), (c); but (a): VIII; (d): sympathetic, such as tachycardia and vasoconstriction

C8. Recover and maintain a stable body and head position (equilibrium) and maintain a stable visual field when the head moves

C9. (a) Semicircular canals
(b) Saccule, utricle
(c) Saccule, utricle
(d) Saccule
(e) Saccule, utricle
(f) Semicircular canals

C10. See text pages 1259–1260.
C11. Not always; see text page 1260.
C12. Do; doll, intact (see Chapter 50, Question A10[f])

Chapter 54

ALTERATIONS IN VISION

A1. (a) Blepharitis
(b) Ptosis
(c) Enophthalmos
(d) Anophthalmos
(e) Dacryocystitis
(f) Stye
(g) Chalazion
(h) Exophthalmos
(i) Keratoconjunctivitis sicca
(j) Sjögren's syndrome

A2. (a) VII, Bell
(b) VII; its pathway through the face makes it more vulnerable to trauma
(c) They protect eyes from microbes by a flushing action and by lysozyme and antibodies; they help to form a protective film over the cornea, which decreases friction over its surface.
(d) Aging, use of antihistamines, prolonged wearing of contact lenses (see text page 1266)

B1. (a), (c); but (b): corneal disease (rather than) conjunctivitis; (d): does not

B2. (a) Bacterial (because of the mucopurulent discharge) and caused by an infection because bilateral
(b) Hyperacute; is; is

B3. (a) Copious, watery
(b) Respiratory infections such as sore throat; swimming pools and crowded military or school sites
(c) Unilateral; antivirals (re antibiotics: not effective; re corticosteroids: not recommended because they can activate the virus)
(d) C. trachomatis A to C; vaginal delivery; 12
(e) (3)

B4. See text page 1268.

B5. (a) Is not; blood vessels do not block light rays from passing through the cornea, but the cornea must depend on adjacent tissues and fluids (such as sclera, aqueous humor, and tears) for oxygen and nutrients; because of its avascularity, the cornea can be transplanted with minimal risk of rejection
(b) Trigeminal; highly; prolonged wearing of hard contact lenses, acute glaucoma, or blunt trauma
(c) In addition to causing severe pain, a traumatized cornea can lead to altered light transmission and visual impairment.
(d) Inflammation of the cornea
(d1) Herpes simplex
(d2) Acanthamoeba
(d3) M. tuberculosis
(e) Irritation (or pain), photophobia (hypersensitivity to light), and tearing
(f) Copper
(g) Elderly persons; does not
(h) The adjacent retina may become inflamed.

C1. (a) Aqueous humor; obstructed outflow; see Chapter 53, Question A3(g)
(b) Noncontact; 10, 17; increase
(c) Wide; (2) (3) (4)
(d) On an eye screening provided at his work site; this condition typically is asymptomatic
(e) Alteration in the trabecular meshwork that should empty aqueous humor into the canal of Schlemm
(f) A leading cause of blindness; the increased intraocular pressure injures the retina and optic nerve and also causes corneal edema and opacification
(g) Funduscopy; it appears more pale and deep (related to atrophy of axons of the optic nerve)
(h) Pharmacologic, topical
(h1) Beta blockers, carbonic anhydrase inhibitors
(h2) Acetylcholine, prostaglandins

C2. (a) Closed; small
(b) Narrow, dilation; any condition that dilates the pupil: sympathetic responses, night vision, or dilator (mydriatic) drugs used to better visualize the retina

(c) Gonioscopy and transillumination

(d) All (1–5)

(e) Removal of part of the iris (iridectomy) to enhance flow of aqueous fluid

D1. (a) Lens; older; common

(b) Aging, genetics, diabetes, smoking, long-term exposure to UVB radiation (sunlight), trauma, and use of certain medications

(c) Genetic defects, environmental agents, and viruses such as rubella

D2. Slowly; the lens enlarges as new fibers form and old ones are altered and fill with vacuoles; concentrations of several electrolytes increase; proteins become less soluble, unfold, and cross link; the lens yellows and has decreased transparency

D3. Blurred vision (Figure 54-1) with glare and loss of visual acuity for both near and far vision

D4. See text page 1275.

E1. (a) Gel-like; five; only at the ciliary body and at the optic disk

(b) Liquefaction of the gel and accumulation of debris within the gel

(c) Growth of new, weakened blood vessels may lead to leakage of blood into the vitreous (see Questions E7 and E8).

E2. (a) Choriocapillaris of the choroid

(b) Central retinal artery branches

(c) Central retinal artery branches (see page 1280)

E3. (a) Retinal blood vessels are the only vessels in the body that can be observed directly, and they reflect health of brain vessels because the retina is an embryonic outgrowth of the brain.

(b) Even temporary ischemia can lead to death of retinal and optic nerve neurons.

(c) Anterior protrusion of the optic cup (of optic nerve) when high intracranial pressure collapses retinal veins and backs up fluid into the optic papilla (papilledema).

(d) A healthy fovea ("macular sparing") as choroid blood supply continues to the macula when occlusion of the retinal artery leads to ischemia of the rest of the retina.

E4. (a) Retinopathy of prematurity

(b) Retinitis pigmentosa

(c) Anopsia

(d) Retinal stroke

(e) Scotoma

(f) Cotton-wool spots or exudates on the fundus

(g) Macular degeneration

(h) Detached retina (See Questions E2[a] and E5[a])

E5. (b), (d); but (a): does because the fovea is deprived of its only blood supply: the choriocapillaris of the choroid; (c): weaker and more leaky

E6. (a) (2)

(b) Year; increase

(c) Is

E7. Proliferative; new vessels grow and leak blood into the vitreous; they also tightly connect the vitreous to the retina and may pull on the retina and detach it

E8. Preretinal → intraretinal → subretinal; preretinal

E9. (a) Scleral buckling

(b) Pneumatic retinopexy

(c) Photocoagulation

(d) Cryotherapy or photocoagulation

F1. Area 17 is the end point of visual pathways for visual reception; association areas ascribe meaning to what has been seen.

F2. Repositioning or shifting gaze to use functional areas of the retina and achieve maximal visual field coverage

F3. (a) One, both

(b) Do not (*Note:* axons do not terminate until they reach the thalamus); nasal

(c) Right, both (See also Chapter 53, Question A9)

F4. (a) Homonymous

(b) Heteronymous

(c) Anopia

(d) Quadrantanopia

(e) Hemianopia

F5. (a) A blow to the anterior of the cranium

(b) Firing of occipital cortical neurons as a result of brief mechanical trauma

(c) Bilateral destruction of visual area 17

(d) Destruction of visual association areas 18 and 19

F6. Ask a client to follow the tip of a pen or a penlight that you move (or to count the number of fingers you hold up) in central and peripheral areas of the visual fields.

F7. (a) Posterior; (3); midbrain

(b) Consensual; parasympathetic, III; mydriasis; miosis. (*Hint:* remember that mydriasis [larger pupil] is a larger word than miosis [constricted pupil]).

G1. By focusing images from the same spot on this page onto corresponding points of the two retinas, you can read with clear, binocular (not double) vision.

G2. (a) Diplopia

(b) Strabismus

(c) Amblyopia

(d) Hypertropia

(e) Cyclotropia

(f) Esotropia

G3. (a) Concomitant (nonparalytic)

(b) Nonconcomitant (paralytic)

(c) Nonparalytic, childhood; months

(d) Paralytic; strokes, inflammation of the central nervous system, muscular dystrophy, multiple sclerosis

G4. See text page 1287.

G5. By age 6 years; see text page 1288.

Chapter 55

ALTERATIONS IN HEARING AND VESTIBULAR FUNCTION

A2. Moist ears (swimming, bathing), allergies (hay fever), irritation (wearing earphones), and scratching itchy ears

A3. (c), (d); but (a): negative; (b): otitis externa

A4. (a), (b), (c)

A5. (a) Tympanic membrane

(b) Eustachian tube

(c) Ossicles

A6. (a) Pars flaccida → handle of the malleus → cone of light
  (b) Tensa
  (c) Umbo, malleus
A7. (a) Equalize pressure on the two sides of the eardrum, drain middle ear secretions into the throat, and protect the middle ear
  (b) Air at higher altitudes (such as in an airplane) exerts less pressure on the outside of the eardrum, so the eardrum gets "stuck" in the outward position. Relief is provided as you yawn or swallow and low-pressure (high-altitude) air enters the eustachian tube and middle ear, equalizing the pressure on the two sides of the eardrum.
  (c) Closed; contraction of the tensor veli palatini (TVP) muscles, such as occurs during swallowing or yawning
  (d) Lack of tube stiffness (related to limited cartilage development) or weakness of TVP muscles; also inflammation within the tube or external compression; for example, by enlarged adenoids
  (e) The eustachian tubes of infants are shorter, wider, and more horizontal; infants spend more of their day lying supine.
A8. His age, gender, being bottle fed, attending a large day-care center, having a sibling with a history of OM, and Evan's own recent history of AOM with antibiotic therapy
A9. (a) (4)
  (b) Do; from nasopharynx through eustachian tube to the middle ear
  (c) (2), (3), (5)
  (d) Tympanocentesis; tympanometry
A10. (a) Because of dramatic increase in drug-resistant *S. pneumoniae* in persons who take antibiotics frequently
  (b) An antibiotic that targets more resistant pathogens is tried.
  (c) To relieve pressure and prevent ragged scarring that would accompany a spontaneously perforated eardrum
  (d) To relieve pressure resulting from recurrent OM infections, and keeping head out of water to prevent entrance of microbes or fluid into middle ears
A11. (c), (d); but (a): 6 months or 4 episodes in 1 year; (b): absent
A12. (a) To develop well linguistically, children need to hear sounds as they watch lips or read words.
  (b) Repeated episodes of reduced hearing by the presence of fluid in the middle ears; damage to the eardrum by pressure or perforation; adhesions of ossicles that cause conductive hearing loss
  (c) Cholesteatoma formed from debris from the injured eardrum, and mastoiditis or infection of other cranial bones by spread of OM microbes
A13. (a) Autosomal dominant
  (b) Reabsorption of bone → bone becomes spongy and soft → overgrowth of hard bone develops

(c) Stapes; stapedectomy with reconstruction of a stapes
  (d) Is (because otosclerosis typically is at least partly a conductive deafness)
A14. (a), (c); but (b): objective; (d): "hard of hearing"
A15. (a) Presbycusis
  (b) Conduction deafness
  (c) Sensineural deafness
  (d) Sensineural deafness
  (e) Sensineural deafness
  (f) Boilermaker's deafness (a form of sensineural deafness)
A16. All answers.
A17. (a) Common; denial related to social embarrassment about hearing aids
  (b) (2)
  (c) Family or friends who are aware of his hearing losses; history of ear trauma and infections, environmental noise exposure, use of toxic drugs, and past use of hearing aids
  (d) Tuning forks; forehead; left
A18. See text page 1300.
A19. Position yourself so your face is in the light; directly face the person as you speak, and articulate clearly in a setting with low background noise; keep your voice tones low (not a high-pitched yell).
A20. See text page 1301.
A21. (a) Left, auditory association
  (b) (3)
  (c) Receptive
B1. (a) Maintain effective posture, and preserve eye fixation on stable objects in the visual field even when head position is changed
  (b1) Facilitate smooth, coordinated movements needed for posture
  (b2) Control eye movements as the head is moved
  (b3) Lead to nausea and vomiting with excessive vestibular stimulation
B2. (a) Nystagmus
  (b) Motion sickness
  (c) Ménière's disease
  (d) Subjective vertigo
  (e) Benign positional vertigo
  (f) Labyrinthitis
B3. (a), (d), (e); but (b): peripheral, such as inner ear; (c): increases (older than 40 years)
B4. (a) Reduce the volume of the endolymphatic space
  (b) Head positioning maneuvers can relocate debris in semicircular canals.
  (c) These chemicals may trigger episodes of vertigo.
B5. Brainstem ischemia, cerebellar tumor, or multiple sclerosis
B6. (a) Romberg test
  (b) Electronystagmography
  (c) Caloric stimulation
  (d) Rotational tests
B7. (a) Antidopaminergics
  (b) Anticholinergics
  (c) Antidopaminergics
B8. See text pages 1306–1307.

Chapter 56

STRUCTURE AND FUNCTION OF THE SKELETAL SYSTEM

A1. (a) Provides protection, support, stability, shape, mineral storage, and blood-forming tissue
  (b) Axial: skull, hyoid, thorax, and vertebrae; appendicular: bones of shoulders, hips, and extremities
  (c) Bone, cartilage, tendons, and ligaments
A2. (a) E
  (b) C
A3. (a) Hyaline
  (b) Hyaline
  (c) Elastic
  (d) Fibrous
A4. (a) Is; chondro; perichondrium
  (b) Do not; by diffusion from vessels in the perichondrium
A5. (a) Two, calcium; collagen
  (b) Cancellous; compact.
  (c) Osteogenic cells → osteoblasts → osteocytes
  (d) Osteoblasts; alkaline phosphatase
  (e) Osteocytes; lacunae, lamellae
  (f) Osteon or haversian system, blood vessels; canaliculi permit communication between lacunae and blood vessels
  (g) Vessels in periosteum travel across bone via Volkmann's canals to reach haversian systems.
  (h) Clasts; monocytes, PTH
A6. It is bound to calcium and can cause discoloration and deformity in the teeth of the developing child.
A7. (a) Contains blood vessels and serves as the point for anchoring tendons and ligaments
  (b) Site of osteogenic cells for new bone growth
  (c) Lines the inside of haversian canals, the marrow cavity, and spaces in spongy bone; formed of osteogenic cells that remodel and repair bone
A8. (a) Parathyroid hormone, vitamin D; calcitonin
  (b) Parathyroid hormone, calcitonin
  (c) All three do
  (d) Calcitonin
  (e) Parathyroid hormone, calcitonin
A9. Bones, intestine (especially the jejunum via stimulating kidney activation of vitamin D), and kidneys (by reabsorption)
A10. (a) Steroid; fish, liver, irradiated milk
  (b) Skin; liver, kidneys
  (c) May have reduced kidney and liver function; if institutionalized, they may not have skin exposed to sunlight
  (d) (3)
  (e) Stimulate, inhibits
A11. (a) Are no
  (b) More; Paget's disease because it involves overactive osteoclasts (Chapter 58, Question B9); it also may be used in a nasal spray form for osteoporosis (Chapter 58, Question B3[k1])
  (c) Decreased
B1. (a) Irregular
  (b) Short

B2. (a) Epiphysis
  (b) Diaphysis
  (c) Metaphysis
B3. (a) Children
  (b) Ligaments, tendons; limited
  (c) Synarthroses; synchondrosis
  (d) Diarthroses; synovial, freely movable
B4. See text page 1318 and Figure 56-6.
B5. (b), (c); but (a): does not; (d): poorly
B6. A case of referred pain because the hip receives some branches of nerves that cross the hip en route to supply the knee joint.
B7. A bunion is a bursa over the metatarsophalangeal joint of the great toe (MTP-1).
B8. Knee; fibrous; cartilage is avascular

Chapter 57

ALTERATIONS IN SKELETAL FUNCTION: TRAUMA AND INFECTION

A1. 70; bones, joints (including capsule, cartilage, tendons, and ligaments), and muscles
A2. (a) Common; high-speed motor accidents
  (b) Unorganized; sudden trauma
  (c) Falls; more; vertebrae, humerus, and proximal femur (hip joint)
A3. (a) Laceration
  (b) Contusion
  (c) Puncture wounds
  (d) Hematoma
A4. (a) Bones, muscles
  (b) Strains; all answers
  (c) Cold
  (d) Ankle, in; 3 and 4
  (e) To reduce pain, swelling, and the risk of muscle contractions pulling injured ends apart
  (f) Partial; more; hip and knee
  (g) Pieces of cartilage and bones
A5. (a) Shoulder; baseball, tennis
  (b) Knee; cartilage; deepen the tibial socket that receives femoral condyles, lubricate and nourish the joint
  (c) Cartilage is avascular; to avoid total joint replacement
  (d) Skiing and tennis; immobilization or bracing, muscle-strengthening exercises, and anti-inflammatory drugs
  (e) Softening
A6. (a) Pathologic
  (b) Fatigue
  (c) Sudden injury
A7. (a), (c); but (b) proximal; (d) children and partial break
A8. (a) Decrease (reduction) of space between broken bone ends so that the bony pieces are returned to their original locations; transverse
  (b) Swelling, loss of function, deformity, and possibly bleeding or bruising from broken vessels

(c) Angulation, shortening, and rotation; muscle pull on bone fragments

(d) A grating sound as bone fragments rub against each other

(e) Nerve function often is lost temporarily.

A9. Hematoma → fibrocartilaginous callus → callus → ossification → remodeling

(a) Hematoma

(b) Fibrocartilaginous callus

(c) Callus and ossification

(d) Remodeling

A10. (a) (1)

(b) (2)

(c) (2)

(d) (1)

(e) (2)

(f) (1)

A11. See text page 1329.

A12. Reduction, immobilization, and preservation or restoration of function; immobilization

(a) Open

(b) Should; joints proximal and distal to

(c) (1) and (2); but (3) must be over 3 sec

(d) Elevated above heart level; swelling during hours following the fracture may further impede circulation

(e) Right, left; to reduce risk of muscle atrophy, joint stiffness, and infections to preserve normal function

(f) Compartment

(g) They stimulate bone growth at about 1 mm/day in areas lacking adequate bone (see page 1330).

(h) (2)

A13. (a) Delayed union

(b) Nonunion

(c) Malunion

A14. They stimulate osteoblasts to lay down new bone.

A15. (a) Fat embolism syndrome

(b) Fracture blisters

(c) Reflex sympathetic dystrophy

(d) Compartment syndrome

(e) Fat embolism syndrome (possibly leading to PE)

A16. (a) Subtle changes in behavior, disorientation

(b) Rapid pulse, sweating, and pallor

(c) That does not blanch upon application of pressure possibly due to thrombocytopenia as platelets stick to fatty globules

A17. Fat particles can release free fatty acids that lead to reduction of surfactant production and acute respiratory distress syndrome (ARDS).

B1. (a) to (d) because infections can spread from bone, joints, skin, or through blood

B2. See text page 1334.

B3. (a) Marrow

(b) See answers to B1.

(c) *Staphylococcus aureus;* because they can bind to bone and can enter osteoblasts where the microbes are sheltered from antibiotic effects

(d) Bone contamination from an open wound

(e) Children; at growing points (metaphyses) of long bones, vertebrae

(f) Bone is so rigid that it cannot expand to accommodate pus, which then accumulates just deep to the periosteum.

B4. See text pages 1334–1335.

B5. (a) Chronic; sequestrum (infected, dead bone) that is surrounded by new bone (involucrum); IV

(b) To remove drainage or release pressure and possibly replace a prosthetic device involved with the infection

B6. Poor circulation to his lower extremity, which leads to the skin infection and ulcer and then to spread of infection to his bone

B7. (a) Spread from its original site (lungs or lymph nodes) to other sites such as bone; globally, increase

(b) Vertebrae

(c) Positive culture for *Mycobacterium tuberculosis*

C1. (a) Death; blood

(b) Subchondral and medullary (marrow), which have a limited blood supply; cortical bone is likely to have collateral circulation.

(c) Yes: the femoral head is composed mostly of spongy bone, and it has poor collateral circulation.

(d) Often, no known cause; fracture or hip surgery, corticosteroid therapy; injury to vessels as by radiation; also sickle cell, Legg-Perthes disease, or rheumatoid arthritis

(e) Rheumatoid arthritis and corticosteroid usage

(f) Pain at the site

(g) Joint (hip) replacement; 10

C2. Medullary necrosis releases both fat and calcium, which form the "soap"; bone lacks the ability to "clean up" the soapy material.

Chapter 58

ALTERATIONS IN SKELETAL FUNCTIONS: CONGENITAL DISORDERS, METABOLIC BONE DISEASE, AND NEOPLASMS

A1. (a), (c); but (b) mesoderm; (d) ninth week

A2. (a) Epiphysis, Metaphysis, Diaphysis

(b) Cartilage; puberty

(c) D; C

(d) Blasts, lamellae; medullary, clasts

A3. (a) Because early interventions are more likely to be successful

(b) Flexion; flexion, months

(c) Ligaments typically are lax in the newborn and are affected by intrauterine position as well as by sleeping or sitting positions of infants.

(d) In, adduction; supple

(e) Internal, multiple; the child's feet are in mild external rotation while in the device

(f) Out, femoral; is.

(g) Internal or medial; anteversion; "W," exacerbates

(h) Is not; dislocation of the head of the femur (slipped capital femoral epiphysis, especially if bilateral: see Question A9)

A4. (a) Bowlegs, varum (*Hint:* draw a large capital "R" for vaRum in the wide space between the child's bowlegs in textbook Figure 58-6; very common; sometimes

(b) Knock-knees, valgum (*Hint:* a capital "R" is too large, but a lower case "l" as in valgum, would just about fit into this narrow space between knees in the child on the right side of Figure 58-6), medial; rarely

(c) These may lead to osteoarthritis or other disorders (text page 1345); early treatment reduces risk of such sequelae

(d) Proximal epiphysis; bowlegs; large, early; uni (see textbook Figure 58-7)

A5. (b), (d); but (a) longitudinal; (c) rigid

A6. (b), (d); but (a) rigid flatfoot; (c) presence of an extra finger or toe

A7. (a) Dominant; recessive, II; is no

(b) Inward; varus; not smoking

A8. (a) She is a first-born white female, and was born breech; joint laxity

(b) Quite common (1 in 100); more

(c1) Barlow's sign

(c2) Ortolani's sign

(c3) Galeazzi test

(d) Dislocated, dislocatable

(e) Waddling (gait)

(f) Abducted

A9. (a) Osteogenesis imperfecta, developmental dysplasia of the hip, and congenital clubfoot

(b) Developmental dysplasia of the hip

(c) Congenital clubfoot

(d) Osteogenesis imperfecta

(e) Osteogenesis imperfecta

(f) Legg-Calvé-Perthes disease, Osgood-Schlatter disease, slipped capital femoral epiphysis

(g) Developmental dysplasia of the hip, Legg-Calvé-Perthes disease, and slipped capital femoral epiphysis

(h) Legg-Calvé-Perthes disease

(i) Osgood-Schlatter disease

(j) Slipped capital femoral epiphysis

A10. (a) (1), (2), (3)

(b) (2) → (1) → (3) → (4)

(c) Uni; yes, in 85% of cases

(d) To reduce deformity of the femoral head; abduction; relieve

(e) Greater because he has more time for remodeling of the femoral head

A11. Lateral, convexity

(a) Girls; 1000; 40

(b) Postural; structural

(c) Not known (idiopathic); laxity; (1)

(d) High shoulder or scapula on the right side (textbook Figure 58-13) with uneven sleeves and hemline, or right shoulder hump when Suzannah bends forward

(e) Scolio; increases; (2)

(f) See text page 1353 and Figure 58-14

(g) Bracing, surgery

B1. (b), (c); but (a) and also (d) trabecular, spongy

B2. (a) Clasts, blasts (*Hint:* remember c for chew up bone, and b for build up bone); progenitor

(b) Months; resorption

(c) Blasts; immobilization

(d) C; citrus fruits; scurvy, more brittle; D

(e) PTH; 6; Paget's

(f) Calcitonin (also estrogens)

(g) Penia; osteoporosis, osteomalacia, certain malignancies, or thyroid disorders

B3. Porous, fine porcelain vase; common, 25 million

(a) 10 (= 0.5%/year × 20 years since peak at age 30 years); 30; 3

(b) (2), (4), (5), (7); but (1), (3), (6) factors that lower risk

(c1) Gwen is well on her way to the "female athlete triad" of disordered eating, leading to amenorrhea (with decreased estrogen) and OP; phosphates in diet soda deplete calcium.

(c2) These antacids and steroids increase calcium excretion. *Note:* her HRT will offset effects of her oophorectomy.

(c3) High protein (steak, cheese), high alcohol, and lack of exercise are all risk factors, and cigarette smoke constricts vessels into bone.

(d) Early, increased; trabecular; vertebrae (textbook Figure 58-16) and the distal end of the radius

(e) Later in life, II

(f) No, not unless fractured; pain resulting from fractures, including vertebral compression fractures

(g) This increased concavity of the thoracic spine is related to osteoporotic wedging of thoracic vertebrae.

(h1) Dual-energy x-ray absorptiometry for assessing bone density

(h2) A system of assessing risk factors for OP: A = age; B = bulk (weight); ONE = never on estrogen

(i) Decreases; (2)

(j) See page 1357.

(k1) Calcitonin

(k2) Biphosphonates

(k3) Fluorides

(k4) Estrogen

B4. (a) Flexible (as a turkey "wishbone" after it sits in a cup of vinegar for a day)

(b) Brittle or ashes (such as postcremation)

B5. (a) Fat, skin

(b) Impaired absorption; China, Japan, northern India

B6. (a) Minerals, calcium, phosphate; softer; rickets

(b) Anticonvulsants, diuretics, muscle relaxants, tranquilizers

(c) Bowlegs, muscle weakness, pain (re hip fractures: not typical as in osteoporosis; re severe hypocalcemia: secondary hyperparathyroidism [see B7] prevents this)

(d) Stress fractures related to OM and seen as fine lines on x-rays

(e) Vitamin D-rich diet; exposure to sun

B7. (a) Activation

(b) Less, more; hypo, increased, resorption; renal

(c) Phosphate; long-term use of antacids that bind phosphates within the GI tract and thus prevent their absorption

B8. (a) Softened, de; 6 months to 3 years

(b) Lack of vitamin D, calcium or phosphate, or inability to absorb these chemicals

(c1) Short body with protruding abdomen

(c2) Prominent rib cartilages in abnormally shaped thorax

(c3) Enlarged with delayed closure of fontanels

(c4) Causes tetany or convulsions and eventual weakness and lethargy

(d) Same as for osteoporosis: vitamin D-rich diet; exposure to sun

B9. A progressive disease involving excessive bone breakdown (by osteoclasts) and abnormal formation of bone (by osteoblasts)

(a) Adults

(b) Thickened skull bone that may compress vessels or nerves. (*Note*: it is thought that Beethoven's deafness, significant by age 28, may have been related to Paget's disease.)

(c) Softening of the femoral neck as well as sacrum and iliac bones

(d) Fractures that occur in diseased bones that can break with even minimal stress

(e) Heart failure due to vasodilation of vessels in bone and overlying skin; this increased circulating blood volume forces the heart into overload.

(f) Yes, if multiple bones are involved in this breakdown-growth process

B10. Osteoporosis

C1. (a), (b), (f); but (c) less as these cancers peak in teen years; (d) benign, cartilage; (e) the most common type

C2. Is not; presence of a mass that can interfere with normal movement

C3. (a) Poorly; high

(b) Magnetic resonance imaging; biopsy

(c) These fractures can cause hematoma formation, which can spread the tumor into the bloodstream.

(d) Chemotherapy

C4. (a) Adolescents, Elderly, 35-year-olds

(b) The most common; is

(c) Sudden

(d) Lungs

(e) Does not; a surgery in which malignant bone and surrounding tissue is excised; the bone is replaced with a combination of donor (cadaver) bone, the client's own bone, and metal plates or rods

C5. (a1) (2)

(a2) Is; (1)

(a3) (1)

(a4) Because fever and weight loss may accompany Ewing's sarcoma and may suggest other diagnoses

(b1) (2)

(b2) (2)

(b3) (1), (2)

C6. (a) 50%; skeletal veins have sluggish blood flow

(b) (2)

(c) Breast, lung, prostate

(d) Stretching of the periosteum or pressure of the tumor on nerves

(e1) This enzyme and this electrolyte are both likely to increase.

(e2) Palliative therapy (to reduce pain and try to prevent fractures)

(e3) As for other bone disorders, these drugs inhibit osteoclasts.

(e4) Stabilize bones that are weakened by cancer

(f) (2)

Chapter 59

ALTERATIONS IN SKELETAL FUNCTION: RHEUMATIC DISORDERS

A1. (a), (c); but (b): very common; (d): many

A2. (a) Women, middle age

(b) Is not; most; much is made by lymphocytes in inflammatory regions of the synovial membrane

(c) Reacts with; complex; the answer is not known, but possibly a virus alters the IgG so it is regarded as foreign, or there may be a genetic predisposition for this alteration

A3. (a) Immune complex formation

(b) Phagocytosis

(c) Lysosomal action

(d) Reactive hyperplasia

(e) Pannus formation

(f) Ankylosis

(g) Extra-articular changes

A4. (a) RA only; destructive to

(b) Pain in

(c) Small, such as in hands and feet; bilateral

(d) Distal interphalangeal

(e) Thumbs (See Figure 59-4); dislocation

(f) Cervical, neck; knee, quadriceps

(g) Nodules, swelling of at least three joints for at least 6 weeks, x-ray changes of hand joints; note that other common signs of RA include anemia and cloudy synovial fluid, but these are not included in the ARA criteria

A5. See text pages 1371–1373.

A6. Joint destruction may be limited with aggressive treatment within 2 years of onset.

A7. (a) Corticosteroids

(b) COX-2 inhibitors

(c) NSAIDs

(d) Corticosteroids

(e) Methotrexate

A8. (a) Arthroplasty

(b) Synovectomy

A9. (a) Polymyositis

(b) Scleroderma

(c) Systemic lupus erythematosus

A10. (a) Higher; androgens; African Americans and Asians
   (b) B-lymphocytes (and T4 or helper lymphocytes), autoantibodies; autoimmune
   (c) Antigens; immune complexes lead to inflammatory responses and tissue injury
   (d) Injury within so many different systems mimics the effects of other diseases that affect these systems; joints, skin, kidneys, lungs, heart, and brain
   (e1, e2) Destruction of red blood cells and platelets by attacking autoantibodies
   (e3) Nephrotic syndrome
   (e4) Vasculitis or hypertension affecting cerebral vessels
   (f) Face (cheeks and nose)
   (g) Many; antinuclear antibodies (ANA)
A11. (a), (b), (e); but (c): very common; (d): do not; (f): skin
A12. All answers
B1. Vertebrae; stiffness of joint
   (a) Axial (including the spine); ligaments that insert into bone; are (note: "-itis")
   (b) Is not; B27, sometimes
B2. (a) Reiter's syndrome
   (b) Ankylosing spondylitis
   (c) Psoriatic arthritis
   (d) Ankylosing spondylitis
   (e) Enteropathic arthritis
   (f) Psoriatic arthritis, Reiter's syndrome
B3. (a-b) The sites where ligaments insert into bone are eroded by inflammation, followed by ossification. As ligaments convert to bony "belts" connecting vertebrae, the spine takes on the bamboo-like appearance; see Figure 59-6.
   (c1) His posture, possible osteoporosis, and diminished vision related to posture (head down) and AS-linked uveitis
   (c2) Chest movements reduced to half of the normal 4 to 5 cm excursions caused by stiffened costovertebral joints and posture
   (c3) Involvement of his sacroiliac joint and lumbar vertebrae; maintenance of his abnormal posture and gait may have led to injury of his hip joints
   (c4) Caused by pain, stiffness, and muscle spasms
   (d) One
   (e) (2), (4), (6); but (1): sleeping on his back; (3): warm bath or heat applications; (5): he is already underweight
B4. Rheumatoid arthritis and systemic lupus erythematosus because the overactive immune responses required to maintain these disorders are reduced in immunodeficiency.
B5. (a) Rheumatoid factor; negative
   (b) Cannot; months
   (c1) Salmonella or Shigella
   (c2) Chlamydia
   (c3) Streptococcus
   (d) Eyes (uvea), intestine, skin, or heart
C1. (a) Metabolic
   (b) Idiopathic

   (c) Anatomic
   (d) Neuropathic
   (e) Post-traumatic
C2. (a) OA
   (b) RA
   (c) RA
   (d) OA
   (e) OA
   (f) RA
   (g) RA
   (h) OA
   (i) RA
C3. (a) Articular cartilage
   (b) Chondrocytes; water, ground substance (a hydrated, semisolid gel), proteoglycans that provide elasticity and some stiffness, and collagen that provides tensile strength and support
   (c) Decrease; normal, maximizes (see Figure 59-8, left side); incongruity of joint surfaces develops so stress is concentrated at limited contact points (see Figure 59-8, right side)
   (d1) Activity overload decreases deformation and damages cartilage.
   (d2) Lack of mechanical loading deprives the avascular cartilage of motion required to squeeze fluids between synovial fluid and chondrocytes, a mechanism that provides nutrients and removes wastes.
   (e) Interleukin-1, protein, collagen, proteoglycans; narrows
   (f1) Eburnation
   (f2) Osteophytes, crepitus
C4. Both large and small
   (a) Hip joint, knee joint
   (b) Cervical vertebrae, lumbar vertebrae
   (c) First carpometacarpal joint, first metatarsophalangeal joint
C5. (a) Knee
   (b) Spine
   (c) Distal interphalangeal joints
C6. Weight loss (if obese), strengthening exercises, and modifying tasks; see text page 1383
C7. Corticosteroids, COX-2 inhibitors, hyaluronate (joint lubricant), NSAIDs; drugs for rheumatoid arthritis include these and also disease-modifying antirheumatic drugs (DMARDs), such as methotrexate or gold salts
D1. Diabetes mellitus, thyroid disease, and AIDS
D2. (a), (c); but (b): middle-aged to older men; (d): monosodium urate
D3. (a) Hyperuricemia; > 7.0
   (b) Monosodium urate crystals cause an inflammatory response in which polymorphonuclear cells phagocytose crystals and then release lysosomal enzymes that attack cartilage and subchondral bone.
   (c) Monosodium urate; about 10 years
   (d) One; may not occur for years; toes and external ears; deposits occur in regions of cooler temperatures

D4. (a) Joint inflammation (which can lead to rapid joint destruction); NSAIDs, because of side effects

 (b) Are not, because they can exacerbate inflammation; they increase renal elimination of uric acid

 (c) Aspirin decreases renal excretion of uric acid.

 (d) This preferred treatment of gout decreases production of uric acid.

 (e) Purines; organ meats such as liver, kidney, brain, and sweetbreads (thymus and pancreas) and certain fish (sardines, anchovies, herring)

E1. To address developmental needs of the child and family issues; see more on text page 1386

E2. (a) Pauciarticular arthritis
 (b) Polyarticular arthritis
 (c) Still's disease
 (d) Juvenile dermatomyositis

E3. (a), (d), (f); (b): good; (c): lower; (e): should not

E4. Common; see text page 1387

E5. Increase

E6. (a) Month, higher
 (b) Days, slower
 (c) Will; they feel better, so think they do not need the therapy; because of side effects
 (d) Gradually; steroids depress ACTH production, which causes atrophy of adrenal glands; gradual weaning provides time for regrowth of adrenal tissue so Mrs. Thielens can produce endogenous corticosteroids.

E7. They are both forms of the same disease; blood vessels (arteries); blindness

E8. So they feel a greater sense of control and may engage more fully in the treatment program.

Chapter 60

CONTROL OF INTEGUMENTARY FUNCTION

A1. See page 1393.

A2. (a), (b), (e); but (c) epidermis; (d) epidermis

A3. (a) Merkel's cell
 (b) Langerhans'
 (c) Melanocyte
 (d) Keratinocyte

A4. Germinativum, spinosum, granulosum, lucidum, corneum
 (a) Corneum
 (b) Lucidum
 (c) Germinativum

A5. (a) Tyrosinase
 (b) Sebum

A6. (a), (d); but (b) do not migrate but instead send out extensions between keratinocytes and deposit melanin in that way; (c) more melanosomes per melanocyte

A7. (a) Thicker; connective, vascular
 (b) Reticular
 (c) Pacinian; dermis, and subcutaneous tissue
 (d) Does
 (e) Eccrine, onto the surface of the skin

 (f) Sebaceous
 (g) Arrector pili muscles
 (h) Dead, keratinized cells

Chapter 61

ALTERATIONS IN SKIN FUNCTION AND INTEGRITY

A1. (a) Elevated and fluid-filled
 (b) Elevated and fluid-filled
 (c) Elevated and solid
 (d) Flat with color change

A2. (a) Petechiae
 (b) Hyper
 (c) Erythematous
 (d) Excoriation

A3. (a), (b); but (c) induce; (d) does not although may give temporary relief; (e) cold

A4. (b), (d); but (a) causes itching; (c) fatty acid-containing

A5. Lower, melanin; acne, sunburn, or other injuries to skin; less

B1. Increased
 (a) (2)
 (b) (1)
 (c) Ozone should absorb UVB and UVC rays, but this layer is diminishing.
 (d) Dilate. Fewer of these immune cells are present to remove sun-damaged cells that could become malignant.
 (e) (1)

B2. (a) 15
 (b) Every 2 hours
 (c) 7 AM to 11 AM

C1. In

C2. (a) Albinism
 (b) Melasma
 (c) Vitiligo

C3. (a) Superficial; other humans, animals, or soil
 (b) Keratin
 (c1) Less
 (c2) More, because of systemic effects
 (d) More, because feet have less exposure to air

C4. Ringworm or superficial mycoses or dermatophytoses, fungal
 (a) Nails
 (b) Scalp or head
 (c) Body (trunk, back, or buttocks)
 (d) Foot
 (e) Corticosteroids

C5. (a) Griseofulvin
 (b) Potassium hydroxide
 (c) Corticosteroids
 (d) Acyclovir
 (e) Tretinoin or isotretinoin
 (f) Tetracycline
 (g) Malathion

C6. (a) The antibiotic "wipes out" not only the agent (*Streptococcus*) that is causing the respiratory problem, but also much of the "normal flora" on any mucous membrane, so *Candida* can then proliferate.
   (b) Frank lacks the CD4 cells that would normally target *Candida*.

C7. (a) Children; superficial, group A β-hemolytic
   (b) Oil; blackheads; 100; androgens; (3)
   (c) Benign, thicker; papilloma; can
   (d) Sensory; burning or tingling (paresthesia); fluid-filled vesicles; do
   (e) (1); (2)
   (f) Is not; acyclovir (or similar drugs); can

C8. (a) Zoster (or varicella), chickenpox; elderly, immunosuppressed
   (b) Uni; weeks
   (c) Can be; blindness; year
   (d) See text page 1415.

C9. (a) Atopic eczema
   (b) Nummular eczema
   (c) Urticaria
   (d) Allergic contact dermatitis
   (e) Irritant contact dermatitis
   (f) Toxic epidermal necrolysis
   (g) Lichen planus
   (h) Psoriasis
   (i) Pityriasis rosea

C10. (a) Bacteria
   (b) Fungi
   (c) Virus
   (d) Virus (warts)
   (e) Arthropod
   (f) Virus

C11. (a) Ticks; Lyme disease; microbes carried by the tick; hours; can
   (b) Mites; commonly; within; can
   (c) Lice
   (c1) Cannot; avoidance of contact with an infected person, or infected sheets, clothing, combs, brushes, hats
   (c2) Head, pubic area, or other areas of the body
   (c3) Along long hair shafts; nits
   (c4) Months

D1. (a), (b); but (c) melanocytes; (d) well; (e) dysplastic

D2. Increased; fair, red or blonde. Increased sun exposure, especially intense, intermittent exposure on weekends and vacations; thinning of the ozone layer so that UV rays reach the earth more readily

D3. Malignant melanoma, squamous cell carcinoma, basal cell carcinoma
   (a) Basal cell carcinoma
   (b) Squamous cell carcinoma

D4. (a) Red hair, freckles on upper back, working outdoors for three or more adolescent years, family history; having a nevus that has changed and visiting tanning salons also increase her risk; 20
   (b) A (asymmetry), B (borders uneven) and D (diameter more than 6 mm)
   (c) Common, are; is

(d) 60; is

D5. Protect against exposure to sun. Detect early by regular, thorough self-examination. (See text page 1432.)

E1. Flame and smoke inhalation; scalding fluids; chemical, electrical, or radiation burns

E2. (a) (4), (2), (3), (1)
   (b) (1)
   (c) (3)
   (d) (2)
   (e) (4)

E3. (a) Yes, because some areas will have second-degree burns that are painful.
   (b) About 42% (18% for each lower extremity plus 6% for about one third of his posterior trunk); major
   (c1) 3, because much of plasma seeps out of burned blood vessels into interstitial spaces, so less circulating blood
   (c2) 56. Loss of fluid from blood plasma → relative polycythemia
   (c3) Polycythemia (thick blood) flows more slowly and increases risk for clot-formation.
   (c4) Increased, because reflex vasoconstriction of vessels into gastrointestinal organs causes gastric mucosa to be ischemic and vulnerable to ulceration
   (c5) Decreased, because reflex vasoconstriction of vessels into kidneys reduces urine formation
   (c6) Interstitial (between cells) areas. Low urinary output contributes to edema, but most of the edema comes from seeping of fluid (and proteins) from burned vessels into spaces between cells.
   (c7) Decreased. Injured airways and lungs cannot function adequately to oxygenate blood, and his hypermetabolic rate increases his need for oxygen.
   (c8) Decreased. The body's first line of defense has broken down.
   (d) Enormous amounts of replacement fluids because he is "third-spacing," and nutrients are needed for healing his injured body

E4. See text pages 1436–1437.

F1. (b), (d); but (a) may develop into malignant melanoma; (c) strawberry hemangiomas

F2. (a) Widely distributed macules to beefy, red, excoriated skin surfaces
   (b) More
   (c) Moist
   (d) Infrequently

F3. See text pages 1439–1441.

F4. Macules on trunk, spreading to extremities and head → vesicle formation → scab formation

F5. (a) Roseola (based on his age and lack of lymph node involvement)
   (b) Scarlet fever (based upon her history of strep throat and her strawberry tongue)

F6. See text page 1441.

F7. (a) Senile angiomas
   (b) Lentigines
   (c) Actinic keratoses

Installing the Student Self-Study Testbank

To install the Self-Study software on your PC, follow these steps:

1. Insert the CD-ROM into your CD-ROM drive
2. Open the Start menu and select Run.
3. In Open box, type d:\setup, where d is the letter representing your CD-ROM drive, and press Enter. (If your CD-ROM drive is a letter other than d, substitute that letter.)
4. Follow the directions on the screen to complete the installation.
5. The program will add a shortcut to your Desktop.
6. To launch the program, double click on the icon on the Desktop.

System Requirements

This program will run on any IBM-PC or compatible computer that *minimally* includes:

A Pentium 100 CPU;
32 MB RAM (64 recommended);
Windows;
SVGA display supporting 256 colors (16 bit recommended);
12X CD-ROM drive;
800 x 600 monitor resolution;
A Microsoft compatible mouse;
5 MB of hard-disk space

Note: In order to run this program, you must have Macromedia Flashplayer installed on your PC. If you do not currently have this program installed, it is a free download available at:
http://www.macromedia.com/software/flashplayer/.

If you still have questions, contact our Tech Support @ 1-800-638-3030, Monday-Friday 8:30 to 5:00 EST, or at techsupp@lww.com.